# Pharmacy Exams

## *- Expert Cracker*

**Quick Review | Solved MCQs | Solved GPAT Papers 2015 -19 & Mock Tests**

**(Useful for GPAT, Pharmacy Competitive Exams and Pharmacy Exit Exam)**

# Pharmacy Exams

## - *Expert Cracker*

**Quick Review | Solved MCQs | Solved GPAT Papers 2015 -19 & Mock Tests**

**(Useful for GPAT, Pharmacy Competitive Exams and Pharmacy Exit Exam)**

**Swati Pandey**
Assistant Professor, Columbia Institute of Pharmacy, Raipur.

**Monika Bhairam**
Assistant Professor, Columbia Institute of Pharmacy, Raipur.

**Amber Vyas**
Assistant Professor, University Institute of Pharmacy, Pt. Ravishankar Shukla University, Raipur.

**Ravindra Kumar Pandey**
Professor, Columbia Institute of Pharmacy, Raipur.

**Shiv Shankar Shukla**
Professor, Columbia Institute of Pharmacy, Raipur.

**PharmaMed Press**
*An imprint of BSP Books Pvt. Ltd.*
4-4-309/316, Giriraj Lane,
Sultan Bazar, Hyderabad - 500 095.

**Pharmacy Exams –** ***Expert Cracker***
**by Swati Pandey, Monika Bhairam, Amber Vyas, Ravindra Kumar Pandey and Shiv Shankar Shukla**



***Published by:***

**PharmaMed Press**

*An imprint of BSP Books Pvt. Ltd.*

4-4-309/316, Giriraj Lane, Sultan Bazar, Hyderabad - 500 095.
Phone: 040-23445688; Fax: 91+40-23445611
e-mail: info@pharmamedpress.com
www.pharmamedpress.com/pharmamedpress.net

**ISBN: 978-93-95039-17-8 (Hardback)**

# PREFACE

This book will provide an in depth knowledge and prepare students to fight competitive exams like GPAT, NIPER, Drug Inspector, Railway Pharmacist etc with much zeal and confidence. This book will provide an opportunity to assemble the diverse knowledge in pharmacy and apply one's ability to grasp the field. The book is well designed and planned with the series consisting of theoretical concept that are denoted in form of short learning points and tables for memorization and last minute revisions followed by the multiple choice questions. As per the modern education system teaching through multiple choice questions is mostly opted. These MCQ's shall enable students to select and plan their learning through continuous inputs.

The syllabus covered in the book includes Pharmaceutics, Medicinal Chemistry and Pharmacology, Pharmacognosy, Pharmaceutical Jurisprudence, Pharmacy Practice that are the areas of focus in the exams of different states. The questions are well designed to suit the level of each type of exam at National/ State/ University at several states with respect to its difficulty levels for improving the skills with multiple choice questions.

The level and state of MCQ's are pleasant and superiority is maintained that comprehend to the all subjects. Another adept/additional benefit/virtue of the book is that each chapter has been divided into sections and sub-sections that enhance the easy of understanding. The book is user friendly and provides information in well structured manner.

We owe a sincere thank to the management of Columbia Institute of Pharmacy for their continued encouragement that helped me to put forth the book in such a comprehensive manner.

A word or suggestion from the reader's side shall add another feather to the crown of subject matter of book. Constructive suggestions and feedback from the readers will always be welcomed, cherished, acknowledged and rightfully included.

With Best Wishes,

**Dr. Shiv Shankar Shukla**
**Raipur**

# CONTENTS

## CHAPTER 3

# Pharmacognosy

### Pharmacognosy



## CHAPTER 4

# Pharmaceutical Jurisprudence

### Pharmaceutical Jurisprudence



## CHAPTER 5

# Microbiology



## CHAPTER 6

# Biochemistry

## Previous years GPAT Solved Question Papers



## Mock Tests

# Chapter 1

# Pharmaceutics

## Pharmaceutics- Theory

### 1.1 Liquid Dosage Froms

Liquid dosage forms Dosage forms are essentially pharmaceutical products in the form which involves a mixture of active drug components and nondrug components (excipients). Liquid form of a dose of a drug used as a drug or medication intended for administration or consumption.

- It may be defined as "A solution is a liquid-preparation that contains one or more soluble chemical substances dissolved in a specified solvent"
- Liquid dosage forms are intended for External, Internal or parenteral use.
- The component of the solution which is present in a large quantity is known as "SOLVENT" where as the component present in small quantity is termed as "SOLUTE"
- They mainly classified in to two category namely as –
  (i) Monophasic Liquid dosage forms.
  (ii) Biphasic liquid dosage forms.

### Monophasic Liquid Dosage Forms

Monophasic dosage form refers to liquid preparation containing two or more components in one phase system; it is representing by true solution. A true solution is a clear homogenous mixture that is prepared by dissolving solute in a suitable solvent.

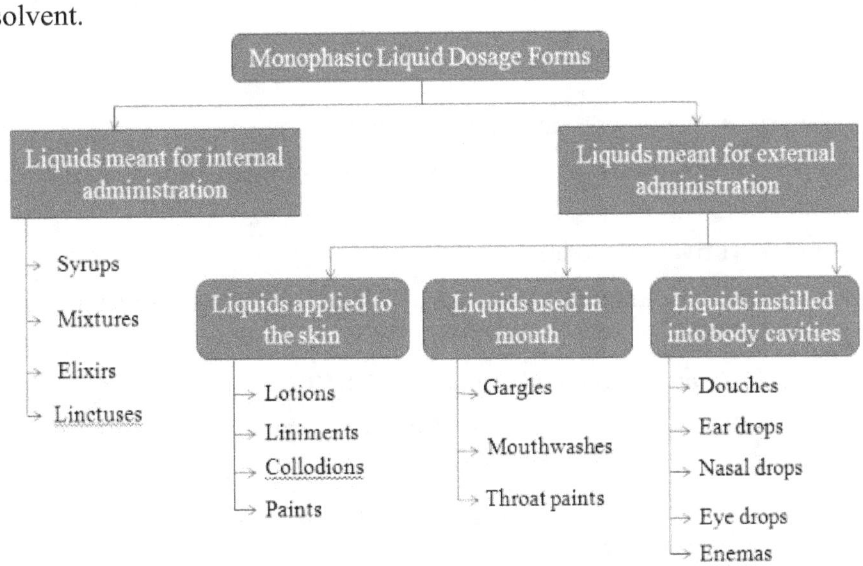

**Solubility:**

| Type | Solubility |
|---|---|
| Soluble | From 10 to 30 part |
| Freely Soluble | From 1 to 10 part |
| Very Soluble | Less than 1 part |
| Slightly Soluble | From 100 to 1000 parts |
| Very slightly Soluble | From 1000 to 10000 parts |
| Sparingly Soluble | From 30 to 100 parts |
| Insoluble | more than 10000 parts |

- A solution should be designed in which the solubility of the solute is not exceeded even at Temperature low as 4°C.
- **pH**: The pH of solution greatly affect the solubility of a solute.
- **Co-solvency**:
  - The mechanism responsible for solubility enhancement through co solvent that it works by reducing the **interfacial tension** between the predominately aqueous solution and the hydrophobic solute.
  - The example of cosolvents is ethanol, Sorbitol, glycerine, propylene, glycol, and several members of polyethylene glycol.
- **Dimethylacetamide** is used as cosolvent in **parenteral** products.
- **Dielectric Constant**
  - The absolute solubility of a solute may vary in two different solvents of the same dielectric constant.
  - Every solute shows a maximum solubility in any given solvent system, at one or more specific dielectric constant
  - The solubility profiles as a function of dielectric constant appears to be similar for a solute in different solvent systems.
- **Solubilizing agent**-The lypophilic surface active agents with HLB value higher than 15 are act best solubilizing agents.
- **Preservatives:**
  - **Acidie preservatives** usually used in oral preparations.
  - **Neutral, mercurial, and quaternary ammonium compounds** widely used in ophthalmic, nasal and parenteral products.
  - The **neutral preservatives** are volatile alcohols.
  - Mercurial, and quaternary ammonium compound are good preservatives but subject to a variety of **incompatibilities.**
  - Methyl and propyl paraben used together in a ratio of **10:1** respectively
  - Syrup containing 85% of sugar act as **self-preservative** by virtue of their exosmotic effect on microorganisms.
  - Syrup containing less than 85% of sugar but having sufficient quantity of polyols also have exosmotic effect on microorganisms.

**Table** Some pharmaceutical used preservatives and their usual concentration

| Class | Preservatives | Concentration |
|---|---|---|
| **Acidic** | Phenol | 0.2-0.5 |
| | Chlorocresol | 0.05-0.01 |
| | O-phenyl of Para benzoic | 0.005-0.01 |
| | Alkyl ester of para benzoic acid | 0.1-0.3 |
| | Benzoic acid and its salts | 0.5-1.0 |
| | Boric acid and its salts | 0.05-0.2 |
| | Sorbic acid and salts | 0.06-0.2 |
| **Neutral** | Chlorobutanol | 0.5 |
| | Benzy alcohol | 1.0 |
| | β-phenyl ethyl alcohol | 0.2-1.0 |
| **Mercurial** | Thimerosal | 0.001-0.1 |
| | Phenyl mercuric acetate and nitrate | 0.002-0.005 |
| | Nitromserosol | 0.001-0.1 |
| **Quaternary** | Benzalkonium chlorides | 0.004-0.02 |
| **AmmoniumCompounds** | Cetylpyridinium | 0.01-0.02 |

- **Sweetening agents:**
  - ➢ Sucrose 85% concentration is widely used as sweetening agents. It is chemically and physically stable in a pH range of**4.0 to 8.0.** It is widely used in conjunction with sorbitol, glycerine, and other polyols to reduce the tendency of sucrose to crystallize.
  - ➢ Liquid glucose is prepared by the partial hydrolysis of **starch with strong acids**. Its main components are **dextrose with small amounts of dextrin and maltose.**
  - ➢ Saccharine is also widely used as sweetening agents and it is approximately **250-500** times sweetener. Than sucrose. It is **having a bitter after taste.**
  - ➢ **Aspartame** is another synthetic sweetening agents and approximately **200 times** sweetener than sucrose and **has no bitter after taste**. It is the **methyl ester aspartic acid and phenylalanine**. It is very stable in dry powder but in aqueous solution it is stable between **pH 3.4 – 5.0** and refrigerated temperature. Its taste property can be improved using sodium **bicarbonate**, **gluconate salt, and lactose**.
- **Viscosity control:** The viscosity of a solution can be improved by a) increasing the sugar concentration b) incorporating viscosity controlling agents like polyvinypyrrolidone or cellulose derivatives like methyl cellulose of sodium carboxy methyl cellulose etc.

## Biphasic Liquid Dosage Forms

- The liquid which consist of two phases are known as a biphasic liquid dosage forms.
- They are sub categorized into two different forms namely as –
  - (i) Emulsion
  - (ii) Suspension

## Emulsion

Emulsion is a biphasic liquid preparations containing two immiscible liquid (Continuous Phase & dispersed phase) made missicible. The liquid which is converted into minute globules is called as dispersed phase & the liquid in which the globules are dispersed is called the continuous phase. An emulsion is a thermodynamically unstable system consisting of at least two immiscible liquid phases one of which is dispersed as globules in the other liquid phase stabilized by a third substance called emulsifying agent.

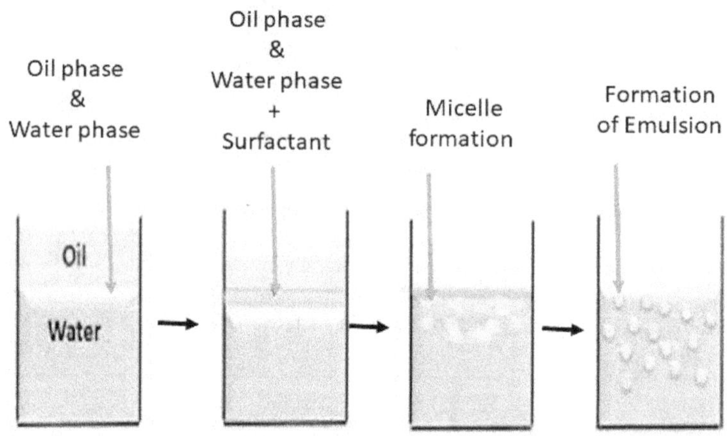


**Fig** Representation of formation of emulsion.

- An emulsion is
  (a) A thermodynamically unstable dispersed system
  (b) Consisting of at least two immiscible liquid phase
  (c) Stabilized by the presence of emulgent (s)
- Ordinary emulsion is white or off-white in colour. This is due to the particle diameter of the dispersed phase generally extends from about 0.1 to 10 µm, and the dispersed globule diameter is higher than the wave length of light.
- An assembly of closely packed monodisperse spherical droplets as the internal phase can occupy no more than approximately 74% of the total volume of the emulsion.
- The dispersed particles having a diameter of less than ¼ the wave length of visible light. i.e less than approximately **120 nm.**
- **Type of emulsion:**
  - Oil-in-water (o/w) type of emulsion e.g. - **Milk & Vanishing cream**
  - Water-in-Oil (w/o) type of emulsion e.g.- **Butter, Cold cream & Salad cream**
  - **Multiple emulsions** or three phase emulsion or emulsion with in emulsion with emulsion. (**o/w /o**)\. Multiple emulsions may be used for prolongation action of drug action, or intramuscular therapy.
  - **-Micro emulsions:** These may be defined as dispersions of insoluble liquids in a second liquid that appear clear and homogeneous to the naked eye. They contain globules of size about **0.01 µm.**
  - **-Fine emulsions:** normally these have milky appearance and the globule size ranges from **0.25-25 µm.**
- **Determination of emulsion type:-**

The following method are used for of determining the type of an emulsion.

**Table** Various methods for determination of emulsion type

| Test | Observation | Comments |
|---|---|---|
| **Dilution test** | Emulsion can be diluted only with external phase | Useful for liquid emulsion only |
| **Dye test** | Water soluble solid dye tints only O/W emulsions and reverse. Microscopic observation usually helpful. | May fail if ionic emulsifier is present. |
| **$CoCl_2$/filter paper** | Filter paper impregnated with $CoCl_2$ and dried, (blue) Changes to **pink** when O/W emulsion is added | May fail if emulsion is unstable or breaks in presence of electrolyte |
| **Fluorescence** | Since oil fluorescence under UV light, O/W emulsion exhibit dot pattern, W/O emulsions Fluorescence throughout. | Not always possible |
| **Conductivity** | Electric current is conducted by o/w emulsions, owing to presence of ionic species in water | Falls in non-ionic w/w emulsions. |

- **Application:**
  - Emulsion may be used as
    - Oral preparation
    - Parenteral preparation
    - Topical preparation
  - Total Parenteral Nutrition (**TPN**), a product recently available in the market to maintain debilitated patients in from of emulsion. When **Bicarbonate** added to TPN formulation it causes an incompatibility problem.
- **Mechanical equipment's used for emulsion:**
  - Mechanical stirrer, Colloidal mill, Homogenisers and used Ultrasonic devices equipment are used in the preparation of emulsion.
  - A homogenizer generally consists of a pump that raises the pressure of the dispersion to arrange of **500 to 5000 psi.**
  - The pressure required range in an ultrasonicator 150 to 350 psi.
  - Given below are ratio of oil: water: gum for preparing primary of different oil
    1. Fixed oil 4:2: 1
    2. Mineral oil 3:2: 1
    3. Volatile oil 2:2: 1
    4. Oleo-resin 1:2: 1
- **Emulsifying agents:**
  - The nature of emulgent is selected for a type of emulsion is based upon Banocraft's rule.
  - Bentonite, veegum, graphite, magnesium, hydroxide are the example of finely divided solid particle used as emulgents.
  - Cetrimide is a synthetic emulsifying agents.
  - Bentonite is an example of inorganic emulsifying agents.
  - Surfactants of HLB range 15 to 18 are ideal solubilizing agent's used to from clear emulsions.
  - Emulsions made with tween are usually o/w.
  - Auxiliary emulsifying agents (Glyceryl monostearate, Stearic acid, CMC sodium, Methyl cellulose, steraryl alcohol) act as thickening agents and help to stabilize the emulsion.

**Table** Emulsifying agents and their mechanism of action

| Emulsifying Agents | Mechanism of Action |
|---|---|
| **Surface active agents (eg. Soaps, Spans, Tweens)** | They reduce interfacial tension |
| **Hydrophilic colloids (Accacia, gelatin)** | They tend to form a multimolecular film around the globules and prevent coalescence |
| **Finely divided solids (Bentonite, vee gum)** | They adsorb at the oil-water interface and form rigid film of closely packed solids and act as a mechanical barrier and prevents the coalescence of globules. |

- **Stability:**
  - ➢ The physical instability of emulsionsis related with phase inversion, creaming or sedimentation, Ostwald ripening and cracking of the emulsion.
  - ➢ For a stable emulsion, the phase volume ratio is generally about 52:48.
- **Physical stability markers**

(a) Flocculation : It is due to interaction of attractive and repulsive forces
(b) Creaming : It is due to density difference between two phases.
(c) Coalescence : Agglomeration of particles in emulsion.
(d) Breaking : Completely separation of oil and aqueous phase
(e) Phase inversion : The change of emulsion type from o/w to w/o or vice versa.

## Points to Remember

The factor responsible for cracking or splitting or breaking of an emulsion are

- Centrifuging
- Addition of electrolytes
- Heat
- Freezing
- Bacterial growth
- Addition of a liquid in which both phases soluble
- Addition of a chemical that is incompatible with the emulsifying agent like calcium and magnesium salts to emulsion stabilized with anionic surfactants.
- Addition of higher percentage of alcohol to an emulsion stabilized with hydrocolloids.
- Creaming may occur upward & downward
- According to Stok's law: -
  - ➢ The creaming of emulsion is indirectly proportional to viscosity of medium.
  - ➢ Rate of settling is directly proportional to particle diameter
- When **sodium chloride** is added to sodium oleate emulsion, the emulsion is destabilized.
- In a macro emulsion the dispersed globules having radius below the range of **10-75nm.**

## Suspension

### Introduction

A pharmaceutical suspension is a type of disperse system in which one (or more) substance (the dispersed phase) is distributed in particulate from throughout another (the continuous phase)

**Formulation additives:**

The additives of a suspension formulation such as –

- Vehicles,
- Thickeners,
- Buffers,
- Stabilizers,
- Preservatives,
- Colours and flavours,

In case of suspension formulation of hydrophobic drugs, it is very difficult to disperse the drug particle in aqueous media. The surface of such drug particles is better wetted by the incorporation of a suitable wetting agent having the HLB value 7 to 9. The wetting agents act by reducing the "contact angle" between the spreading liquid and the solid surface of the drug particles help in wetting the particle with vehicle. The contact angle between a liquid and solid may be 0° signifying complete wetting for it may approach to 180°, at which wetting is insignificant.

**Dispersing Agents**

The agents help in causing the dispersion of the solid particles to be evenly distributed in the suspension. Especially in deflocculated suspension, the individual particle should remain dispersed. In some materials where the quantum of surface charger is not sufficient, the particles tend to come together. To overcome this tendency some material which carry good charge and can get easily absorbed into the

- Dispersed phase particle can be added. These are dispersing agents. Eg. **Darvans, Daxods** etc. They increase the "Zeta potential" considerably, thus discouraging the particles in the suspension to come together.
- The surface of the dispersed drug particles may be charged due to preferential adsorption of a particular ion (cation or anion) or due to ionization of a particular ionisable group attached to the solid surface of the drug particles.
- Naturally a potential known as "Nernst potential" or electro thermodynamic potential is developed at the surface of the solid, which will attract oppositely charged counterion or gegenion in the tightly bound solvent layer around the surface of the solid.
- Now depending upon the number of ions adsorbed at as the surface of the solid and the counterian in the tightly bound solvent layer, the surface of the tightly bound layer may charge.
- The zeta potential is defined as the difference in potential between the surfaces of the tightly bound layer and the electro neutral region of the solution.
- This may be positive, zero or negative Good dispersing agents increase the magnitude of zeta potential there by help the individually dispersed solid particles to retain their individually due to the repulsive force experienced between two approaching particles.

**Method of Preparation of Suspension**

There are several methods of preparing flocculated suspension. For instance in the preparation of the oral suspension of a drug, clays such as diluted bentonite magma are commonly employed as the flocculating agent. Electrolytes can also act as flocculation agents, apparently by reducing the electrical barrier between the particles of the suspension and forming a bridge so as to link them together.

Levigation (wet grinding) process followed in small scale lmanufacturing of suspension where as in industry the mixture is passed through colloid mill to break the clumps and to produce a homogenous suspension.

**Suspension containing diffusible Solids**

Some insoluble powders are light and easily wetable, hence they readily mix with water and, on shaking, diffuse evenly through the liquid for long enough to ensure even distribution in each dose, such substances are known as diffusible of dispersible solids. Eg. Calcium carbonate, Light kaolin, Magnesium carbonate, Magnesium trisilicate, rhubarb powder etc.

**Suspension Containing Indiffusible Solids**

Indiffusible solids will not remain evenly distributed in a vehicle long enough to ensure uniformly of dose. The simplest way of correcting the problem is to increase the viscosity of the vehicle by adding a thickening agent. Some examples of indiffusible solids are aspirin, chalk, phenobarbitone, succinylsulphathiazole, sulphadimidine, calamine, hydrocortisone, sulphur, zinc oxide etc.

**Suspensions Produced by chemical Reactions**

Very occasionally the insoluble active constituent of a lotion etc. is formed by a chemical reaction. A Filner precipitate is obtained if dilute solutions of the reactants are mixed, hence, the reacting substances

Should be dissolved separately in approximately half volumes of the vehicle and the two parts mixed prepared in the manner the precipitate is diffusible and no suspending agents is necessary. An official example of this kind of preparation is zinc sulphide location B.P.C which is used to treat acne and scabies.

**Physical Stability of Suspension**

In most cases suspension formulation are not physically stab le due to the sedimentation of the dispersed particles. Hydrocolloids used as suspending agents are very susceptible to microbial growth resulting in gas and color formation. Discoloration and loss of viscosity along with others. Therefore suitable preservative should be incorporated along with other necessary stabilizers.

The factors influencing the rate of sedimentation is expressed by **Stoke's law** as follows

$$V = \frac{d^2(\rho_1 - \rho_2)g}{18\eta} = \frac{2r^2(\rho_1 - \rho_2)g}{9\eta}$$

Where,

V = Velocity of the settling particles

g = Acceleration due to gravity

d = Average diameter of the particle

r = Average radius of the particle

$\rho_1$= Density of the particle

$\rho_2$= Density of the liquid / dispersed mediums

$\eta$ = The viscosity of the dispersion medium

## Points to Remember

- A wetting agent is included in the formulation of a suspension, particularly when the suspended particles are **hydrophobic.**
- When charcoal powder is dusted on the surface of water, the contact angle that the charcoal exhibits is **108°**

- Suspension and emulsion are coarse dispersion when particle size is usually 1-100 micron
- **Electrolyte, Surfactant & polymer** are used to make flocculated suspension are stability of suspension can be predicated by measuring **Zeta potential.**
- The most commonly used flocculating agents is **bentonite magma.**
- A suspension is not suitable dosage for **intravenous** type of injection.
- **Pseudo plastic flow &Thixotrophy** are the properties are desirable in a pharmaceutical suspension.
- A suspension is said to be colloid able when particle size is usually **1-500 micron.**
- The characteristics of particles in an ideal suspension are, **particle should be aggregated.**
- Brownian movement of particle in suspension depends upon density of the particle, density of the medium and viscosity of the medium.
- Suspensions containing high concentration (50% or more) of deflocculated particles represents **Dilatant flow.**
- The initial rate of setting of particle is determined by floc size & porosity of aggregated mass.
- The ratio of volume of the sediment and original volume of suspension is called **Sedimentation volume.**
- The pH of an antacid suspension is around 8.
- Sorbitols, Menitol, Potassium citrate, Sodium Citrate are the agents added to **prevent gelling.**
- **Magnesium hydroxide** is used along with aluminium hydroxide gel in the antacid preparation because magnesium hydroxide has **laxative action** which counters the **constipation action** of aluminium hydroxide.
- The antioxidants like sodium formaldehyde sulfoxylate USP is added in suspension with high solids content because **it prevent the color** formation during storage.
- The suspension made by dispersion process is achieved by **Pulverization** of solid by **micro ionization** technique.
- The suspensions made by controlled crystallisation, a supersaturated solution should be formed and then quickly cooled with rapid stirring.
- The suspension stability can be evaluated by a) Sedimentation volume b) Rheological method c)Electro kinetic technique d)Particle size determination.

  The **silicon is coated** glass is used for packing the suspension products due to

  (a) Improve drainage of suspension

  (b) Minimize the leaching of alkali from glass in to the product.
- **Polyacrylic acid(Carbopol),** a pure synthetic polymer is widely used in preparation of external lotion and gel.
- Clay suspension and gels contains non-ionic preservatives like paraben esters and benzoates. But quaternary preservatives are ineffective.
- A maximum sedimentation volume will be obtained when zeta potential is **Zero.**
- When aluminium chloride or Calcium hydrogen phosphate is dissolved in water, the suspension exhibits a **negative apparent zeta potential.**
- When is dissolved in water? The apparent zeta potential initially is **negative.**
- Protective colloids differ from surfactant. In respect that

  (a) They do not **reduce interfacial tension** like surfactants

(b) They are used in **higher concentration** than surfactants.

(c) They have ability to **increase the Zeta-potential**

- **Hydrophilic** colloidal material is used commonly in the preparation of a structured vehicle.
- The isoelectric point of insulin is **pH 5**
- The isoelectric point of protamine zinc insulin is **pH 6.9 to 7.3**
- The protamine zinc insulin suspension is prepared by a method like **altered pH precipitation.**

## 1.2 Pharmaceutical Engineering

### Size Reduction

Size reduction is a process of reducing large solid unit mass (vegetable or chemical substances) into small unit mass, coarse particles or fine particles. This is also termed as communication or diminution or pulverization.Size reduction can be achieved by two processes-

- Precipitation method,
- Mechanical process.

**Precipitation Process:**

The substance is dissolved in appropriate solvent. Subsequently, it is finely precipitated by the addition of another solvent, which is immiscible with the first, but in the later the substance is insoluble. Inorganic chemical such as calcium carbonate, magnesium carbonate and yellow mercuric oxide, are prepared by precipitation method.

**Mechanical process:**

In this process the substances is subject to mechanical forces using grinding and cutting equipment.

**Table** General Characteristics of Various Types of Mills

| Name of the Mill | Action | Product size | Uses | Not for used |
|---|---|---|---|---|
| **Cutter mill** | Cutting | 20-80 mesh | Fibrous, crude animal and vegetable drugs | Friable material |
| **Roller mill** | Compression & attrition | 20-200 mesh | Fine grinding of abrasive material | Abrasive material |
| **Hammer mill** | Impact | 4-325 mesh | All most all drugs | Abrasive material |
| **Ball mill** | Attrition & Impact | 20-200 mesh | Brittle drugs | Soft material |
| **Fluid energy mill** | Attrition & Impact | 1-30 | Moderately hard & friable material | Soft & sticky material |
| **Edge runner mill** | Crushing & shearing | 20-80 mesh | All most all the drugs | Sticky material |
| **End runner mill** | Crushing & Shearing | 20-80 mesh | All most all the drugs | Sticky material |
| **Colloid mill** | Shearing | 3-75 μm | All most all the drugs | Dry milling |
| **Disintegrator** | Impact & grinding | | Hard drugs | |
| **Pin mill (Reddrop-periflo mill)** | | | Fine grinding substances with low melting points such as resin, soap, sugar etc. | |

**Table** Some of mill used for size reduction and their specifications

| Name of the mill | Action | Use | Variants |
|---|---|---|---|
| **Cutter mill** | The cutting action is attained by two sets of stationary and rotating knives.<br>The rotor disc is allowed to rotate **200-900** revolutions per minute | Medicinal plants, Plant parts, and animal tissues are normally converted into small parts. | Double runner disc mill<br>Single runner disc mill |
| **Roller mill** | The degree of the size reduction can be attained by adjusting the gap between the two follers. | It is used for crushing and cracking of seeds before extraction of fixed oils.<br>It is also used to crush soft issues to help in the penetration of solvent during extraction process. | |
| **Hammer mill** | The hammers are made up of **stainless steel** and the impact surface is made of **haystellite and carbaloy.**<br>The hammers are to be in a continueous motion **8000-15000 r**evolution per minute. | It is used to mill dry materials, wet filter press cakes, ointments, slurries etc. | 1.Fitzpatrick communicating machine (Fitz mill)<br>2. Stokes tornado mill<br>3. Micro pulveriser |
| **Ball mill (Tumbling mill)** | The cylinder contain ball that occupy **30-50%** of the mill volume. The drug to be reduced in size should fill in the cylinder of **60%** volume. | Brittle drugs | Harding mill<br>Continuous ball mill<br>Vibrating ball mill |
| **Fluid energy mill/ Jet mill/ micronizer/ ultrafine grinder** | It consists of an elliptical pipe, which has a height of about 2 meter long and diameter ranging from **20 to 200** millimetres.<br>Normally compressed air is used at **600 kilopascal to 1.0 mega pascals.** | It is mostly used to reduce the particle size of most of the drugs such as **antibiotics and vitamins.** | 1.Centrifugal impact pulveriser |
| **Edge runner mill** | The size reduction done by crushing (compression) due to heavy weight of stones. | It is used for plant based products. | |
| **End runner mill** | The size reduction done by crushing (compression) due to heavy weight of steel pestle. | It is used for fine grinding products. | |
| **Colloid mill** | The clearance between rotor and stator can be adjusted from **0.05-0.75mm.**<br>The rotor is moving at **3000-20000** revolution per minute.<br>During milling heat is generated and may rise the temperature up to **40°C** hence cold water circulation is provided to reduce the temperature up to **20°C.**<br>The capacity of mill ranging from **2-3L/min** for small mills to **440L/min** for the large mills. | Usually suspension and emulsion are placed in this mill. | |

- **Griffith theory** -The amount of force to be applied depends on the crack length and focus of stress at the atomic bond of the crack apex.
- **Hooke's law-**Stress is proportional to strain
- **Young modulus**-Express the stiffness or softness in dyne per square centimetre
- **Kick's law**-The energy required for size reduction is directly related to the reduction rati
- **Bond low**-The energy required for size reduction

## Points to be Remembered

- The size of micro ionized particle is typically **less than 10μm.**
- Micro calorimetry process, Dynemic vapour sorption process, inverse gas chromatography process (IGC) are used to detect the **change in crystallinity of the drug** particle & other surface property of powder during size reduction.
- Laser light scattering technique is used, to detect distribution of particle sizes.
- Malvan Masersizer is used to measure particle sizes.
- Malvan Masersizer works on the principal of laser **diffraction.**
- Fraunhofer& Mie's light scattering theory is applied to determine to **measure particle size.**
- Aerosizer is used to measure particle sizes. It works on the technique of **light scattering.**
- The sizer of colloid particles are preferably determined by **quasi elastic light scattering** technique.
- Couter determines particle size by Electrical Zone sensing technique.
- Photon correlation spectroscopy (PCS) and single particle optical sizing (SPOS) technique are used to measure **particle sizes.**
- Krypton & gas is used to determine surfaces area of drug particles by gas adsorption method
- $S_t = \frac{V_{mom} N A_{cs}}{M}$ is the equation is used for surface area determination of the drug particles for the BET isotherm for Type –II adsorption methods.
- **Displacement of liquid** method is most commonly used method in the pharmaceutical industry for measuring true density.
- **Helium** is taken as references during the true density measurement by Gas picnometry method

**Table** Particle size range and their specifications

| Technique | Size range |
|---|---|
| Laser light scattering (Quasi elastic) | 0.001 – 1 μm |
| Electrical Zone sensing | 1 – 200 μm |
| Electron microscopy | 0.001 – 5 μm |
| Woven wire sieving | 20 – 125, 000 μm |
| Sedimentation by centrifugation | 0.01 – 5 μm |
| Optical microscopy | 5 – 150 μm |
| Sieving by perforated plate | 1000 – 125000 μm |

## Size Separation

Size Separation is a pharmaceutical process by which the particles of different sizes are separated from a mixture. Also called as,

- Sifting.
- Sieving.
- Classifying.
- Screening.

**Table** Official standard for powders

| Grade of powder | Sieve size all particles pass through | Nominal mesh aperture size | Sieve through which 40% particles pass | Nominal mesh aperture size |
|---|---|---|---|---|
| **Coarse** | #10 sieve | 1.7 mm | #44 sieve | 355 µm |
| **Moderately coarse** | #22 sieve | 710 µm | #60 sieve | 250 µm |
| **Moderately fine** | #44 sieve | 355 µm | #85 sieve | 180 µm |
| **Fine** | #85 sieve | 180 µm | - | - |
| **Very fine** | #120 sieve | 125 µm | - | - |

**Table** The list of method of size reduction and the particle size related to it:

| Match the method of size separation | Particle size |
|---|---|
| **Microscopy** | 0.4 to 150 µm |
| **Sieving** | 10 to 50 µm |
| **Sedimentation** | 1 to 200 µm |

**Types of sieves:**

1. Woven wire sieves : These sieves are included in roller mill, ball mill.
2. Blotting cloth sieves : Silk, nylon, and cotton are generally woven from twisted multi-trend fibres. These are used for separation of fine powders. Hum-mer screen uses this type of screens.
3. Bar screen : These are used handling large and heavy pieces of materials. Grizzlies use this type of screens.
4. Punched plate : These types are used for coarse sizing. And used in hammer mill.
5. Herringbone design : This is the punched plate type of sieve. It consists of a series of slotted holes repeated across the surface of the seven. These are made at an angle of degree to the length of the screen.

**Sieve number**: Sieve number indicate the number of meshes per liner length of 25.4 millimetres.

**Nominal mesh aperture size**: It indicates the distance between the two adjacent wires. It represents the side of a square aperture. It is expressed in mm or µm.

**Sieve shaker machine**: It is a mechanical shaker apparatus and the standard sieves of different mesh numbers are fixed vertically. A sample of 50 gm of powder is placedon the top sieve and shaken for 20 minutes of time. After the powder retained in each sieve is weighed and the percentage retention is calculated.

**Cyclone separator**: In cyclone separator centrifugal forces is used to separate the solids from fluids. It's also used to separate solids from gases.

**Elutriation**: This is a size separation method based on sedimentation principle it may be used to separate the coarse and fine particle present in a paste after levitation.

## Mixing

**Mixing** is defined as the unit operation that combines two or more components together by agitation, shear or mixers. The final product of mixture contains uniform distribution of both components of mixture.

Example of mixers: Blenders, Planetary mixtures, Propellers etc.

**Table** Mechanism of mixing

| Method | Mechanism |
|---|---|
| **Trituration** | Rubbing or grinding a substance in a mortar |
| **Spatulation** | Small amount of powder is blended |
| **Levigation** | Adding a suitable agent to form a paste & then rubbing |
| **Pulverization** | Reducing & sub diving a substance by adding as easily removed |
| **Tubling** | Process of mixing powder in a large container rotated by electric motor |
| **Geometrical mixing** | Method used when potent substances are to be mixed |

**Table** Various instruments and their specification which are used for mixing

| Equipment's | Rate of rotation | Mechanism | Mixing materials |
|---|---|---|---|
| **V cone blender** | Smaller – 35 rpm<br>Larger – 15 rpm | Tumbling | |
| **Double cone blender** | 30 -100 rpm | Tumbling | Powder |
| **Fluidized mixture** | | Air supported blending | Wet granulation of tablet |
| **Barrel type of continuous mixture** | | Rotating shell and rotating blade | |
| **Zig-zag continuous mixture** | | Rotating shell and rotating blade | |
| **Ribbon blender** | | Stationary shell and rotating blade | Mixing of glident with tablet granules before punching |
| **Sigma blade mixture** | | Stationary shell and rotating blade | Wet granulation of tablet Stiff paste and ointment |
| **Planetary mixture** | Varied as per desireness | Shear | Wet granulation of tablets |
| **Emulsifier (Silver son mixer)** | | Shear & Turbulence | Emulsion and cream of fine particle size |
| **Colloid mill** | | | Emulsion |
| **Ultrasonic emulsifier** | | Ultrasonic vibration | Emulsion |
| **Triple roller mill** | | | Suspension, paste & ointment |

## Filtration

Filtration is a separation technique used to concentrate or purify substances based on their physical or chemical properties. It is a simple and routine method used in many laboratories to remove insoluble particles from solutions and to prepare samples for analysis. Filtration is used to reduce sample complexity, improve clarity of viscous samples, and reduce background signals resulting in increased signal-to-noise ratios in analytical tests.

**Table** Filtration according to particle size

| Pore size (micron) | Particle removed |
|---|---|
| 0.22 μm | All bacteria |
| 0.45 μm | All coliform group bacteria |
| 0.2 μm | All bacteria |
| 0.8 μm | All airborne particle |
| 1.2 μm | All non-living particles considered dangerous |
| 0.45 μm | All coliform group bacteria |

**Table** List of material and their filtration performance

| Fibres used for filter | Temperature recommends | Performance |
|---|---|---|
| | Safe limits °F | |
| Catton | 210 | Poor |
| Polyester | 200 | Very Good |
| Dynelmodacyclic | 300 | |
| Acrylic | 475 | Excellent |
| Saran | 160 | |
| Polyethylene | 165 | |
| Polypropylene | 175 | |
| Polyvinylchloride | 165 | Good |
| Wood | 210 | |
| Teflon | 475 | |
| Rayon & acetate | 210 | Poor |
| Glass | 750 | Excellent |
| Nylon | | Fair |
| Wool | | Very Good |

**Mechanism of filtration:**

(a) Straining : The particles larger cannot pass through the smaller pore size of the filter medium.

(b) Impingement : Solids having the momentum move along the path of streamline flow and strike the filter medium. Thus the solids retained on the filter medium.

(c) Entanglement : Particles becomes entwined in the mass of fibres due to smaller size of particles then the pore size.

(d) Attractive force : Solids are retrained on the filter medium as a result of attractive forces between particles and filter medium, as in case of electrostatic precipitation.

**Theory of filtration:**

Darey's equation: $$V = \frac{KA\Delta P}{\eta L}$$

Poiseuille's equation: $$V = \frac{\pi \Delta P r^2}{8\eta L}$$

Kozeny- Carman equation: $$V = \frac{A}{\eta S^2}, \frac{\Delta P}{KL}, \frac{\varepsilon^2}{(1-\varepsilon)^2}$$

## Drying

- **Bond moisture:** It is the minimum moisture held by the material that exerts an equilibrium vapour pressure less than the pure water at the same temperature.
- **Unbound moisture:** It is the amount of moisture held by the material that exerts an equilibrium vapour equal to that of pure water at the same temperature.
- **Equilibrium Moisture content (EMC):** It is the amount of water present in the solid which exerts a vapour pressure equal to the vapour pressure of the atmosphere surrounding it.

- For **zero humidity, EMC** of **all material is zero.** As the temperature of air increase, the EMC of solid decreases.
- **Free Moisture content (EMC):** It is the amount of moisture that is free to evaporate from the solid surface.

**Table** Type of dryer and their mechanism

| Type of dryer and mechanism | Example | Use |
|---|---|---|
| Static Bed Dryer<br>**System in which there is no relative movement among the solid particle being dried, although may be bulk motion of the entire drying mass.** | Tray dryer and freeze dryer | Sticky material, Plastic substance, granular mass or crystalline material, precipitates and pastes can be dried in a tray dryer. |
| Moving Bed Dryer<br>**System in which the drying particles are partially separated so that they flow over each other.** | Drum dryer | It is useful for drying solutions, suspension, slurries etc. Usually the products dried are milk products starch products etc. |
| Fluidised Bed Dryers<br>**System in which the solid particles are partially suspended in an upward moving heated gas system** | Fluidised bed dryer | It is used for drying of granules in the production of tablets.<br>I can be useful for three operations such as mixing, granulation and drying. |
| Pneumatic Dryer<br>**System in which drying particles are entrained and conveyed at a high velocity gas stream.** | Spray dryer | |
| Freeze Dryer<br>**Freeze drying, is also known as lyophlization. In freeze drying, water is removed from the frozen state by sublimation.** | Freeze dryer | It is used in the production of blood plasma, and its fractioned products, Bacterial and viral cultures, Antibiotics and plant extracts, steroids, Vitamins and enzymes, Human tissue etc. |
| Vacuum Dryer<br>**In vacuum dryer, material is dried by the application of vacuum is created; the pressure is lowered so that water boils at a lower temperature. Hence water evaporates faster.** | Vacuum dryer | It is used for heat sensitive materials, Dusty and hygroscopic materials, Drug containing toxic solvents, Drugs which are required as porous end products and friability dry extracts. |

## 1.3 Semisolid Dosage Froms

- Semisolid dosage forms meant for external application
- Semisolid dosage forms subcategorized are as-
  - ➢ Creams
  - ➢ Paste
  - ➢ Jellies
  - ➢ Ointment
  - ➢ Suppositories
- The suppositories are also included in this category but it is a unit dosage forms.

### Creams

- ➢ These are viscous semisolid emulsions, which are meant for external use.
- ➢ Cream is divided in to two types namely as
  - (i) Aqueous creams
  - (ii) Oily creams

- In case of aqueous creams the emulsions are o/w type & it is relatively non greasy. The emulsifying waxes are anionic, cationic & non –ionic used. Generally polysorbate, triethanolamine soap are used as emulsifying agent.
- In case of oily creams w/o type & it is relatively greasy. The emulsifying agent such as wool fat, wool alcohols, and beeswax & calcium soap is used.
- The cream should be store in collapsible tube & supplied in well closed container to prevent evaporation & contamination.

## Pastes

- Pastes are semisolid preparations intended for external application to skin.
- The pastes are generally very thick & stiff.
- They do not melt at ordinary temperature & thus forms a protective coating over the area where they are applied.
- Pastes are differ from ointment as they contain a high proportion of finely powdered medicaments.
- They are mainly used as a antiseptic, protective, soothing dressings.
- Pastes should be stored & supplied in containers made of materials which do not allow absorption or diffusion of content.

## Jellies

- Jellies are transparent or translucent, non greasy, semi solid preparations mainly used for external application to skin.
- These are also used for lubricating catheters, surgical gloves & rectal thermometer.
- The substance like gelatin, starch, tragacanth, sodium alginate & cellulose derivatives are used for the formulation of jellies.
- Jellies are of three types namely as
- Medicated jellies
- Lubricating jellies
- Miscellaneous jellies

## Ointments

- Ointments are semisolid preparation meant for application to skin or mucous membrane.
- The ointments are mainly used for their protective or emollient properties
- It may be defined as a medicament or medicaments dissolved, suspended or emulsified in ointment base.
- There is no single ointment base which possesses all the qualities of ideal ointment base, so it become necessary to use more than one ointment base in the preparation of ointment.

**Table** Base for the Ointments and ointment types

| Name of base | Ointments |
|---|---|
| **Hydrocarbon base** | Soft paraffin, Hard paraffin, Liquid paraffin |
| **Absorption base** | Wool fat (Anhydrous lanolin), Wool alcohol, Bees wax, Cholesterol, Lanolin (Hydrous wool fat) etc. |
| **Water-Miscible bases** | Anionic, cationic non-ionic emulsifying base |
| **Water soluble base** | Polyethylene glycol |

**Table** Other Ingredients of Ointment bases

| Name | Example |
|---|---|
| **Vegetable oils** | Arachis, castor, coconut, olive etc |
| **Synthetic esters oil fatty acid** | Isopropyl myristate |
| **Higher fatty alcohols** | Cetyl, sterayl, cetosteary alcohols etc. |
| **Silicons** | - |
| **Propylene glycols** | - |

- Determination of iodine value depends upon addition of iodine at the **double bond of fatty acids.**
- **Plastibase** is a common ointment vehicle. It is a mixture **of mineral oil and hydrocarbon waxes.**
- The following procedures help to improve the absorption of a drug into the skin-
  - Application of the ointment and covering the area with an occlusive bandage or saran wrap
  - Incorporating an oil-soluble drug in polyethylene glycol ointment rather than white ointment.
  - Appling the medicated ointment on the back of the hand rather than on the palms.
  - Increasing the concentration of the active drug in the ointment base.
- The substances which have been shown to increase the permeability of the skin are sodium lauryl sulphate, Chloroform, Benzene, Dimethyl sulfoxide etc.
- The substances which have been shown to **increase the permeability** of the skin are sodium lauryl sulphate, Chloroform, Benzene, Dimethyl sulfoxide etc.
- **Aqueous solutions** may be incorporated in to the entire following ointment base like lanolin, Aquaphor Unibase, polysorb etc.
- Silicones are useful in ointment formulas since they are good water repellents.
- Lassar's paste is a zinc oxide paste with salicylic acid.
- Hudrophlic petrolatum contains Cholesterol as an emulsifier.
- Petrolatum rose water ointment is a synonym for cold cream USP.
- Iodine **value** may be defined as the weight of iodine absorbed by **100 parts by weight** of the sample of fat of oil.
- The liberation of oil or water from ointment base is called bleeding.
- The term greasiness is suitable used for water dispersible base & o/w base.
- The effect of temperature on the consistency of an ointment base can be analysed by rotational viscometer.
- Melting point range of paraffin wax is 35-75°C
- Crup testing is applied to analyse the viscoelastic property of Ointment.
- Ceresin is a mixture of Ozokerite (mined wax) & Paraffin wax.
- Stearic acid is used in water removable creams as an emulsifier.
- Promulgen G is a mixture of Stearyl alcohol & Ethoxylated cetearyl alcohol.
- During prepration of a topical ointment, the preservative efficacy of the formulation is determined by using Tat broth.
- AS per the microbiological guideline, the limit for the raw material used for Baby product is Not more than (nmt) 500 microorganisms per gram of millilitre.

- About the eye- nmt 500 microorganisms per gram or millilitre.
- Oral products – nmt 1000 microorganisms per gram or millilitre.
- All other products nmt 10500 microorganisms per gram or millilitre.
- Methyl paraben and propyl paraben are tend to irritate to eye or nasal passage, So quaternary ammoniym compounds or phenyl mercuric salts are suitable preservatives for ophthalmic and nasal preparations.
- The paraben esters of p-hydroxybenxoic acid is less effective against gram negative bacteria.
- Germall II (Imidazolidine urea) (0.1-0.5%) is used in combination to increase the activity.
- Liqa per is an emulsion of p-hydroxybenzoic acid esters. A 50% by weight oil-in-water emulsion. The oil phase is a mixture of p-hydroxybenzoic acid esters –n-butyl, isobutyl and iso propyl. The aqueous protion contains water with emulsion stabilizers.
- Dowicil, chemically cis isomer 1-(3chlorollyal)-3, 5, 7-triaza-1-azoniaadimanteane is IA broad spectrum anti-microbial agent and not inactivated by non-ionic, anionic, or cationic formulation ingredients.

**Table** Various type of base and their example with composition

| Base | Example and their water number with composition |
|---|---|
| Oleaginous base | Lanolin |
| Absorption base | Kersolin, Wool fat, Aquaphor |
| Emulsion base | Mineral oil |
| Water soluble base | Polyethylene glycol |
| Petrolatum | 9 to 15 water number |
| Wool fat | 185 water number |
| Cocoa butter | Mixed glycerides |
| Cotmar | Partially hydrogenated cotton seed oil |
| Dehydag | Hydrogenated fatty alcohol & esters |
| Wecobee R | Glycerides of saturated fatty acid |
| Wecobee SS | Triglycerides derived from coconut oil |
| Eitpsol | Triglycerides of saturated fatty acid |

| **Different values** | **Definition** |
|---|---|
| Iodine value | Number of grams of iodine that treacts with 100 g of fat |
| Water number | Amount of water in grams that can be incorporated in 100 g of fat |
| Acid value | KOH required to neutralize the free acid |
| Saponification value | KOH required to neutralize th free acids &saponify the easters |
| Hydroxyl value | Measuring un esterified position of glyceride molecules |

## Gels

- Gels may be defined as semisolids, being either suspension of small inorganic particles or large organic molecules interpenetrated with liquid.
- On the basis of the nature of the colloidal phase the Gels may be classified into-
  1. **Inorganic gels**: Bentonite magma.
  2. **Organic gells**: Natural gum (Accacia, caragreen xanthan gum, anionic polysaccharide)
     Polyethylenes
     Metalic stearates

Polypeptides (Gelatin)
Synthetic block polymers (ploxamers)

- On the basis of the nature of the solvents the Gels may be classified into –
- **Hydrogel**: Bentonite megma&Gelatin
- **Organogels (With non-aqeous solvent)**: Low molecular weight polyethylene dissolved in mineral oil and shock cooled metallic stearates in oils.
- Solid gels with very low solvent concentration are known as **xerogels.**Eg. Dry gelatin, tragacanth ribbons and acacia tears.
- Liquid of the gel is pressed out naturally after standing for sometimes. This process is called **Syneresis.**
- Sometimes the gel structure would converted to solution structure, which again in a undisturbed stage converted to gel structure. This phenomenon is known as **Thixotrophy.**
- The stability of visco elastic material of gel can be measured by **penetrometer.**
- When gels can accommodate small amount of liquid without measurable increase in the volume, the process is known **imbibition.**
- Pectin paste is a **Jelly.**

**Table** Different type gels and their example

| Different types of gels | Definition / example |
|---|---|
| **Gel** | Solid or semisolid system in which at least two constituents condensed in which liquid is interpenetrated |
| **Jelly** | Coherent matrix is rich in water |
| **Xerogel** | Frame work of gel in fee from liquid |
| **Hydrogels** | Water containing gels |
| **Organogels** | Organic liquid containing gels |
| **Organic hydrogel** | Tragacanth jelly |
| **Inorganic hydrogels** | Bentonite gel |
| **Animal organogel** | Theobroma oil |
| **Soap base organogel** | Mineral oil gel |
| **Hydrocarbon type organo-gel** | Petrolatum |
| **Hydrophillicorgano-gel** | Carbowax base |

## Suppositories & Pessaries

**"Suppositories"** are solid medicated preparations designed for insertion in the rectum where they melt, dissolve or disperse and exert a local or systemic effect.

**"Pessaries"** are similar solid medicated preparation designed for insertion into the vagina, usually to exert a local effect.

**"Bougies"** are urethral suppositories.

- **Suppository bases:** There are two main classes of suppository base.
  - ➢ Fatty base designed to melt at body temperature. : eg. Theobroma oil, Synthetic hard fat.
  - ➢ Water soluble or water miscible base designed to dissolve or disperse with the body eg. Glycero-Gelatin, Macrogels (PEG) like Macrogel- 400, 1000, 1540, 4000, 6000.

**Displacement value:** The number of parts by weight of medicaments that displace one part by weight of the base-

- Glycerin suppositories contain 92% glycerine and are solidified by the use of sopdium stearate.
- A group of substances used as suppository bases that dissolve rather than melt are carbowaxes
- Most commercial vaginal suppositories use a base of Polyethylene glycol.
- Suppositories may be used as a deodorant.

**Table** Cocoa butter and their boiling point

| Cocoa butter form | Boiling point |
|---|---|
| α – form | 24°C |
| β – form | 28 to 31°C |
| β' – form | 34 to 35°C |
| γ – form | 18°C |

**Table** Represents different values for ideal suppository

| Different values for ideal suppository | |
|---|---|
| Acid value | 0.2 |
| Saponification value | 200 to 245 |
| Iodine value | 7 |

## 1.4 Cosmetics

### Lipstick

Lipsticks are the lip cosmetic molded into sticks are essentially dispersion of colourings matter in a base consisting of suitable blends of oil, fats, and waxes.

**Ingredients of Lipstick**

**1. Colouring material:**

(i) Eosin

(ii) Halogenated fluorescein (Tetrachlorotetrrabroimo fluorescein, di-iodoflorescein)

- Eosin produces purple red stain above pH4
- Halogenated fluorescein produces brilliant bluish stain.

**2. Pigments:**

(i) Titanium dioxide (It is the most effective white pigment used as opacifying agent.)

(ii) D&C Red No.36, and D&C Orange No.17 (These are insoluble in both water & oil used as pigments)

(iii) Lakes (Calcium lakes, Barium lakes, Aluminum lakes)

**3. Base:**

(a) Natural oil – Castor Oil (30-40%)

(b) Fatty alcohol (Lauryl - $C_{12}$, Steryl - $C_{18}$, Myristyl- $C_{14}$, Oleyl- $C_{18}$, Cetyl - $C_{16}$,

(c) Hexadecyl alcohol)

(d) Easter (Adipic, Sebcic)

(e) Polyethlene glycols (Carbowaxes)

(f) Monoakanolamide (Loramine)

(g) Polychol-5 (It is an ethylene oxide derivate of lanolin alcohol)

(h) Valpoa-3 (It is a polyoxethyleneoleyl ether)

**4. Other base ingredients:**

- Carnumba wax – It is used for raising melting point and providing contraction properties in the molding process.
- Candeilla – It serves some function as carnauba wax but having low melting points and less brittle.
- Ozokeriatic wax- It gives short – fibred texture to the products.
- Microcrystalline wax – It is used to modify the rheology of the products.
- Bees wax – It is used as shifting agent for castor oil.
- Lanolin – They have eosin solvent property. They act as binding agent for other ingredient and acting as plasticizer.
- Petroleum jelly – They have eosin solvent property. They act as binding agent for other ingredient and acting as plasticizer.
- Lecithin – It act as dispersing agent for pigments.
- Silicon wax- These are used as cosmetic solvent & colouring agents. eg. Organosilicon block Polymer, hydrocarbon silicon polymer, Silphenylene co-polymer.

**5. Perfumes: (2-4%)** e.g. Rose oil, Aniseed oil, cinnamon Oil, Clove oil, lemon oil, orange oil Etc.

- **Manufacture of lipsticks**

  The lipstick manufacture involves three stages.

  - The preparation of component blends, that is oil blend, color dispersion, and wax blend.
  - Blending of the intermediates too form the lipstick mass.
  - The molding of lipstick mass into the sticks.

- **Transparent lipsticks**

  - These type of lipsticks does not contain any insoluble opaque pigment or lakes but instead uses soluble or solubilized dyes.
  - This allows light to shine through it.
  - Giving sparkle.
  - The staining action of these days is enhanced by the use of suitable solvent such as Loramine OM-101 or dipropylemne glycol methyl ether.

- **Liquid lipstick**

  The liquid lipstick consists of

  - Alcoholic solution of alcoholic soluble dyes-e.g. - Alcoholic soluble halogenated fluorescins.
  - Suitable film forming resins- e.g. – Ethyl cellulose, polyvinyl alcohol and polyvinay acetate.
  - Plasticizers - e.g – Triethylcitrtate, dioctyl acetate, methyl abietate or Polyethylene.

- **Evaluation of lipsticks**

  Lipsticks are evaluated by means of following tests:

  1. Droop point test – The temperature at which the lipstick starts oozing out oil or flatten out from within the case is known as droop point.
  2. Breaking point test – This determines the strength of lipstick. The lipstick is held horizontally in a socket and a gradually increasing weight is applied on the lipstick half an inch away from the base, and the weight at which breaks is taken as breaking point.

3. Test for penetrability – This test indicates the rheological property of the lipstick. A needle of specific diameter is allowed to penetrate the lipstick and depth of penetration is noted.
4. Test for force of application – Lipstick is applied on the piece of paper (kept in a balance at an angle of 45°, and the force required for applying is read from the balance.
5. Stability test – Stability of lipsticks can be determined by means of accelerated stability test in which lipstick formulation is kept at higher temp. (Say 45°C) and assessing the lipstick for surface defects, perfume, color and application characteristics.

## Shampoos

Shampoo is a preparation meant for cleaning hairs of dust, grime, crust and to impart gloss to hairs.

Characteristics of a Good Shampoo-

- Effectively remove soil, sebum, and residues of hair setting lotions or oils from the scalp
- Good amount of foam to satisfy psychological needs of the customer.
- Easily removed on rinsing of hairs.
- Makes the hair soft, lustrous and manageable.
- Pleasant fragrance.
- Non-toxic and non-irritant.

**Formulation of shampoos**

1. Surfactants
2. Conditioning agents
3. Thickening agents
4. Chelating agents
5. Antidandruff agents
6. Colours
7. Perfumes
8. Preservatives

- **Surfactants:** These are principle surfactants used in shampoo. Cationic surfactants are only used as conditioners and not as principle surfactants because of their irritation potential. Non-ionic are also used but they do not good foaming ability. Soaps were used earlier as they are cheap but they ae highly alkaline and they make hair dull. Further they also leave deposits of calcium and magnesium with hard water. Examples of surfactants used include **Sodium lauryl sulphate, Triethanolamine lauryl sulphate, monoethanol lauryl sulphate etc.**
- **Conditioning agents**: These agents improve manageability, feel lustier of the hairs. Various materials used as conditioning agents include lanolin, mineral oil, egg albumin, amino acids, lecithin and herbal extracts like shikakai and henna.
- **Thickening agents:** This make shampoo viscous so that they are easy to poor and handle. Example of thickening agents employed in shampoos include natural gum like gum karaya, gum tragacanth, cellulose derivatives like **CMC, HPMC**, polymers kuje**Polyvinylalcohol, carbopol 934P** etc.
- **Chelating agents:** These are used to prevent the deposition of calcium and magnesium salts of soaps on hairs eg. **Disodium edentate, polyphosphates, citric acid etc.**

**Types of Shampoo**

1. Liquid shampoo
2. Liquid shampoo

3. Cream based shampoo
4. Powder Shampoo
5. Aerosol shampoo
6. Antidandruff shampoo
7. Baby shampoo

**Table** Some important material used in Antidandruff shampoo for the treatment of Dandruff

| Name of the material | Usual conc. % |
|---|---|
| Thymol | 0.05-0.2 |
| Selenium sulphide | 0.1-2.5 |
| Quaternary Ammonium compound | 15-20 |
| 1,2 Bithional | 0.5-1.0 |
| 2-pyridinethiol-oxide | 2 |
| Zink pyridinethiol-oxide (ZPTO) it is used in Head& Shoulder the popular anti dandruff shampoo | 2 |
| 2-mercapto-quinoxaline-1-okide | |
| 2-mercapto-quinoline-1-oxide | |

- **Baby Shampoo**: The baby shampoo's mild ness is provided by choosing non-irritant surfactants that produce limited detergency. The most common surfactants are amphoteric imidazoline dervatives and the fatty sulphosuccinate esters and amides are usually combined with ethoxylatedsorbitan or mannitan ester to give sting free composition.
- Tween 20 is combined with a complex obtained from tridecyltrilethoxy sulphate and N-(2-cocoamidoethyl) diethanolamine is used in the **Johnson & Johnson's** popular baby shampoo **'no more tears'**

## Nail Preparations

**Nail polish/ Nail enamels:** A distinction is drawn between those polishes which by abrasive action bestow a gloss on the nail surface & a nail varnish.

The formulation includes as-

1. Film former
2. Solvent
3. Plasticizers
4. Colours
5. Pearlescent pigments
6. Perfume

- **Film former:** Cellulose nitrate, Cellulose acetate, Cellulose acetobutyrate, ethyl cellulose, Stannic acid, powered silica, methacrylate and vinyl polymers are used as film formers in nail lacquers. But ethyl cellulose is most widely used film formers.
- **Solvent:** Usually a mixture of high boiling, medium boiling, and low boiling solvents are employed in nail enamels. The mixture of solvents is so balanced that precipitation of cellulose nitrate is prevented. The example of solvents are-
- High boiling – butyl lactate, ethyl oxalate, isoamyl acetate etc.
- Medium boiling – Isopropylacetate, touene, methyl acetate, ethyl acetate etc.

- Low boiling – Ether, Carbon disulphide, acetone, methyl acetate, ethyl acetate etc.
- **Plasticizers:** These impart flexibility and gloss to the film, and also help in adhesion of fill to the nails e.g. Dibutyl phthalate, resorcinol diacetate, castor oil, butyl acetyl ricinolate etc.
- **Pearlescent:** These impart pearly appearance to the film. E.g. 2-amino, 6-oxypurine (crystalline guanine), bismuth oxy chloride coated pigments.
- **Enamel Remover:** These are the preparations intended to remove enamel from the nails and basically consists of simple mixture of solvents such as acetone, amyl acetate of ethyl acetate. Gamma-Valera tone (GVL) is used as strong enamel remover.

## Dentrifices

Dentifrices are the preparations intended to clean the teeth of food debris, prevent calculus and plaque formation, polish to import lustre for the teeth and to leave a refreshing feeling in mouth. They are two types tooth powder and tooth paste.

**Formulation of the Tooth Powder:**

1. Abrasives and polishing agents: (Calcium carbonate (2-20 μmparticle size), Dicalcuim phosphate, sodium metaphosphate etc.
2. Detergent and foaming agents: Sodium lauryl sulphate, Sodium lauryl sarcosinate, Sodium lauryl sulphosuccinate and soap like sodium palmitate etc.
3. Saccharine sodium is the most commonly used sweetening agents.
4. Flavouring agent: Anise oil, peppermint oil, cinnamon oil etc.

**Table** Formulation of tooth paste with example

| Ingredients | Example | | Composition |
|---|---|---|---|
| **Abrasives and polishing agents** | Calcium carbonate (2-20μm particle size).<br>Dicalcium phosphate<br>Sodium metaphosphate | | 15-56% |
| **Detergent and foaming agents** | Sodium lauryl sulphate,<br>Sodium lauryl sarcosinate,<br>Monoglyceride sulphate | | 1-2% |
| **Gelling or binding agents** | Hydrophillic colloids which disappears in aqueous medium are mainly used. | Gum tragcanth,<br>Karaya gum,<br>Sodium alginate,<br>SCMC<br>Hydroxy ethyl cellulose<br>Irish moss | 1.0% |
| **Humectants** | Glycerine, propylene glycol, sorbitol | | 10-30% |
| **Preservatives** | Methyl paraben or propyl paraben<br>Tricoslan (It is now a days most widely used in tooth paste) | | 0.1-0.2% |
| **Flavouring agent** | Anise oil, Peppermint oil, cinnamon oil, eugenol | | 1-1.5% |
| **Anti caries agent** | Sodium fluoride, Sodium lauryl sarcosinate | | |
| **Desensitizers** | Potassium nitrate ans strontium chloride are used to reduce the sensitivity of teeth to hot and cold | | |

- When the fluorides like sodium fluoride or sodium mono fluorophosphates is added to tooth paste the abrsive must be chosen carefully because the free calcium ions present in calcium carbonate will quickly precipitate as calcium and the characteristic activity will be lost.
- In this case the abrasive like sodium metaphosphate and special grade of calcium pyrophosphate is used.
- Evaluation of dentifrices:
  1. **Abrasive action**- A very techniques are commonly used to test abrasive action.
     - Shadograph method
     - Surface profile method
     - Interference microscopy,
     - Replication technique
     - Radio tracer method (This is the most widely accepted method in the world)
  2. **Particle size**: The particle size should be remain with a range of 2-20μm
  3. **pH**
  4. **Consistency**

## 1.5 Novel Drug Delivery System

The main objective of sustained/controlled/prolonged release formulation

The formulation is designed ion such a way that minimum effective plasma concentration (MEC) level drug should attain quickly and thereafter the rate of entry of drug to the body should equal with the rate of total eliminator or inactivation of drug from the body, as a result the plasma drug concentration curve will run parallel to the time axis just above the MEC level.

**Few Latest Delivery Systems**

1. **Mocroenca[sulation:** In this technique the drug along with a suitable polymer (s) are transformed to numerous micro- capsules. Few hundreds of such a solid microcapsules containing a definite amount of drug is then taken in hard gelatine capsule shell of compressed into a quickly disintegrating tablet for administration to the patient. This formulation now-a-days is widely used as sustained release formulation as the entrapped drug release slowly from the microcapsule.
2. **Nano-particles:** In this case also the entrapped or adsorbed drug is released slowly giving sustained action and the sizes of the particles permit.
3. **Transdermal drug delivery system:** Our skin can absorb a considerable amount of a drug to initiate and continue physiological response. The drug with moderate lipid water partition co-officiant (not too hydrophilic or too lipophilic) can be delivered as transdermal patch along with pressure sensitive adhesive. The patient is directed to fix up the patch when the drug action is not required.

   **Examples include:**

   (a) Transdermal scopolamine control motion sickness

   (b) Transdermal testosterone

   (c) Transdermal oestrogen to female during post-menopausal period

   (d) Transdermal antianginal preparation.
4. **Liposomal drug delivery system.**
5. **Multiple emulsions.**
6. **Monoclonal antibody tagged drug delivery system.**

7. **Drug loaded erythrocytes.**
8. **Iontophretic techniques.**
9. **Controlled release suppositories.**
10. **Prodrug for sustained drug action.**

**Table** Some terminologies related to novel delivery system and their definition

| Type of release | Definition |
|---|---|
| **Delayed release** | Use of repetitive, dosing of drug from one or more immediate release unit incorporated into a single dosage from |
| **Sustained release** | Drug delivery system that achieves slow release of drug over an extended period of time |
| **Controlled release** | Successfully maintained constant drug level in the blood or target tissue. |
| **Prolonged release** | unsuccessfully maintained constant drug levels but extend the duration of action over that achieved by conventional delivery |
| **Site-specific release** | Targeting of a drug directly to a specific biological location |
| **Reservoir release** | the target is a certain organ or tissue for receptor release |
| **Reservoir device for sustain release** | A core of drug is surrounded by a polymeric membrane |
| **Matrix device for sustain release** | Drug dissolved or dispersed drug is distributed uniformly throughout an inert polymeric matrix |

| **Different type of products** | **Name of the products** |
|---|---|
| Reservoir diffusion products | Measurin tablet, Bronkodyl SR capsule, Nitrospan tablet |
| Matrix diffusion products | PBZ to SR, Choleadyl SA tablets, Dospan tablet, Fero-Gard 500 |
| Encapsulated dissolution products | Hispril, Diamox, Artane |
| Matrix dissolution products | Nicobid, Mestinon |
| Ion exchange products | Lonamin capsule, Tussiones, Biphetamine capsule |

- **Osmotic Pump** a pharmaceutical technology utilized to achieve rate controlled & sustained released solid dosage forms.
- **Galactomannose** a hydrophilic polymer is used as a retardant in matrix tablet formulation.
- The most common mechanism utilized in rate controlled pharmaceutical products is **Erodible system** controlled by the erosion of a polymeric matrix.
- The half-life a drug is suitable for formulated in to a sustained release dosage from is **2 to 4 hours**
- **KCI** is the osmotic active substance is used in osmotic pressure controlled release system.
- **PVC** is an insoluble, insert polymer, used as a retardant in matrix tablet formulations.
- The release of drug from a reservoir device is governed **by Ficks 1st law of diffusion**.
- Absorption of poorly soluble drug is dissolution rate limited.
- The flux of diffusion constant decreases with increasing of partitioning, particle size and molecular weight.
- Phase separation **concertation** is used in **Microencapsulation** process.
- **ZYO** is referred to Modified release tablet.
- **Liposomes** interest with cell membrane by Fusion, Adsorption and Endocytosis.
- Release of drug is the first rate limiting step for controlled drug delivery system.

- **Scopolamine &Nitroglycerine** drug can be introduced by transdermal drug delivery system
- Liposomes are **Uni or multi layred vesicles of phosphonolipds**.
- **Propylene glycol** is a non-ionic surfactant used as a penetration enhancer in the preparation of mucoadhesives.

**Table** Micro encapsulation and approximate particle size

| Approximate Particle Size | Approximate Particle Size (μM) |
|---|---|
| Air suspension | 35 to 5000 |
| Conservation phase separation | 2 to 5000 |
| Multiorifice centrifugal | 1 to 5000 |
| Pall coating | 600 to 5000 |
| Solvent evaporation | 5 to 5000 |
| Spray drying and congealing | 600 |

**Table** List of various material used in encapsulation

| Core Material | Purpose of Encapsulation |
|---|---|
| Acetaminophen | Taste masking |
| Activated charcoal | Selective Absorption |
| Aspirin | Taste masking and reduction of gastric irritation |
| Progesterone | Sustained release |
| Potassium chloride | Reduced gastric irritation |
| Urease | Permeability of enzyme |
| Vitamin A palmitate | Stabilization of enzyme |
| Islet of Langerhans | Sustained normalization of diabetic condition |

## 1.6 Pharmaceutical Calculation

**Calculation based on density**

Density = weight / Volume

Volume = weight / density

Weight = Density × Volume

Example: Calculate the volume of 5 kg of glycerine. The density of glycerine is 1.25g/ml.

Volume = weight / density

= 5000/1.25g/ml

= 4000 ml

Example: Calculate the weight of 1 liter of fixed oil whose density is 0.9624g/ml

Weight = Density × Volume

= 0.9624 × 1000

= 962.4 g

**Alcohol dilution**

**Formula:** Volume of stronger alcohol used = $\frac{\text{Volume required} \times \text{Percentage required}}{\text{Percentage used}}$

**Example**: What volume of 50% v/v alcohol could be prepared from on liter of 95% v/v alcohol?

**Formula:** Volume of stronger alcohol used = $\frac{\text{Volume required} \times \text{Percentage required}}{\text{Percentage used}}$

$$1000 \text{ ml} = \frac{\text{Volume required} \times 50}{95}$$

$$\text{Volume required} = \frac{1000 \times 95}{50} = 1900\text{ml}$$

**Example:** What is the percentage of alcohol in a mixture obtained by mixing 5L of 25% , 1L of 50% and 2L of 95% alcohol?

500ml × 25% = 1250

1000ml × 50% = 500

2000ml × 95% = 1900

8000ml 3650

3650:8000:: X:100

$$X = \frac{3650 \times 100}{8000} = 45.6\%$$

Therefore the percentage strength of the mixture is 45.6

**Example:** What is the strength of ZnO in an ointment prepared by mixing 400g if 10% of 20% and 50g of 5% ointment?

| | | |
|---|---|---|
| 400g | 10% = | 40 |
| 100g | 20% = | 20 |
| 50g | 5% = | 2.5 |
| 550g | | 62.50 |

62.50:550:: X : 10

$$X = \frac{62.50 \times 100}{550} = 11.36\%$$

Therefore the percentage strength of the mixture is 11.36

If a diluent is to be added along with the component of known quantity and strength to obtain mixture the diluent is generally taken to be zero % strength.

**Example:** What is the % strength of an alcoholic mixture obtained by mixing 500ml of 40% alcohol, 2L of 20% alcohol and 500 ml of water?

| | | | |
|---|---|---|---|
| 500ml | X | 40% | = 200 |
| 2000ml | X | 20% | = 400 |
| 500ml | X | 0% | = 0 |
| 300ml | | | 600 |

$$X = \frac{600 \times 100}{3000} = 20\%$$

Therefore the percentage strength of the mixture is 20%

**Allegation method:**

When the calculation involves mixing of two similar preparation of different strength, to produce a preparation of intermediate strength, the allegation method is used.

For calculation purpose the figures are written as given below:-

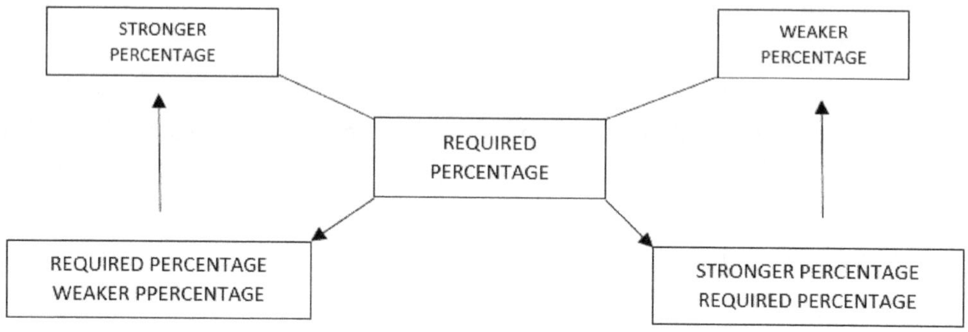


**Example:** Calculation the volume of 95% alcohol required to prepare 600 ml of 70% alcohol.

Volume required = 600 ml

% of alcohol required = 70

% of alcohol used = 95

By using allegation method

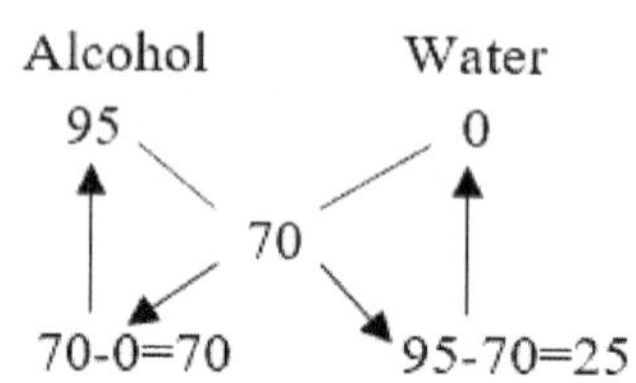


70 parts of 95% alcohol and 25 part of water will produce the required percentage alcohol.

$$\text{Quantity of 95\% alcohol required} = \frac{600 \times 70}{95} = 442.10 \text{ ml}$$

$$\text{Quantity of water required} = \frac{600 \times 25}{95} = 157.9 \text{ ml}$$

**Example:** Calculation the amount of 70%, 60%, 40%, 30% alcohol should be mixed to get 50% alcohol.

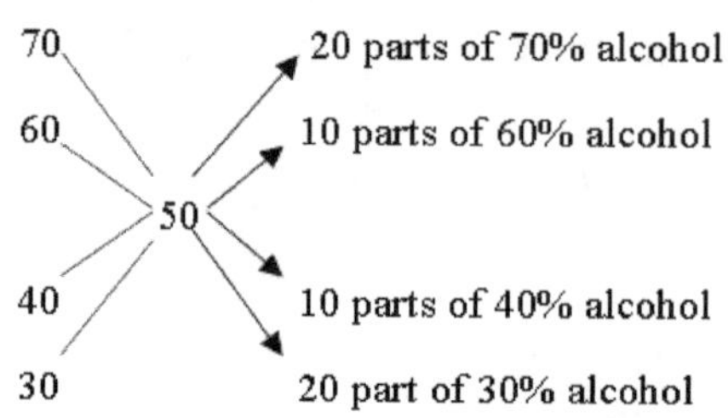

Therefore when 20 parts of 70% alcohol, 10 parts of 60% alcohol, 10 parts of 40% alcohol, and 20 parts of 30% alcohol are mixed together the resulting solution will produce 50% alcohol.

**Example:** Calculation the volume each of 90%, 60%, 30% and water are required to produce 500ml or 50% alcohole.

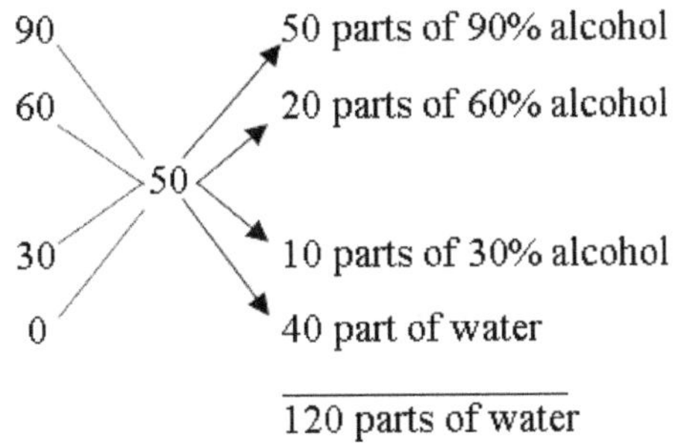


Therefore when 50 part of 90% alcohol, 20 parts of 60% alcohol, 10 part of 30% alcohol and 40 part of water are mixed together the resulting solution will produce 50% alcohol

1. Volume of 90% alcohol required

   = 120part: 500 ml :: 50 part : v

$$V = \frac{500 \times 50}{120} = \frac{2500}{12} = 208.33$$

2. Volume of 60% alcohol required

   = 120part: 500 ml :: 20 part : v

$$V = \frac{500 \times 50}{120} = \frac{1000}{12} = 83.33$$

3. Volume of 30% alcohol required

   = 120part: 500 ml :: 10 part : v

$$V = \frac{500 \times 10}{120} = \frac{500}{12} = 41.67$$

4. Volume of water required

   = 500-208.33 + 83.33 + 41.67 = 166.67ml

### Proof Spirit

Proof means pure or absolute alcohol b means of proof degrees. It means 100 proof spirit contains 50% (by volume) or 42.49% (by weight) of ethyl alcohol and specific gravity is 0.91976.
In India 57.1%v/v alcohol is 100 volume of proof spirit.

- The term 10° UP (under proof) signifies that 100 volumes of spirit contains 90 volumes of proof spirit + 10 volume of water.
- 30° OP indicates that 100 volumes diluted with water yields 130 volume of spirit.

Proof spirit = % strength of alcohol X 1.7530

Proof spirit in USA = % strength in alcohol X 2

Proof strength = (% strength of alcohol X 1.7530) – 100

**Example:** Find out proof spirit of an elixir containing 30% v/v alcohol.

Proof spirit = % strength of alcohol X 1.7530

= 30 × 1.753

= 52.59 proof spirit

**Example:** Find out the proof strength of an alcoholic product containing 55% v/v alcohol solid at U.S.A

Proof spirit in USA = % strength in alc0hol x 2

= 55 × 2

= 110 proof spirit

**Example:** Find out the proof strength of an alcoholic product containing 25% v/v

Proof strength = (% strength of alcohol x 1.7530) – 100

= (25 × 1.7530) – 100

= 43.8 – 100

= -56.2 or 56.2° U/P (since negative number)

**Example:** Find out the proof strength of an alcoholic products containing 65% v/v alcohol sold in U.S.A

Proof strength in USA = (% strength in alcohol x 2) – 100

= (65 × 2) – 100

= 130 – 100

= 30°O/P

**Example:** Calculate the real strength of 30° O.P and 40°U.P

30 Over proof means 100 = 3

Alcohol strength = 130/ 1.753 = 74.15% v/v

40 U.P means 100 – 40 = 60. Alcohol strength = 60 / 1.753 = 34.23% v/v

## Calculation of Doses

### 1. Young's formula

$$\text{Dose of child} = \frac{\text{Age in years}}{\text{Age} + 12} \times \text{Adult dose}$$

This is formulation is used for calculating the doses for children under 12 years of age.

**Example:** If the adult dose of a drug is 200mg. whit will be the dose for a child of 8 years.

According to the young's formula, the dose will be

$$\frac{8}{8+12} \times 200 = 80\text{mg}$$

### 2. Dilling's formula

$$\text{Dose of child} = \frac{\text{Age in years}}{20} \times \text{Adult dose}$$

This formula is used for calculating the doses for children in between 4-20 years of age.

**Example:** 25 mg of ephedrine hydrochloride can be given to an adult. What will be the dose for a boy of 16 years?

According to the Dilling's formula, the dose will be

$$\frac{16}{20} \times 25 = 20\text{mg}$$

**3. Cowling's formula**

$$\text{Dose of a child} = \frac{\text{Age in years} + 1}{24} \times \text{Adult dose}$$

**Example:** If the adult dose of a drug is 25mg, what will be the dose for a boy of 15 years.

According to the Cowling's formula, the dose will be

$$\frac{15+1}{24} \times 25 = 17\text{mg}$$

**4. Clark's formula**

$$\text{Dose of a child} = \frac{\text{Wdight in pounds}}{150} \times \text{Adult dose}$$

**Example:** If the adult dose of a drug is 100mg, what will be the dose for a child of weighing 15 pounds.

According to the Clark's formula, the dose will be

$$\frac{15}{150} \times 100 = 10\text{mg}$$

**5. Bastedo's formula**

$$\text{Dose of a child} = \frac{\text{Age in years} + 3}{30} \times \text{Adult dose}$$

**Example:** If the adult dose of a drug is 300mg, what will be the dose for a boy of 12 years old?

According to the Bastedo' formula, the dose will be

$$\frac{12+3}{30} \times 300 = 150\text{mg}$$

**6. Fried's Formula**

According to the Fried's formula, the dose will be

$$\text{Dose of a child} = \frac{\text{Age in month}}{150} \times \text{Adult dose}$$

This formula is used for calculating the doses for children under 2 years of age.

**Example:** If the adult dose of a drug is 100mg what will be the dose for a infant of 10 month old?

According to the Fried's formula

$$\frac{10}{150} \times 100 = 6.7\text{mg}$$

**Milliequivalents**

1 equivalent = 1000 miliequivalent

Ie. 1 mEq = 1Eq. wt. / 1000

e.g. one mEq of $<^{+}$ (ion) combines with 1mEq of $Cl^{-}$ to give 1mEq of KCI

The eq. wt of KCI ≅ 74.5 g of KCI ≅ 74500 mg of KCI

∴ 1mEq of KCI ≅ 74.5 g pf KCI (1mEq $K^{+}$ is 39mg + 1 mEq $CI^{+}$ is 35.5mg)

**Example:** A solution that contains 409.5 mg of NaCI / 100 ml has how many mEq of Na and CI?

***Ans:*** 1 mEq of NaCI = 58.5mg

i.e. 58.5 mg = 1 mEq of NaCI

1 mg = 1/58.5 mEqwt of NaCI

∴ 409.5 mg = 409.5 / 58.5 mEq wt

= 7

∴ 7 mEq wt/ of NaCI is to be dissolved to make 500 ml solution containing 500 mEq of$Na^{+}$.

## Isotonic Solutions

Calculation of Isotonicity based on Freezing point method: The lachrymal secretion contains several solutes in I and has a freezing point of -0.52°C. All solution which freeze at -0.52°C will be isotonic with the lachrymal fluid. Human blood plasma also freezes at this temperature and hence solution having freezing point at -0.52°C. Will be isotonic with blood plasma as well. Adjustment of tonicity is simplified if the freezing point of the medicament and the inert salt (Adjusting substance) are known for various strengths of their solution. Freezing points are usually expressed in terms of 1% solution and on can calculate the quantity by multiplying the freezing point with the factor.

Freezing point of tear secretion or human or human blood plasma = freezing point of drug + Freezing point of the adjusting substance.

Therefore the amount of adjusting substance required may be calculated from the equation.

$$W = \frac{0.52 - a}{b}$$

Where

W = the weight in gram of the added substance in 100 ml of the final solution.

a = the depression of the freezing point produced by the medicament already present in solution.

Calculated by multiplying the value for the medicament by the strength of the solution expressed as a percentage w/v

b = the depression of the freezing point of water produced by 1% of the adjusting substance.

**Example:** Find the concentration of sodium chloride required to render a 1.5% solution of procaine hydrochloride iso-osmotic with blood plasma. (The freezing point of a 1% (w/v) solution of procaine hydrochloride is -0.122°C, and that of a 1% (w/v) solution of NaCI is -0.576°C.

**Ans:**

$$\frac{0.52 - (0.122 \times 1.5)}{0.576} = 0.585\%\ \text{w / v}$$

Calculation of Isotonicity based on Molecular concentration:

The osmotic pressure of blood plasma and lachrymal secretion as approximately 6.7 atmosphere; hence, the molarity of these fluids is 6.7 / 22.4 = 0.3 M approximately. Consequently, a 0.3 M solution of any non-ionizing solute will be iso-omatic with plasma and tears.

**Example:** Find the concentration of anhydrous dextrose needed to produce a solution iso-osmotic with blood plasma.

**Ans:** The molecular weight of dextrose is 180 and it is non-ionising.

Therefore 0.3 x 180 = 54g per its required.

If the solute ionizes in solution this is assumed to be complete and the following formulation is used.

$$W = \frac{0.3M}{N}$$

Where, W = Amount required in g per litter.

M = Molecular weight of solute

N = No. of ions produced from each molecule of the solute.

**Example:** Find the concentration of Sodium chloride needed to produce a solution iso-osmotic with blood plasma.

**Ans:** The molecular weight of sodium chloride is 58.5 and it dissociates into 2 ion.

Therefore $W = \frac{0.3M}{N} = \frac{0.3 \times 58.5}{2} = 8.8g$ per litre (0.88 w/v)

**Calculation of HLB of a Blend of Emulsifying Agents**

When a blend of emulsifying agents is used, the total HLB of the mixture is the arithmetic addition of the contribution of ach part.

**Example:** What is HLB of mixture of 50% of Span 80 and 50% of Tween 80?

(HLB of span 80 = 4.3 and HLB of Tween 80 = 15.0)

HLB X % of mixture

Span 804.3 X 50% = 2.15

Tween 80 X 15.0 = 7.50

HLB of the mixture = 9.65

**Calculation of Relative Amount of emulsifier to obtain a Required HLB value**

The calculation involves the use of allegation alternate.

**Example:** In what proportion should Tween 60 and Span 60 to be blended to obtain a required HLB of 12.0 (HLB of Span 60 = 4.7 and HLB of Tween 60 = 14.9)

By allegation

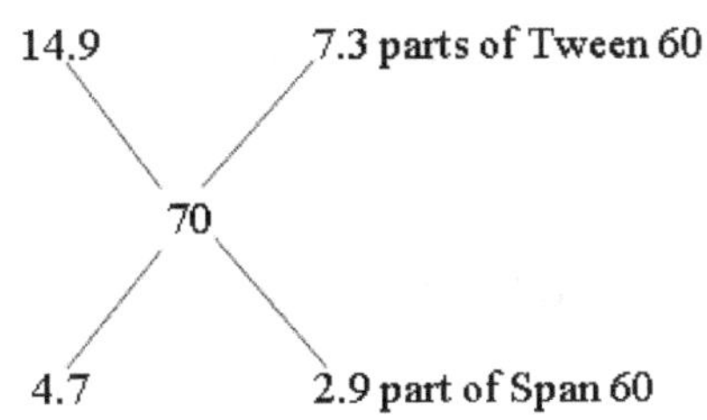

Relative amount of Tween 60: Span 60
7.3: 2.9
Or 71.5% : 28.5%

### Displacement Value of Medicaments

This displacement value of medicament is defined as that proportion which displace on part of the standard calibrating substance. (oil oi Theobroma or cocoa butter) This displacement values (butter known as density factor i.e density of a medicament relative to cocoa butter) as reported in books are with reference to the oil of Theobroma and hence when other bases e.g. gelato-glycerine, polyethylene glycols etc. are used, the displacement values are to be calculated accordingly.

**Example:** Supply 12 suppositories of boric acid each weighing 4 gm and containing 300 mg of boric acid (the displacement value of boric acid = 1.5)

12 suppositories require 12 × 300mg = 3600 mg of boric acid.

The displacement value of boric acid = 1.5

The total amount of cocoa butter displacement by 3.6 gm of boric acid = 3.6/1.5 = 2.4 gm

Hence the quantity of base required = (12 × 4) – 2.4 = 45.6g

The formula for 12 suppositories would be

Boric acid = 3.6g

Cocoa butter = 45.6g

**Conversion Formula**

1. Conversion of mEq to mmol per litre

$$\text{mmol} = \frac{\text{mEq}}{\text{Vaiency}}$$

2. Conversion of % w/v strength to mmol per litre

$$\text{mmol per litre} = \frac{\text{\% w / v strength} \times 10000}{\text{mg of substance containing 1 mmol}}$$

3. Conversion of mmol per litre to % w/v strength

$$\text{\% w/v strength} = \frac{\text{1 mmol} \times \text{mmol per litre}}{10000}$$

4. Conversion of mg per litre to mmol per litre

$$\text{mmol per litre} = \frac{\text{mg per litre}}{\text{mg of substance containing 1 mmol}}$$

5. Conversion of mmol per litre to mg per litre

   Mg per litre = mmol per litre x mg of substance containing 1 mmol

6. Conversion of °C (degree centigrade) into °F (degree Fahrenheit)

$$F = 32 + \frac{9}{5}C$$

7. Conversion of °F (degree Fahrenheit) into °C (degree centigrade)

$$C = (F - 32) \times \frac{5}{9}$$

## 1.7 Aerosols

- Aerosol or pressurized package is defined as a system that depends upon the power or a compressed or liquefied gas to expel the contents from the container.
- The aerosol products consists of
  1. Propellant
  2. Container
  3. Valve & actuator
  4. Products concentrate

1. **Propellant**
   - The propellant is responsible for the development of proper pressure within the container and it expel the products when the valve is opened.
   - The fluorinated hydrocarbon such as trichloromonofluoromethanne (propellant 11), dichloro-difluoromethane (propellant 12), and dichlorotrtrafluoroethane (propellant 114) are widely used in oral and inhalational aerosol.
   - Hydrocarbons like propane, butane, and isobutene and compressed gases like nitrogen, nitrous oxide and carbon dioxide are used in topical pharmaceutical aerosols.
2. **Container**
   - The aerosol containers which must withstand pressure as high as 140 to 180 psig at a 130 °F
   - Aluminium used to manufacturing seamless aerosol container. It has les chances of incompatibility due to its seamless nature.
   - The combination of ethanol and propellant 11 in an aluminium container has been shown to produce hydrogen acetyl chloride, propellant 21, aluminium chloride and other corrosive product.
   - Stainless steel container has been used for a large number of aerosols pharmaceutical. It is available in with or without plastic coating.
   - Glass container – If the total pressure of the system is below 25 psig and there is not more than 15% of propellant, a glass can be safely used, pressure up to 33 psig can be utilized if the glass container having a double plastic outer coating.
3. **Valve**
   (a) An aerosol valve consists of many different parts like
   (b) Ferrule or mounting cap
   (c) Valve body or housing
   (d) Stem
   (e) Gasket
   (f) Spring
   (g) Dip tube

   **(a) Ferrule or mounting cap**
   - The mounting cap is used to attach the valve proper to the container. The cup is made from teen plate steel, at the aluminium also can be used. In the underside of the valve cup a single or double epoxy or vinyl coating can be added to increase resistance of corrosion.

   **(b) Valve body or housing**
   - The housing is generally made up of Nylon or Delrin. It has a opening at the point of the attachment of the dip tube is about 0.013 to 0.080 inch. The housing may or may not

containanother opening that is vapour tap which prevent valve clogging with product containing insoluble material. The vapour tap opening is about 0.013 to 0.08 inch.

- A recent development that is useful for pharmaceutical is the aquasol valve. It is used in water based aerosol system where only active ingredient and water dispensed (Propellant is in vapour state and present only extremely small quantity). There is no chilling effect as occurs with hydrocarbon propellant.
- The chief difference between the Aquasol system and three phase system is that the fromer dispenses a fairly drug spray with very small particles.

**(c) Steam**

- It is also made up of Nylon or Delrin. But metal such as brass and stainless steel also used. One or more orifice is set into the stem. They range from one orifices of about 0.013 inch to 0.030 inch to three orifices of 0.040 inch each.

**(d) Gasket**

- Buna- N and Neoprene rubber are commonly used for gasket.

**(e) Spring**

- Spring is made up of stainless steel. The spring folds the gasket in place and return the valve to its closed position.

**(f) Dip tube**

- Dip tube are made from polyethylene or polypropylene. The inside diameter of commonly used dip tube is about 0.120 to 0.125 inch. Capillary dip tubes are 0.050 inch. For highly viscous products it may 0.195 inches.
- Metered valves are applicable to the dispensing of potent medication. Approximately 50 to 150 mg $\mp$10% of liquid can be dispended at one time with the use of such valves.

**(g) Actuator**

- Actuator is an integral part of almost every aerosol package to ensure that the aerosol product is delivered in the proper and desired from.

**4. Products concentrate**

- Product having low pH and containing water utilize organic lining of epoxy and vinyl resins. As compared to vinyl resin the epoxy resin has greater degree of heat stability. The vinyl resin forms a tough film and cannot be utilized for products that must be heat sterilized.

- **Manufacture of pharmaceutical aerosols utilize**
  - ✓ Pressuring filling apparatus
  - ✓ Cold filling apparatus
  - ✓ Compressed gas filling apparatus

  Pressuring filling apparatus: This cannot be used fill inhalation aerosol where as cold filling apparatus should not be used to fill hydrocarbon aerosols.

  Cold filling apparatus: This method requires to chilling of all components including concentrate and propellant of temperature−40°F, whereas the pressure filling method is carried out room temperature.

- **Evaluation**
  - Testing of pharmaceutical aerosol include flame projection, flash point, vapour point, vapour pressure density, moisture content etc.

- The flash point is determined by use of the standard Tag open cup apparatus, this aerosol products is chill to temperature of about−25°F,
- A can punching device is available for accurately measuring vapour pressure.
- The density of aerosol system can be accurately determined through the use of a hydrometer or a pycnometer.
- The moisture content can determined by Karl Fisher method and Gas chromatography.
- Gas chromatography and infrared spectrophotometer have been used to identify the propellant.
- Particle size of aerosol is determined by the cascade impactor and light scatter decay method.

## Calculation (Naming)

### 1. Propellant 114

Propellant 114

- 1st number + 1 = Carbon number
- 3rd number = Florine number
- 2nd number -1 = Hydrogen number

So,

C => 1+1 = 2

H => 1-1 = 0

F =>4

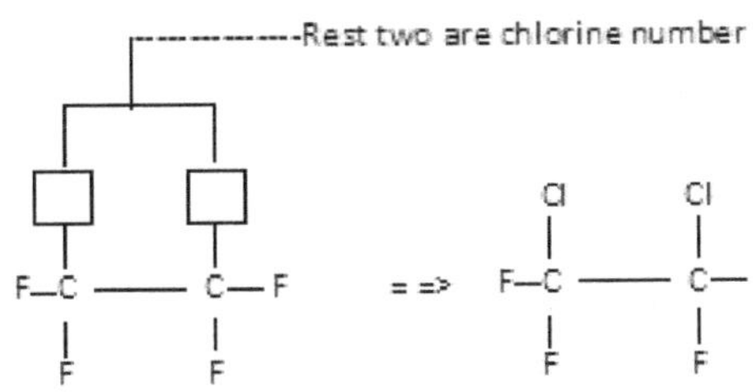


Naming- Dichloroterafluoro ethane (Propellant 114)

### 2. Propellant 12

Propellant 12 =Propellant 012

- 1st number + 1 = Carbon number
- 3rd number = Florine number
- 2nd number -1 = Hydrogen number

So,

C => 0+1 = 2

H => 1-1 = 0

F =>2

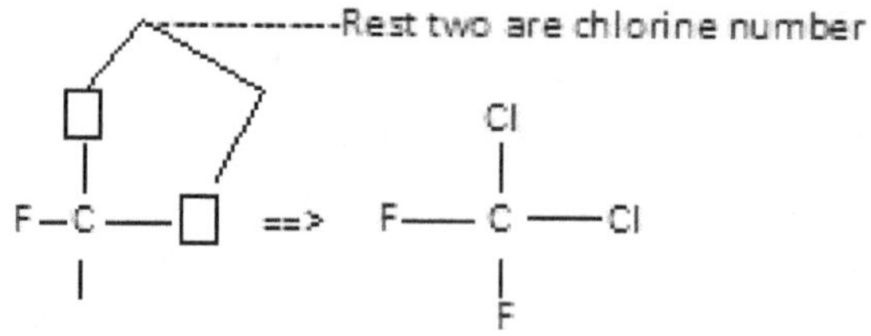


Naming- Dichlorodifluro methane (Propellant 12)

## 1.8 Solid Dosage Forms

### Tablet

Tablets are solid dose pharmaceutical preparation containing drug substances usually prepared with the aid of suitable pharmaceutical excipients. They may vary in size, shape, weight, hardness, thickness, disintegration, and dissolution characteristics and in other aspects, depending on their intended use and method of manufacture.

**Important characteristics**

- Tablet is essentially tamperproof dosages from
- They offer the greatest capabilities of all oral dosage forms for the greatest dose precision & the least content variability.

### Evolution

**1. Size**

At the constant compressive load, tablet thickness varies with

(i) Changes in die fill

(ii) With particle size distribution

(iii) Packing of particle mix being compressed.

(iv) Total weight

- With a constant doe fill thickness varies with comprehensive load.
- ***The crown thickness of a tablet is measured with micrometre.***
- ***The total crown thickness of tables is measured with Side calliper.***
- Tablet thickness should be controlled with in a $\pm 5\%$ variation of standard value,

**2. Shape**

- Shaped tablet required slotting punches
- Round tablet requires conventional punches
- ***More convex the tablet surface, the more likely it is to cause capping problems.***

**3. Colour**

- The quantities colour evaluation may be done with
  - (a) Reflectance spectrophotometry
  - (b) Tristimulus calorimeter
- To measure the colour uniformity and gloss on a tablet surface – Micro reflectance photometer.

4. **Hardness & Friability**

The hardness of a tablet can be determined by

(a) Monsato tester

(b) Strong cobb tester

(c) Pfizer tester

(d) Erweka tester

(e) Schleuniger tester

(f) At a constant die fill a hardness increase and thickness decreases.

(g) At a constant compression force (fixed distance between upper & lower hardness increases with increasing die fills & decreasing with lower die fills.

(h) Vickrs, Brinell Static test and dynamic tests associated to determine hardness.

(i) Brinell hardness can be calculated by the equation $BHN = \dfrac{2F}{\pi D_1 \sqrt{(D_1 - D_1^2 - D_1^2)}}$

(j) Vickers hardness can be calculated by the equation. $Hv = \dfrac{2F \sin 68^\circ}{d^2}$

**Factors effecting for harder of tablet**

- Tablets are harder after several hour of compression than after immediately compression.
- Lubricants if used in a high concentration or mixed for a prolonged period of time can affect hardness.
- Large tablets requires greater force and therefore less harder than small tablets.
- In a given granulation a Flat bevelled tool produces a tablet more harder than a deep cup tool.

5. **Friability Test**

- The laboratory friability tester is known as **Roche friabilator.**
- This works in the principal of **abrasion and shock.**
- It revolves at **25 RPM.**
- It drops at a distance of **6 inches.**
- During test it is operated for **100 revolutions.**
- Conventional compressed tablets that lose less than **0.5 to 1 %** of their weight are generally considered acceptable.
- Usually **chewable tablets** have higher friability value.
- **Very dry granulation** result high friability value.
- In a large scale industry, where the large no. of tablets are products, the friability evaluation is performed by **Rough handling test**. This test includes a. **Vibration test, b. Drop test, c. Incline plate impact test**
- **(When concave or deep concave punches are used they produce whispering at the tablet edge.)**
- **2 to 4 % moisture in granules act as binder.**

6. **Weight Variation Test**

- 20 tablets to be weighed individually an calculate average weight than compare with the individual tablet weight with the average weight.
- If no more than **2 tablets** are outside the percentage limits and if no tablet differs by more than **2 times** the percentage limit then the tablets are accepted.

**Table** Weight variation tolerance for uncoated tablets

| Average wt. of a table in (mg) | Maximum percentage difference allowed |
|---|---|
| <130 | $\pm 10$ |
| 130 – 324 | $\pm 7.5$ |
| > 324 | $\pm 5$ |

**7. Disintegration Test**

- The height of disintegration tube is **3 inch long.**
- The temperature maintained during disintegration is **37°C ± 2°C**
- During the test the tablets remain 2.5 cm below the surface of liquid on their upward movement & descend not closer than 2.5 cm from the bottom of the beaker.
- 28-32 cycles are maintained per minute.
- Perforated plastic disc may be placed on the top of the tablet which imports an abrasive action to the tablets.
- **Un coated tablets** have disintegration time below **5 to 30 minutes.**
- For **enteric coated tablets** the disintegration time is **1 hour** in gastric fluid, then in intestinal fluid for **2 hour.**
- Disintegration test mesh size **10 mesh.**
- Disintegration test basket mesh size is **40 mesh.**
- Croscarmellose sodium Sodium starch glycolate &Crospovidone are super disintigrants. Among all **Crospovidone**is having **high wicking activity.**

**8. Dissolution Test**

- The temperature of the medium **37°C ± 0. 5°C**
- AS per IP the dissolution apparatus type 1 is **basket type.**
- **Electronic devices such as a Thomas Tablet Sentinel, Pharmakontroll and the Kilian Control System – MC, Monitor the tablet weight.**

## Tablet Diffect

**Capping:** It is a term used to describe the partial or complete separation of the top or complete separation of the top or bottom crown of a tablet from the main body of tablet.

**Lamination:** It is the separation of a tablet into two or more distinct layers.

**Cause**: Deformational property of the formulation during & immediately following compression.

**Table** Formulation defects

| Capping & Lamination cause | Solution |
|---|---|
| **Rapid decompression** | - Precompression.<br>- Slowering the tabletting rate<br>- Reducing the final compression pressure |
| **Deep concave punch (Capping)** | Use of flat punch |
| **Too dry granulation** | Addition of hygroscopic substances such as sorbitol, methyl cellulose or PEG- 4000 |
| **Die develops a wear " ring " the area of compression** | To turn the die over so that compression occurs in an unknown are over the ring. |
| **Incorrect set up at the press** | Correct set up at the press. |

- **Brittle Fracture Index test (BFI)** is used to measure capping and lamination.
- In a tablet batch manufacturing process the lamination for BFI **is NOT more than 0.8**
- **Strain Index and Bonding Index** is associated **with Capping of a tablet**
- In a tablet batch manufacturing process the limitation for BFI is a **not more than 0.8**

### Picking & Sticking

- Packing is a term used to describe the surface material from a tablet that is sticking to and being removed from the tablet surface by a punch. It is particularly concern with punch tips above engraving or embossing with letter 'B', 'A', 'O'.
- Sticking refers to the tablet materials adhering to the die wall.
- Chipping refers to the serious sticking at ejection of tablets cause chipping of tablet edges and can produce rough edge.

### Remedies

- ➢ Lettering should be designed as large as possible.
- ➢ Platting of the punch faces with chromium is a method of avoiding picking and sticking.
- ➢ Colloidal silica may be added as polishing agents and make the punch faces smooth.
- ➢ Sometimes low melting point such as stearic acid & PEG may soften from the heat of compression to cause sticking. This can be avoided by either reducing low melting point ingredients or adding the ingredient with high melting point.
- ➢ When a low melting point medicaments are present high concentration. Refrigeration of the granulation may the made.
- ➢ Excess moisture may cause sticking. This may avoid by further drying of the granulation.

### Mottling

- ➢ It is an equal distribution of colour on a tablet.
- ➢ Cause: The drug colour differs from the colour of tablet excipients.
- ➢ The drug whose degrading product are coloured both can be avoided by using colorants.
- ➢ A dye can cause mottling by migrating to the surface of granulation during drying. This can be overcome by changing solvent system, binding system, reducing the drying temperature.
- ➢ Coloured adhesive gel solution may not be distributed well because they must be hot & may lead to mottling. This can be overcome by incorporating fine powder adhesive such as acacia and tragacanth into the products before adding the granulating fluid or to disperse a drug colour additive during the powder blending step.

### Orange Peel Effect

**Cause:** Inadequate spreading of the coating solution before drying.

### Bridging

**Causing:** The film may shrink & pull away from the sharp corner

## Weight Variation

**Cause:**

1. Granule size and size distribution before compression.
   - The apparent volume in the die is essentially same if the size of granules is filled inside the die. The void spaces between the granules ma cause weight variation of tablets.
   - This can be avoided by filling the die with different size of granules so that the void space is minimized and hence the variation minimized.
2. Poor flow
   - Arching or bridging and Rat- holing at Hooper side are the prime cause of poor flow. It may be controlled with the vibrato attached with it.
   - Recent a patent is issued for a new feed frame design that accommodated excessive flow from the Hooper without compromising uniform weight variation.
3. Poor mixing
   - Inadequate mixing cause unsatisfactory granulation flow.
4. Punch variation
   - When lower punches are unequal length, they cause weight variation.
5. Hardness variation
   - If the volume of the martial or the distance between punch varies, hardness varies and hence weight also varies.
6. Double impression
   - This involves only punches that have monogram of other engraving on them.

**Table** Tablet weight variation test

| Average Weight (MG) | Wt. Variation |
|---|---|
| 130 or less | 10% |
| 130 to 324 | 7.5% |
| More than 324 | 5% |

## Tablet Granulation

- Granulation is in part of pharmaceutical process that attempts to improve the flow of powdered materials by forming sphere like regularly shaped aggregate called granules.

$$\text{The shape Co-officient of } (a_{vs}) = \frac{a_s \text{ (surface shape factor)}}{a_v \text{ (volume shape factor)}}$$

- The shape co-efficient of a sphere is 6
- The shape co-efficient of a cubic is 6.8

## Determination of Granulation Characteristics

- Particle size and shape (By microscopic method)
- Surface area (By gas adsorption and air permeability method)
- Density (By pycnometer)
- Strength & Friability (By compression strength or friability measurement)

## Flow Properties

- Fine powders ≤ 150μm, the magnitude of the frictional and vender walls forces usually predominate.
- The larger particles ≥ 150μm, such as granules produced by wet granulation process frictional forces normally predominate over Vander wall force.
- Repose angle and Hopper flow measurement are common methods to determine flow properties.
- Value of angle of repose ≤ 30° usually indicate free flow and ≥ 40° indicate poor flow.
- Shear cell method, Hausner ratio method & Carry index method are used to measure powder flow properties.

## Compaction

- Transducers are used to measure the forces applied during compression process.
- Avalanching Behaviour is associated with powder flow property.
- Hackel equation is mostly used to describe Compaction of pharmaceutical powder.
- Hackel equation is in $\left[\frac{1}{1-Dr} = k\,p + A\right]$

## Manufacture of Granules

**By dry manufacturing method**

- Roller compactor is used in large scale for compression granulation.
- In this compactor first the material are formed in to ribbon like structures, which can than screened or milled into a granulation suitable for compression into tablets.
- Slugging is a process by which compacted mass (slug) are produced by a tablets press or by a special designed machinery followed by milling an screening to produce granules.

**Wet granulation**

These can be prepared by

1. LittelfordLodige mixture
2. Diosna mixture
3. Littelford MGT mixture
4. Gral mixture

## Tablet Design & Formulation

**Excipients**

1. Diluent 2. Binder 3. Disintegrate 4. Lubricant 5. Colorant 6. Flavors 7. Sweeteners

**Diluent**

- Round tablets are in a size of 3/16, to ½ inch. And weight about 120 to 700mg.
- Oval tablets are up to 800 mg.
- Tetracycline product made with a calcium phosphate diluent has less than the half of the bioavailability of standard product.
- Divalent and trivalent cations form insoluble complexes and salts with a number for amphoteric or acid functionally antibiotics greatly reduces absorption.

- When amine drugs prepared commonly with lactose diluents in presence of magnesium stearate or any metal stearate (lubricant), the resultant tablets were discoloured.
- The diluents which exist in their common salt of hydrate contain water as water of crystallization. These are not excellent diluents for water sensitive drugs because during storage condition at elevated temperature the products might be exposed. However the diluents like Dibasic calcium phosphate & calcium sulphate even contain water of crystallization, the water content does not release until the temperature is approximately 80°C is reached. Such excipients have low remaining moisture and superior to any anhydrous diluent.

**Table** Specification of lactose

| Types of Lactose | Property | Disadvantages |
|---|---|---|
| **Lactose** | It is commercially available in 60 to 80 meshes (coarse) and 80 to 100 mesh (Regular) grades. | - |
| **Anhydrous lactose** | It does not undergo Maillard reaction which may lead to browning and discoloration of certain drugs. | - |
| **Hydrous lactose** | It is used in wet granulation process | It undergoes Maillard reaction which may lead to browning and discoloration of certain drugs. |
| **Spray dried lactose** | It is used for direct compression | It is prone to darkening in presence of moisture, amines and other compounds owing to the presence of a furaldehyde.<br>A neutral or acid lubricant is used when spray dried lactose is used. |
| **Corn, wheat, Potato starch** | It contains a moisture of **11 to 14%** | |
| **Sta Rx 1500** | It is used in direct compression<br>It contains a moisture of **10 to 15%**<br>**It is used as binder, diluent, and disintegrating agent.**<br>It has self-lubricant action but during preparation of little amount of drug (5 to 10 %), It is mixed with **0.25%** of **colloidal silicon dioxide**. | |
| **EM dex & Celutab** | These are hydrolysed starches and used as direct compression<br>It contains a moisture of **8 to 10%**<br>They contains basically **90 to 92 % of dextrose & 3 to 5 of maltose**<br>They are used in place of mannitol in chewable tablets because of their sweetness and smooth feeling in mouth. | |

**Dextrose**

- It is available in hydrous and anhydrous from.
- Dextrose is combined with spray dried lactose **to reduce the tendencies** of tablets resulting darkness.

**Mannitol**

- It has a characteristic of **negative heat of solution**, low solubility and **pleasant testing** hence widely used in chewable tablets.
- It is non hydroscopic and used in vitamin formulation.
- These are having poor flow properties and require high lubrication labels.

**Sorbitol**

- It is optical isomer of **mannitol**.
- It is combined with mannitol to reduce its cost.
- It is hygroscopic at humidites **above 65%**

**Sugar tab**

- It is used in direction compression
- It contains 90 to 93 % sucrose + 7 to 1 % invert sugar.

**Di pac**

- It is used in direct compression.
- It contains 95% sucrose + 3% modified dextrin

**Nu tab**

- It is used in direct compression.
- It contains 95% sucrose + 4% invert sugar with small amount of corn starch and magnesium stearate.
- **Avice (Microcrystalline cellulose)** it is used in direct compression.
- It exists in two tablet grades **PH (101) – Powder & PH (102) – granules**.
- IT is a **unique diluent in that while producing cohesive compact**.
- These materials also act as **disintegrant.**

## Points to Remenber

- Jivrajet al (2000) is usually used as **filler for direct compression.**
- **Ludipres** is lactose monohydrate + Polyvinylphyrrolidone + Crospovidone
- **Cellactose** is Microcrystalline cellulose + Lactose
- **Cel-O-Cal** is Clcium sulphate + compressed microcrystalline cellulose.

**Table** Example of various binder & adhesives with their properties

| Binder & Adhesives | Properties |
|---|---|
| Acacia &Trangacanth | - These are natural gums<br>- They are added in dry or liquid form in a solution ranging from 10% to 25% concentration.<br>- They are more effective when added in form a solution.<br>- They often contaminated with bacteria and in wet granulation masses should be quickly dried at a temperature above 37° to reduce microbial proliferation. |
| Gelatin | It is a natural protein and used in combination with acacia. |
| Starchpaste | During preparation starch undergo hydrolysis to dextrin & glucose |
| Liquid glucose (50%) | It is also used as binding agent. |
| Modified natural polymer<br>**a. Alginate**<br>**b. Methyl cellulose**<br>**c. Hydroxy propyl methyl cellulose**<br>**d. Hydroxy propyl cellulose** | - In **dry form** all are used as **binder** and in **aqueous solution** they have **adhesive** properties.<br>- HPMC is used an alcoholic solution to provide and anhydrous adhesive<br>- **Ethyl cellulose is used only as alcoholic solution**. They also **retard the disintegration & dissolution time of drugs**. |
| Polyvinylpyrolidone | - I is a **synthetic polymer** and used as adhesive in either aqueous or alcoholic solution. |

### Disintegrant

1. Starch USP - 5 to 10 % of tablet weight
2. Primogel & Explotab (Low substituted carboxy methyl cellulose) - 1 to 8 % (4% is optimum)
3. Pregelatinised starch - 5% concentration
4. Vegum V and bentonite - 10%
5. Microcrystaline cellulose -
6. Ac – Di- Sol - (it is an internally cross linking form of sodium cmc)
7. Super disintefrant - Sodiunm starch glycolate, Cross povidone, carmelos

### Lubricant

These are intended to reduce the friction during tablet ejection between the walls of tablet and the wall of die cavity in which the tablet is formed.

1. Steraic acid : It is salt and dervatives.
2. Talc : Due to presence of iron in it, sometimes the drug whose breakdown is catalysed by iron.
3. PEG : Used as water soluble lubricant.

### Antiadherant

- These reduce sticking or adhering of any tablet granulation or powder to the faces of punches or to the die wall.
- All water insoluble lubrication usually act as antiadharent.
- Talc, Management state, starch and starch derivative also act as antiadharent.

### Glident

They promote the flow of the tablet granulation or powder materials by reducing fraction between particles.

1. Talc – 5%
2. Corn starch - 5 to 10 %
3. Colloidal silica

   Cab-O-Sil - 0.25 to 3%
   Syloid - 0.25 to 3%
   Aerosil - 0.25 to 3%

**Colours** – FD & C and D&C days

**Flavours** – Flavour oils added with 0.5 to 0.75%

### Sweetners

1. Mannitol - 72% AS sweet as Sucrose
2. Sacchrrine - IT is only an artificial sweetner.
   - It is 500 times sweetener then sucrose
   - It is major disadvantage is that it has bitter after taste and it is carcinogenic.
3. Aspartane - It is largely replaced to saccharine.
   - It is disadvantage is lack of stability due to presence of water.

## Type of Tablets

### Compressed Tablets

- The category referred to standard uncoated tablets

### Multiple Compressed Tablets

These are

1. Layered Tablets
2. Compressed coated tablets

- These are unusually prepared to separate physically or chemically incompatible ingredients or to produce repeat action or prolonged action products.

### Repeat action tablets

- In this preparation the core tablet is usually coated with shellac or enteric polymer so that it will not release its drug load in the stomach. The second dose of drug is than added in the sugar coating which is allowed to coat on the surface of tablets. This coat is allowed to its drug load in the stomach. Ultimately the tablet produces repeat action in stomach & intestine.

### Enteric coated tablet / Delayed action tablet

- All the enteric coated tablets remain intact in the stomach but quickly release in the duodenum.
- In the disintegration test the enteric coated tablets are immersed in water at room temperature for 5 minutes.
- Cellulose acetate phthalate or polyvinyl acetate phthalate or Hydroxypropyl methylcellulose phthalate are commonly used for enteric coating.
- The pH gastric fluid is – up to 4
- The pH of duodenum is – 4 to 6
- The pH of intestine is - 7 to 8
- The drug like erythromycin is prepared as enteric coated because it destroys in low pH.

### Sugar coating tablets

- These types of tablets permit separation of incompatible ingredients between coating and core.
- The above principle helps for the preparation of multivitamin & multi mineral or vitamin combination.
- Water soluble polymers are often incorporated in sugar coating solution to reduce the coat weight of tablets (may be 50% less).
- Automation spray coating equipment is used in this coating process.

### Film coated tablets

- An article spray coating procedure is typically for film, coating composition.
- This is the coating preparation where drug is not required coating.
- Polymers such as Hydroxypopyl cellulose, HPMC is dissolved in water with an appropriated plasticizer are used to produce immediate release film coating.
- The colloidal dispersion of Ethyl cellulose in water makes it possible to produce slow or controlled release film coating without the use of organic solvents.
- Aqua coat trade name of 30% Ethylcellulose dispersion is marketed under FMC Corporation.
- The film coated tablets have better mechanical strength of the coating based on the elasticity & flexibility of the polymer coating.

**Chewable tablet**

- The antacid tablets are prepared in chewable form because the dose of antacid is too large to swallow and if the tablet chewed prior to swallowing better acid neutralization may be possible

## Tablet Classes

**Buccal & Sublingual tablets**

- When these preparation held in the mouth, they release their drug for absorption through oral mucosa an intended to produce systemic circulation.
- They avoid to first pass metabolism
- They are designed not to disintegrate but to slowly dissolve typically over a 15 to 30 minute period.

**Troches & Lozenges**

- The y designed not to disintegrate in mouth but to dissolve slowly over a period of 30 minutes or less.
- Lozenges are formed by fusion or by candy molding process.
- Troches are formed by direct compression.

**Dental cones**

- The usually vehicle for the preparation is sodium bicarbonate, sodium chloride, or an amino acid.
- The drug content of the tablet is dissolved slowly for 20 to 40 minute period.

**Implantation tablet**

- They are typically shaped and not more than 8mm length.
- Keron injector is used to implant the tablet.
- They are restricted to use month to a year.
- They are restricted to use in humans because of surgical technique and tissue toxicity at the site of application.
- They usually applied to administration of growth hormones to food producing animals.

**Effervescent tablet**

- The tablet is typically prepared by compressing the active ingredients with a mixture of organic acid such as citric acid or tartaric acid and sodium bicarbonate.
- The effervescent tablet is specially packed in Hermetic-type-foil and various acid anhydrides may be used in combination with sodium glycine carbonate and various sesquicarbonates

## Important Chart to Remember

| **Ingredient** | **Use** |
|---|---|
| Calcium phosphate | Adsorbent diluent |
| Calcium hydrogen phosphate | Used for direct compression |
| Colloidal silica | Improve granular flow |
| Anhydrous dextrose | Adsorb moisture at high relative humidity |
| Dextrose (spray dried) | direct compressible but absorbs moisture at high |
| Lactose | Inexpensive & gives granules by moist granulation |
| Lactose (Spray dried) | useful for direct compression & incompatible with primary amine |
| Lactose anhydrous | direct compressible but prevent moisture uptake |

| | |
|---|---|
| Starch | Direct from used as absorbent & used as disintegrate |
| Mannitol | Gives cooling defect in the mouth |

| **Material** | **(Lubricant)** |
|---|---|
| Boric acid | External lubricant + Lubricant die wall |
| Colloidal silica | Lubricant + Glidant |
| Hydrogenated vegetable oil | Internal Lubricant + Lubricant die wall |
| Magnesium stearate | External Lubricant + Lubricant die wall |
| Polyethylene glycol | Internal Lubricant + Lubricant die wall |
| Stearic acid | die wall |
| Talc | Lubricant + Glidant |

## Tablet Coating

**Objective**

- To make the taste, odor, or colour of the drug.
- To provide physical and chemical protection.
- To control the release of the drug.
- To protect the drug gastric environment.
- To improve the pharmaceutical elegance.
- To incomplete another drug or formula adjuvant in the coating to avoid chemical incompatibility.

**There are three primary component involved in table coating**

1. Tablet preparation.
2. Coating process (Coating equipment)
3. Coating material or composition.

**There are three types of equipment are generally used for tablet coating**

1. The standard coating pan
2. The perforated coating pan
3. The fluidized bed (air suspension coater)
    - The standard coating pan consist of a circular metal pan of **8 to 60 inches** in diameter and rotated on
    - It is horizontal axis.
    - The improved standard coating pans are Pellegrini pan, immersion sword an immersion tube.
    - The perforated pan system consists of a perforated or partially perforated drum that is rotated on its horizontal axis. The perforated pan system includes.
        (a) Acclacota
        (b) Hi-coater
        (c) Dria coater
    - The **Glatt coater** is the latest perforated pan coater.
    - The fluidized bed to basic types of system is used.
        1. High pressure, air less
        2. Low pressure, air atomised.

- In the air less system liquid is pumped at high pressure (250-3000psig) through a small orifice ( 0.009-0.020inch in diameter)
- In the low pressure air atomized system liquid is pumped at low pressure i.e. **5-50 psig** through a somewhat larger orifice (0.02 inch to 0.060 inch in diameter)
- **Air capacity**: - This value represents the quantity of water or solvent that can be removed during the coating process.
- There are two type of tablet coating process.
  1. Sugar coating
  2. Film coating
     - Sealing
     - Sub coating
     - Syruping (Smoothing)
     - Finishing
     - Polishing

**Sealing**

- Seal coating prevent the moisture penetrating into the tablet core.
- Shellac is an effective seal coating agent but the disintegration and dissolution times increased because polymerization of shellac.
- Zain is an alcohol soluble protein derivative from corn which is also used for seal coating.

**Sub coating**

- The sub coating is done to increase the tablet weight and to round the edges.

**Syruping (Smoothing)**

- The purpose of syrup coating is to cover and fill the imperfection of the tablet surface caused by the sub coating step and to impart the desired colour.

**Polishing**

- Polishing is the final step and is done by canvas – lined polishing pan or clean standard coating pans. The bees wax or cornouba wax or worm wax or worm solution of these waxes in naptha.

The film fottmers are two types-

1. Non enteric material
2. Enteric material

**The non-enteric materials are:**

Hydroxy propyl methyl cellulose.

Methyl hydroxyl ethyl cellulose

Ethyl cellulose

Hydrox propyl cellulose

Povidine

Sodium carboxy methyl cellulose

Acrylate polymers

- HPMC is a material of choice for air suspension and pan coating system. HPMC is ideal polymer for film coating.
- Ethyl cellulose is completely insoluble in water and gastrointestinal fluid. This material is available as Aqua coat (30% ethyl cellulose)
- Povidone is a synthetic polymer available as four different viscosity grades. I.e. K-15, K-30, K-60 and K-90. The most commonly used povidone is K-30. Povidone is soluble in both acidic and basic medium.
- Acrylate polymer i.e.EudragitE is a cationic polymer which is only Eudrazit material freely soluble in gastric fluid up to pH 5.

**The enteric materials:**

- They deliver drug included for local action in the intestine and by pass systemic absorption in the stomach, they are resistant to gastric fluid.
- Example: Cellulose Acetate phthalate (CAP)
  Acrylate polymers
  Hydroxy propyl methyl cellulose
  Polyvinyl acetate phthalate
- CAP is most widely used acrylate polymer and has and disadvantages. i.e. dissolve only above pH 6.
- Two forms of acrylic resins are Edragit L and Edragit S. Edragit L and S are soluble in pH 6 and 7.
- Plasticizers used in tablet coating are castor oil, Propylene glycol, glycerine, low molecular weight PEG and surfactant i.e. Tweens and Spans.
- Colorants: - The inorganic materials (iron oxides) and the natural colouring materials (Anthocyanin, Carmel, Carotenoids, Chlorophyll, Indigo turmeric) are also used to prepare coating solution.
- Opalux: - opaquant colour concentrate for sugar coating.
- Opaspray:-Opaquant colour concentrate for film coating.
- Opaquant extenders:- The most commonly used material is titanium dioxide. Some other material is silicates, carbonates, sulphate oxide and hydroxides.
- Extrusion &Spheronisation are the process used to obtain spherical particles, suitable for coating to produce controlled are the process used to obtain spherical particles, suitable for coating to produce controlled release formulation.
- Side vented pan is mostly used for film coating.
- A polymer which has optimal dissolution profile for enteric coating is HPMCP

## Film Defect

Sticking and Picking: - Over weighting or excessive film thickness causes tablet to stick to each other, or to the coating pan.

Orange peel effect: - Inadequate spreading of the coating solution before during causes a bumpy of orange peel effect on the coating.

Bridging and filling: - During drying the film may shrink and pull away from the sharp corners resulting in a bridging of the surface depression.

Filling is caused by applying too much solution resulting in a thick film that fills and narrow the monogram or bisect.

Blistering: - When coated tablets required further drying, too rapid evaporation of the solvent from the core results in blistering.

Hazing / Dull film: - This is sometimes called bloom. It can occur when too high processing temperature is used for a particular formulation.

Cracking: - Cracking occurs if internal stress in the film exceeds the tensile strength of the film.

**Table** Some important solution with example

| Different Solutions | Name |
|---|---|
| **Seal coating solution** | Dextrin, PEG-4000 |
| **Sub coating solution** | Gelatine, Sugar cane |
| **Polishing solution** | Naphtha |
| **Sub coating powder** | Dextrin |
| **Syrup solution** | Syrup USP |

**Table** Some example with their trade name and composition

| Trade Name | Composition |
|---|---|
| **Methocel** | Methyl cellulose |
| **Carbomer** | Carboxypolymethylene |
| **Povydone** | Polyvinyl pyrolidone |
| **Atlas** | Sorbitsan esters |
| **Calgon** | Polymetaphosphate |

**Table** Some of polymeric powder with their specification

| Types of Polymer | Example | Characteristic |
|---|---|---|
| **Water soluble polymer** | Hydropropyl cellulose<br>Hydroxyprop cellulose Povidone | - |
| **Water insoluble polymer** | Ethyl cellulose,<br>sodium alginate | - |
| **Homo polymers** | - | consist of a single monomer |
| **Copolymers** | - | consists of more than two monomer |
| **Natural polymer** | Cellulose, proteins | - |
| **Synthetic polymer** | Dacron, Cellulose | - |
| | | |

**Table** Polymer and their trade name with their specification

| Trade Name | Extended to Release products type |
|---|---|
| Disintergrants | Avicel & Explotab |
| Lubricant | Talc |
| Coating agent | Castorwax |
| Enteric coat | CAP |
| Sustained release agent | Keltrol& Ethyl cellulose & HPMC |

**Table** pH range inside body fluid

| Fluid | pH |
|---|---|
| Stomach | 6.5 to 8.0 |
| Duodenum | 5.0 to 6.0 |
| Jejunum & large Intestine | 1.2 to 3.5 |

## Capsule

- **Capsules** are solid dosage forms in which medicinal agents and / or inert substances are enclosed in a small of gelatine.
- Mother & Dublin invented single place of gelatine capsule.
- Murdock invited two piece telescopic capsule.

## HRAD Capsules

- The capsule are mainly made of **gelatineblends** and may contain small amount of certified dyes.
  - Opaquing agents, plasticizers and preservatives.
- Gelatine is a heterogeneous predicts derived by irreversible hydrolytic extraction of treated animal collagen.
- Common sources of collagen are animal bones, hide portions and Frogen pork skin.
- **Blends of bone** and **pork skin**gelatins normally used for hard capsule production.
- The pork skin gelatin contributes **plasticity and clarity** to the bend and thereby reducing haze and clarity to the bend.
- **Type Agelatin** is derived from an acid treated precursor and exhibits an isoelectric point at **pH 9.0**
- **Type B gelatin** is derived from an alkali treated precursor an exhibits an isoelectric point at **pH 4.7**
- **'Green" (Fresh)** bones are used for the preparation of a gelatin of the **Type "B".**
- **"Acid bones"** are used for the preparation of a gelatin of the **Type "A".**
- Titanium dioxide **is used as** Opacifier for **gelatin mass (0.2 to 1.2%)**

## Preparation of Capsule Shell

- Gelatin capsule are formed by dipping cool stainless steel mould pins & by centrifugal casting method.
- Automatic capsule production machine include the steps like dipping, spinning, drying, tripping, trimming and joining.
- The stainless steel mould pins are used to form the capsules and the tolerance is held with in fractions of a thousand of an inch.
- A number of (About 150) pair on pins is dipped in to a molten gelatin solution aform caps and bodies separately. The capsules are striped from the pins by bronze jaws and trimmed to definitive length. The cap and body sections are joined and finally ejected from the machine.
- The entire cycle is completed by 45 minutes.
- Thickness of the capsule wall is controlled by the viscosity of the gelatin solution and the speed and time of dipping.
- The size of the empty capsule may be varied due to variation of moisture content.
- Empty capsule usually receive the moisture of 12% to 15%
- Below 10% moisture content in gelatin shell caus brittle and may shrink to the point.
- Above 16% moisture content in gelatin shell cause size problem in the filling equipment.
- The solubility limit for empty capsules are
  (a) Water resistant fails to dissolve in water at 20 to 30 °C in 15 monute.
  (b) Acid solubility – dissolves in less than 5 minuts in 0.5% aqueous HCI (w/w) at 36 to 38 °C

**Table** List of filling equipment with their capacity and specification

| Company | Model | Filling Capacity | Filling Material | Specific Feature |
|---|---|---|---|---|
| Eli-Lilly | ROTOFIL | 1200 Capsule/minute | Pellets | |
| Farmatic | 2000/15 | 40000/hour | Powder | It's function is based in a continues motion with dosator- type powder feeding units |
| | 2000/30 | 80000/hour | | |
| | 2000/60 | 160000 / hour | | |
| Hofiger and Karg | GKF - 303 | 303 / Minute | Pallets, Powder, Tablets Thixotropic liquids (The first three models) | |
| | GKF - 602 | 602 / Minute | | |
| | GKF - 1500 | 1500 / Minute | | |
| | GKF - 2500 | 2500 / Minute | | |
| Mocofar | MT- 12 | 35000 / hour | Powder | It is function is based in a rectification and filling. |
| | MT – 13/1 | 5000 / hour | | |
| | MT – 13/2 | 10000 / hour | | |
| mG2 | G36/2 | 300 / minute | Powder<br>Granule<br>Pellete | It is function is based in a rectification and filling. |
| | G36/4 | 150 / minute | | |
| | G36 | 600 / minute | | |
| | G37N | 1600 / minute | | |
| | G38 | 1000 / minute | | |
| Osaka | R-180 | 70000 to 135000 / minute | Powder granule | |
| Perry | CF ACOFIL | 600000 / hour | Powder | It has a powder dose control capacity which is a unique feature |
| Zanasi | LZ-64 | 4000 / hour | Powder, Pallet and Tablet | |
| | AZ-20 | 9000 to 20000 / hour | | |
| | BZ-40 | 30000 / hour | Powder, Pallet and Tablet (BZ-72 & BZ-40) Powder & Granule (BZ-110) Powder (BZ-150) | |
| | BZ-72 | 60000 / hour | | |
| | BZ-110 | 110000 / hour | | |
| | BZ-150 | 150000 / hour | | |
| | Z-5000R1 | 70000 / hour | Powder, Granule and tablet | |
| | Z-5000R2 | 110000 / hour | | |
| | Z-5000R3 | 150000 / hour | | |

## Capsule Filling

- The empty capsules can be handled in the area having humidity level of 30-45%
- Capacity of hard gelatin capsules ranges from numbers 000 to 5 9600 to 30 mg)
- Approximately capacity of empty gelatin capsule areas follows-

| Size | 000 | 00 | 0 | 1 | 2 | 3 | 4 | 5 |
|---|---|---|---|---|---|---|---|---|
| Vol. | 1.40 | 0.95 | 0.68 | 0.50 | 0.37 | 0.30 | 0.21 | 0.13 |

- During the filling by Eli-Lilly (Rotofil), Hofiger and Karg (GKF), Oskar (R-180) and Perry (CIACOFIL) models, the powder must have flow characteristics. For example when the acetyl salicylicacid is filled by the above model, the excipient should be flow able corn starch. The ideal lubricant is metallic stearate.
- During the filling by Zanasi ,(LZ, BZ, ZR,) Macofar(MT), Farmatic (2000) and mG2 (G) models the powder must have sufficient cohesiveness to retain its slug form during delivery to the capsules. For example when the acetyl salicylic acid us filled by the above models the excipient should be microcrystalline cellulose. The ideal lubricant is mineral oil.
- The glidants usually used (less than 2%) during filling a capsule are glycol esters, silicones, silicon dioxide, Metallic stearate, stearate acid and talc.

## Evaluation

1. **Weight variation test**
   - 20 intact capsules are individually weighed and the average weight is determined. If none of the individually weights are less than 90% or more than 110% of the average the it meets the test requirements.
   - If the above test does not meet the requirements, then the individual net weight is determined and these are averaged. Then the difference is determined. If the difference does not exceed 10% of the average in more than 6 of 60 capsules, and if in no case any difference exceed 25% then it meets the test requirement.
   - ROTOWEIGHT is high speed capsule weighing machine. The capsules are gravity – fed onto vacuum Pins which measure the reflected energy (backscatter) of a low power X-ray beam directed at each capsule.
   - This reflected energy is proportional to the weight of the filled capsule. The machine operates 73000 capsules per hour.
   - VERICAP 2000 is a high speed capsule weight machine. It operated by detecting capacitance variation, as filled capsules are propelled at high speed by compressed air between two charged plates. The measured change in dielectric constant thus produced is correlated to the weight of the capsule. The machine operates 73000 capsules per hour.

## Capsule Dusting / Polishing Machine

The following method is used for Polishing of capsules.

1. **Pan polishing:** Accelacota tablet coating pan may be used to polish the capsule. A polyuthrane

   Or Cheese cloth liner is placed in the pan and the liner is used to trap the removed dust as well as to impart to gloss to the capsule.
2. **Cloth dusting:** In this method bulk filled capsule arte rubbed with a cloth.
3. **Brushing:** In this method capsules are fed under rotating soft brushes.
4. **Rotosort:** This is equipment used for dedusting and polishing of capsules. It is also used t oseparate unfilled capsules. Filled or unfilled bodies and loose caps. The machine handles 15000 capsules per hour.
5. **Erweka KEA:** This is equipment used for polishing of hard gelatin capsules. It moves the capsules between soft plastic tassels against a perforated plastic sleeve, under vacuum.
6. **Seidenader model:** This is an equipment offers two units may be used separately or may be combined in the (PM-60) finishing of the filled gelatin capsules. If removes unfilled capsules. The PM-60 unit used to polish the finished capsules. It consists of two lamb wool belts moving in the opposite direction. The capsules are carried on the lower belt and both belts are under suction.

## Special Techniques

**Imprinting:** This is the process by which the company print the products and identification information on capsules surfaces. The different companies which provide the machines are as follows.-

| Company | Capacity | Types of Printing |
|---|---|---|
| Ackely | 50000 / hour | Straight line and circumference |
| Markem | 60000-250000 / hour | Straight line but not circumference |
| Harnet | 500000 / day | Straight line and circumference |

- Fluidised bed drier is used in the pharmaceutical industry for the drying of powders before filling.
- Capsule all liquid. Solution and suspension for capsulation should be homogeneous, air free and flow by gravity at room temperature.
- Water soluble and volatile constituents can migrate into the hydrophilic shell and volatilize from its surface.
- The products cost of capsule is directly proportional to **shell thickness.**

**Table** Ingredients used in preparation of capsules shell

| Purpose | Ingredients used in Preparation of Capsules Shell |
|---|---|
| Preservative | Propyl paraben (0.2%) |
| Aids solubility | Fumeric acid |
| Organoleptic additive | Essential oil |
| Opacifier | Titanium dioxide |

**Table** List machine used in capsule preparation

| Name of the machine | Use |
|---|---|
| **a. Rotosort** | 1. Capsule sorting machine |
| **b. Erweka KEA** | 2. Capsule dedusting and polishing machine |
| **c. Seidenader model PM-60** | 3. Capsule polishing machine |
| **d. 0.2% Markem model 280 A** | 4. Capsule imprinting machine |
| **e. Vericap 1200, Rotoweigh** | 5. Capsule weighing machine |
| **f. Hartnett Model** | 6. Capsule imprinting machine |
| **g. Osaka, Accofil** | 7. Capsule filling machine |

**Table** Disintegration time of capsules

| Capsule | Disintegration Time |
|---|---|
| **Hard capsule** | 30 minutes |
| **Soft capsule** | 60 Minutes |

## Soft Capsule

- The custom manufacturers are specialist in production of these soft gelatins.
- The soft gelatins are useful in oral, suppository, topical, ophthalmic and otic preparations.

## Method of Manufacture

| **Method** | **Weight variation in the net content** |
|---|---|
| Plate process | 20-40% |
| Rotary die process | ±3% |
| Reciprocating die process | Negligible |
| Accogel machine | Negligible |

## Nature of Capsules Shell

- The capsules shells principally composed of Gelatin, Plasticizer, and water. It mayalso contain preservatives, colorants, opacifyingagent's flavourings, sugars and acids.

**Gelatin strength**

- The bloom strength or gel strength of gelatin is the cohesive strength of the cross – linking that occurs between gelatin molecules and this strength is proportional to the molecular weight of the gelatin.
- Bloom is determined by measuring the weight in grams required to move a plastic plunger that is 0.5 inches in diameter 4 mm into a $6\frac{2}{3}$ % gelatin gel that has been held at 10°C for 17 hours.
- The normal bloom strength of a gelatin is usually 150-250g.
- The higher bloom strength becomes more physically stable capsule shell.
- The cost of the gelatin is directly proportional to bloom strength.

**Viscosity of gelatin**

- The viscosity of gelatin determined on a $6\frac{2}{3}$ % concentration of gelatin in water at 60°C.
- The viscosity of gelatin is 38±2 milipoise (25 – 45 milipoise).
- Low viscosity (25-32 milipose) with high Bloom (180 to 250g) gelatins are used for the capsulation of gygroscopic vehicles or solids.

**Iron content**

- The iron content present in gelatin used for manufacturer of soft capsules should not more than 15 ppm.

**Plasticizers**

- ➢ The role of plasticizer in capsule is tit determines the hardness of shall.
- ➢ Gelatin is plasticized by addition of glycerine. Sorbitol or other polyol.
- ➢ The ratio by weight of water to dry gelatin is, Water (0.7-1.3) : dry gelatin (1.0)
- ➢ Gelatin and glycerine are used for the preparation of lamellas in specified ratio 5:1.

**Table** Specification for hardness of capsules

| Ratio of dry glycerine and dry gelatin | Types of hardness |
|---|---|
| 0.4: 1 | Hard |
| 0.6: 1 | Medium |
| 0.8: 1 | Soft |

- ➢ Usually medicaments to the gelatin mass are not added. But benzocaine is added (3mg / capsule shell) in chewable cough capsules)

**Colorants**

- Usually darker colour are used large size capsules (14 to 20 minim oblong).
- Clear type colour is used in clear type filling materials and opaque colours are used in suspensions.
- Before the colour is chosen, mixture should be checked by addition of water to ascertain.
- In the preparation of vitamins and minerals, as the iron is present in the gelatin, the water soluble iron sensitive ingredients migrated from the filling material in to shell an cause darks sports.
- FD & C and D&C water soluble dyes, certified lakes pigments, and vegetable colour alone or in combination is used as colorants.

**Table** Additional component of gelatin mass

| Use | Name | Concentration |
|---|---|---|
| **Preservative** | Methyl paraben and propyl paraben In ratio of 4:1 | 0.2% |
| **Opacifier** | Titanium dioxide | 0.2 to 1.2% |
| **Flavoring agent** | Ethly vanillin Essential oils | (0.1%) |
| **To produce chewable shell and taste** | Sucrose | (up to 2%) |
| **Aids solubility (Reduces aldehydes Tanning of gelatin)** | Fumaric acid | 5% |

**Table** The nature of the capsule content

| Soft gelatin capsule size and shapes | Maximum volume for human intake |
|---|---|
| Oblong | 20 minim |
| Oral | 16 minim |
| Round | 9 minim |

## Liquids

### Full volume

- The minimum fill volume may be calculated from the specific gravity of liquid.
- The size of capsule depends on the dosage required.
- The die size and shape may be chosen from the nominal capacities in minims.
- The content of the soft gelatin capsule is liquid or a combination of miscible liquids, solutions suspension, etc.
- Liquids those are water miscible and volatile in nature cannot be included as a major constituent of capsule because they can migrate into the hydrophilic gelatin shell and volatize from its surface.
- Gelatin plasticizer like glycerine and polyethylene glycol cannot also be the major constituent of the capsule because they will make the capsule softer. However water an alcohol up to 5% if capsule content can be used as co-solvent to aid in the preparation of solutions.
- The plasticizer like glycerine and propylene glycol up to 10% of capsule content can be used as co-solvents with polyethylene glycol.
- The most widely used liquid for human use are as follows-

| Oil Active ingredients | Vegetable oils | Non-ionic suffocative agents | Fish oil |
|---|---|---|---|
| Clofibrate | Soyabin oil | Polysorbate 80 | Shark liver oil |
| | | Polyethylene glycol 400 | |
| | | Polyethylene glycol 600 | |

- The viscosity of liquids ranging from 0.222 cp to 3000 cp (at 25°C) is allowed to encapsulated but the liquid like glycerine (954cp at 25°C) can notbe encapsulated because it can cause binding of slide valves and pumps filling machine.
- The pH of liquids to be encapsulated should have been between 2.5 to 7.5
- The organic or inorganic solids which is to be encapsulated in suspension from should be 80 mesh or finer particles.

- The formulation of suspension for soft gelatin encapsulation depends upon the technique base adsorptions of the solids to be suspended. Base adsorption is expressed as the number of grams of liquid base required to produce a capsulatable mixture when mixed with one gram of solid.
- The base adsorption is used o determine the "minim per gram" factor (m/g) of the solid. The minim per gram factor is the volume in minims that is occupied by one gram of the solid plus the weight of liquid base required to make a capsulatble mixture.

## Capsule Manuracturer Processing and Control

- Except the gelatin preparation area the temperature range of manufacturer are is 20-22°C and the humidity level in is a maximum of 40% in the operating areas and a range of 20-30% in drying areas.

### Gelatin Preparation

- The gelatin is weighed on a printomatic (most accurate) scales and mixed with the accurately metered an chilled (7°) liquid constituents in a pony mixer. The mixing process requires about 25 minute for 270 kg of mass.
- The resultant fluffy mass is transferred to melting tanks a melted under vacuum (29.5"HG) at 93 for 3 hours.
- The mass is then maintained at a temperature of 57-60 before an during capsulation process.

### Material Preparation

1. **Weighing-** All materials used for preparation for encapsulation must be weighed with. Printomatic scales for exact measurement and control record.
2. **Blending-** All weighed ingredients are kept in a mixture like Cowells for initial blending of solids with the liquids base.
3. **Milling-** After initial blending the materials are put through a milling or humanizing process. The equipment used in this process such as the homoloid mill, stone mill hopper mill or the Urschel Comitrol. The purpose of milling operation is to break up the agglomerates of solid and to make certain that solids are ''wet'' with the liquid carriers so as to achieve a smooth and homogenous mixture.
4. **Deaeration-** Then all mixture are subjected to deaeration. This is necessary to achieve uniform capsule fill weights and this also protects against loss of potency through oxidation prior to and during capsulation. This is the process by most liquids and suspension may be deaerated by means of equipment designed to expose thin layer of material continuously to vcuum (29.5''Hg) and at the same time transfer the material from the mixing tank to the container that will be used at the capsulation machine.

### Capsulation Rotary Die Process

- The gelatine mass is fed by gravity to a metering device,this device control the flow of the mass onto air cooled (13-14°C) rotating drums.
- Gelatine ribbon of controlled (± 10%) thickness are formed. The wet shell thickness may very from 0.022 to 0.045 inch.
- The ribbons are feed through a mineral oil lubricating bath, over guide rolls, and down between the wedge and the die rolls.
- The materials to be capsulated flow in to the gelatine ribbons between die rolls.
- Now the filled, shaped and hermetically sealed capsule cut from the gelatine ribbon.
- The sealing of the capsule achieved by mechanical pressure on the die fills and the heating (37 to 46°C) of the ribbons by the wedge.
- The capsules are now conveyed through neptha wash unit to remove mineral oil.

- The capsules are now dried by infrared drying steps or allowed to come equilibrium with forced air condition of 20-30% relative humidity at 21-24°C, capsules at equilibrium with 20-30% RH at 21-24°C are considered dry and the shell of such a capsule contains 6-10% water.
- The moisture content of the shell is determined by toluene distillation method.
- The capsules thereafter sent for heat branding or ink printing or ink printing for purpose of identification.

**Physical Stability**

- Physical stability of capsule product depends upon –

  a. Types of gelatine b. Gelatine formulation
- The physical stability soft gelatine capsule is associated primarily with the pick-up or loss of water by the capsule shell.
- The capsule shell is dried at the equilibrium with 20-30% at 21-24°C
- The ratio between dry glycerine to dry gelatine is 0.5:1
- The ratio between water and dry gelatine is 1:1
- The low humidifies (>20%RH), low temperature (<2°C) and high temperature (>38°C) or combination of these condition have only transient effects.
- The accelerated physical stability test is strictly relevant to the integrity of the gelatine shell and should not be constructed as stability of test ingredients.
- The resultant of ''soft spot'' pm a capsule is dee to slower drying.
- The rotating- bottle method is used for dissolution study of capsules.

**Important Point to Remember**

- Ingredient used for capsulation is soft capsule should flow by gravity at a temperature not exceeding 350.
- The soft gelatine capsule is soft, globular having gelatine shell is thicker than hard gelatine capsule.
- The type of soft gelatine is discarded are a. overfills b. underfills c. foregin
- Equipment which are used in capsulation for milling or homogenization a. Homoloid mill b. stone mill c. urchelcomitrol mill
- The scaling temperature of soft gelatine capsule is usually in therange of 37 to 40°C.
- While making soft gelatine capsules, gelatin mass is fed by gravity to a metering device known as spreader box which controls the flow of mass on to air cooled rotating drum.
- The thickness of wet shell of soft gelatine capsules is between 0.025-0.032 inches.
- The ideal bloom strength for manufacturer of hard gelatin shells is 230-275.
- The viscosity of the solution used to manufacturer hard gelatin shells is 3.3-4.7 mpas.
- The water content permissible in hard gelatin is 13-15%.
- The relative humidity where the hard gelatin capsule filed are 30-50%
- Cross linking of gelatin which is sometimes present at trace level in excipients is catalysed by formaldehyde.
- Auger method, piston temp method, Dosator methods are the independent method for powder and granulate filling in capsules.
- Osaka machine is used for powder & granulate filling method by dependent method.
- Zanasi machine is used to examine lubricity requirement of formulations being filled with dosator machine.
- In liquid encapsulation microscopy sealing (LEMS) process, 50% water + 50% ethanol is the sealing fluids which sprayed on the joint between the cap & body.

- The alternative material for gelatine offered by capsule manufacturer is Starch & HPMC.
- During manufacturer of soft gelatin capsules, the oxygen sensitive drug can be protected by filling under Nitrogen.

### Microencapsulaton

- Microencapsulation provides the desired coating properties such as-

  a. Strength and flexibility b. Imermebility c. Optical prooertues d. stabilising and sustained release
- The method which are suitable for microencapsulation are
- Air suspension b. Pan coating c. Polymerization d. Coacervation
- Microencapsulation is a process by which solid, liquid or even gases may be encapsulated into microscopic size particles.
- Blisters are made up of **Polyvinyl chloride.**
- Polychlorotrifluoroethylene film is laminated to protect the content in Blister package from moisture
- A water soluble substance used as coating material in microencapsulation process is Hydroxy ethyl cellulose

| Ingredients in Gelatin | Concentration |
|---|---|
| Methyl Paraben and propyl paraben | 0.2% |
| Titanium dioxide | 0.2 to 0.2% |
| Ethyl vanillin | 0.1% |
| Essential oil | 2.0% |
| Sugar | 5% |
| Fumaric acid | 1% |

## 1.9 Sterile Products

Parenteral drug products are the dosage forms intended for administration by a route that does not involve the gastrointestinal (GI) tract (thus, parenteral). Most of the parenteral drug products are injectable dosage forms that are intended for administration by injection using a syringe and a needle.

### Vehicle

- The most common vehicle for sterile product is water for injection. Sometimes non-aqueous solvents are also used.
- The conductivity of WFI is 0.99 micromhos.
- The total solid content of WFI is 10 ppm.
- The non-aqueous solvents are two types. 1. Water miscible, 2. Water immiscible.
- The solvent which is miscible with water usually used in combination with water as vehicle. These are for example dioxolanes, dimethyklacetamide, butyl glycol, polyethylene glycol 400 and 600, propylene glycol, glycerine, ethyl alcohol, N-(β-hydroxyethyl) -lactamide, etc.
- The solvent which is not miscible with water includes fixed oils, ethyl oleate, isopropyl myristate, benzyl benzoate.
- The most frequently used non aqueous solvent is polyethylene glycol, propylene glycol, and fixed oils.

- In non-aqueous injection the oil used as solvent are sesame oil cotton seed oil, corn oil and peanut oil.
- The most suitable vehicle for cardiac glycosides is 40% Ethyl alcohol.
- The capacity of buffer for parenteral preparation should be Moderate.
- Most suitable vehicle for Amylobarbitone sodium is WFI free from CO2.
- Most suitable vehicle for progesterone injection BP is a sterile solution in Ethyl oleate.
- Water for injection differs from sterile distilled water as it is free from pyrogens.
- Bacteriostatic water for injection should be packed in containers of 30 ml.
- For aseptic processing Class 100-room process is used.

## Pyrogens

- Pyrogens are water soluble & non-volatile in nature. Chemically they are Lipo polysaccharides. The main source of pyrogens is Gram-ve bacteria.
- I hour after injection the pyrogens produce clinical symptoms in human body.
- The containers used for the preparation of parenteral products may be rendered free from pyrogens.
- By heating usually at 210 or 3-4 hours or 650 for 60 second.
- The limits endotoxin content in WFI 0.25 units/ml.

## Solutes

(a) Antioxidants

The antioxidants are three types.

(a) Reducing agents Eg. Ascorbic acid, Sodium bisulfite, Sodium metabisulfite, Sodium formaldehyde, sulfoxylate, Thiourea

(b) Blocking agents. Eg. Ascorbic acid ester, Butylhydroxytoluene (BHT), Tocophenols

(c) Synergestics Eg. Citric acids, Citranoic acid, Phosphoric acid, Tartaric acid.

(b) Tonicity

- The compounds contributing to the isotonicityof products reduce the pain of injection in areas.
- They also contribute to the colligative properties of the preparation.
- Dextrose 5%, sodium chloride 0.9%, serve as tonicity contributors.
- The isotonicity of the solution can be determined by a. freezing point depression method, haemolytic method by using red blood cell.

**Table** Classes and example of parenteral additives

| Additive class | Example of parenteral additives | Usual concentration (%w/v) |
|---|---|---|
| **Antimicrobial** | **Benzalkonium chloride** | 0.01 |
| | Benzyl alcohol | 1-2 |
| | Chlorobutanol | 0.25-0.5 |
| | Phenol | 0.25-0.5 |
| | Butyl p-hydroxybenzoate | 0.015 |
| **Antioxidant** | Ascorbic acid | 0.01-0.5 |
| | Cysteine | 0.1-0.5 |
| | Sodiumbisulfide | 0.1-1.0 |
| | Tocopherols | 0.05-0.5 |

**Table** *Contd...*

| Additive class | Example of parenteral additives | Usual concentration (%w/v) |
|---|---|---|
| **Buffers** | Acetates<br>Citrates<br>Phosphates | 1-2<br>1-5<br>0.8-2.0 |
| **Bulking agents** | Lactose<br>Mannitol<br>Sorbitol | 1-8<br>1-10<br>1-10 |
| **Chelating gents** | Salts of ethylene diaminetetra acetic acid | 0.01-0.05 |
| **Solubilising agents** | Ethyl alcohol<br>Glycerine<br>Lecithin<br>Polythene glycol | 1-50<br>1-50<br>0.5-2.0<br>1-50 |
| **Surfactants** | Polyoxy ethylene sorbitan monooleate<br>Surbiton monooleate | 0.1-0.5<br>0.5-0.25 |
| **Inert gases** | Nitrogen or carbon dioxide | |

## Container

### 1. Plastic Container

- The principal ingredient of the various plastic containers is the thermoplastic polymer.
- All of the thermoplastic polymer can be autoclaved during parenteral preparations except

**Polyethylene and Polystyrene**

- A new group of plastic **propylene** and the copolymer **polyethylene – polypropylene** belonging to polyolefin is most widely now days used. Polypropylene is a liner polymer that can be produced to be highly crystalline. Because of its crystallinity, it has high tensile strength, a high melting point **of 165°C,** and relatively low permeability to gases and water vapour. It is transulant, abrasion- resistant and high surface gloss.
- **Flexible polyethylene containers** are used **for ophthalmic containers** and flexible polyvinyl chloride bags used **for intravenous solutions.**

**Evolution of plastic materials:**

The test procedure for evaluating the toxicity of plastic material consists of following phases

(a) Implanting shall pieces of plastic material IM in rabbits

(b) Injecting elutes using sodium chloride injection, with or without alcohol IV in mice.

(c) Injecting elutes using PEG – 400 and sesame oil intraperitoneally in mice.

(d) Injecting all four elutes subcutaneously in ribbits.

Result: The reaction from the test samples must not be significantly greater than non-reactive control samples.

### 2. Glass Container

- The two general types of glasses are Soda lime and borosilicate. They are also divided in to various type like Type – I, Type – II, Type – III, NP, depending on chemical resistance.

## Chemical Resistance

- The most chemical resistant glass is composed entirely of the Silicon dioxide.
- The brittleness and high melting point characteristic of chemical resistance glass can be modified by Boric oxide.
- The chemical resistance of glass is evaluated by powder glass test and water attack test. The test result measures the amount of alkaline constituents leached from the glass.
- The borosilicate glasses are Type – 1 type and they are highly resistance to chemicals. They are preferred for most sterile products. Buffered and unbuffered aqueous solutions. Powder glass test is used to evaluate the chemical resistance of glass.
- The treated soda lime glasses are Type -11 type. They are preferred for the product has a non-aqueous vehicle or the period of contact with the aqueous vehicle is less. They may be used for buffered aqueous solutions with pH less than 7, dry powder and oleaginous solutions. Water attack test is used to identify the alkalinity of the glass.
- The general purpose soda-lime glasses are **NP type**. They **are least resistant** to chemicals. They are not used for parenteral. They are used for tablets oral solutions, and suspensions, ointments, and external liquids.
- Soda-lime glasses are **Type- III type;** they are preferred for the products of dry powders and oleaginous solutions. Powder glass test is used to evaluate the chemical resistance of glass.

## Physical Characteristics

- Glass containers are sometimes coated internally with silicone fluid to produce a hydrophobic surface. To achieve permanency, the silicon must be baked at a temperature of approximately **150°(300°F)**
- Volume of container: For single dose not more than **1000 ml** and for multiple dose not more than **30 ml**

## Rubber Closers

- Rubber closers are made-up of principle, natural rubber (latex) or by synthetic polymer.
- The elastomer used in rubber stopper formulation is butyl neoprene, Polysoprene, and silicon
- The other ingredients present are sulphur (**vulcanizingagents**), accelerator, 2-mercaptobenxothiazol (active organic compound), zinc oxide **(activator)** lime stone (**filters**), antioxidants, lubricants etc.

## Evaluation

Bioburden test is done to determine

a. number of microorganism present in a parenteral products
b. Type of microorganism present in parental products

**Leaker test**

It is intended to detect incompletely sealed ampoules. Tip sealed ampoules are most likely to be incompletely sealed than that of pull – sealed**. 0.5 – 1.0%methylene blue dye** is used in leaker test. It is usually detected by producing negative pressure within an incompletely sealed ampoule. **The vacuum 27 inches Hg**. For is released for **30 minutes** to carry out the test. **A spark tester probe** is applied to for the leaker test of vials and bottles.

**Clarity test**

- The limitation permitted for particles in the larger volume of infusions are 50 particles of 10 µm or larger and 5 particles of 25 µm and larger per millimetre.

- The particulate count and size distribution of a liquid in a parenteral product can be done by utilizing. The principles of light
- Scattering, light absorption, and electrical resistance.
- A video image projection coupled with electronic circuit detector is used for the clarity test of 1-5 ml containers.

**Pyrogen test**

The different method used for pyrogen testing is a. Ribbit test b. LAL test

- The veins of rabbits are selected to perform this test.
- If pyrogen is injected to the vein of a rabbit, an elevation temperature occurs within 3 hours.
- Minimum volume of preparation above which pyrogen test should be performed is **15ml.**
- Limulus amebocyte lysate test is rapid in vitro test for parenteral to detect the **presence of Pyrogens.**
- During the test, in the presence of pyrogenic endotoxins from gram negative bacteria, a firm gel is formed within 60 minutes when incubated at **37°C.**

**Table** Important charts to remember

| Material | Additive present | Water vapour permeation | Gas permeation ($O_2$) | Physical Properties |
|---|---|---|---|---|
| **Polyethylene** | Low | High | Low | Translucent + Flexible |
| **PVC** | High | High | | Translucent + Flexible |
| **Polypropylene** | Low | Moderately | | |
| **Butyl rubber** | Moderately | Low | | Opaque + Flexible |
| **Soda lime glass** | High | No | | Optically clear + rigid |
| **Borosilicate glass** | Low | No | None | Optically clear + rigid |
| **Silicone rubber** | Moderately | Very high | Very high | Translucent + Flexible |
| **Neoprene rubber** | High | Moderately | | Opaque + Flexible |
| **Polyvinyl chloride** | | High | | |
| **Polyamide** | | High | | Translucent + rigid + tough |
| **Natural rubber** | | Moderately | Moderately | Opaque + Flexible |
| **Polyisoprene rubber** | | Moderately | Moderately | Opaque + Flexible |
| **Polystyrene** | | | High | Translucent + rigid |
| **Teflon** | | | Low | |
| **Polycarbonate** | | | | Translucent + rigid |

**Important Points to remember:**

- The pH range for a parenteral preparation by subcutaneous route is **3-6.**
- Citrate buffer is preferably selected for parenteral products whose pH is restricted within **2.1 – 6.2.**
- The osmolality of parenteral products should be between **280-290 mOsm/L.**
- **Cardarone IV & Etoposide IV**is used as surfactants used in parenteral products.
- **Cardarone IV** is 10% of Polysorbate 80.
- **Hydroxypropyl β – cyclonextrin** is suitable for parenteral use.
- **Un substituted α & β cyclodextrin** are not suitable for parenteral preparation because they cause **Nephrotoxicity.**
- **Lypholization** is a process applied in pharmaceutical industry to remove unwanted water portion from a parenteral products.

- The concentration of antioxidants like disodium edetate, Ascorbic acid, & sodium metabisulfite used in parenteral preparation is **0.005, 1, and 0.003 present respectively**.
- The most popular excipient combinations used for aqueous suspension in parenteral products is PEG/ Tween -80 & CMC /Tween – 80.
- The size of Liposomes used in parenteral is **less than 3000nm**

**Table** Important chart to remember

| Ingredients | Use |
|---|---|
| **Calcium phosphate** | Adsorbent diluent |
| **Calcium hydrogen phosphate** | Used for direct compression |
| **Colloidal silica** | Improve granular flow |
| **Anhydrous dextrose** | Adsorbs moisture at high relative humidity |
| **Dextrose (spray dried)** | Direct compressible but absorbs moisture at high |
| **Lactose** | Inexpensive & gives granules by moist granulation |
| **Lactose (spray dried)** | Useful for direct compression & incompatible with primary amine |
| **Lactose anhydrous** | Direct compressible & but prevent moisture uptake |
| **Starch** | Dried from used as absorbent & used as disintegrate |
| **Mannitol** | Gives cooling effect in the mouth |
| **Barium sulphate** | Used in roentgenography |
| **Propyliodone** | A radio-opaque medium for broncho graphic use |
| **Ethiodizedoid** | Used in emphography |
| **Ipodate sodium** | Used in roentgenography |
| **Iophendulate** | For myclography |
| **Ipodate calcium** | Used as a contrast medium for cholecystography |
| **Indocyanine green** | To determine cardic output, hepatic function & live blood flow |
| **Methiodal sodium** | A radio – opaque medium for retrograde pyelography |
| **Ndigotindisulfonate sodium** | In a kidney function test |
| **Insulin** | Diagnostic agent for evaluation of glomerularfiltration |
| **Phenol sulfonphthalein** | For determining kidney function |
| **Evans blue** | A diagnostic agent used in blood volume estimation |
| **Azuresin** | An ion to exchange resin used as indicator |
| **Congo red** | Used in th detection of amyloidosis |
| **Povidone** | Non enteric material |
| **Cellulose acetate phthalate** | Enteric material |
| **Ingredients** | Purpose |
| **Titanium Dioxide** | Opacifier |
| **Ethyl vanillin** | Flavouring |
| **Methyl Paraben and propyl paraben** | Preservative |
| **Essential oils** | Flavoring agent |
| **Ethrosine sodium** | Dental disclosing agent used to identify areas of plaque on the teeth |
| **Fluorescein sodium** | As an ophthalmic diagnostic aid |
| **Ascorbyl Palmitate** | An antioxidant used in food &pharmaceuticals |
| **Butylated hydroxyanisole** | An antioxidant in cosmetics |
| **Butylated hydroxytoluene** | As oxidant employed to rtard oxidative degradation of oils & fats |
| **Chlorobutanol** | It has antibacterial &germicidal properties |
| **Sodium bisulfate** | Antioxidant & stabilizer |

**Table** *Contd...*

| Ingredients | Use |
|---|---|
| **Monothioglycerol** | Used as a preservation |
| **Sorbet acid** | Mold& yeast inhibitor |
| **Chlorobutanol** | Antibacterial & germicidal |
| **Potassium sorbate** | To inhibit the growth of mould & yeast |
| **Sulphur dioxide** | A – bleaching agent |
| **Carmel** | Colouring agent |
| **Ginger** | Flavouring agent |
| **Ethyl vanillin** | Flavouring agent |
| **Sodium metabisulfite** | Preservative |
| **Vanillin** | Only as a flavour |
| **Compressible sugar** | Tableting excipient & sweeting agent |
| **Calcium sulphate** | Diluent |
| **Carnauba wax** | Polishing agent |
| **Calcium stearate** | Lubricant |
| **Micro crystalline cellulose** | Diluent & Disintegrate |
| **Cellulose acetate phthalate** | Enteric tablet coating material |
| **Citric acid** | Anticoagulant |
| **Dextrin** | An excipient & emulsifier |
| **Dextrose** | As a supplement to milk for infant feeding |

## 1.10 Interfacial Phenomena

- Surface tension is defined as the force in dynes, acting on the surface of the liquid at right angles to any line of length of surface 1 cm.
- The units of surface tension are dyne / cm in CGS systems and Newton's / meter in MKS systems.
- The inter molecular attraction between similar molecules is called as **cohesive forces**& the inter molecular attraction between dissimilar molecules is called as adhesive forces.

**Example of liquids and Intermolecular Interaction**

| | |
|---|---|
| Polar (Water) | Hydrogen bonding |
| Semi Polar (Benzene) | Landon and inductive forces |
| Non Polar (Carbon tetrachloride) | London type forces |

**Table** Determination of surfaces & Interfacial tension

| Methods | Equation | Instruments used |
|---|---|---|
| 1. **Capillary rise method** | $\gamma = \frac{1}{2}$ rphg | Capillary tube |
| 2. **DuNouy Ring method** | $\gamma = \frac{\text{dial reading (dynes)}}{2.2\pi}$ x Correction factor | Du Nouytensiometer |
| 3. **Drop count method** | $\frac{n(\text{liquid}) x\ \rho\ (\text{liquid})}{n\ (\text{water}) x\ \rho(\text{water})}$ x $\gamma$ (water) | Stalgmometer |

- Surface free energy is defined as the work required to increase the area of a liquid by 1sq.cm.

## Surface Active Agents

Surface active agents are defined as the substances which preferentially get adsorbed at the interface

And exhibits self-association in the bulk of solution at a specific concentration. These substances reduce interfacial tension. They have hydrophilic and lipophilic portions in their structure. The functional

Groups such as alcoholic (-OH), carboxylic acid (-OOH), Sulphate (-SO4) and quaternary

Ammonium (-NH4 ) contribute to the hydrophilic portion. Alkyl chain contribute to the lipophlic nature

### Application of Surface active agents

1. Pharmaceutical adjuvant (Solubilizing, Wetting, Suspending, Emulsifying, Foaming agents and Detergents)
2. Influence on the drug action. (Surfactants on **low concentrations** enhance the penetration of hexylresorcinol into pinworms, round worms etc.)
3. Antibacterial activity Ionic surfactants adsorb on the cell surface by **electrostatic interaction**. Both ram negative and tram organisms are susceptible to the action of **cationic quaternary compounds**. Whereas the gram positive organisms are attacked more easily by **anionic agents** than gram negative organisms.

### Hydrophilic – Lipophilic Balance (HLB)

- The HLB system used to classify surfactants.
- HLB of sodium lauryl sulphate is 40.0
- Tween 20 is a hydrophilic surfactant.

**Table** The HLB range of different agents are given below

| Different Agents | HLB Value |
|---|---|
| Antifoaming agents | 1.5 to 8 |
| W / O emulsifying agents | 3 to 6 |
| Emulsion o/w | 8 to 18 |
| Wetting and spread agent | 7-9 |
| Antifoaming agents | 1-3 |
| Foaming agents | 8 |
| Solubilizing agents | 16-19 |
| Detergents | 13-16 |
| No dispersion | 1.5 to 3.7 |
| Poor dispersion | 3.8 to 5.5 |
| Clear solution | 13.1 to 20.0 |
| Milky dispersion (stable) | 9.5 to 10.3 |
| Milky dispersion (unstable) | 6.1 to 8.6 |
| Translucent to clear dispersion | 10.5 to 13.0 |

**Table** HLB values of different surfactants

| Different Agents | HLB Value |
|---|---|
| Span 20 (SORBIRTAL MONOLAURATE) | 4.5 |
| Span 40 (SORBIRTAL MONOPALMITATE) | 6.7 |
| Span 60 (SORBIRTAL MONOSTEARATE) | 4.7 |
| Span 80 (SORBIRTAL MONOOLEATE) | 4.3 |
| Tween 20 (PolyoxyethylensorbitalMonolaurate) | 13.3 |
| Tween 40 (PolyoxyethylensorbitalMonopalmitate) | 15.6 |

**Table** *Contd...*

| | |
|---|---|
| **Tween 60 (PolyoxyethylensorbitalMonosterarate)** | 9.6 |
| **Tween 80 (PolyoxyethylensorbitalMonooleate)** | 15.0 |
| **Propylene glycol monostearate** | 3.4 |
| **Propylene glycol monolaurte** | 4.5 |
| **Polyoxyethylene glycol monosterate** | 11.5 |
| **Polyozyethylene glycol monooleate** | 11.2 |

| Type of surfactant | Example |
|---|---|
| Nonionic | Sodium lauryl sulphate, Polyoxyethylene lauryl ether, Sorbian mono-oleate, Polyoxyethylenesorbitan mono-oleate Sorbianmonopalmitate |
| Cationic | cetyltrimethyl ammonium bromide N-cetyl-N-ethyl morpholiumethosulfate Benzalkonium chloride |
| Ampholytic | Dimethly dodecyl ammoniym propane sulfonate, Lecithin |
| Anionic | Trethanolamine |

| Dispersed Phase | Dispersion Medium | Example |
|---|---|---|
| Solid | Liquid | Solution |
| Solid | Gas | Smoke |
| Liquid | Liquid | Emulsion |
| Liquid | Gas | Fog |
| Gas | Liquid | Foam |
| Gas | Solid | Pumice |

## Wetting Phenomenon

- Wetting is an **adsorption process** in which intimate contact of the solid with liquid phase is achieved
- For the proper wetting of solids by liquids, the contact angle should by nearly **Zero.**
- The efficacy of wetting activity can be detected by **Draves test.**
- **Washburn equation**: It states that the distance that a liquid penetrates into a bed of powder in time is proportional to the square of Cosθ. This is used to evaluate the wetting ability of powder by different vehicles.

## Contact Angle

- Contact angle can be defined as an angle between the liquid droplet and surface over which it spreads.
- Wetting ability of a vehicle can be detected by observing **contact angle.**
- A low contact angle indicates that adhesive forces between the liquid and the solid predominate and wetting occurs, while a high contact angle indicates that cohesive forces of the liquid predominate
- The basic equation that applies to wetting is young's equation.

  Contact angle $\cos\theta = \frac{-\gamma_{sl} + \gamma_s}{\gamma_s}$

## Detergency

- The HLB requirement for detergency is about 13 – 16.
- Cationic type of detergent are Zephiran (benzyldimethylcetyl ammonium chloride and **Cetrimide** (cetyltrimethyl ammonium chloride)
- **Anionic** type of detergent are Soaps, Sodium lauryl sulphate etc.

## Electrical Properties of Interfaces

- **Nernest potential (Electro thermodynamic potential):** It is defined as the difference in potential between the actual surface and the electro neutral region of the solution.
- **Zeta potential (Electro Kinetic potential):** It is defined as the difference in the potential between the surface of the tightly bound layer (shear plane) and the electro neutral region of the solution.
- If the zeta potential **falls below a particular value**, the attractive forces exceed the repulsive forces and this result in the **aggregation** of particles.
- Zeta potential decrease more rapidly when the concentration of electrolytes is increased or the valency of counter ions is higher.

## Miscellaneous Points to Remember

- **Marasperse** is a deflocculating agent
- When non polar substances are dissolved in a polar solvent using surfactants, the process is called **solubilisation**.
- Ostwald pipette is used to measure **viscosity**
- The munsell system is associated with **colours**.
- The Crocker – Henderson system is used to classify **odours**
- Povan could be classified as **cyaninedye**.
- **Couldpoint**: The temperature above which cloudiness suddenly appears for non-ionic surfactants in solution is known as **Cloudpoint**.
- **Kraftpoint**: The rapid increase in solubility of a surfactant solution above definite temperature is known as **Kraftpoint**.
- **Spreadingcoefficient**: The difference in the work of adhesion and the work o cohesion of liquids ion the surface of other liquid is known as **Spreadingcoefficient**.
- **Micellarsolubilisation**: The phenomenon of increasing the solubility of non-polar drugs by addition of surfactants is known as **Micellarsolubilisation**.
- Stalagometer is used for the measurement of **Surfacetension**.
- At critical temperature the surface tension is **Zero**.
- Electrolytes are added to **decrease** the Zetapotential.
- **Antonlff's rule** is applicable to slightly polar liquids against water.
- The HLB range for lipophilic surfactants is **2 to 9.**
- **Gegenions** mean ion having a charge opposite to the potential determining ions.
- In the thermodynamic treatment of dispersion of hydrophilic solids, **the Gibb's free energy change** and the **entropy change**, respectively, are negative and positive.
- Near critical micelle concentration, micelles of the surfactant molecules assume the shape of spherical.

**Important Equations related to surface and interfacial phenomenon**

| Name | Equation |
|---|---|
| Kelvins equation | $\left(\frac{P}{P^0}\right) = \frac{2yv}{rRT}$ |
| Gibb's equation | $T_2^1 = -RT\frac{dy}{dlna_2}$ |
| Langmuir equation | $\frac{c}{x/m} = \frac{1}{b} + \frac{c}{b}$ (It is used to describe the adsorption from solutions) |
| Freundich equation | I/k = $\left(\frac{DkT}{2ne2z2}\right)^{\frac{1}{2}}$ |
| Debye length | $\frac{x}{m} = Kc^{1/n}$ |
| Vant Hoff | II = CRT |
| Vanderwalls force | F = Ad (Ad / $12x^2$) |

- **Schulze Hardy rule:** It states the strong effect of the valence of electrolyte on the double – layer repulsive force.
- **DLVOR theory:** It is considered only the balance between electrostatic repulsive and Van der walls attractive forces.
- **Gibb's equation:** It states that a solute that concentrates in the interfacial region causes decrease in surface tension as the concentration of the solute is increased.
- **PZC:** Point of Zero change (PZC), which represents the pH at which the net surface charge is zero.
- **Mechanism of crystal growth:** The size distribution of dispersed systems may increase during aging, owing to three principle mechanisms. 1. Ostwald repining 2. Polymorphic transformation 3. Temperature cycling
- **Taub's rule**: The rule is that a polar adsorbent preferentially adsorb's the more polar component of a non-polar solution.

## 1.11 Micromeritics

### Particle Size

- Micromeritics involve the study of small particles and of the order of a few microns size.
- One micrometer (μm) = $10^{-3}$ mm or $10^{-6}$ m.
- One Milimicrometer = One nanometer (nm) = = $10^{-6}$ mm = $10^{-3}$ μm =$10^{-9}$ m.

**Table** Particle size diameter and their specification

| Surface diameter | **Diameter of a sphere having the same surface area as that of the asymmetric particles** |
|---|---|
| **Volume diameter** | Diameter of a sphere having the same volume as that of the asymmetric particles |
| **Projected diameter** | Diameter of a sphere having the same area of the asymmetric particles observed under microscope |
| **Stroke's diameter or equivalent sphere diameter** | Diameter of an equivalent sphere undergoing sedimentation at the same rate as the symmetric particles |
| **Sieve diameter** | Diameter of a sphere that passes through the same sieve aperture as the asymmetric particles |
| **Volume-surface diameter** | Diameter of the sphere having the same volume to surface area ratio as the asymmetric particles |

## Particle shape

The shape factor of a particle can be expressed as the ratio of surface to volume factors.

$$\text{Shape factor} = \frac{a_s}{a_y}$$

- The minimum possible value for shape factor is **6 for a sphere**. If the ratio value **exceed 6**, it is considered as **asymmetric.**

## Powder Characteristics

- If the powder contains particles of one size then it is called **monodisperse.**
- If the powder contains particles of different size then it is called **polyisperse.**
- Arithmetic mean of a powder is defined as the sum of the **particle** sizes divided by the **number** of particles.

$$\text{Volume surface mean diameter } d_{vs} = \frac{\Sigma nd\,3}{\Sigma nd\,2}$$

$$\text{Surface number mean diameter } d_{sn} = \sqrt{\frac{\Sigma nd\,3}{\Sigma n}}$$

**Determination of particle size:** The methods to estimate particle size are

1. Optical microscopy (Particle size of 0.2 – 100 μm can be measured. Particle in suspension, emulsion, aerosol can be determined)
2. Sieving method (Particle size range of 50 – 1500 μm)
3. Sedimentation method (Particle size range of 1 – 200 μm)
4. Conductivity method (Particle size range of 0.5 – 500 μm)

**Powder surface area**

- **Air permeability method** is used to determine **particle surface diameter**. **The Kozeny-Carman equation** is used to determine the surface area by this method.
- The Kozny-Carman equation $V = \frac{A}{\eta S_{w2}} \frac{\Delta Pt}{KI} \frac{\varepsilon}{(1-\varepsilon)^2}$

**Derived properties of powder**

$$\text{True density} = \frac{\text{Weight of powder}}{\text{True volume of powder}}$$

$$\text{Bulk density} = \frac{\text{Mass of powder}}{\text{Bulk volume}}$$

$$\text{Consolidation index} = \frac{\text{Tapped density} - \text{fluff density}}{\text{Tapped density}} \times 100$$

$$\text{Angle of repose } \theta = \tan^{-1}\frac{h}{r}$$

**Relation between angle of repose and powder flow**

| Angle of repose | Flow |
|---|---|
| <25 | Excellent |
| 25 – 30 | Good |
| 30 – 40 | Passable |
| >40 | Very poor |

| % compressibility | Flow ability |
|---|---|
| 5 to 15 | Excellent |
| 12 to 16 | Good |
| 23 to 35 | Poor |
| <40 | Very poor |

### Points to Remember

- **Surface area** of a particle significantly affects the physical, chemical and biological properties of the drug
- Due to the particles in a powder are irregular in shape it is difficult to express the size of particles in a meaningful diameter.
- When cumulative percent frequency on a probability scale is plotted against logarithm of the particle size, 50 percent on the probability scale gives the **geometric mean**.
- **Stoke's diameter** is important in the formulation development of emulsions and suspensions.
- Stoke's law cannot be used, if Reynolds number is **more than 0.2.**
- **Fisher subsieve sizer** is used to determine the surface area of the powder, The surface area is measured based on the change weight of powder when air is passed through the powdered pack
- **When Coulter-counter** apparatus is employed for powder analysis, **dispersion medium** should be in **conducting** stage
- In Coulter-counter, as the particles travel through the orifice, **resistance between the electrodes increases.**
- **High repose angle** of the granules **indicates roughness** of the granule surface.
- The term **'light'** as applied to pharmaceutical powders means: low granule density.
- Porosity of a porous powder is defined as **void volume/ bulk volume.**
- Shear cell method, Hausner ratio method, Carr Index method are used to **measure powder flow properties**
- **Avalanching Behaviour** is associated with Powder flow property.
- Hackle equation is mostly used to describe **compaction of pharmaceutical powder.**
- Hackle equation = In $\left[\frac{1}{1-Dr}\right]$ = **K p +**

## 1.12 Rheology

### Viscosity

**Coefficient of viscosity**

It is defined as the force per unit area required to maintain unit difference in velocity between two parallel layers in the liquid, one centimetre apart.

Kinematic viscosity- It is defined as ratio of viscosity of the dispersion to that of the solvent

Specific viscosity- It is defined as relative increase the viscosity of the dispersion over that of the solvent alone.

Reduced viscosity- It is defined as ratio of specific viscosity to the concentration.

- The units of viscosity is **poise or centipoise**
- The CGS units for poise are **dy.sec/$cm^2$. Or** $g.cm^{-1}.sec^{-1}$
- In SI system, one unit of poise is equal to $\mathbf{0.1Nsm^2}$

- The unit of kinetic viscosity is **stokes** (s)centistokes (cs)
- The unit of Shear stress is **dy/cm$^2$**

## Flow of Liquids

**Newtonian flow:** Simple liquids exhibit Newtonian flow eg: Water, glycerine, Solution or syrup, Chloroform etc.

**Non-Newtonian flow:** The heterogeneous dispersions such as emulsion, suspensions ad semisolids exhibit Non-Newtonian flow.

**Non-Newtonian flow are three types**

1. Plastic flow (Expressed in terms of Bingham equation) $U = \frac{F-f}{G}$

   Where F = Shear stress, f = yield value, G = rate of shear.
2. Pseudo plastic flow: The viscosity of pseudo plastic follow cannot be expressed by a single value.
3. Dilatant flow: This viscosity exhibits where there is high concentration of solids.

**Determination of flow properties**

| Types of flow | Types of viscometer | Example | Equation |
|---|---|---|---|
| Newtonian | Single Point viscometer | Ostwald viscometer | $\eta_1 = \frac{\rho_{1}t_{1}}{\rho_{2}t_{2}}\eta_2$ |
| | | Filling sphere viscometer | $\eta_1 = t(S_b - S_F)B$ |
| Non-Newtonian | Multi point viscometer | Cup and bob viscometer | $\eta = K_v \frac{W}{V}$ |
| | | (Rotational Viscometer) | |
| | | Cone and plate viscometer | $U = C_1 \frac{T-T_1}{V}$ |

- **Brookfield viscometer** is also a **rotational** viscometer. The construction of this instrument is similar to as the Cup and bob viscometer.
- **Plug flow** is not observed in cone and plate viscometer.

## Points to Remember

- Flocculated suspensions exhibit the **plastic flow.**
- Plug flow is NOT related to the **falling sphere viscometer.**
- A corresponding expression in Non-Newtonian fluids (in terms of viscosity) is **apparent.**
- Fluidity is a term associated with Newtonian fluids. An equivalent term in plastic flow fluids is **mobility.**
- -Dilatant flow is characterized as a reverse phenomenon of **pseudo plastic flow.**
- Deflocculated suspension with high concentration of the dispersed solids exhibits the **dilatant** type of flow
- In antithixotropy, the down-curve is frequently positioned to **right side** (with respect to up-curve)
- The pseudo plastic flow behaviour can be explained by **apparent viscosity.**
- Creep testing is applied to analyse the viscoelastic property of **ointment.**
- The system that undergoes gel-to-sol transformation is known as **shear thinning.**
- The type of viscosity specified in I.P. (Ostwald viscometer) is **kinematic viscosity.**
- After giving the I.M. injection of procaine penicillin G, the process of forming a depot in the muscle is due to **rapid thixotropic recovery.**

- Plug flow is NOT observed in cone and plate viscometer. The reason is **shear can be maintained uniformly.**
- Poiseuille's equation $\eta = \frac{\Delta P \pi 4}{8LQ}$

## 1.13 Colloids

**Kraft Point:** It is defined as the temperature at which solubility of the surfactant is equal to cmc.

**DLVO theory:** According to this theory, the distance between two dispersed particles mainly influences Particle-particle interactions.

**Gold number:** It is defined as the minimum weight in milligrams of a protective colloid (dry weight or dispersed phase) required to prevent t a color change from red to violet in 10ml of gold solution on addition of 1ml of 10% solution of sodium chloride. Basically gold solution is a hydrophobic colloid and has a red color. When at electrolyte like sodium chloride is added. Coagulation of colloids is observed indicating the violet color. When protective colloid is observed indicating the violet color. When protective colloid is added these stabilize the gold solution and prevent the change to violet color. Lower the gold number, greater the protective action.

**Lyophilic colloid:** Dispersed phase consists of large organic molecules.

Dispersions are stable in the presence of electrolytes.

**Amphiphilic colloids:** Dispersed phase consists of aggregates of small organic molecules

**Lyophobic colloid:** Unstable in the presence of small concentration of electrolytes

| Protective colloid | Gold number | Products | Particle size |
|---|---|---|---|
| Gelation | 0.005 to 0.01 | Molecular dispersion | a. Less than 1.0 nm |
| Albumin | 0.1 | Colloidal dispersion | b. 0.5 µm to 1.0 nm |
| Acacia | 0.1 to 0.2 | coarse dispersion | c. more than 0.5 µm |
| Tragacanth | 2 | | |

## Some Essential Chart of Physical Pharmacy

| Mineral | Structural type |
|---|---|
| Kaolinite | Layer lattice non-expanding |
| Mont morillonite | Layer lattice expanding |
| Analcite | Zeolite open network lattice |
| Synthetic permutite | Amorphous alumina silicate gel |

| Material | Flowability |
|---|---|
| Celutab | Excellent |
| Star X-1500 | Fair passable |
| Maize starch | Poor |
| Dicalcium-Phosphate dehydrate (fine) | Very Poor |
| Titanium dioxide | Very Poor |

| Temperature | Degree centigrade |
|---|---|
| Cool | $8^0$ to $15^0$c |
| Cold | $2^0$ to $8^0$c |
| Warm | $30^0$ to $40^0$c |
| Room temperature | does not exceed $25^0$ c |
| Excessive heat | above $40^0$c |

| Character | Humidity |
|---|---|
| Non-hydroscopic | No increase of humidity |
| Slightly hydroscopic | The increase of relative humidity but less than 40% |
| Moderately hydroscopic | Moisture increase may occur less than 50% |
| Very hydroscopic | Moisture increase at relative humidity's as low as 50% |

# Pharmaceutics MCQs

1. Humectants added in cosmetic preparations generally act by
   (a) Hydrogen bond formation
   (b) Covalent bond formation
   (c) Complex formation
   (d) The action of London forces
2. In the mixing of thymol and menthol the following type of incompatibility occurs:
   (a) Chemical incompatibility
   (b) Therapeutic incompatibility
   (c) Physical incompatibility
   (d) Tolerance incompatibility
3. Bloom strength is used to check the quality of
   (a) Lactose (b) Ampoules
   (c) Hardness of tablets (d) Gelatin
4. The characteristic of non-linear pharmaco-kinetics include:
   (a) Area under the curve is proportional to the dose
   (b) Elimination half-life remains constant,
   (c) Area under the curve is not proportional to the dose
   (d) Amount of drug excreted through remains constant
5. Thioglycolic acid-like compounds have applications in following type of cosmetic formulations :
   (a) Depilatory preparations
   (b) Epilatory preparations
   (c) Vanishing creams
   (d) Skin tan preparations
6. Which one of the following is a flocculating agent for a negatively charged drug?
   (a) Aluminium chloride
   (b) Bentonite
   (c) Tragacanth
   (d) Sodium biphosphate
7. The healing agent used in hand creams is
   (a) Soft paraffin (b) Urea
   (c) bees wax (d) Stearyl alcohol
8. Which one of the following is the commonly used bulking agent in the formulation of freeze dried low dose drug products?
   (a) Sodium chloride (b) Mannitol
   (c) Starch (d) HPMC
9. The applicability of Noyes-Whitney equation is to describe
   (a) First order kinetics
   (b) Zero order kinetics
   (c) Mixed order kinetics
   (d) Dissolution rate
10. Which filler can NOT be used for the preparation of tablets for amine containing basic drugs to avoid discoloration of the tablets?
    (a) Dicalcium phosphate
    (b) Microcrystalline cellulose
    (c) Starch Lactose
11. What quantities of 95 % v/v and 45 % v/v alcohols are to be mixed to make 800 mL of 65 % v/v alcohol?
    (a) 480 mL of 95 % and 320 mL of 45 % alcohol
    (b) 320 mL of 95 % and 480 mL of 45 % alcohol
    (c) 440 mL of 95 % and 360 mL of 45 % alcohol
    (d) 360 mL of 95 % and 440 mL of 45 % alcohol

12. The role of borax in cold creams is
    (a) Anti-microbial agent
    (b) To provide fine particles to polish skin
    (c) *In-situ* emulsifier
    (d) Antioxidant
13. Drugs following one compartment open model pharmacokinetics eliminate
    (a) Bi-exponentially
    (b) Tri-exponentially
    (c) Non-exponentially
    (d) Mono-exponentially
14. Drugs in suspensions and semi-solid formulations always degrade by
    (a) First order kinetics
    (b) Second order kinetics
    (c) Zero order kinetics
    (d) Non-linear kinetics
15. In nail polish, following polymer is used as a film-former:
    (a) Nitrocellulose
    (b) Polylactic acid
    (c) Hydroxypropyl methylcellulose
    (d) Cellulose acetate phthalate
16. A drug (200 mg dose) administered in tablet form and as intravenous injection (50 mg dose) showed AUG of 100 and 200 microgram hr/mL, respectively. The absolute availability of the drug through oral administration is:
    (a) 125% (b) 250 %
    (c) 12.5% (d) 1.25%
17. How many mL of a 1:500 w/v stock solution should be used to make 5 liters of 1:2000 w/v solution?
    (a) 750 mL (b) 1000 mL
    (c) 1250 mL (d) 1500 mL
18. The Volume of distribution of a drug administered at a dose of 300 mg and exhibiting 30 microgram/mL instantaneous concentration in plasma shall be
    (a) 10 L (b) 100 L
    (c) 1.0 L (d) 0.10 L
19. It is required to maintain a therapeutic concentration of 10 microgram/mL for 12 hours of a drug having half life of 1.386 hr and Vd of 5 L. The dose required in a sustained release product will be
    (a) 600 mg (b) 300 mg
    (c) 30 mg (d) 60 mg
20. In which of the following techniques the sample is kept below triple point?
    (a) Lyophilization (b) Spray drying
    (c) Spray congealing (d) Centrifugation
21. Which of the following is not a semisolid dosage form
    (a) Paste (b) Creams
    (c) Ointments (d) Suspensions
22. Generally pastes contain
    (a) High percentage of insoluble solids
    (b) Low percentage of insoluble solids
    (c) Both
    (d) None
23. Most widely used hydrocarbon in semi-solid dosage forms
    (a) Petrolatum (b) Mineral oil
    (c) Both (d) None
24. Which of the following hydrocarbon waxes are employed in the manufacture of creams and ointments?
    (a) Paraffin wax (b) Ceresin
    (c) Both (d) None
25. Which of the following is not a vegetable oil
    (a) Peanut oil (b) Almond oil
    (c) Olive oil (d) Petrolatum
26. Which of the following fatty acid used in water removable creams as emulsifier
    (a) Stearic acid (b) Palmitic acid
    (c) Both (d) None
27. Combination of a surfactant with oilsoluble auxiliary emulsifier is known as
    (a) Simple emulsifier system
    (b) Mixed emulsifier system
    (c) Both
    (d) None

28. Promulgen means
    (a) Anionic emulsifiers composed of fatty alcohols & their ethoxylates
    (b) Non-ionic emulsifiers com-posed of fatty alcohols & their ethoxylates
    (c) Cationic emulsifiers composed of fatty alcohols & their ethoxylates
    (d) All the above

29. Promulgen D contains
    (a) Cetyl alcohol & Ceteareth-20
    (b) Stearyl alcohol & Ceteareth-20
    (c) Both
    (d) None

30. Promulgen G contains
    (a) Cetyl alcohol & Ceteareth-20
    (b) Stearyl alcohol & Ceteareth-20
    (c) Both
    (d) None

31. With promulgen D, which type of emulsion generally obtained?
    (a) Liquid emulsion
    (b) Thick consistency emulsion
    (c) Both
    (d) None

32. With promulgen G, which type of emulsion generally obtained?
    (a) Liquid emulsion
    (b) Thick consistency emulsion
    (c) Both
    (d) None

33. Which of the following polyols used as humectants in creams
    (a) Glycerine (b) Propylene glycol
    (c) Sorbitol 70% (d) All the above

34. The choice of humectants is based on
    (a) Rate of moisture exchange
    (b) Viscosity and texture of preparation
    (c) Both
    (d) None

35. Which of the following is more hygroscopic at low concentration?
    (a) Sorbitol 70% (b) Glycerine
    (c) Both (d) None

36. Due to which factors, petrolatum is most widely used as a hydrocarbon basic in ointments
    (a) Its consistency
    (b) Its neutral characteristics
    (c) Its ability to spread easily on the skin
    (d) All

37. Water number means
    (a) Maximum amount of water that can be added to 100 g of a base at given temperature
    (b) Maximum amount of water that can be added to 10 g of a base at given temperature
    (c) Maximum amount of water that can be added to 5 g of a base at given temperature
    (d) All

38. Lanolin is which type of base
    (a) Hydrocarbon base (b) Absorption base
    (c) Both (d) None

39. In the preparation of vanishing creams, which types of bases are used generally?
    (a) Absorption bases
    (b) Water removable bases
    (c) Hydrocarbon bases
    (d) None

40. In the preparation of cold creams, which types of bases are used generally?
    (a) Absorption bases
    (b) Water removable bases
    (c) Hydrocarbon bases
    (d) None

41. Water soluble bases are also known as
    (a) Greasy ointment bases
    (b) Greaseless ointment bases
    (c) Both
    (d) None

42. In pastes, the concentration of insoluble powder substances in
    (a) 20%-50% (b) 50%-100%
    (c) 50%-75% (d) None

43. Jellies are generally
    (a) Water-soluble bases
    (b) Water-insoluble bases
    (c) Both
    (d) None

44. As per USP XX, the term "objectionable" means
    (a) An organism can cause disease or the presence may interrupt the function of the drug or lead to deterioration of the product
    (b) Pathogens if they produce disease or infection, in the newborn or debilitated persons
    (c) Organisms or their toxins that is responsible for human disease or infection
    (d) None

45. The success or failure of a preservative in protecting a formulation against microbial spoilage depends on
    (a) Interaction between preservative with surfactant
    (b) Interaction between preservative with active substances
    (c) Sorption by packaging materials
    (d) All the above

46. A suppository is generally intended for use in
    (a) Rectum (b) Vagina
    (c) Urethra (d) All the above

47. Vaginal suppositories also called as
    (a) Pessaries
    (b) Simple suppositories
    (c) Bougies
    (d) None

48. "Oleum theobromae" was first recommended by
    (e) Taylor (b) Griffin
    (c) Stocks's (d) None

49. Weight of rectal suppository for adults is
    (a) 1 g (b) 2 g
    (c) 5 g (d) None

50. Weight of rectal suppository for children is
    (a) 1 g (b) 2 g
    (c) 5 g (d) None

51. Urethral suppositories also called as
    (a) Pessaries (b) Bougies
    (c) Both (d) None

52. Urethral suppositories having which shape
    (a) Oviform shape (b) Torpedo shape
    (c) Pencil shape (d) None

53. Weight of urethral suppository for males & females respectively
    (a) 4 & 2 (b) 2 & 4
    (c) 4 & 6 (d) 6 & 4

54. Shape of vaginal suppositories is
    (a) Oviform shape (b) Torpedo shape
    (c) Pencil shape (d) None

55. Rectal suppositories mainly used for the treatment of
    (a) Constipation (b) Hemorrhoids
    (c) Both (d) None

56. The number of milligrams of KOH required neutralizing free acids & saponify the esters contained in 1 g of fat is known as
    (a) Iodine value
    (b) Saponification value
    (c) Water number
    (d) Acid value

57. The number of grams of iodine that reacts with 100 g of fat is known as
    (a) Iodine value
    (b) Saponification value
    (c) Water number
    (d) Acid value

58. The number of milligrams of KOH required neutralizing free acids in 1 g of fat is known as
    (a) Iodine value
    (b) Saponification value
    (c) Hydroxil value
    (d) None

59. The number of milligrams of KOH required neutralize the acetic acid used to acetylate 1 g of fat is known as
    (a) Iodine value
    (b) Saponification value
    (c) Hydroxil value
    (d) Acid value

60. Which of the following method is used to manufacture suppositories
(a) Hand molding
(b) Compression molding
(c) Pour molding
(d) All the above

61. Which of the following is most commonly used suppository base
(a) Cocoa butter (b) PEG 1000
(c) PEG + Hexanetriol (d) None

62. Cocoa butter available in following forms
(a) α-form (b) β-form
(c) γ-form (d) All

63. The solidification point of cocoa butter lies between
(a) 12 – 13o (b) 20 – 30o
(c) 5 – 10o (d) None

64. Which of the following method is simple & oldest method of preparation of suppositories?
(a) Hand molding
(b) Compression molding
(c) Pour molding
(d) All the above

65. Most commonly used method for producing suppositories on both a small & large scale is
(a) Hand molding
(b) Compression molding
(c) Pour molding
(d) All the above

66. Which formula can be used to calculate the amount of base that is replaced by active ingredients?
(a) f = 100 (G – E) +1(G) (X)
(b) f = 100 (E – G) +100 (G) (X)
(c) f = 100 (E – G) +1 (G) (X)
(d) f = 100 (E – G) +10 (G) (X)

67. Rancidity generally results from
(a) Auto oxidation
(b) Decomposition of unsaturated fats
(c) Both
(d) None

68. Which of the following is not antioxidant
(a) BHT (b) BHA
(c) Tocopherol (d) Theobroma oil

69. Suppositories are generally evaluated by
(a) Melting range test (b) Breaking test
(c) Liquefaction (d) All the above

70. 3. Major 1. Which of the following materials are used in pharmaceutical packaging?
(a) Glass (b) Plastic
(c) Metal (d) All the above

71. Which of the following packaging material is protect the drug content against light
(a) Plastic containers
(b) Amber colored glass containers
(c) Both
(d) None

72. disadvantages of glass as a packing material are
(a) Fragility (b) Weight
(c) Both (d) None

73. Composition of glass is
(a) Sand
(b) Soda ash
(c) Lime stone & Cullet
(d) All the above

74. Soda ash also known as
(a) Pure silica
(b) Sodium carbonate
(c) Lime stone
(d) Calcium carbonate

75. Which of the following one is a broken glass & acts as fusion agent
(a) Cullet (b) Soda ash
(c) Lime stone (d) Sand

76. Which of the following methods are used in the production of glass
(a) Blowing (b) Drawing
(c) Pressing & casting (d) All the above

77. To produce molten glass, which of the following method is used
(a) Blowing (b) Drawing
(c) Pressing (d) Casting

78. To protect the contents of a bottle from the effects of sunlight by UV rays, which glass is used?
    (a) Amber glass (b) Red glass
    (c) Both (d) None
79. To evaluate the chemical resistance of glass, which of the following tests are conducted?
    (a) Powder glass (b) Water attack test
    (c) Both (d) None
80. Which of the following test is performed on crushed grains, to evaluate the chemical resistance of glass?
    (a) Powder glass (b) Water attack test
    (c) Both (d) None
81. Which of the following test is performed on whole container?
    (a) Powder glass (b) Water attack test
    (c) Both (d) None
82. Type I glass is also known as
    (a) Borosilicate glass
    (b) Regular soda-lime glass
    (c) Treated soda-lime glass
    (d) None
83. The advantages of plastic containers over glass containers are
    (a) Easy formation
    (b) Resistance to breakage
    (c) Freedom of design
    (d) All the above
84. Plastic containers are generally made from the following material
    (a) Polyethylene (b) Polypropylene
    (c) Polystyrene (d) All the above
85. Which of the following ingredients are present in rubber stopper?
    (a) Vulcanizing agent (b) Softner
    (c) Antioxidant (d) All the above
86. Which of the following packaging systems are identified by the FDA?
    (a) Blister pack (b) Strip pack
    (c) Bubble pack (d) All the above
87. Which of the following packaging is commonly used for packaging of tablets & capsules?
    (a) Blister pack (b) Strip pack
    (c) Both (d) None
88. Which of the following materials offer moisture barrier properties?
    (a) Aclar (b) Cellophane
    (c) Polyester (d) All the above
89. Which of the following mechanism is responsible for release of encapsulated core materials?
    (a) By disrupting the coating by pressure
    (b) By offering permeability facilities
    (c) By leaching of permanent fluid
    (d) All the above
90. Pre - formulation studies mainly focus on
    (a) Physical properties of new compound
    (b) Chemical properties of new compound
    (c) Physico-chemical properties of new compound
    (d) None
91. Which of the following information is helpful in designing the preformulation evaluation of a new drug?
    (a) Structure of a compound
    (b) Formula & molecular weight of a compound
    (c) Therapeutic indication of a new compound
    (d) All the above
92. Which of the following problems commonly encountered in evaluating salt forms are
    (a) Poor crystallinity (b) Hygroscopicity
    (c) Instability (d) All the above
93. Which of the following salts generally used in pharmaceutical products?
    (a) Acetate (b) Gluconate
    (c) Lactate (d) All the above
94. Description of the outer appearance of a crystal is known as
    (a) Crystal habit (b) Internal structure
    (c) Both (d) None

95. Which of the following techniques used to prepare amorphous forms?
   (a) Rapid precipitation (b) Lyophilization
   (c) Rapid cooling (d) All the above

96. Amorphous forms generally having
   (a) Low thermodynamic energy & low solubility
   (b) High thermodynamic energy & high solubility
   (c) Both
   (d) None

97. Which of the following compound possess high aqueous solubility's?
   (a) Hydrates (b) Anhydrates
   (b) Both (d) None

98. Which of the following properties may change with changing of the internal structure of a solid?
   (a) Melting point (b) Density
   (b) Optical properties (d) All the above

99. Which of the following methods generally used for studying solid forms?
   (a) DSC (b) XRD
   (b) TGA (d) All the above

100. Which of the following methods generally used to measure heat loss or gain within a sample?
   (a) DSC (b) DTA
   (b) Both (d) None

101. Which of the following co-solvent can be used to increase the solubility of poor soluble drugs?
   (a) Ethanol (b) Propylene glycol
   (b) Glycerin (d) All the above

102. Partition co-efficient generally measures
   (a) Drug's lipophilicity
   (b) Ability of drug to cross cell membrane
   (c) Both
   (d) None

103. Dissolution of a drug particle is described by
   (a) Noyes-Whitney equation
   (b) Stock's equation
   (c) Drag's equation
   (d) None

104. The effect of temperature on drug stability can be described by
   (a) Noyes-Whitney equation
   (b) Stock's equation
   (c) Arheneous equation
   (d) None

105. Unequal distribution of color on a tablet, refers to
   (a) Picking (b) Mottling
   (c) Capping (d) Sticking

106. Match the following and find out the correct combination
   1. Capping
      (P) Separation of a tablet into 2 or more layers
   2. Lamination
      (Q) Unequal distribution of color on a tablet
   3. Mottling
      (R) Separation of top/bottom crowns of a tablet from the main body
   4. Sticking
      (S) Adherence of tablet material to the die wall
   (a) 2-P, 3-Q, 1-R, 4-S
   (b) 1-P, 2-Q, 3-R, 4-S
   (c) 3-P, 1-Q, 2-R, 4-S
   (d) 4-P, 1-Q, 3-R, 2-S

107. Which of the following one is responsible for sticking?
   (a) Excessive moisture (b) Low moisture
   (c) Both (d) None

108. Which of the following mixer is a first high shear powder blender/mixer
   (a) Diosna mixer
   (b) Littleford lodige mixer
   (c) Plow mixer
   (d) Gral mixer

109. If the dose of a drug is inadequate, then it generally requires the following one, to make up its bulk
   (a) Binders (b) Disintegrants
   (c) Lubricants (d) Diluents

110. The first and most widely used diluents in tablet formulation is
(a) Dextrose (b) Lactose
(c) MCC (d) Starch

111. Anhydrous lactose has the advantage over hydrous lactose
(a) Improved flow
(b) Absence of millard reaction
(c) Improved compressibility
(d) High microbial load

112. Which of the following is not a commercially available starch product?
(a) Sta-Rx 1500 (b) Celutab
(c) Emdex (d) Sugar tab

113. Which of the following is a synthetic adhesive?
(d) PVP (b) MC
(c) HPMC (d) HPC

114. Which of the following is a water soluble lubricant?
(a) Stearic acid
(b) Mineral oil
(c) PEG
(d) Magnesium stearate

115. Find out the correct statements regarding a sweetener, saccharin
(P) It is 500 times sweeter than sucrose, but it is carcinogenic
(Q) It is 500 times sweeter than sucrose, but it has bitter taste
(R) It is sweeter than sucrose, but it is safe
(S) It is sweeter than sucrose, but it is unstable
(a) P, S (b) P, R
(c) P, Q (d) R, S

116. Aerosil is used as
(a) Glidant (b) Lubricant
(c) Antiadherant (d) None

117. What is the pH of duodenum?
(a) 2-3 (b) 7-8
(c) 4-6 (d) 10

118. Tablets, which are placed between cheek and teeth, are known as
(a) Buccal (b) Sublingual
(c) Lozenges (d) Troches

119. Which statement is not correct?
(a) Buccal routes avoids first pass metabolism
(b) Parenteral route avoids first pass metabolism
(c) Sublingual route avoids first pass metabolism
(d) Oral route avoids first pass metabolism

120. Match the following ingredients according to their purpose in the formulation of tablets and find out the correct set
(i) Glidant (P) Pre- gelatinized starch
(ii) Diluent (Q) Pyramine
(iii) Adherent (R) Colloidal silica
(iv) Disintegrant (S) Calcium sulphate
(v) (T) Sodium alginate
(a) 1-R, 2-S, 3-P, 4-T
(b) 1-S, 2-R, 3-Q, 4-P
(c) 1-R, 2-S, 3-T, 4-Q
(d) 1-Q, 2-T, 3-R, 4-P

121. Enteric coating is achieved by using
(a) HPMC (b) CMC
(c) CAP (d) Povidine

122. The disintegration time for sugar coated tablets is
(a) 30 minutes (b) 45 minutes
(c) 60 minutes (d) 75 minutes

123. Flow rate of granules from the hopper can be improved by adding
(a) Disintegrant (b) Glidant
(c) Binder (d) Lubricant

124. Given below are equipment used in the manufacture of following products PT. Match them and find out correct answer
(i) Zenasi (P) Tablet granules
(ii) Hepa filter (Q) Tablet coating
(iii) Chilsonator (R) Emulsion
(iv) Accela cota (S) Injectables
(v) (T) Capsule
(a) 1-T, 2-S, 3-P, 4-Q
(b) 1-P, 2-Q, 3-S, 4-R
(c) 1-T, 2-R, 3-Q, 4-P
(d) 1-S, 2-R, 3-P, 4-Q

125. Match the ingredients according to their purpose in the formulation and find out correct set
   (i) Film coating (P) Sodium benzoate
   (ii) Syrups (Q) Ethyl cellulose
   (iii) Emulsification (R) Eudragit
   (iv) Enteric coating (S) Sucrose
   (v) (T) Sodium oleate
   (a) 1-P, 2-Q, 3-R, 4-S
   (b) 1-R, 2-S, 3-T, 4-Q
   (c) 1-T, 2-P, 3-S, 4-Q
   (d) 1-R, 2-S, 3-Q, 4-T

126. Match the following regions in GIT with the pH levels indicated from P-T and find out correct answer
   (a) Mouth (P) 5-6
   (b) Stomach (Q) 6.8-7.5
   (c) Deodenum (R) 6.8-7
   (d) Large intestine (S) 3-5 (T) 1.5-3
   (a) 1-Q, 2-T, 3-S, 4-R
   (b) 1-P, 2-R, 3-S, 4-T
   (c) 1-S, 2-T, 3-Q, 4-R
   (d) 1-R, 2-S, 3-T, 4-P

127. In sugar coating of tablets, sub- coating is done
   (a) To prevent moisture absorption
   (b) To round the edge & build tablet size
   (c) To smoothen the surface
   (d) To prevent the tablet from breaking due to vibration

128. Some possible causes are mentioned in P-T, for the following defects during the film coating of tablets. Match them
   (a) Chipping (P) Poor spreading during spraying
   (b) Cracking (Q) Over heating during spraying
   (c) Orange peel (R) Higher internal stresses in film
   (d) Blistering (S) Excessive coating process
   (e) (T) Precipitation of polymer due to high temperature/poor solvent
   (a) 1-S, 2-R, 3-P, 4-Q
   (b) 1-T, 2-S, 3-R, 4-P
   (c) 1-P, 2-Q, 3-R, 4-S
   (d) 1-R, 2-P, 3-Q, 4-T

129. Sub coating is given to the tablets
   (a) To increase the bulkiness
   (b) To avoid deterioration due to microbial attack
   (c) To prevent the solubility in acidic medium
   (d) To avoid stickness

130. The following ingredients are commonly used as coating agents for film coating except
   (a) CAP
   (b) Carnauba wax
   (c) HEC
   (d) Sodium CMC

131. The ingredients mentioned in P-S are used in various stages of sugar coating of tablets. Match them and find out correct answer
   (a) Seal coating (P) Gelatin
   (b) Sub coating (Q) Carnauba wax
   (c) Syrup coating (R) PEG 4000
   (d) Polyshing (S) Cane sugar
   (a) 1-S, 2-P, 3-R, 4-Q
   (b) 1-Q, 2-S, 3-R, 4-P
   (c) 1-P, 2-Q, 3-R, 4-S
   (d) 1-R, 2-P, 3-Q, 4-S

132. The courster process can be used to
   (a) Coat tablets
   (b) Determine the disintegration time
   (c) Gas sterilize parenteral solution
   (d) Automatic filling of capsules

133. Which of the following is the first process that must occur before a drug can become available for absorption from a tablet dosage form?
   (a) Dissolution of the drug in GI fluids
   (b) Dissolution of the drug in epithelium
   (c) Ionization of the drug
   (d) Disintegration of the drug

134. Tablets are placed into coating chamber & hot air is introduced through the bottom of the chamber. Coating solution is applied through an atomizing nozzle from the upper end of the chamber. This technique is called
   (a) Sealing before sugar coating
   (b) Coating by air suspension
   (c) Spray-pan coating
   (d) Chamber coating

135. A synthetic sweetening agent which is approximately 200 times sweeter than sucrose & has no taste is
(a) Saccharin (b) Aspartame
(c) Cyclamate (d) Sorbitol

136. Shellac is used the purpose of coating tablets as
(a) Polishing agent
(b) Film coating agent
(c) Enteric coating agent
(d) Sub-coating agent for sugar coating

137. Dose dumping is a problem in the formulation of
(a) Compressed tab
(b) Suppository
(c) Soft gelatin capsules
(d) Controlled release drug products

138. Select the equation that gives the rate of drug dissolution from a tablet
(a) Fick's law
(b) Henderson-Hasselbatch equation
(c) Noyes-Whitney equation
(d) Michelis Menton equation

139. Which of the following substance is used as muco adhesive
(a) Acacia (b) Sodium CMC
(c) Burnt sugar (d) Saccharin

140. In the preparation of multi layer tablets, one of the following is used for hydrophilic matrix coating
(a) Shellac (b) CMC
(c) Stearyl alcohol (d) Bees wax

141. The diameter of the mesh aperture in the I.P. disintegration apparatus is given below. Choose the correct size
(a) 2 mm (b) 4 mm
(c) 1mm (d) 1.50 mm

142. Diclofenac tablet with CAP has been administered to a patient. Where do you expect the drug to be released?
(a) Stomach (b) Oral cavity
(c) Small intestine (d) Liver

143. Which of the following flavour is used in a formulation containing sour taste?
(a) Wild cherry (b) Vanilla
(c) Citrus (d) Chocolate

144. Durability of a tablet to combined effects of shock & abrasion is evaluated by using
(a) Hardness tester
(b) Disintegration test apparatus
(c) Friabilator
(d) Screw guage

145. A retardant material that forms a hydrophilic matrix in the formulation of matrix tablets is
(a) HPMC (b) CAP
(c) Polyethylene (d) Carnauba wax

146. A water soluble substance used as coating material in micro encapsulation process is
(a) Polyethylene (b) Silicone
(c) HEC (d) Paraffin

147. One of the following is used as a pH dependant controlled release excipient
(a) Carnauba wax
(b) HPMCP
(c) MC
(d) Glyceryl mono stearate

148. In the tablet coating process, inadequate spreading of coating solution before drying causes
(a) Orange peel effect (b) Sticking effect
(c) Blistering effect (d) Picking effect

149. Crown thickness of a tablet is measured by
(a) Micrometer (b) Pychnometer
(c) Hydrometer (d) All the above

150. Friabilator is operated at
(a) 100 RPM (b) 75 RPM
(c) 50 RPM (d) 25 RPM

151. Enteric coated tablet disintegrate in……hours in simulated intestinal fluid
(a) 1 (b) 2
(c) 3 (d) 4

152. In dissolution test, flask is maintained at
(a) 37°C ± 0.5°C (b) 41°C ± 1°c
(c) 39°C ± 0.6°C (d) 40°C ± 1°C

153. Capping is prevented by using one of the following punches
(a) Flat (b) Circular
(c) Square (d) Rectangular

154. Plating of punch faces are done by
(a) Chromium (b) Zinc
(c) Iron (d) All

155. Sta-Rx-1500 contains ……% of moisture
(a) 15 (b) 10
(c) 18 (d) 50

156. Acacia trgacanth is used in the concentration of
(a) 10%-25 % (b) 60%-70 %
(c) 40%-50 % (d) 90%

157. Starch on heating hydrolyze into
(a) Glucose
(b) Fructose & Sorbose
(c) Fructose & Mannose
(d) Dextrin & Glucose

158. PH of the small intestine is
(a) 1-2 (b) 3-4
(c) 6 (d) 7-8

159. Aqua coat is a
(a) 30% w/v of ethyl cellulose dispersion
(b) Solution of HPMC
(c) 2% w/v of methyl cellulose dispersion
(d) None

160. Lozenges were originally named as
(a) Capsule (b) ODT
(c) Pastillies (d) Sustained axn tab

161. Implantation tab are NMT……..mm in length
(a) 20 (b) 100
(c) 40 (d) 8

162. Seal coating is done by using
(a) Shellac (b) Acacia
(c) Gelatin (d) None

163. Sub coating is done to
(a) Round the edges
(b) Increase the bulk of tablet
(c) Both a & b
(d) Make water resistant 60. CAP dissolves at PH
(a) Above 6 (b) Below 6
(c) 4 (d) 2

164. Which of the following one is used as opacifier
(a) TiO2 (b) Mgo
(c) Siliactes (d) All of the above

165. Green bone is a source of
(a) Type A Gelatin (b) Type B Gelatin
(c) Both (d) None

166. Empty capsule has moisture content in the range of
(a) 60% (b) 12%-15 %
(c) 50%- 70% (d) 30%

167. Which treatment is used for solubility of gelatin
(a) Heat (b) Formalin
(c) Water (d) Alcohol

168. Which of the following is used to fill powdered dry solid into soft gelatine capsule
(a) Aceo gel (b) Rotobil
(c) Rotosort (d) Rotoweigh

169. Sealing of capsule is achieved by
(a) 100°C (b) 20°C
(c) 37°C-40°C (d) 70°C

170. Moisture content is determined by
(a) Gas Chromatography
(b) K-F Method
(c) Both
(d) None

171. Foam stability is measured by
(a) IR Spectroscopy
(b) UV Spectroscopy
(c) Rotational viscometers
(d) All

172. Particle size is determined by
(a) Gas Chromatography
(b) Cascade impactor
(c) Light scatter decay
(d) Both b & c

173. Chewable tablet contains the following base
(a) Manitol (b) Glucose
(c) Lactose (d) None

174. Which of the following is not added in lozenges?
   (a) Sweetener (b) Binder
   (c) Disintegrant (d) All

175. Enteric coated tablet is disintegrated in
   (a) Stomach (b) Liver
   (c) Intestine (d) Mouth

176. The ability of a substance dissolves in a given solvent system is depends on
   (a) Nature and intensity of the forces present in the solute
   (b) Nature and intensity of the forces present in the solvent
   (c) Interactions between solute and solvent
   (d) All the above

177. Which of the following substances having poor water solubility
   (a) Weak electrolytes
   (b) Non-polar molecules
   (c) Both
   (d) None

178. The solubility of weak electrolytes & non-polar substances can be increased by adding water miscible solvents. This process is known as
   (a) Co-solvency (b) Complexation
   (b) Both (d) None

179. How co-solvents increase the solubility of poorly soluble drugs?
   (a) By reducing the interfacial tension between the predominant aqueous solution and hydrophobic solute
   (b) By reducing the interfacial tension between solute and solvent
   (c) Both
   (d) None

180. Which of the following co – solvents are used to increase the solubility of a drug
   (a) Ethanol (b) Sorbitol
   (c) Glycerin (d) All the above

181. Which of the following co – solvent is accepted as a co – solvent in parenteral products, but its use in oral liquids is limited
   (a) Glycerol formal (b) Glycerol
   (b) Dimethyl acetamide (d) None

182. Due to which factor, dimethyl acetamide is not been used as a co-solvent in oral liquids
   (a) Due to objectionable odor
   (b) Due to objectionable taste
   (c) Both
   (d) None

183. Thiomersal is belongs to which category preservative
   (a) Acidic
   (b) Neutral
   (c) Mercurial
   (d) Quaternary ammonium compounds

184. Which of the following are widely used and excellent preservatives
   (a) Mercurial
   (b) Quaternary ammonium compounds
   (c) Both
   (d) Acidic

185. Benzalkonium chloride is categorized as
   (a) Acidic preservative
   (b) Neutral preservative
   (c) Mercurial preservative
   (d) Quaternary ammonium compounds

186. At which concentration, phenol act as preservative
   (a) 0.2 – 0.5 (b) 0.5 – 0.8
   (c) 0.05 – 0.1 (d) None

187. Which of the following sugar has bitter taste
   (a) Glucose (b) Sucrose
   (b) Saccharine (d) None

188. Which of the following is a synthetic sweetener
   (a) Glucose (b) Sucrose
   (c) Sorbitol (d) Aspartame

189. To increase the viscosity of liquid, which of the following agents are used
   (a) PVP
   (b) Methyl Cellulose
   (c) Sodium Carboxy Methyl Cellulose
   (d) All the above

190. Which of the following agents are used as flavoring agents
   (a) Menthol (b) Chloroform
   (c) Both (d) None

191. Most widely used flavoring agent in food industry
(a) Menthol
(b) Chloroform
(c) Mono sodium glutamate
(d) None

192. Which of the following flavor is not responsible for sour taste
(a) Citrus flavours (b) Liquorice
(c) Raspberry (d) Mint spice

193. The filling method of a pharmaceutical liquid depends on the following factors
(a) Viscosity of the liquid
(b) Surface tension of the liquid
(c) Compatibility with the materials used in the construction of the filling machine
(d) All the above

194. Which of the following methods are generally used in liquid filling
(a) Gravimetric
(b) Volumetric
(c) Constant level method
(d) All the above

195. In the formulation of suspensions, generally which types of drugs are selected?
(a) Hydrophilic (b) Hydrophobi
(c) Both (d) None

196. In the formulation, to facilitate the wetting of insoluble solids, which of the following agents used
(a) Suspending agents (b) lavoring agents
(c) Wetting agents (d) None

197. How surfactants will facilitate or aid wetting of hydrophobic materials in liquid
(a) By decreasing the solid-liquid interfacial tension
(b) By increasing the solid-liquid interfacial tension
(c) Both
(d) None

198. Stoke's equation is expressed as
(a) 2V = 2r (d1 – d2 )g 9η
(b) 2V = 2r (d1 – d2 )g 18η
(c) Both
(d) None

199. The stability of suspensions can be evaluated by
(a) Sedimentation volume
(b) Degree of flocculation
(c) Re-dispersibility
(d) All

200. To identify the emulsion type, which of the following tests are conducted?
(a) Dilution test (b) Dye test
(c) Conductivity test (d) All

201. The temperature at which the inversion occurs depends on emulsifier concentration is known as
(a) Phage temperature
(b) Inversion temperature
(c) Phase inversion temperature
(d) All

202. Which of the following mechanical equipment can be used for emulsification?
(a) Homogenizers
(b) Mechanical stirrers
(c) Ultra sonifiers
(d) All

203. Which of the following is not used as a emulsifying agent?
(a) Surfactant
(b) Hydrophilic colloids
(c) Electrolytes
(d) Finely divided solids

204. HLB system was developed by
(a) Griffin (b) Stock's
(c) Dalla Valle (d) None

205. Gum Arabic is a
(a) Anionic polysaccharide
(b) Cationic polysaccharide
(c) Neutral polysaccharide
(d) None

## Answer Key Pharmaceutics

1. a
2. c
3. d
4. c
5. a
6. a
7. a
8. b
9. d
10. d
11. b
12. a
13. d
14. c
15. a
16. c
17. c
18. a
19. b
20. a
21. d
22. a
23. c
24. c
25. d
26. a
27. b
28. b
29. a
30. b
31. b
32. a
33. d
34. c
35. a
36. d
37. a
38. c
39. b
40. a
41. b
42. a
43. a
44. a
45. d
46. d
47. a
48. a
49. b
50. a
51. b
52. c
53. a
54. a
55. c
56. b
57. a
58. d
59. c
60. d
61. a
62. d
63. a
64. a
65. c
66. c
67. c
68. d
69. d
70. d
71. b
72. c
73. d
74. b
75. a
76. d
77. a
78. c
79. c
80. a
81. b
82. a
83. d
84. d
85. d
86. d
87. b
88. d
89. d
90. c
91. d
92. d
93. d
94. a
95. d
96. b
97. b
98. d
99. d
100. c
101. d
102. c
103. a
104. d
105. b
106. c
107. a
108. b
109. d
110. b
111. b
112. d
113. a
114. c
115. c
116. a
117. c
118. a
119. d
120. a
121. c
122. c
123. b
124. a
125. b
126. a
127. b
128. a
129. d
130. b
131. a
132. a

133. d
134. b
135. b
136. c
137. d
138. c
139. b
140. a
141. a
142. c
143. c
144. c
145. a
146. c
147. d
148. a
149. b
150. a
151. b
152. a
153. a
154. a
155. b
156. a
157. d
158. d
159. b
160. c
161. c
162. a
163. c
164. a
165. a
166. b
167. c
168. b
169. a
170. c
171. b
172. c
173. d
174. a
175. c
176. a
177. c
178. a
179. a
180. d
181. c
182. c
183. c
184. c
185. d
186. a
187. c
188. d
189. d
190. c
191. c
192. d
193. d
194. d
195. b
196. c
197. a
198. b
199. d
200. d
201. c
202. d
203. c
204. a
205. c

# Chapter 2

# Pharmacology and Pharmaceutical Chemistry

## Pharmacology & Pharmaceutical Chemistry Theory

### 2.1 Drugs Acting on Autonomic Nervous System: Introduction

The autonomic nervous system (ANS) functions largely below the level of consciousness and controls visceral functions. The major differences between the somatic and autonomic nervous systems.

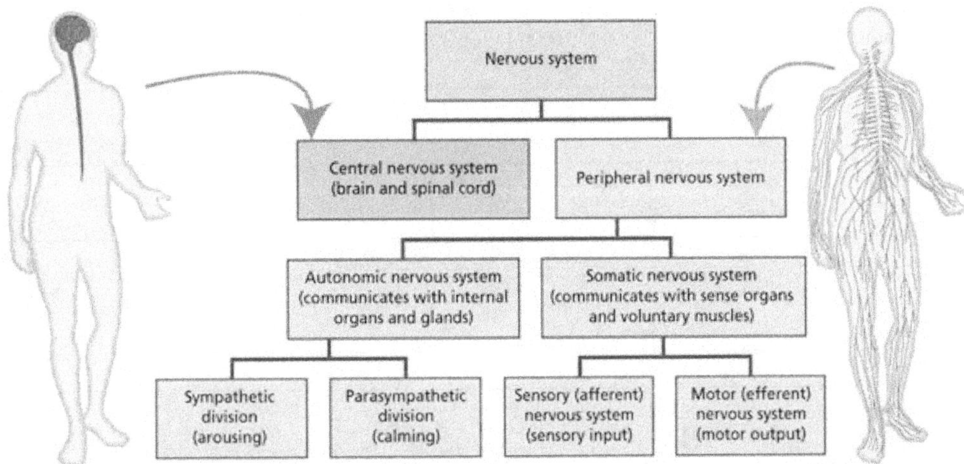


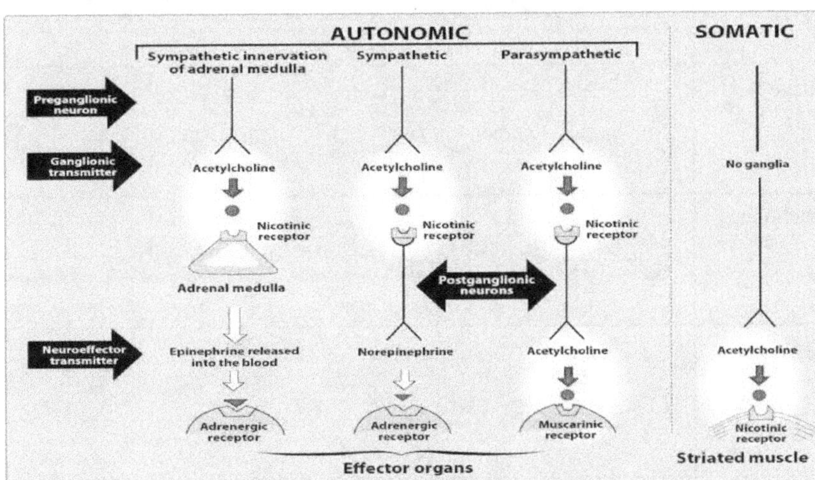

| **Organ and their Sympathetic Effect** | | | | |
|---|---|---|---|---|
| Organs | Sympathetic effect | Adrenergic Receptors | Parasympathetic effect | Cholinergic Receptors |
| Heart | ↑ Rate and force of contraction | β1 | ↓ Rate and force of contraction | M2 |
| Blood vessels | Arterioles: Constriction<br>Veins: Dilatation | α | No effect | - |
| Bronchi smooth Muscle | Dilatation | β2 | Constriction | M3 |
| Glands | No effect | - | Secretions | M3 |
| GI Tract : | ↓ Motility | α1, α2, β2 | ↑ Motility | M3 |
| Spincters | Constriction | α2, β2 | Dilatation | M3 |
| Gastric acid secretion | No effect | - | Secretions | M1 |
| Uterus | Pregnant - Constriction<br>Non-pregnant - Relaxation | α<br>β2 | - | - |
| Male sex Organ | Ejaculation | α | Erection | M3 |
| Eye | Pupil - Dilatation | α | Constriction | M3 |
| Sweat Glands | Secretion - Choinergic Transmission | α | - | - |
| Salivery Glands | Secretion | α, β | Secretion | M3 |
| Lacrimal glands | - | - | Secretion | M3 |
| Kidney | Renin Secretion | β2 | No effect | - |
| Liver | Glycogenolysis<br>Gluconeogenesis | α, β2 | No effect | - |

| | |
|---|---|
| Acetylcholine | 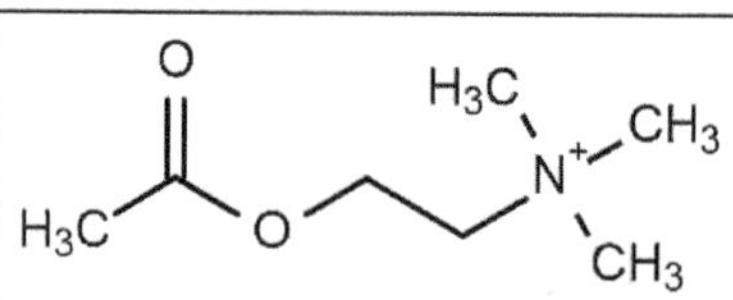 |
| Carbachol | 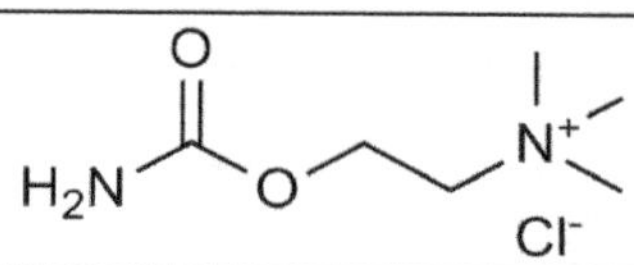 |
| Methacholine | 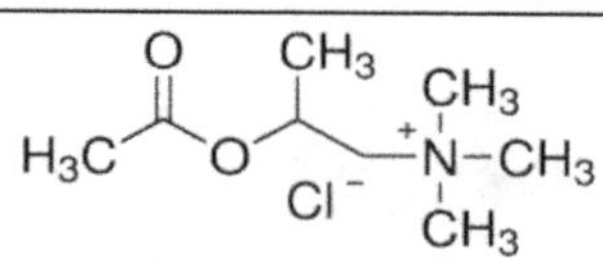 |
| Pilocarpine | 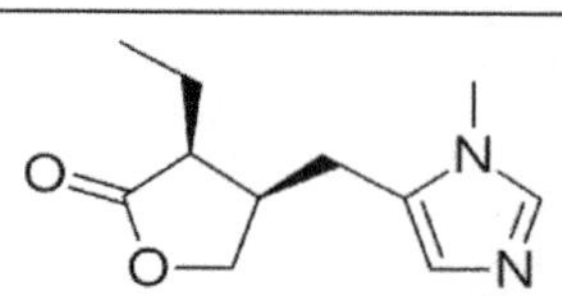 |

**Table** *Contd...*

| | |
|---|---|
| Physostigmine | 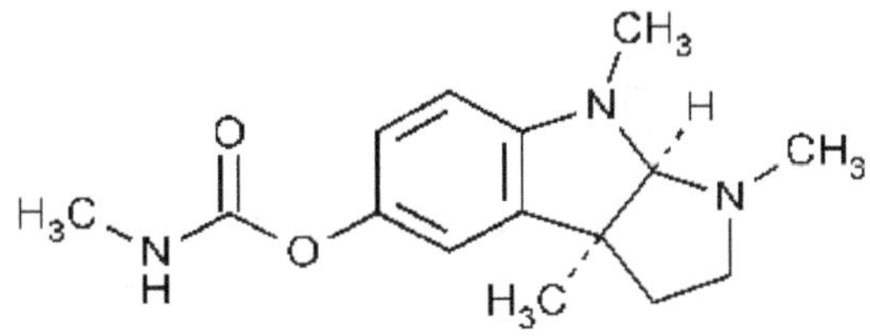 |
| Neostigmine | 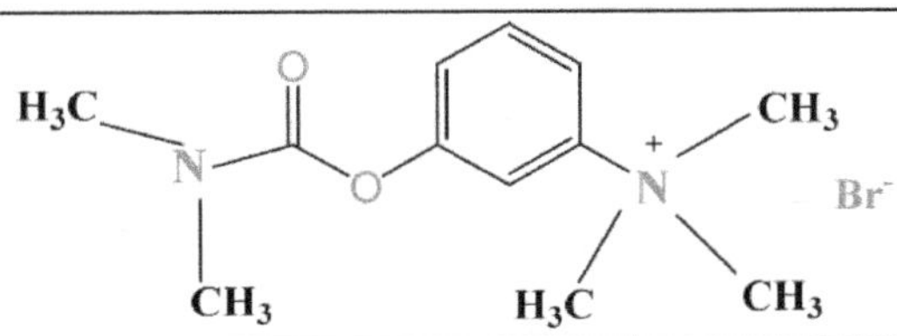 |
| Tacrine | 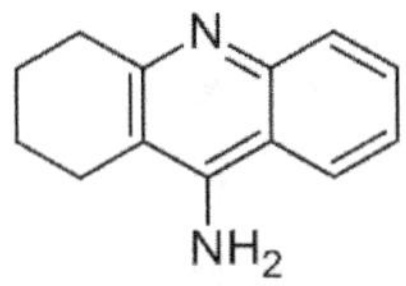 |
| Malathion | 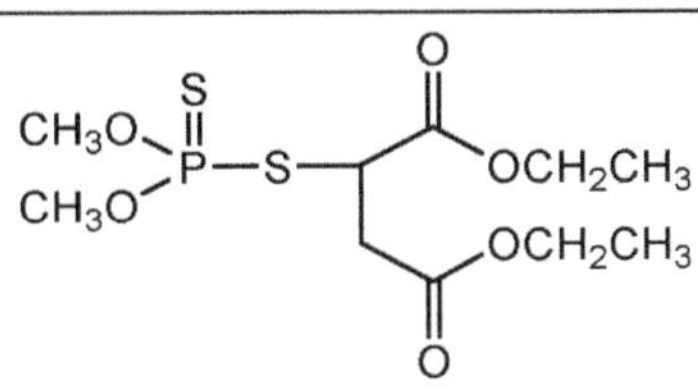 |
| Diazinon | 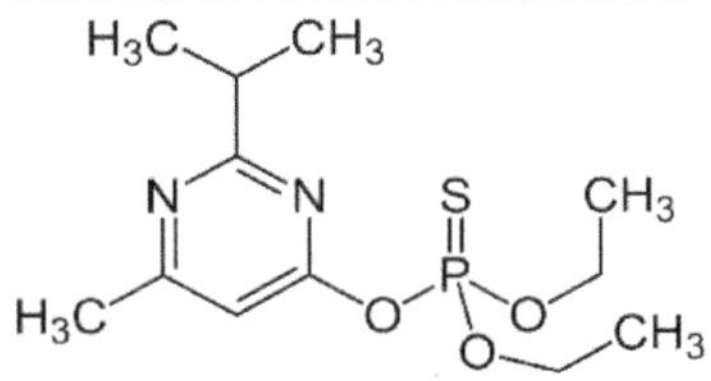 |

**ANTICHOLINERGIC DRUGS**
**(Muscarinic antagonists, Atropinic drugs, Parasympatholytics)**

- **Natural alkaloids**
  - Atropine
  - Hyoscine (Scopolamine)
- **Semisynthetic derivatives**
  - Atropine methonitrate
  - Homatropine
  - Hyoscine butyl bromide
  - Ipratropium bromide
  - Tiotropium bromide
- **Synthetic compounds**
  - **Mydriatics**
    - Cyclopentolate
    - Tropicamide
  - **Vasicoselective**
    - Oxybutynin
    - Flavoxate
    - Tolterodine
  - **Antiparkinsonian**
    - Trihexyphenidyl (Benzhexol)
    - Procyclidine
    - Biperiden
  - **Antisecretory-antispasmodics**
    - **Quaternary comps.**
      - Propantheline
      - Oxyphenonium
      - Clidinium
      - Pipenzolate methyl bromide
      - Isopropamide
      - Glycopyrrolate
    - **Tertiary amines**
      - Dicyclomine
      - Valethamate
      - Pirenzepine

| | |
|---|---|
| Atropine | 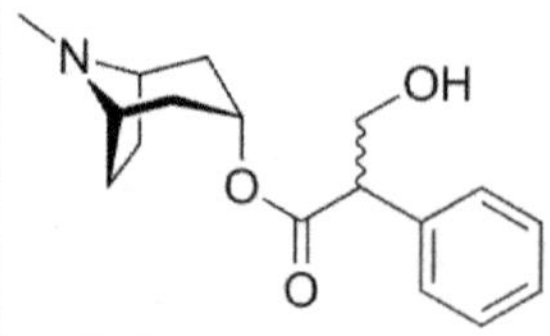 |
| Hyoscine | 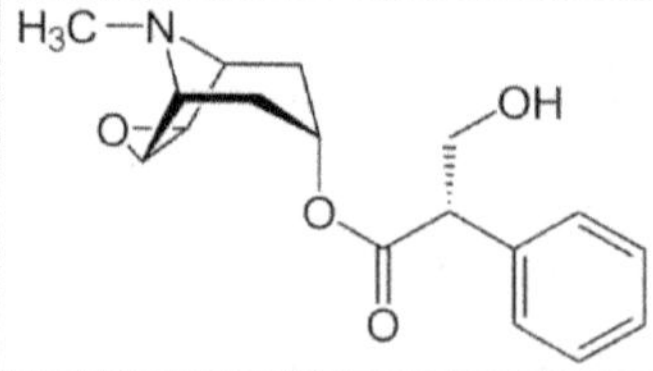 |
| Atropin Methonitrate | 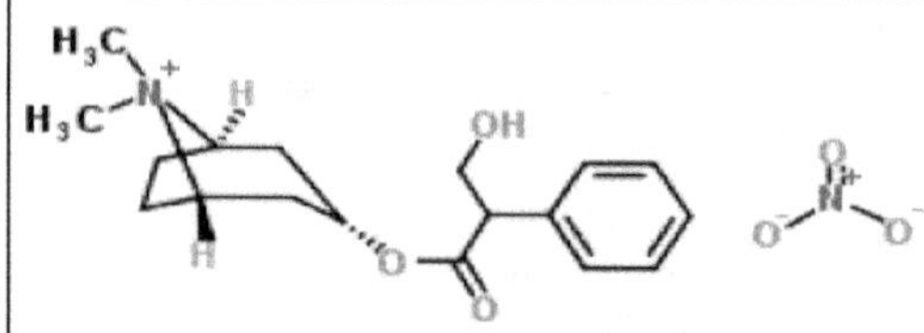 |
| Clidinium | 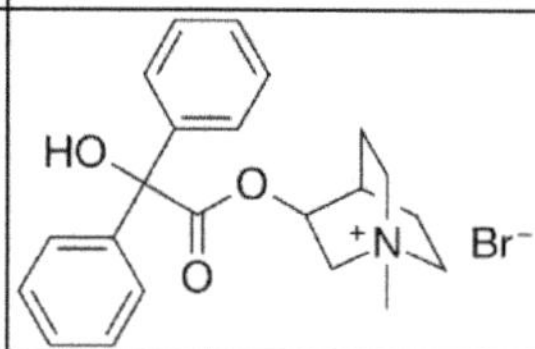 |
| Pirenzepine | 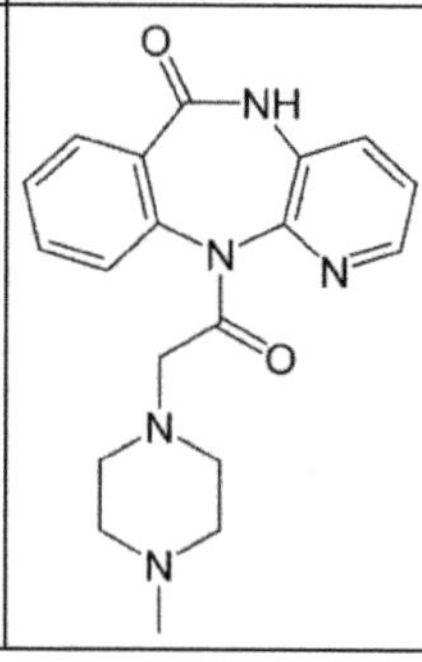 |

**GANGLIONIC STIMULANTS**

- **Selective nicotinic agonists**
  - Nicotine (small dose)
  - Lobeline
  - Dimethyl phenyl piperazinium (DMPP)
  - Tetramethyl ammonium (TMA)
  - Varenicline
- **Nonselective/muscarinic agonists**
  - Acetylcholine
  - Carbachol
  - Pilocarpine
  - Anticholinesterases
  - MCN 343-A

**GANGLIONIC BLOCKING AGENTS**

- **Competitive blockers**
  - **Quaternary ammonium comps.**
    - Hexamethonium
    - Pentolinium
  - **Amines**
    - Mecamylamine
    - Pempidine
  - **Monosulfonium comp.**
    - Trimethaphan-camforsulfonate
- **Persistent depolarizing blockers**
  - Nicotine (large dose)
  - Anticholinesterases (large dose)

| | |
|---|---|
| Nicotine | 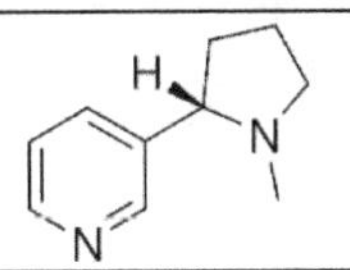 |
| Dimethyl phenyl piperazinium | 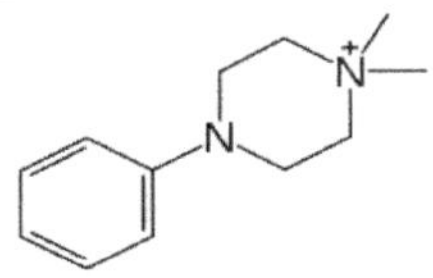 |
| Tetramethylammonium | 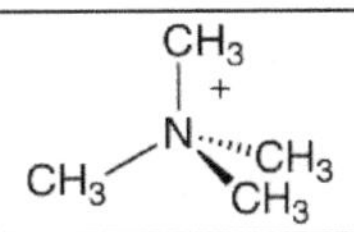 |
| Varenicline | 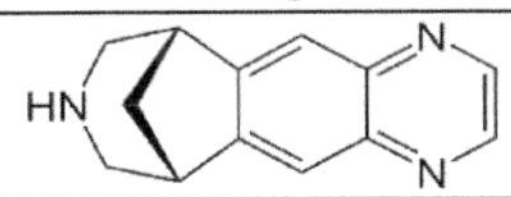 |
| Carbachol | 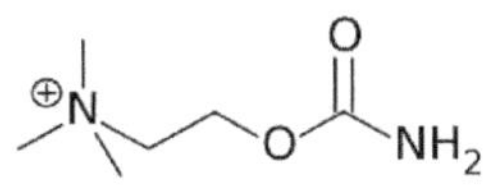 |
| Pilocarpine | 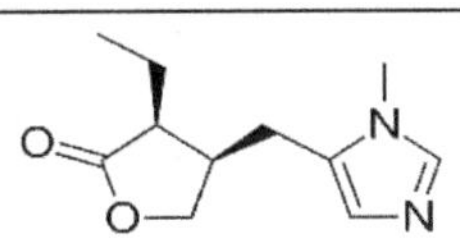 |
| Pentolinium | 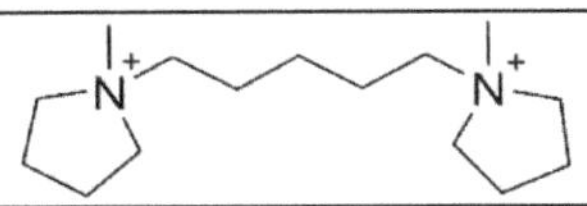 |
| Pempidine | 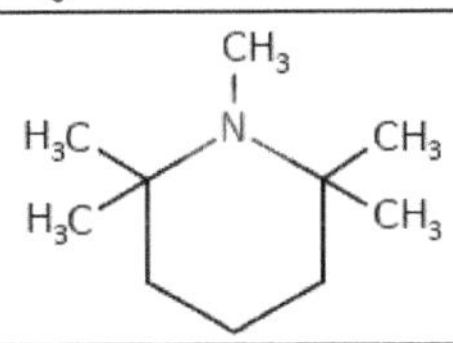 |

## ADRENERGIC DRUGS (Sympathomimetics)

**Pressor agents**
- Noradrenaline (Norepinephrine)
- Ephedrine
- Dopamine
- Phenylephrine
- Methoxamine
- Mephentermine

**Bronchodilators**
- Isoprenaline
- Salbutamol (Albuterol)
- Terbutaline
- Salmeterol
- Formoterol
- Bambuterol

**CNS stimulants**
- Amphetamine
- Dexamphetamine
- Methamphetamine
- Methylphenidate

**Uterine relaxants**
- Ritodrine
- Isoxsuprine
- Salbutamol
- Terbutaline

**Cardiac stimulants**
- Adrenaline
- Isoprenaline
- Dobutamine

**Nasal decongestants**
- Xylometazoline
- Oxymetazoline
- Naphazoline
- Phenylephrine
- Phenylpropanolamine
- Pseudoephedrine

**Anorectics**
- Amphetamine
- Fenfluramine
- Dexfenfluramine
- Sibutramine

| | |
|---|---|
| Norepinephrine | 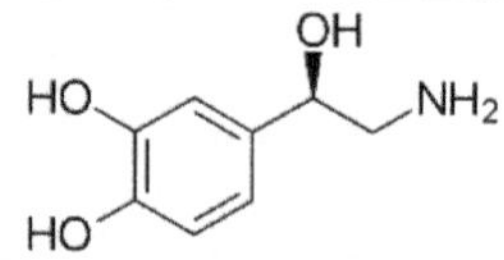 |
| Ephedrine | 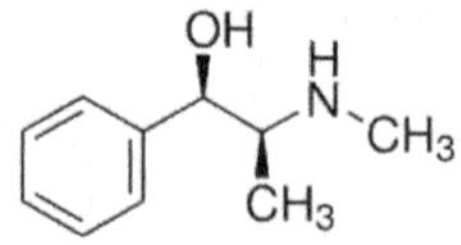 |
| Dopamine | 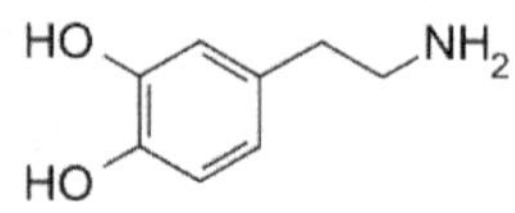 |
| Phenylephrine | 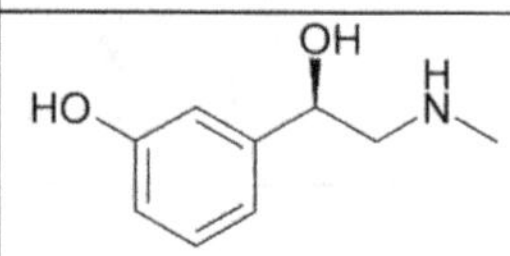 |
| Salbutamol | 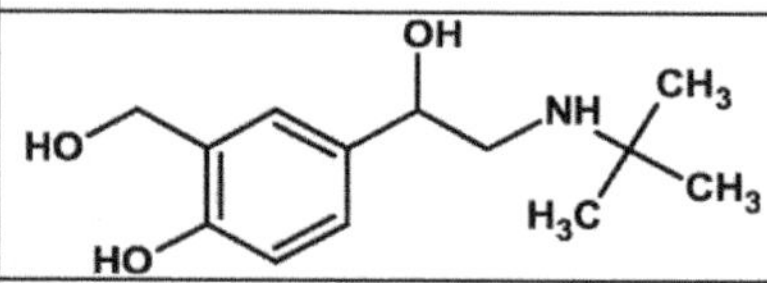 |
| Isopranaline | 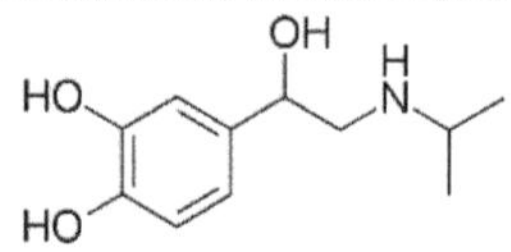 |
| Terbutaline | 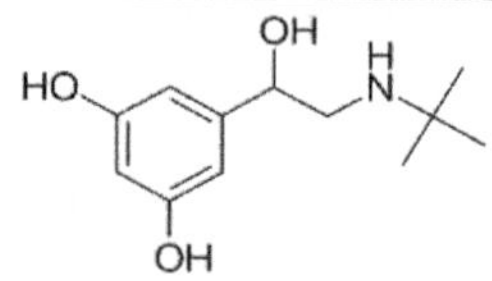 |
| Dobutamine | 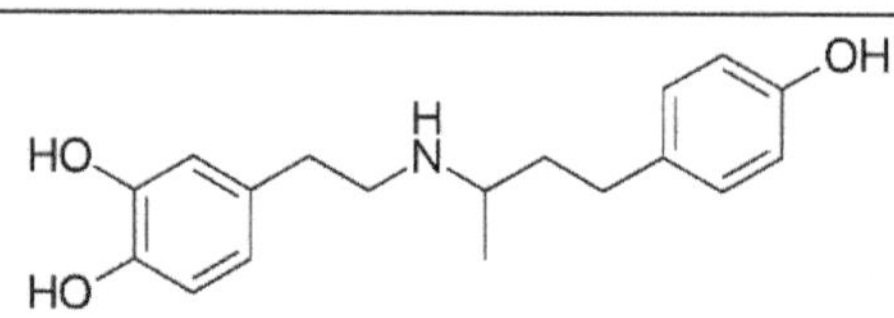 |
| Nephazoline | 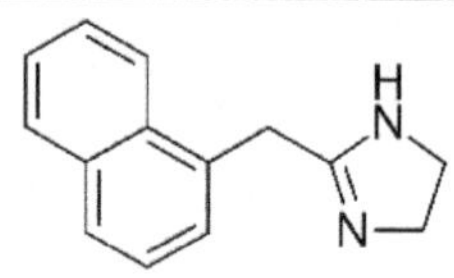 |
| Phenypherine | 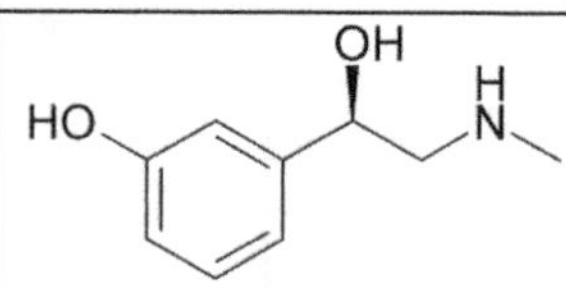 |
| Amphtamine | 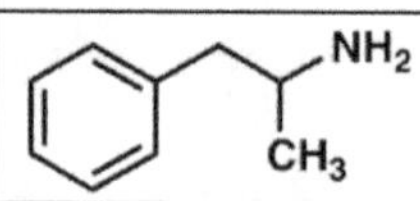 |
| Methylphenidate | 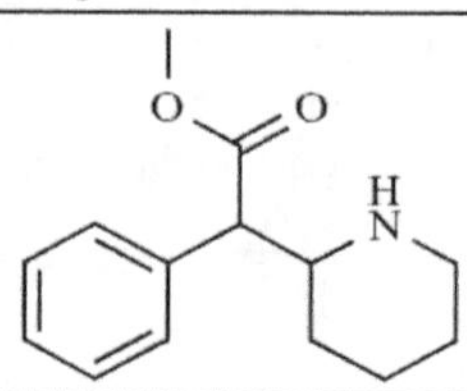 |

**Table** *Contd...*

| | |
|---|---|
| Ritodrine | 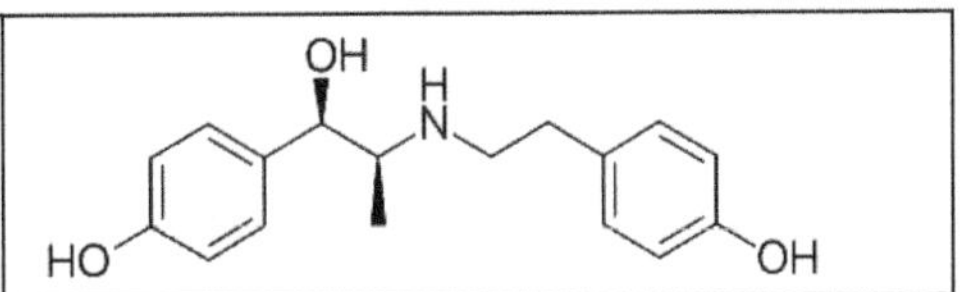 |
| Fenfluramine | 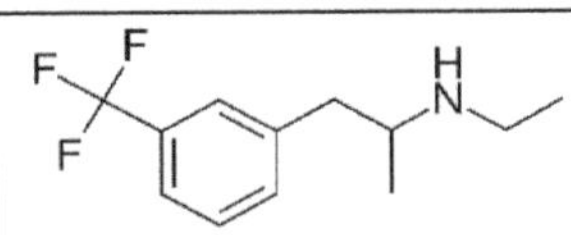 |

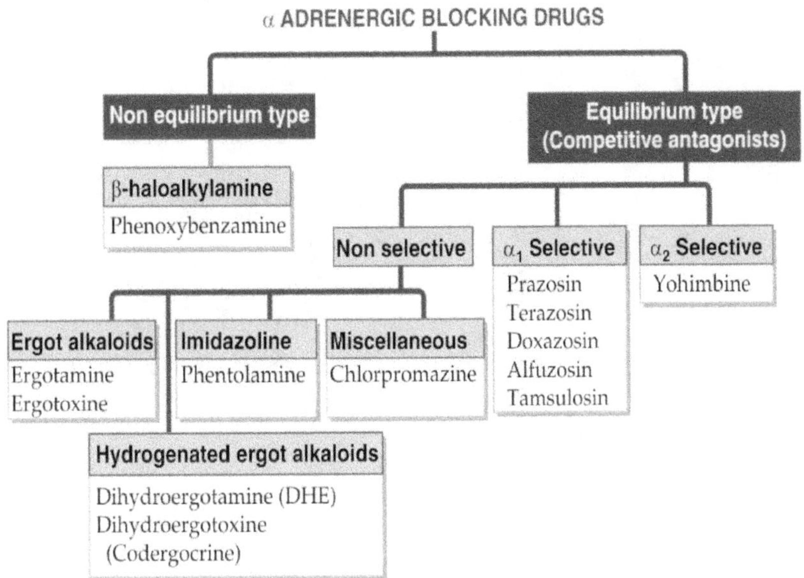


| | |
|---|---|
| Phenoxybenzamine | 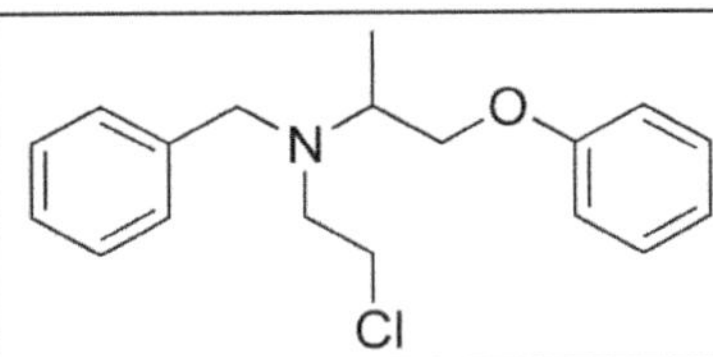 |
| Ergotamine | 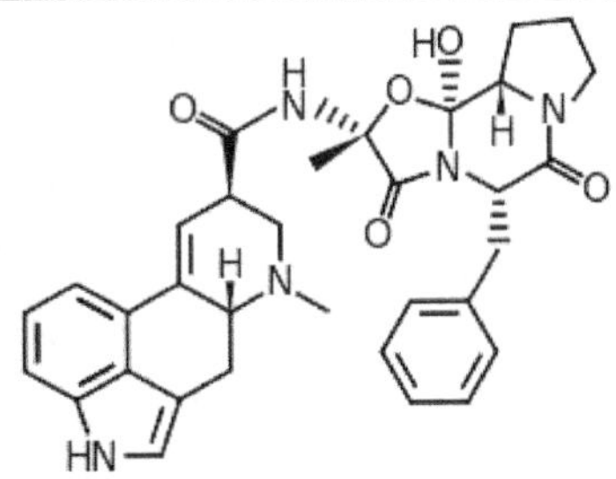 |
| Phentolamine | 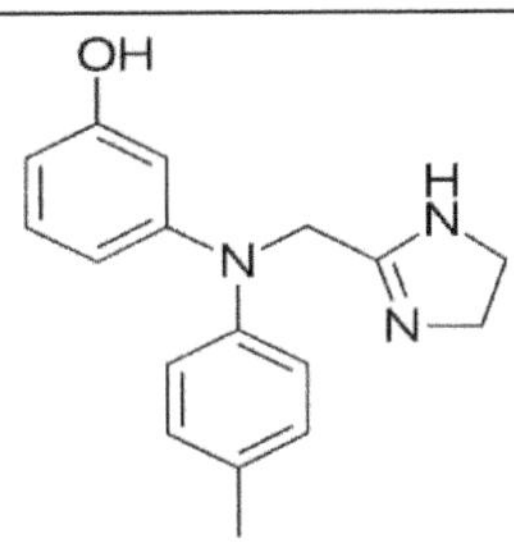 |

**Table** *Contd...*

| Dihydroergotamine | 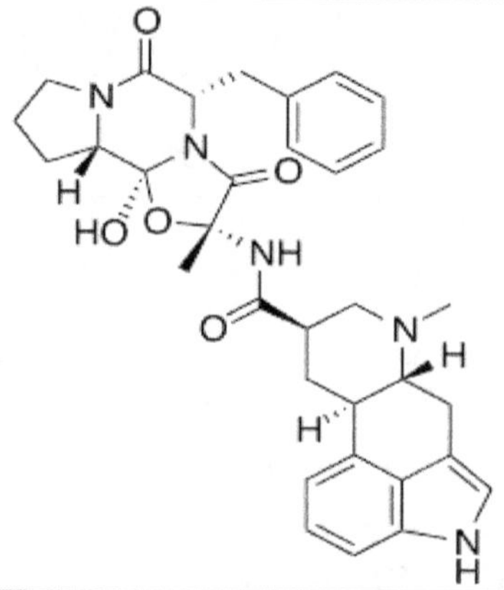 |
| --- | --- |
| Chlorpromazine | 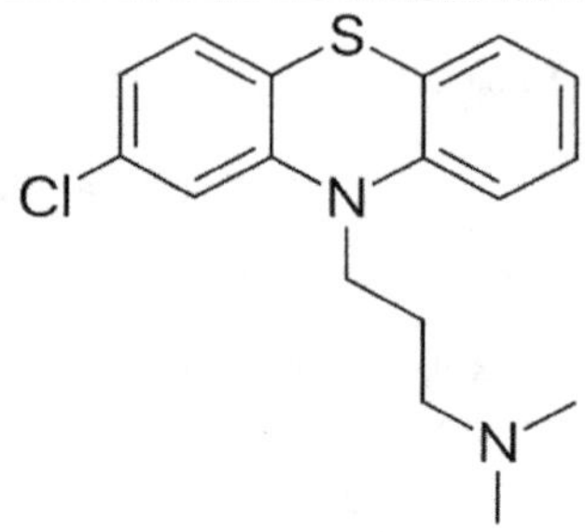 |
| Prazocine | 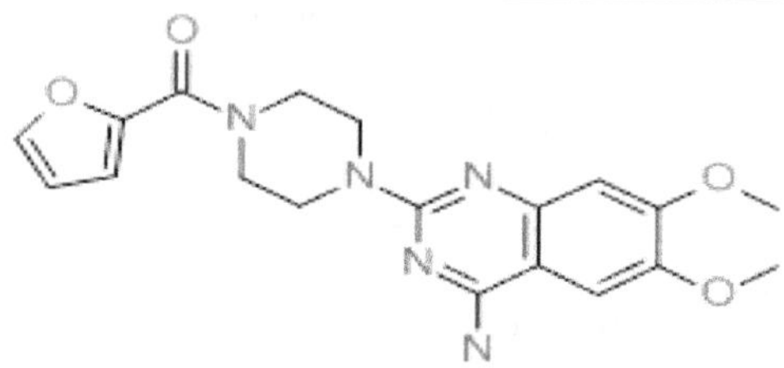 |
| Terazocine | 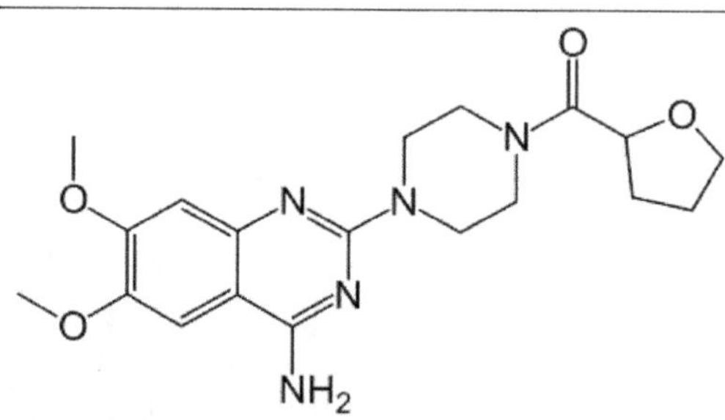 |
| Yohimbin | 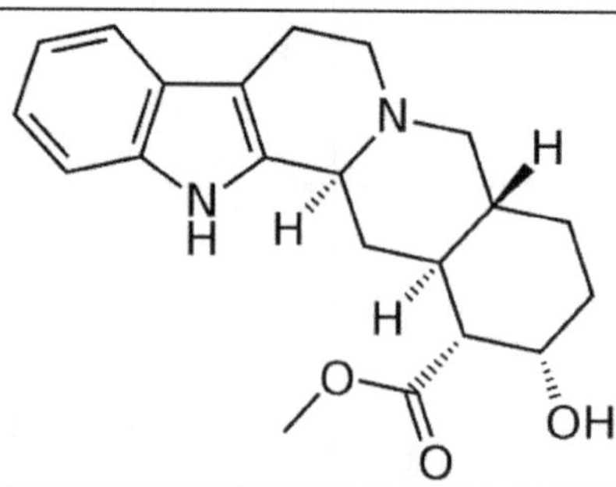 |

## TOPICAL DRUGS FOR GLAUCOMA

| β-Adrenergic blockers | α-Adrenergic agonists | Prostaglandin analogues | Carbonic anhydrase inhibitors | Miotics |
|---|---|---|---|---|
| Timolol<br>Betaxolol<br>Levobunolol<br>Carteolol | Dipivefrine<br>Apraclonidine<br>Brimonidine | Latanoprost<br>Travoprost<br>Bimatoprost | Dorzolamide<br>Brinzolamide | Pilocarpine<br>Physostigmine<br>Echothiophate |

| | |
|---|---|
| Timolol | 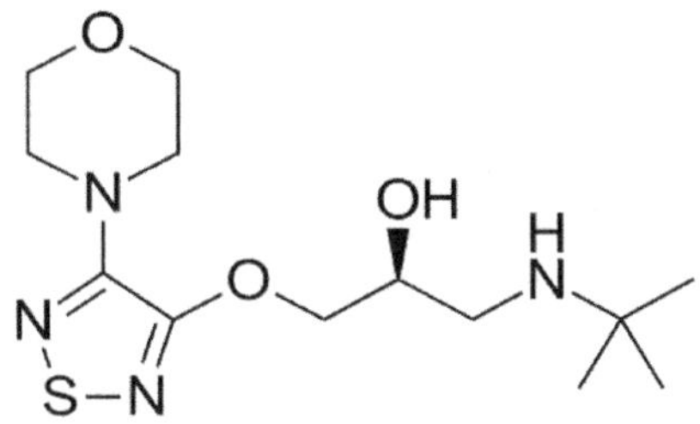 |
| Betaxolol | 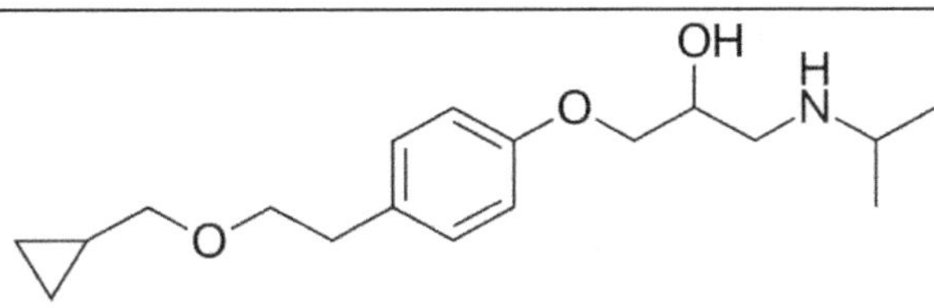 |
| Carteolol | 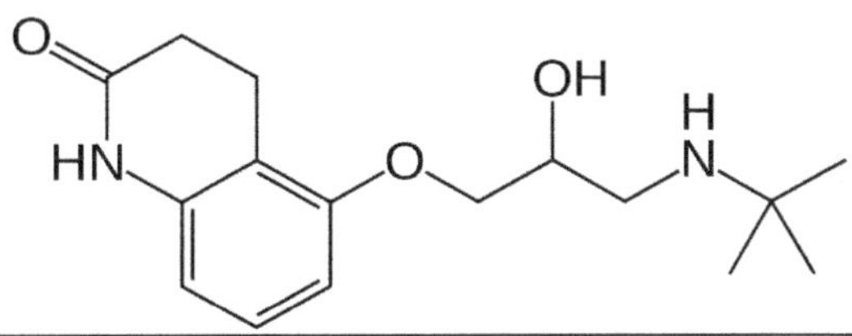 |
| Dipivefrine | 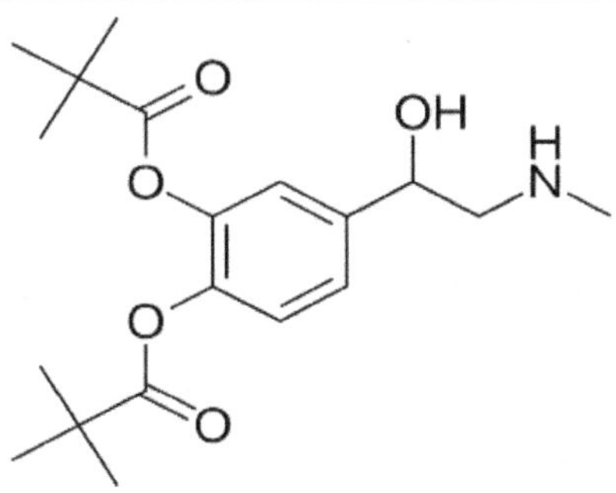 |

**Table** *Contd...*

| | |
|---|---|
| Latanoprost | 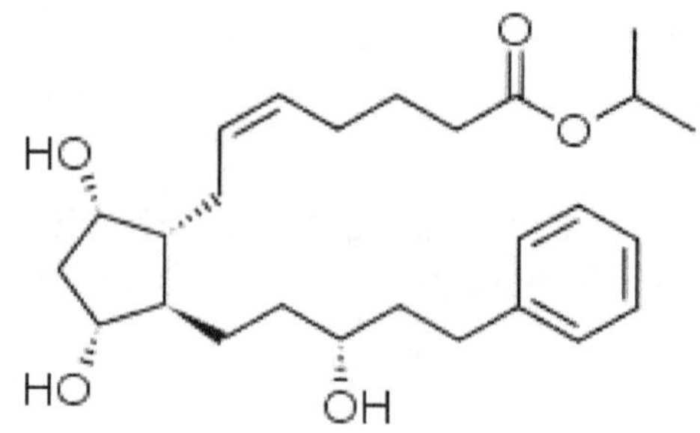 |
| Dorzolamide | 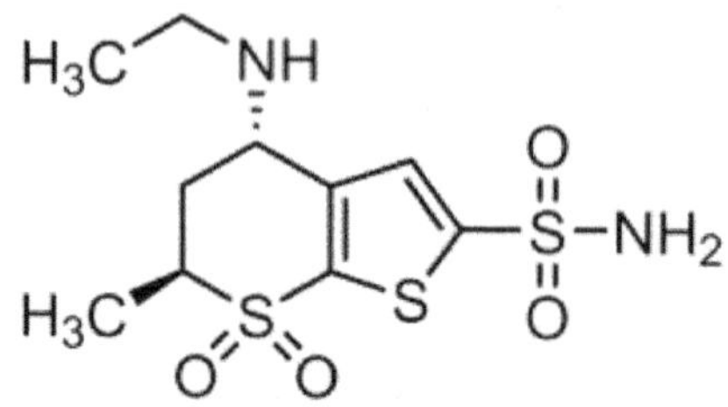 |
| Brinzolamide | 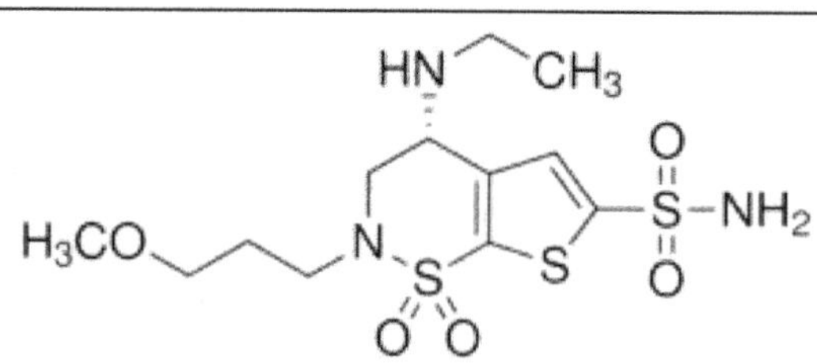 |
| Pilocarpine | 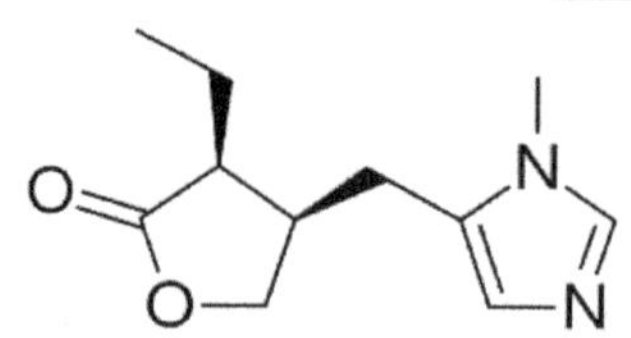 |
| Physostigmine | 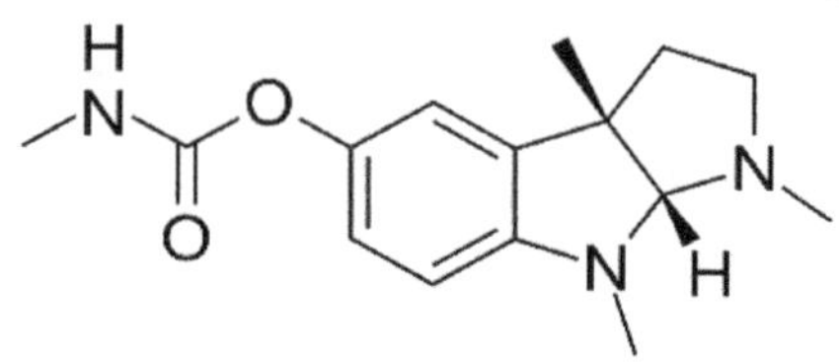 |

## 2.2 Drugs Acting on Somatic Nervous System

Skeletal muscle relaxants are drugs that act peripherally at neuromuscular junction/muscle fiber itself or centrally in the cerebrospinal axis to reduce muscle tone and/or cause paralysis. The neuromuscular blocking agents are used primarily in conjunction with general anesthetics to provide muscle relaxation for surgery, while centrally acting muscle relaxants are used mainly for painful muscle spasms and spastic neurological conditions.

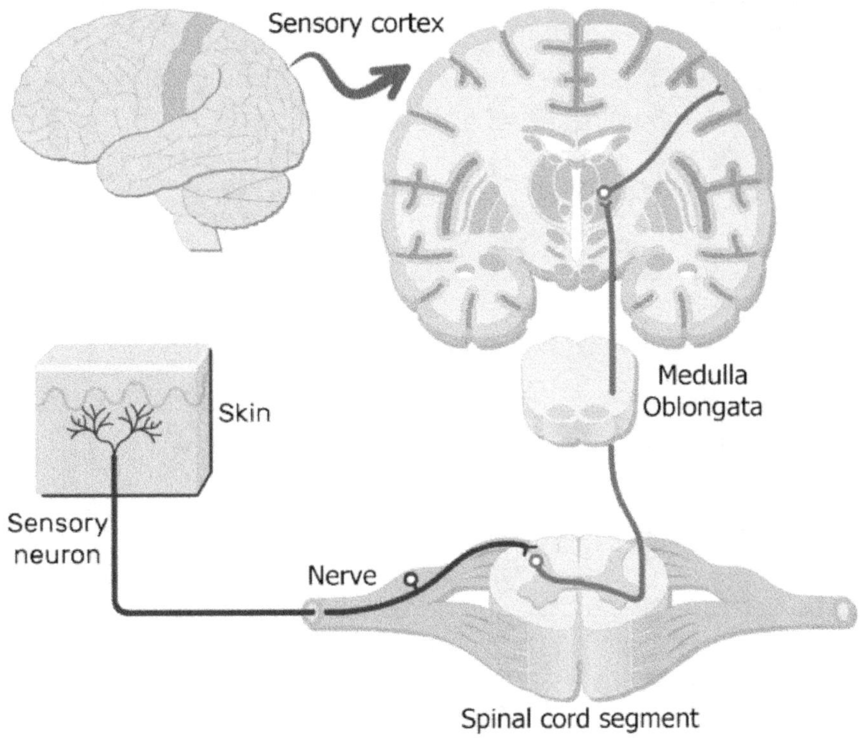


**SKELETAL MUSCLE RELAXANTS**

- **Peripherally acting**
  - **Neuromuscular blocking agents**
    - **Nondepolarizing (competitive) blockers**
      - **Long acting**: d-Tubocurarine, Pancuronium, Doxacurium, Pipecuronium
      - **Intermediate acting**: Vecuronium, Atracurium, Cisatracurium, Rocuronium, Rapacuronium
      - **Short acting**: Mivacurium
    - **Depolarizing blockers**: Succinyl choline (suxamethonium), Decamethonium
  - **Directly acting agents**: Dantrolene sodium, Quinine
- **Centrally acting**
  - **Mephenesin congeners**: Carisoprodol, Chlorzoxazone, Chlormezanone, Methocarbamol
  - **Benzodiazepines**: Diazepam, etc.
  - **GABA mimetic**: Baclofen, Thiocolchicoside
  - **Central $\alpha_2$ agonist**: Tizanidine

**Fig.** Representation of reflex arch.

| | |
|---|---|
| Succinylcholine | 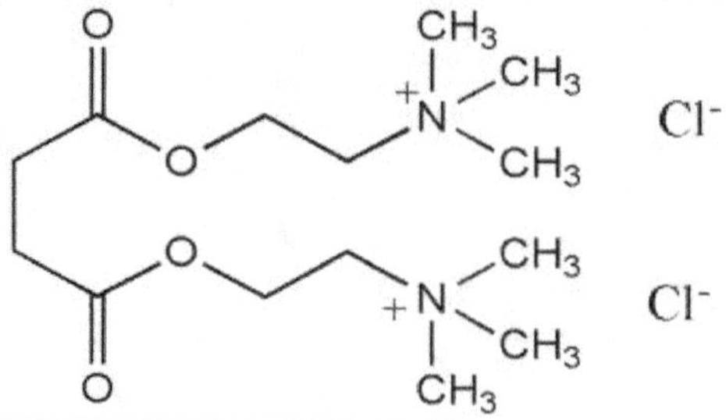 |
| D-Tubarculine | 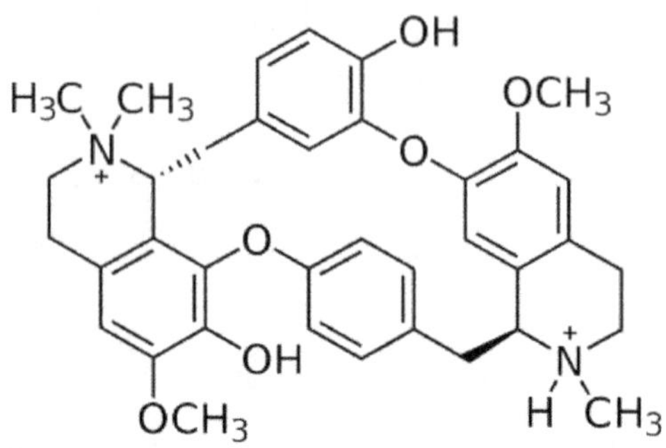 |
| Vecuronium | 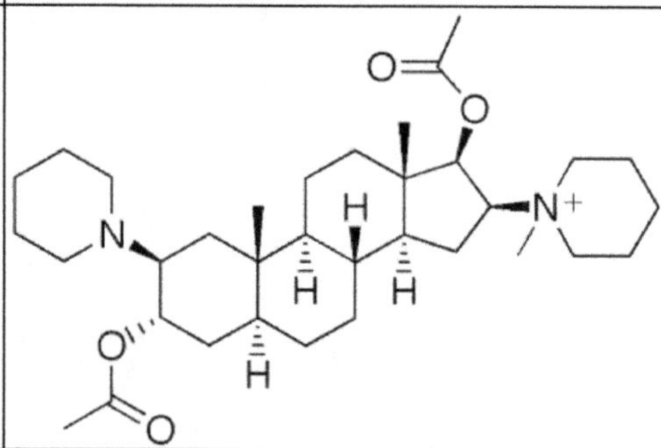 |
| Mivacurium | 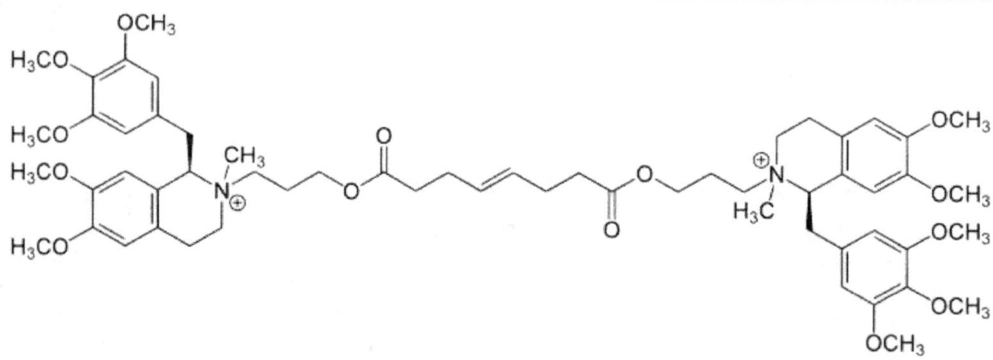 |
| Quinine | 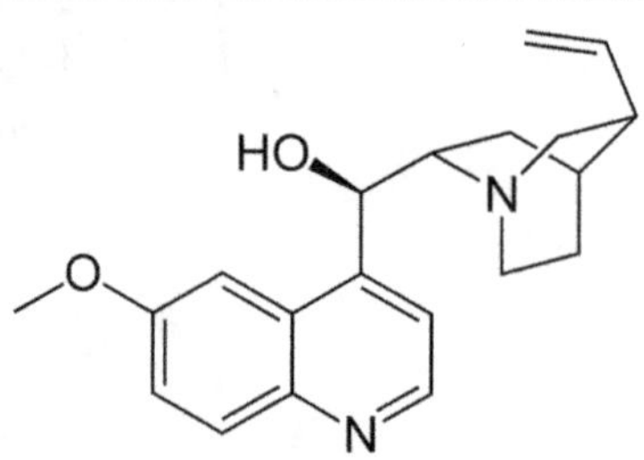 |

**Table** *Contd...*

| | |
|---|---|
| Carisoprodol | 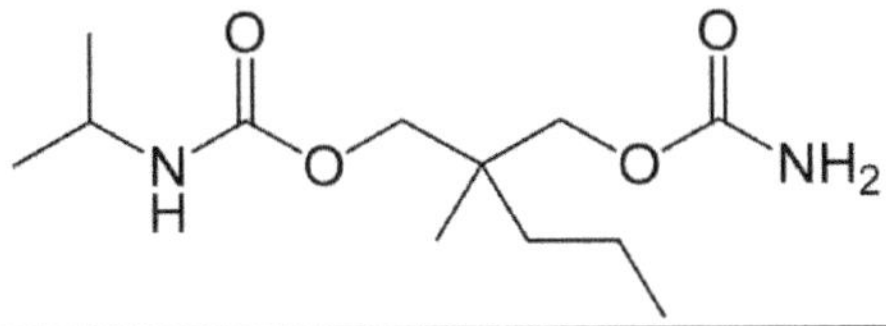 |
| Diazepam | 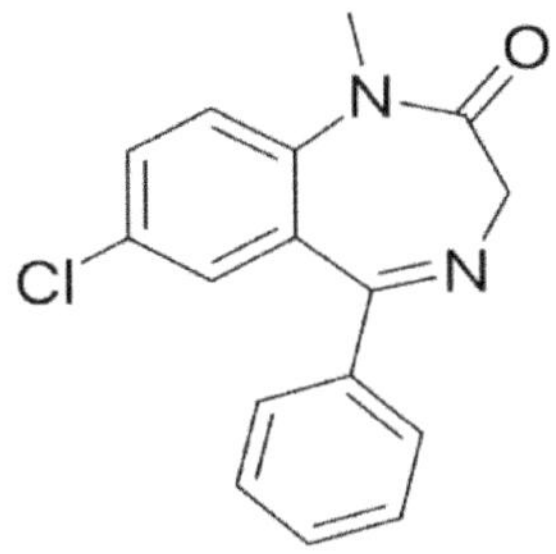 |
| Baclofen | 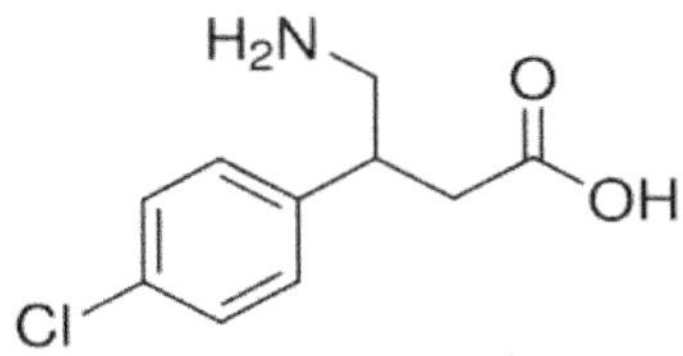 |

LOCAL ANAESTHETICS

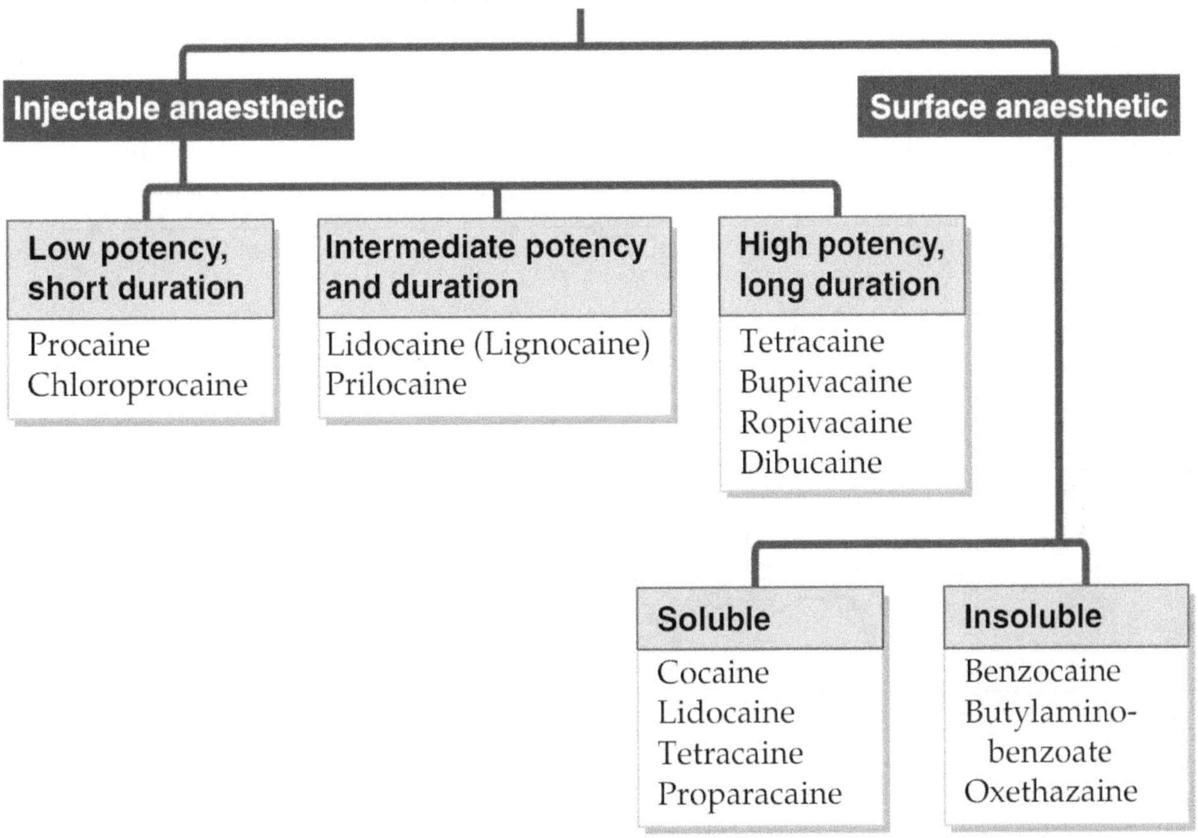

| | |
|---|---|
| Procaine | 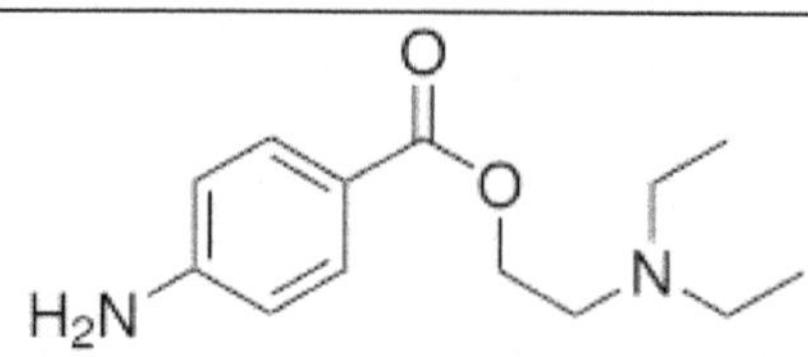 |
| Chloroprocaine | 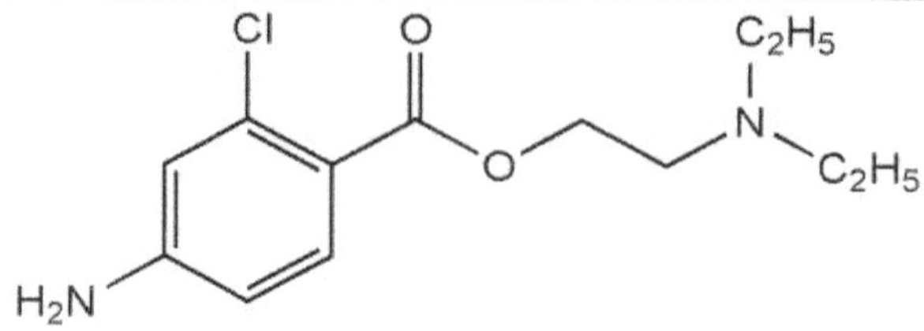 |
| Lidocaine | 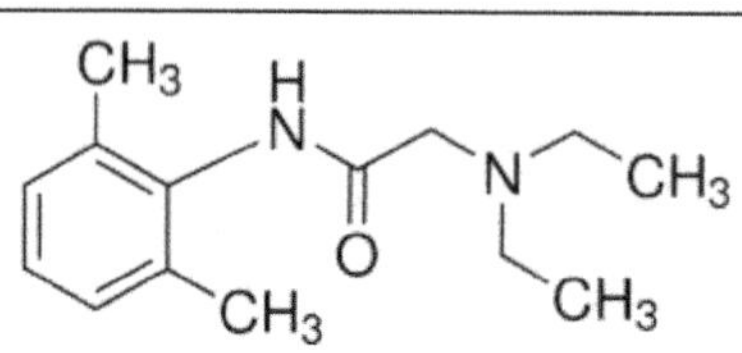 |
| Prolocaine | 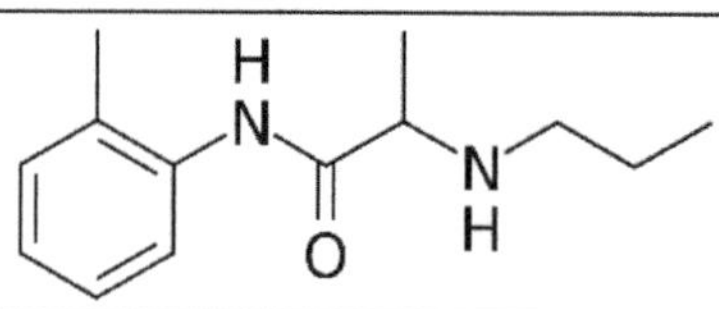 |
| Tetracain | 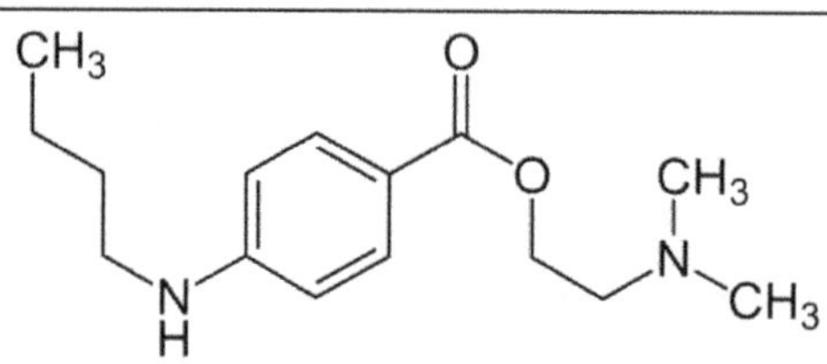 |
| Ropivacaine | 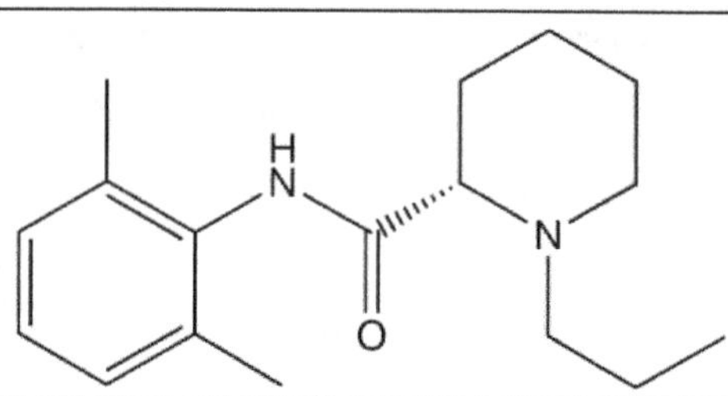 |
| Cocain | 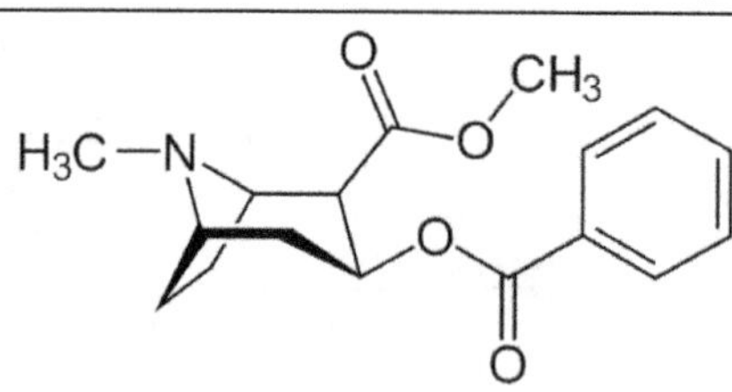 |
| Benzocain | 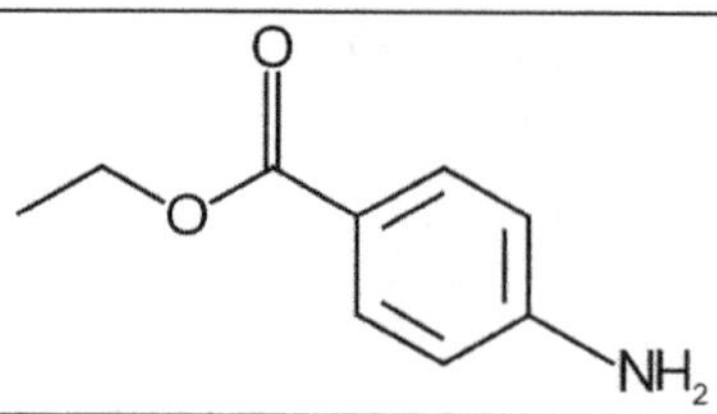 |

**Table** *Contd...*

| Oxethazaine | 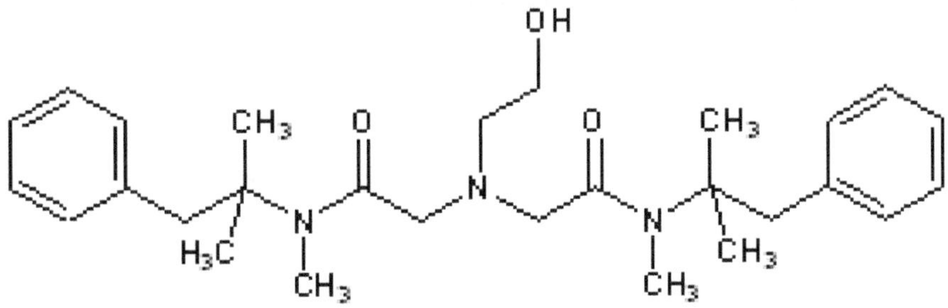 |
|---|---|

## 2.3 Drugs Acting on Central Nervous System

### Sedatives and Hypnotics

**Sedatives** – reduce anxiety and exert a calming effect

**Hypnotics -** produces drowsiness and facilitates the onset and maintenance of a state of sleep.

**Classification**

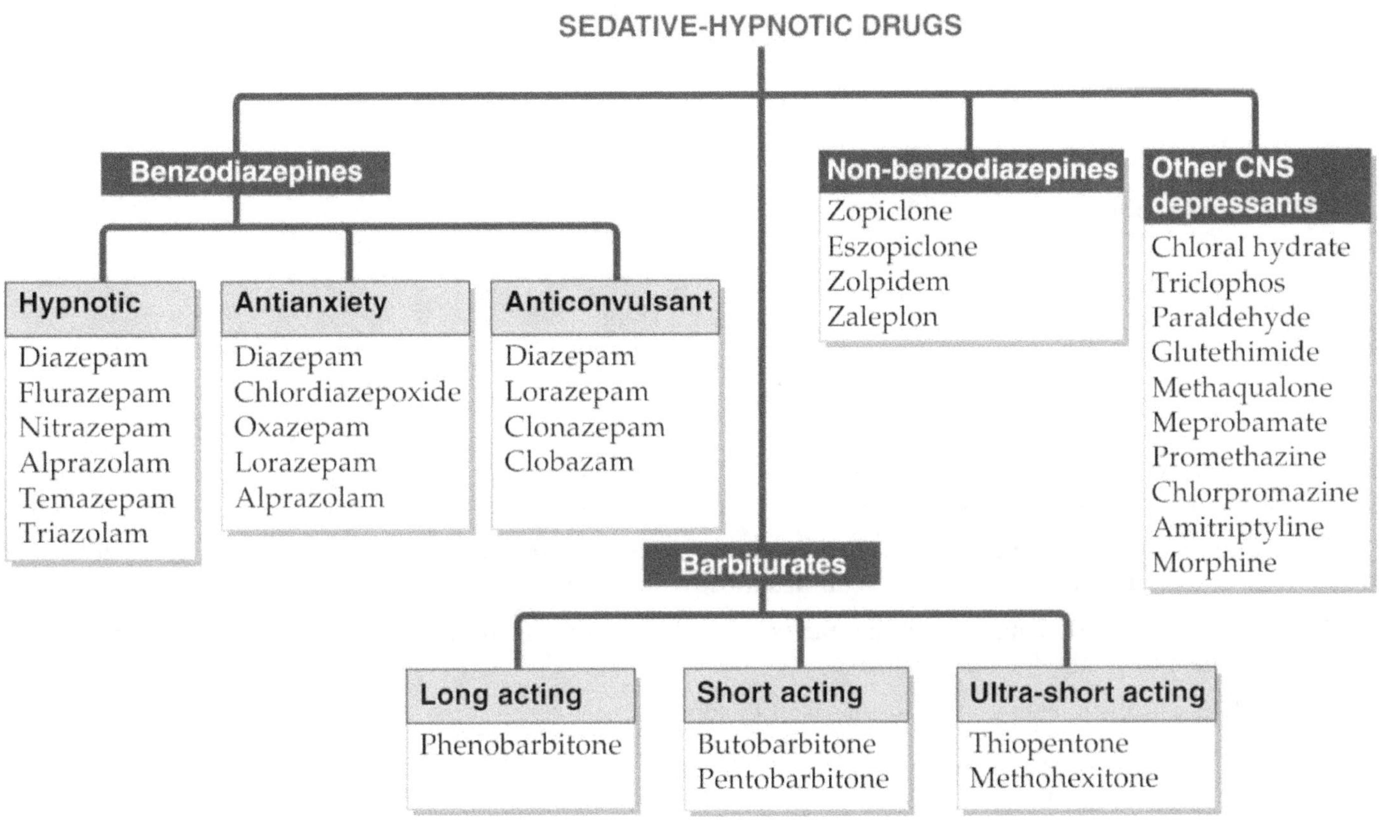

**Mechanism of Action of Barbiturates and Benzodiazepines-**

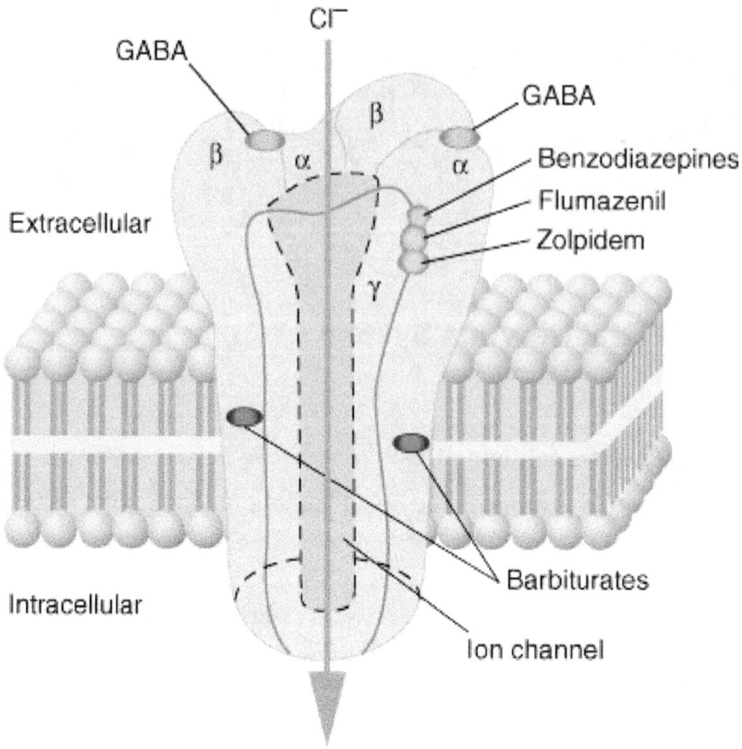


**SAR of Barbiturates**

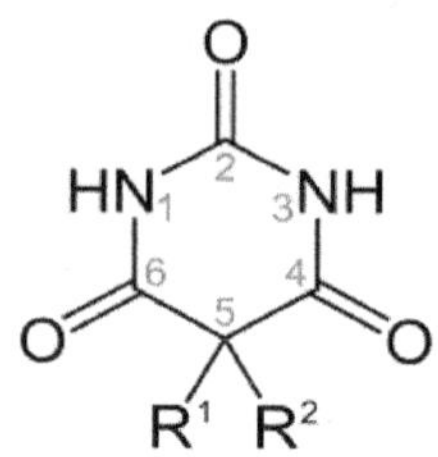


1. Barbituric acid itself does not possess any hypnotic properties.
2. Activity requires a balance of acidic and lipophilic properties.To make the drug sufficiently acidic, both or at least one of the two nitrogen must be unsubstituted.
3. To make drug sufficiently lipophilic, the two hydrogen atoms at position 5 : 5 must have the appropriate substituent (e.g., alkyl or aryl groups)
4. The type of substituent's control 2 aspects of the drug
    - Potency
    - Duration of Action.
5. The total number of carbon atoms present in the two groups at carbon 5 must not be less than 4 and more than 10 and influences onset of action and duration.
6. Only one of the substituent groups at position 5 may be a cyclic group.

**Barbituric Derivatives Structures**

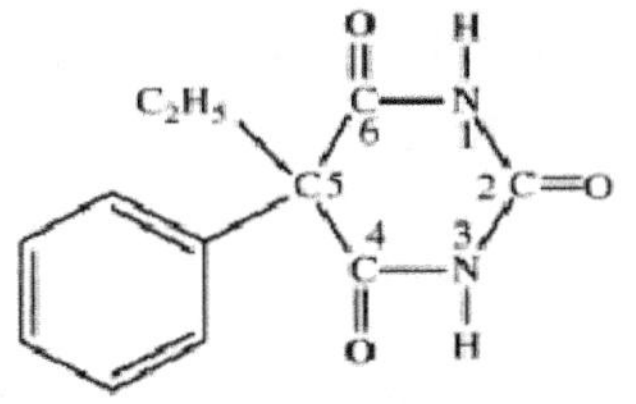

**Phenobarbital**

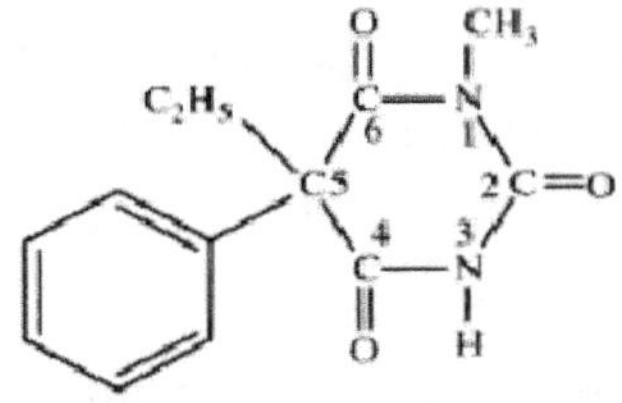

**Mephobarbital**

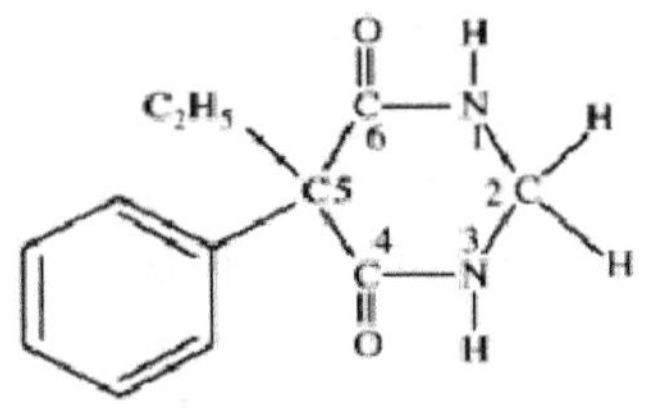

**Primidone**

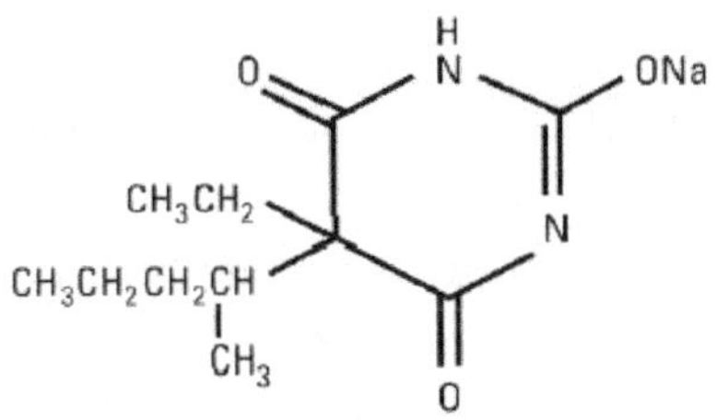

**Pentobarbitone**

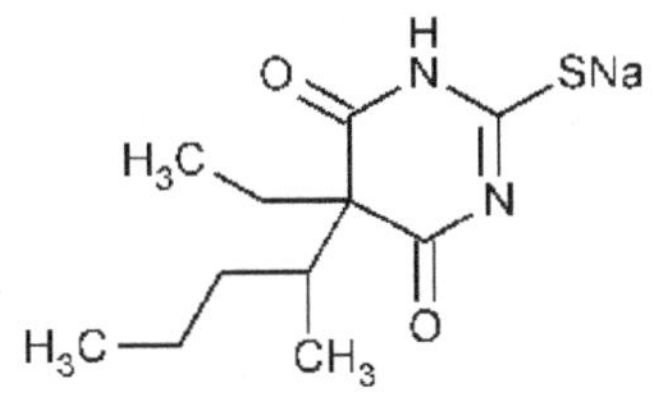

**Thiopentone**

## Gaba Alpha 1 Selective Hypnotics – MOA of Zaleplon and Zolpidem

- The GABAA receptor contain 6 different alpha subunits
- Benzodiazepines bind to four of GABAA alpha subunits: alpha 1, alpha 2, alpha 3 and alpha 5.
- Each of these subunits is associated with different effects, and thus benzodiazepines not only cause sedation but are also anxiolytic, cause muscle relaxation, and have alcohol potentiating actions.
- The hypnotics zaleplon and zolpidem bind selectively to GABA-A receptors that contain the alpha 1 subunit (sleep).

## SAR of Benzodiazepine

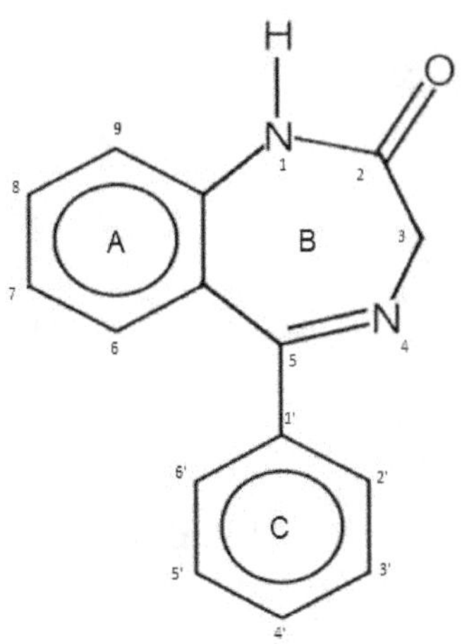

1. All benzodiazepines have a benzene ring attached to a diazepine ring.
2. In benzene rings and diazepine ring, with the whole 1,4-benzodiazepine system
3. The electron attractive substituents on ring A enforce the activity

   NO2>Br>CF3>Cl
4. Ring B is necessary for activity.
5. The electron attractive substituents with small volume on benzene ring of C-5 will enforce the activity
6. The hydrolysis of amide and imine
7. **Ring A:** The minimum requirement for 5-phenyl 1,4 benzodiaipin 2one derivatives to BZR include an aromatic or hetroaromatic ring
8. The substitution on this ring produces varied effect on binding with the receptor, however such effects are not predictable on the basis of electronic and stearic properties.
9. **Ring B:** A proton accepting group (carbonyl oxygen) at 2-position of ring B is necessary to interact with receptor histidine residue that act as proton donor and help in ligand binding Electron donating group must be in the same plane with electronegative group on ring A, favoring a coplanar spatial orientation of two moieties
10. Substitution of O with S effect selective binding GABA BZR sub-populations but anxiolytic activity is maintained.
11. Substitution 3-position methylene or imine nitrogen is sterically unfavourable
12. Ring C: The 5-phenyl ring C is not required for binding to the BZR in vitro, however, this aromatic ring contribute favorable hydrophobic or steric interactions to receptor binding and its relationship to ring A
13. Substitution at 4' (para position) is unfavorable for activity, however, ortho substitution is not detrimental to agonist activity

**Benzodiazepines Derivatives Structures**

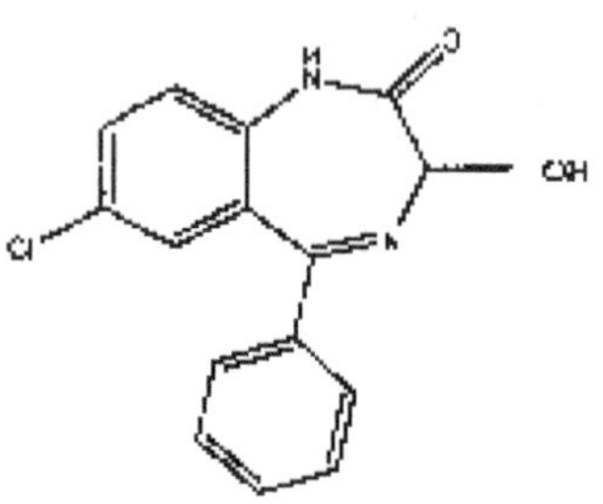

Oxazepam

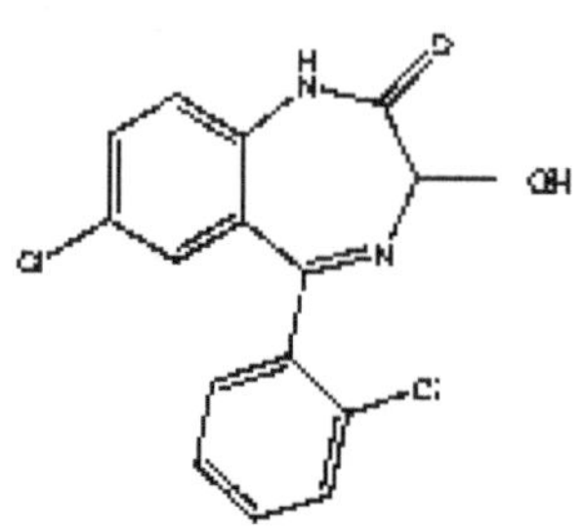

Lorazepam

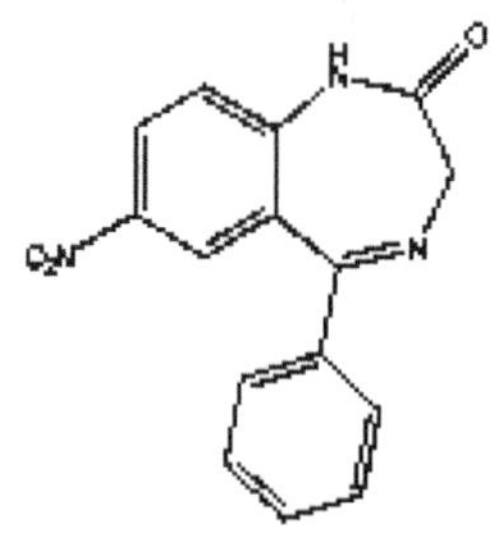

Nitrazepam

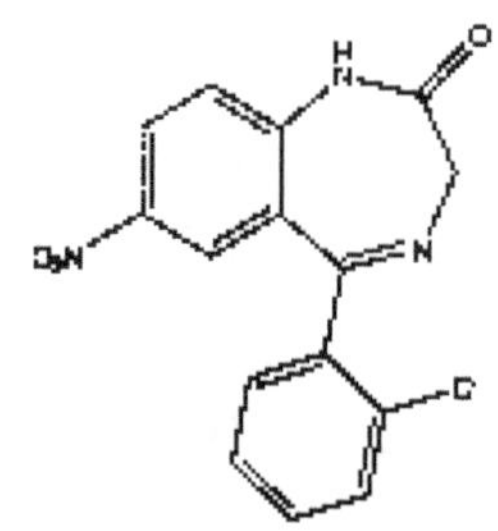

Clonazepam

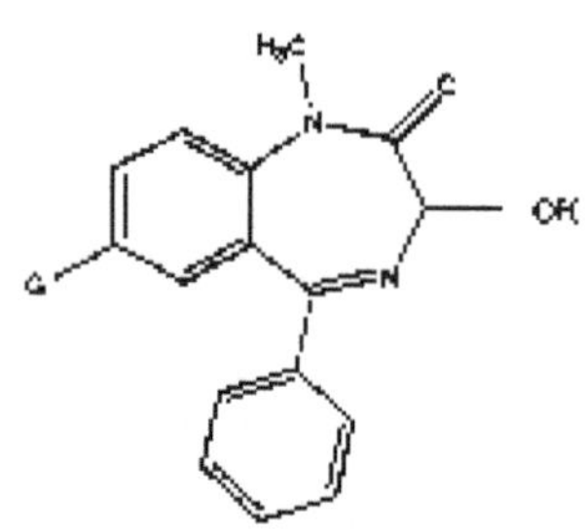

Temazepam

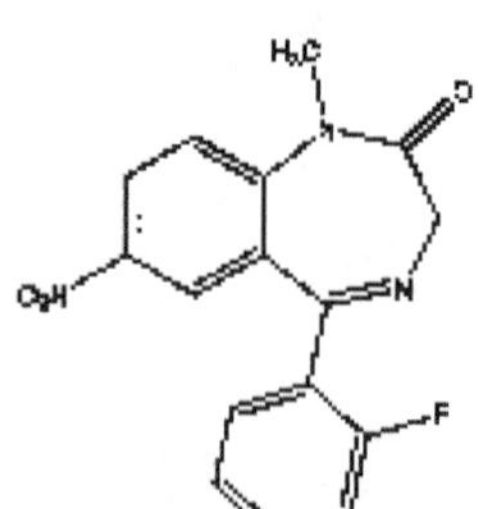

Flunitrazepam

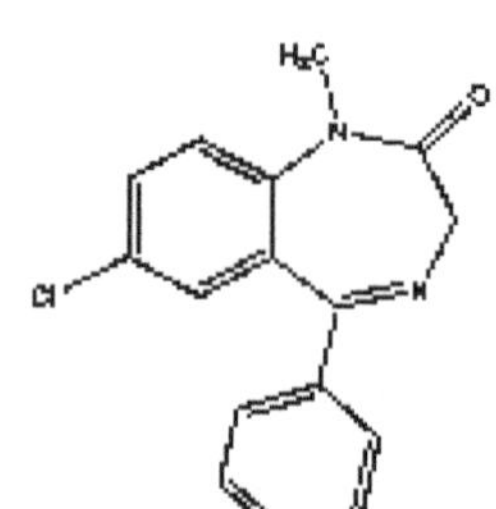

Diazepam

## Flumazenil: A Benzodiazepine Receptor Antagonist

**Primary Indications for the use of Flumazenil are -**

- Management of suspected benzodiazepine overdose.
- Reversal of sedative effects produced by benzodiazepines administered during either general anesthesia.
- The administration of a series of small injections is preferred to a single bolus injection.
- A total of **1 mg** flumazenil given over 1-3 minutes usually is sufficient to abolish the effects of therapeutic doses of benzodiazepines.
- Patients with suspected benzodiazepine overdose should respond adequately to a cumulative dose of 1-5 mg given over 2-10 minutes;
- A lack of response to 5 mg flumazenil strongly suggests that a benzodiazepine is not the Major Cause of Sedation.

## Melatonin Congeners

**Ramelteon**

- Synthetic Tricyclic Analog Of **Melatonin**.
- It Was Approved For The Treatment Of Insomnia, Specifically Sleep Onset Difficulties.

**Mechanism of Action**

- Melatonin levels in the suprachiasmatic nucleus rise and fall in a circadian fashion

↓

concentrations increasing in the evening as an individual prepares for sleep, and then reaching a plateau and ultimately decreasing as the night progresses.

**Mechanism of Action**

- Two **GPCRs** for melatonin, **$MT_1$** and **$MT_2$,** are found in the suprachiasmatic nucleus, each playing a different role in sleep.
- **RAMELTEON** binds to both **$MT_1$** and **$MT_2$** receptors with high affinity.
- Binding of **Melatonin** to **$MT_1$** receptors **promotes the onset of sleep**.
- Binding of **Melatonin** to **$MT_2$** receptors shifts the timing of the circadian system.
- **RAMELTEON** is efficacious in combating both transient and chronic insomnia

**Anti Anxiety/Anti Psychotic Drugs/Neuroleptics**

A syndrome of chronic disordered thinking and disturbed behavior (schizophrenia, mania, depression)

The most important types of psychosis are:

- Schizophrenia
- Affective disorders (e.g. depression, mania)
- Organic psychoses (mental disturbances caused by head injury, alcoholism, or other kinds of organic disease).

Schizophrenia results from excess activity of dopamine neurotransmission in Mesolimbic and Mesocortica Pathways because all antipsychotic drugs block dopamine receptors.

**Mechanism of Action:** There are many type of DA-receptors. The antipsychotic drugs probably owe their therapeutic effects mainly to blockade of D2 receptors. The main groups, phenothiazines, thioxanthines and butyrophenones, show preference for D2 over D1 receptors; whereas clozapine is relatively nonselective between D1 and D2, but has high affinity for D4.

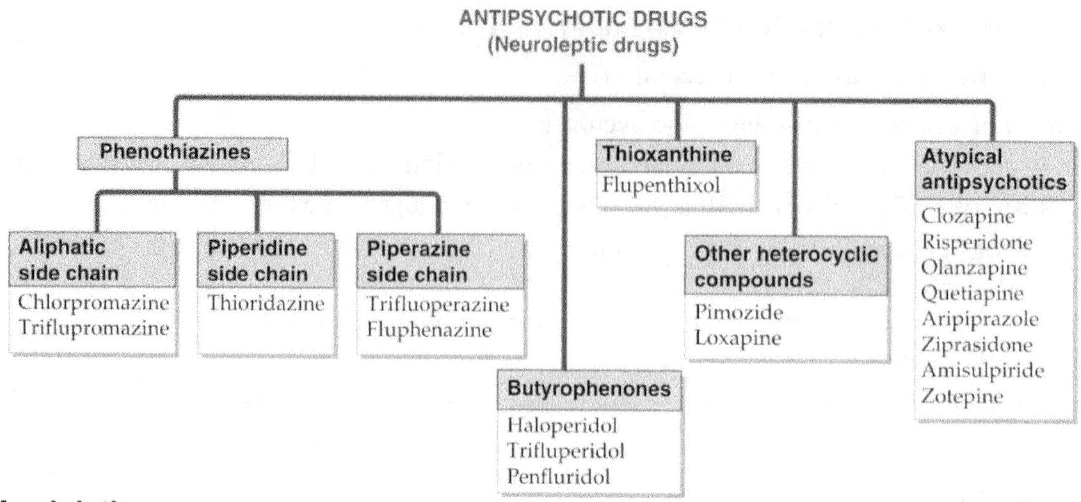


## Atypical Anxiolytics

Buspiron, Ipsapirone, Gepirone

Buspirone relieves anxiety

- without causing marked sedative, hypnotic, or euphoric effects.
- no anticonvulsant or muscle relaxant properties.

Buspirone does not interact directly with GABAergic systems.

Anxiolytic effects of buspirone is by acting as a partial agonist at brain 5-HT1A receptors.

- the anxiolytic effects of buspirone may take more than a week
- unsuitable for management of acute anxiety states
- no rebound anxiety or withdrawal signs on abrupt discontinuance
- The drug is not effective in blocking the acute withdrawal syndrome resulting from abrupt cessation of use of benzodiazepines or other sedative-hypnotics
- Buspirone has minimal abuse liability
- The drug is used in generalized anxiety states but is less effective in panic disorders.

**Antipsychotic Drugs Structures**

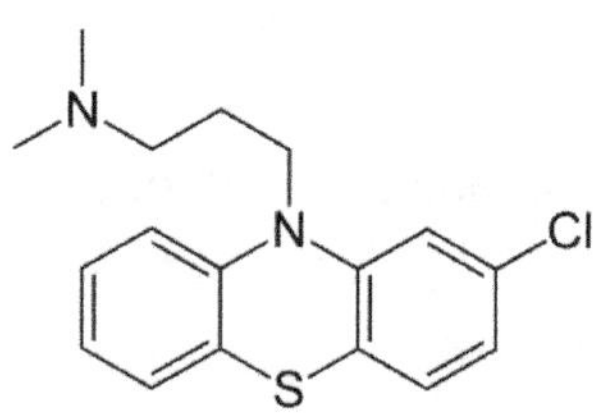

**Chlorpromazine**

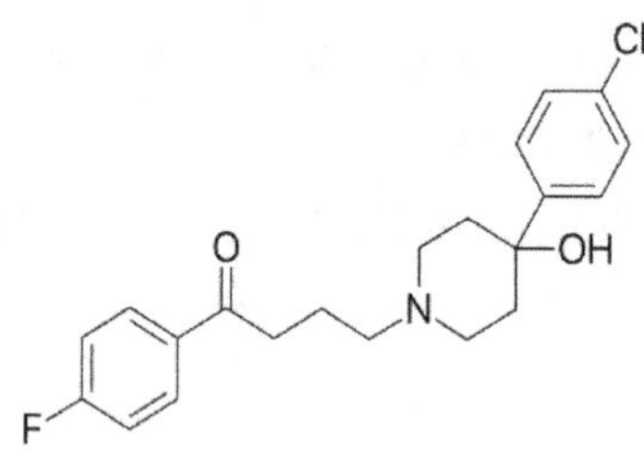

**Haloperidol**

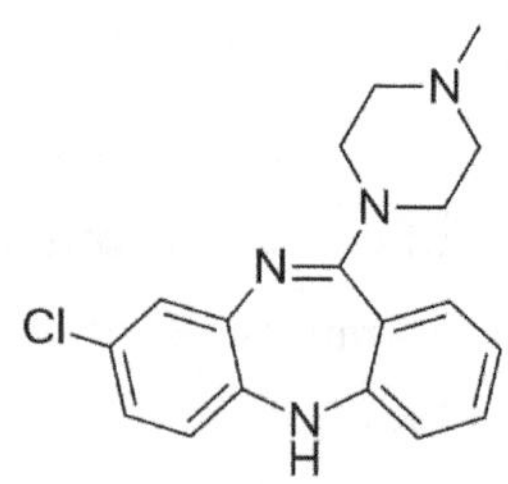

**Clozapine**

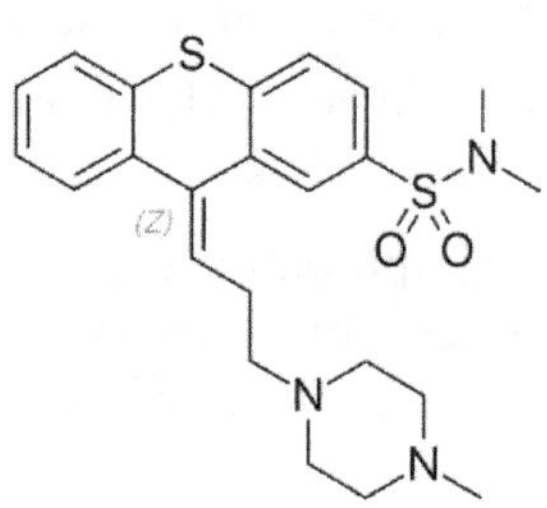

**Thiothexine**

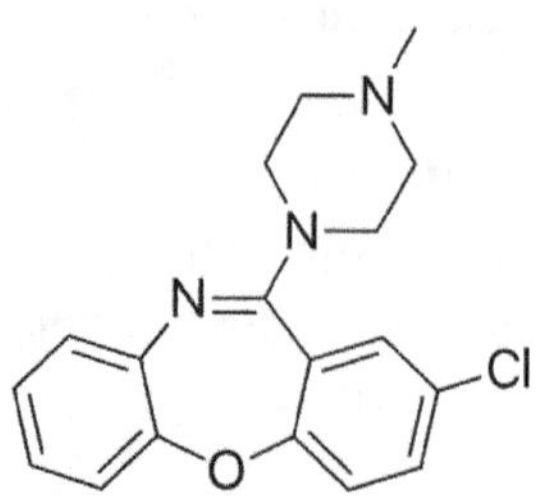

**Loxapine**

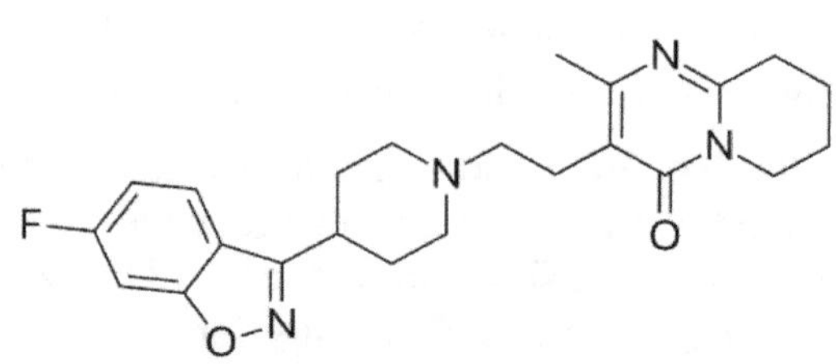

**Resperidone**

### Anti Convulsant /Anti Epileptic Drugs

Anticonvulsants, sometimes also called antiepileptics, used in prevention of the occurrence of epileptic seizures.

- The goal of an anticonvulsant is to suppress the rapid and excessive firing of neurons that start a seizure.
- Anticonvulsant drug decreases the frequency and/or severity of seizures in people with epilepsy.
- They treat the symptom of seizures, not the underlying epileptic condition Anticonvulsants

### What are seizures?

- Seizures are episodes of neurologic dysfunction arising from abnormal synchronous activity of neurons.
- Epilepsy is a disease characterized by spontaneous recurrent seizures. It is a group of disorders characterized by excessive excitability of neurons within the central nervous system (CNS) and is common, affecting about 1% of the population.

### Classification

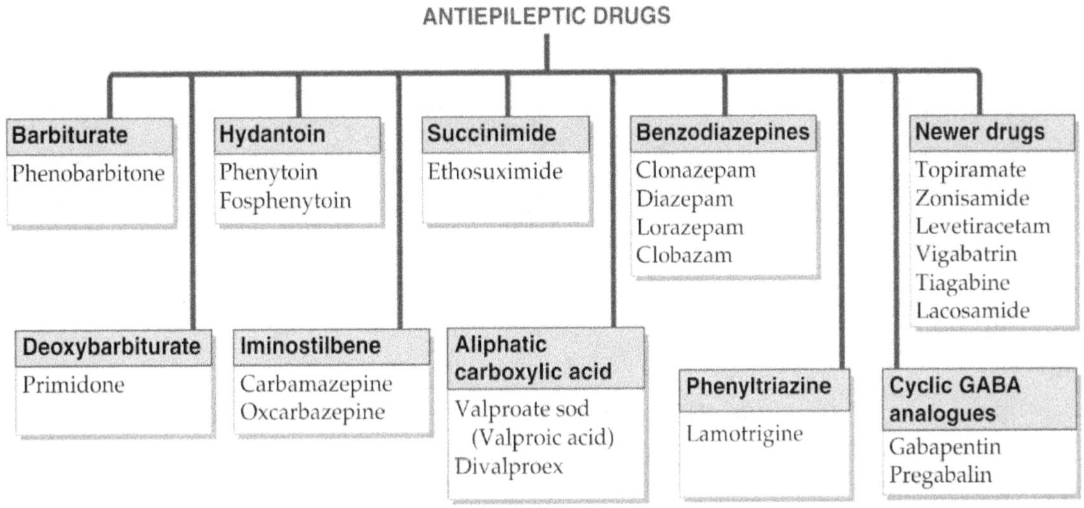


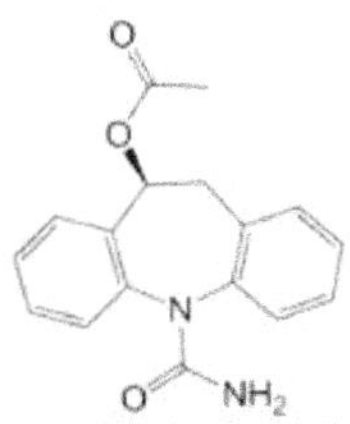

Eslicarbazepine acetate

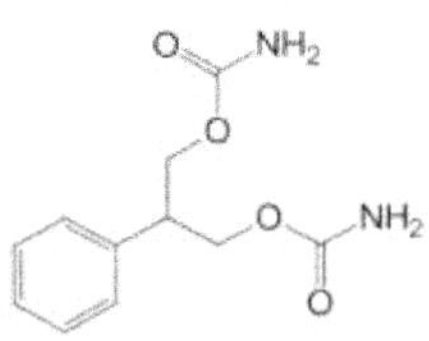

Felbamate

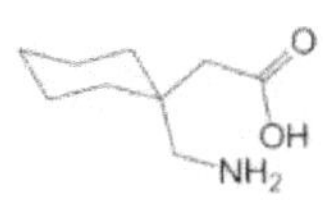

Gabapentin

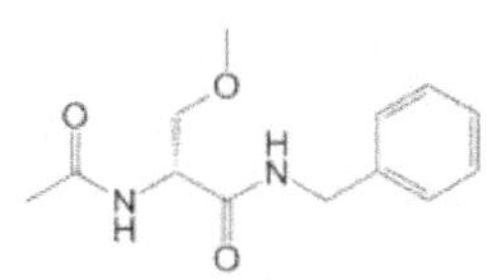

Lacosamide

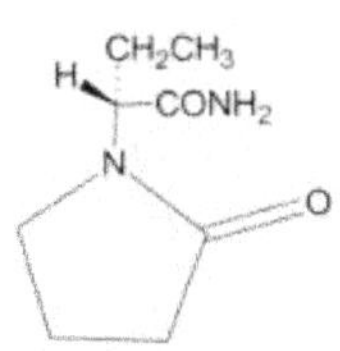

Levetiracetam

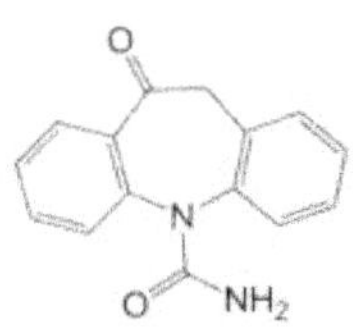

Oxcarbazepine

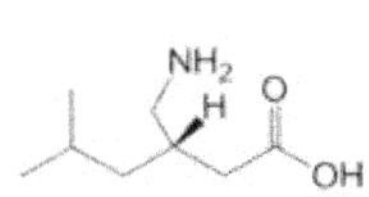

Pregabalin

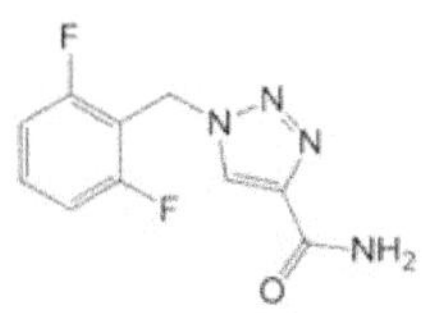

Rufinamide

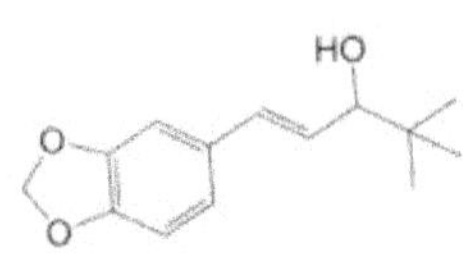

Stiripentol

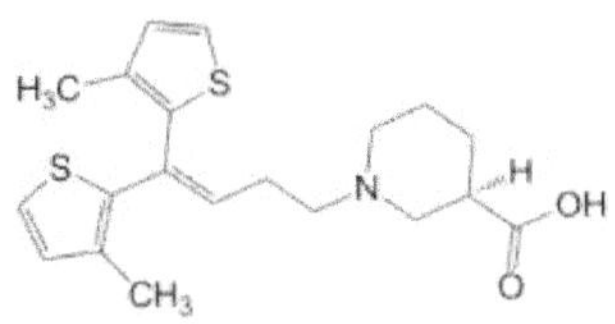

Tiagabine

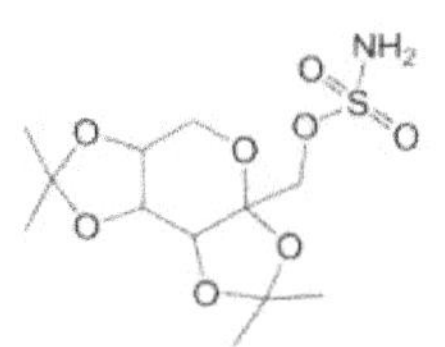

Topiramate

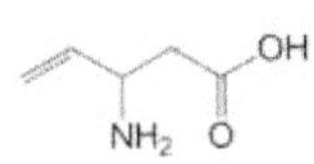

Vigabatrin

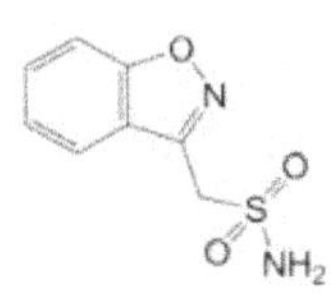

Zonisamide

### New Anticonvulsants

- ✓ Because they are new, the clinical indications for these agents are not yet completely defined, and none are currently used as the first treatment for epilepsy.
- ✓ Many of them are used as an "add-on" medication
- ✓ These newer anticonvulsants have good efficacy, fewer toxic effects, better tolerability, and no need for blood level monitoring were developed.
- ✓ Examples: Felbamate Lamotrigine Gabapentin Topiramate Tiagabin Levetiracetam Vigabatrin Zonisamide
- ✓ Gabapentin (Neurontin) is a pharmaceutical drug, specifically a GABA analog. It was originally developed to treat epilepsy, and currently is also used to relieve neuropathic pain.
- ✓ Vigabatrin (Sabril) is an antiepileptic drug that inhibits the catabolism of gamma-aminobutyric acid (GABA) by irreversibly inhibiting GABA transaminase. It is an analog of GABA.

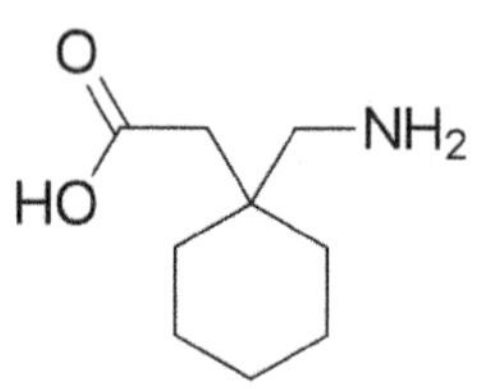


**Gabapentin**

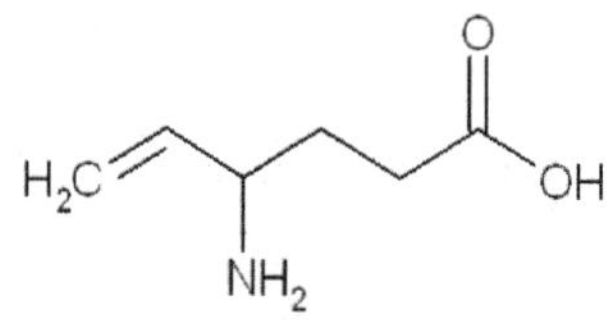


**Vigabatrin**

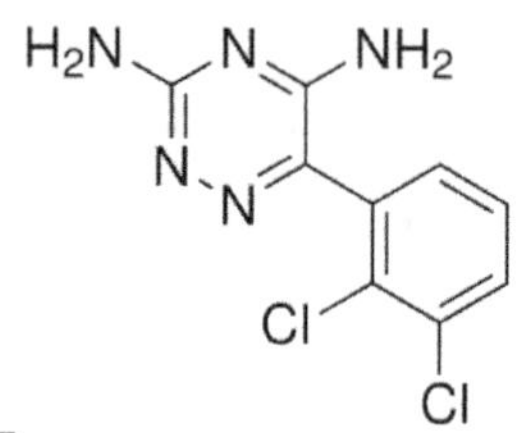


**Lamotrigine**

## General Anesthetics

### Classification

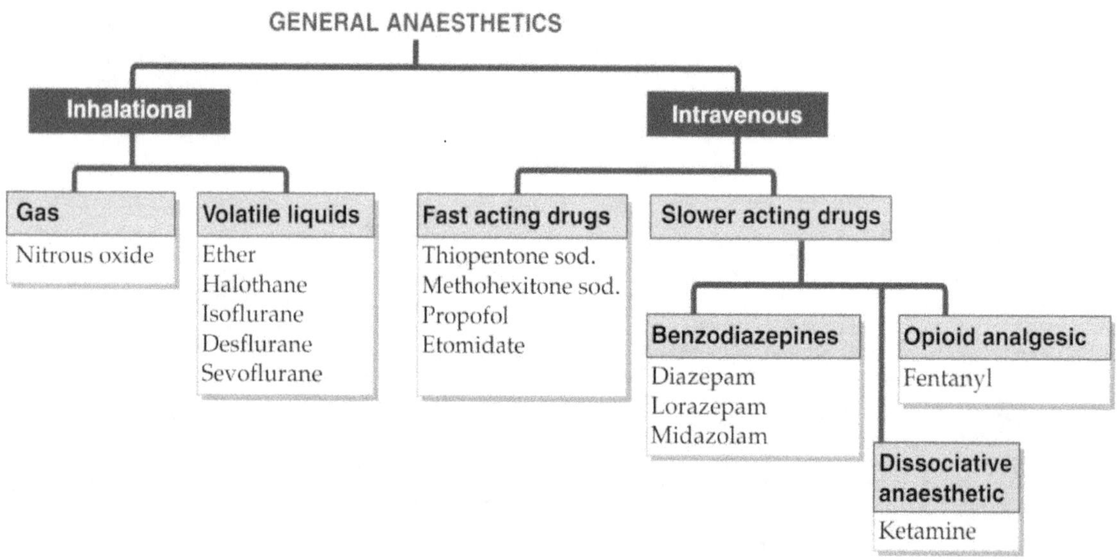


### Anaesthesia

- Hypnosis – Loss of consciousness
- Reversible loss of sensations
- Amnesia – Loss of memory
- Analgesia – Loss of perception of pain
- Immobility – Loss of motor reflexes

- Skeletal muscle relaxation
- Quick acting and rapid eliminated
- No toxic effects – Large margin of safety

**Stage of Analgesia**

- Stage of Delirium
- Surgical Anaesthesia
- Medullary Paralysis

**Important Terms**

**Minimal Alveolar Concentration (MAC):** Smaller the MAC value more potent is the anaestheti and vice versa.

**Arteriovenous concentration Gradient(ACG):** Smaller the ACG value faster will be the onset of action and vice versa .

**Blood – Gas partition coefficient:** Smaller the B/G partition coefficient value faster will be the onset of action and vice versa.

**Anti Parkinsonian Drugs**

- Parkinsonism is a extrapyramidal motor disorder characterised by rigidity, tremor and hyperkinesias
- other secondary effects like dementia, defective posture, mast like face and after several years person enable to breath properly.
- It occurs due to degeneration of neuron in SNPC (substantia nigra pars compacta), dopaminergic tract lead to deficiency of DA(Dopamine) in striatum, therefore activity become dominant.

**Classification**

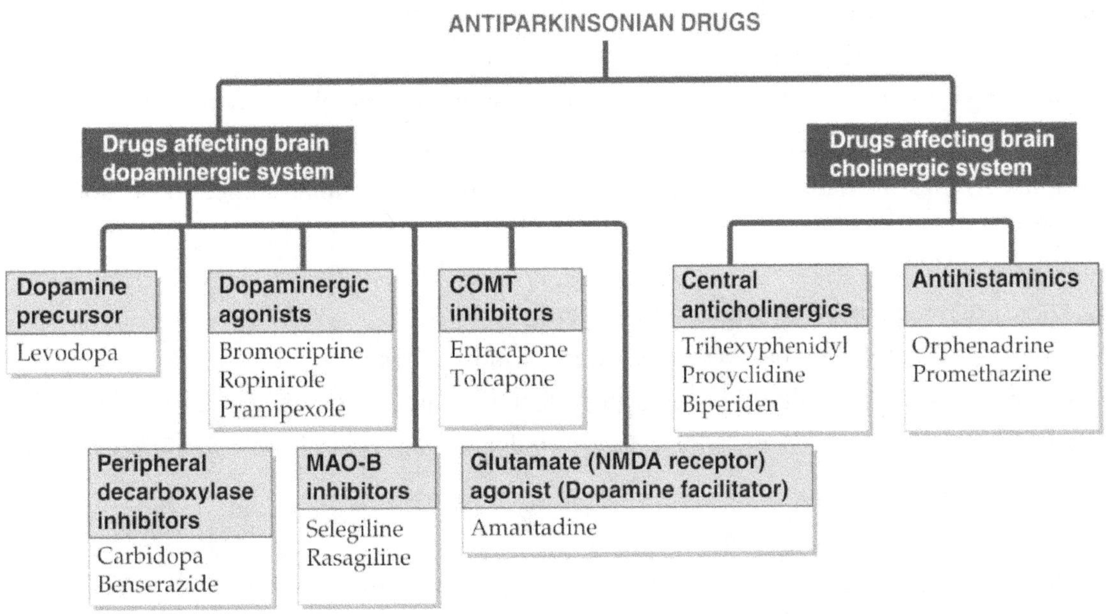


- Parkinson's disease is degeneration neuron in SNPC and it lead to deficiency of DA in striatum.
- Imbalance between dopaminergic (inhibitory) and cholinergic (excitatory) system.
- Oxidation of DA by Mao-B and Aldehyde Dehydrogenase generates hydroxyl free radical (OH) which damage DNA results in neuronal degeneration.

## Metabolic Pathway of Levadopa

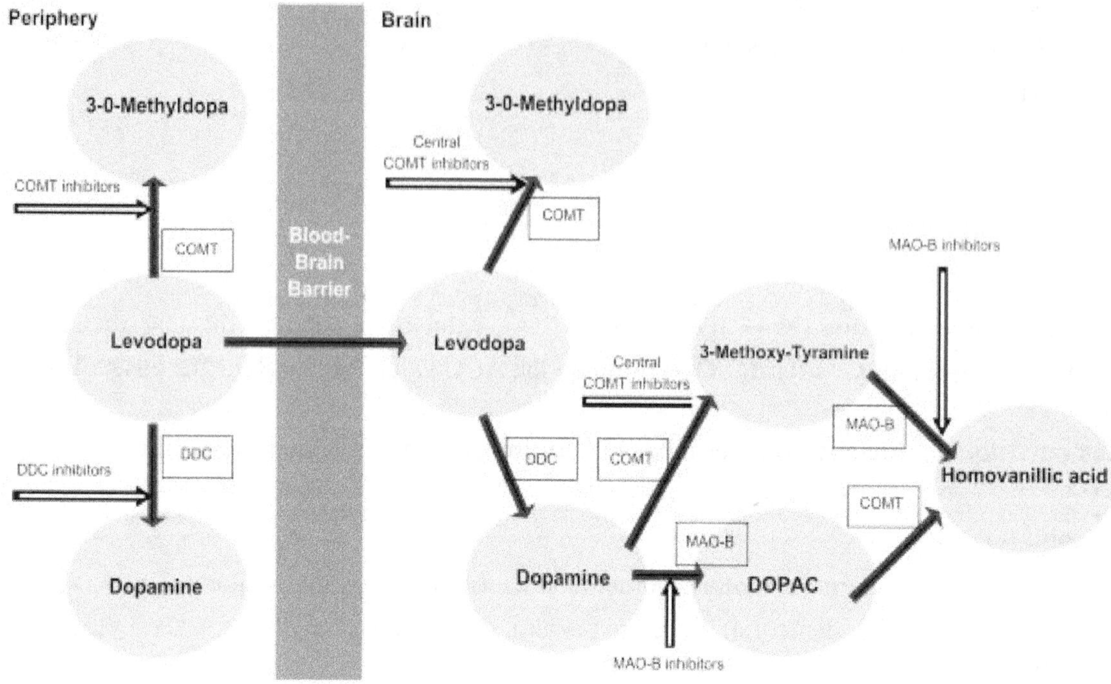


## OPIOD Analgesics/Narcotic Analgesics

- Analgesics- substance that relieves pain
- Narcotic analgesics are drugs that can relief pain without causing narcosis (loss of consciousness)
- Choice of drugs for managing chronic pain as with cancer or RA
- Used as inducing agent (fentanyl) or analgesic supplement with General anesthetics
- They have clinical use as anti-diarrheal and antitussive eg Loperamide and Dextromorphan
- Some opioids such as methadone and buprenorphine are used to counter addiction of more potent opioids such as heroin
  - ➢ Analgesic receptors
    - There are three types in brain and spinal cord
    - μ (mu) --> most widely occurring and target of most drugs
    - K (kappa) --> lack respiratory depressing effect and can counter analgesic effect of μ agonist
    - δ (delta) --> reduced GIT motility, respiratory depression, convulsant effect limited clinical use
    - Only μ and K have clinical use
  - ➢ Mechanism of Action
    - Opiod analgesic agonize opiod receptors μ,κ and δ which are G-protein couples receptors. This leads to a series of event which ultimately block neuronal pain transmission by:
      1. Inhibition of activation of voltage gated Ca+2 channels which depresses NT release
      2. Increases K+ conductance outside the cell to cause hyper polarization of cell thus reducing it's excitability
      3. Inhibtion of adenyl cyclase (adenyl cyclase--> cAMP --> PKA --> phosphorylation of ion channels --> increase chances of channel opening)

**Classification**

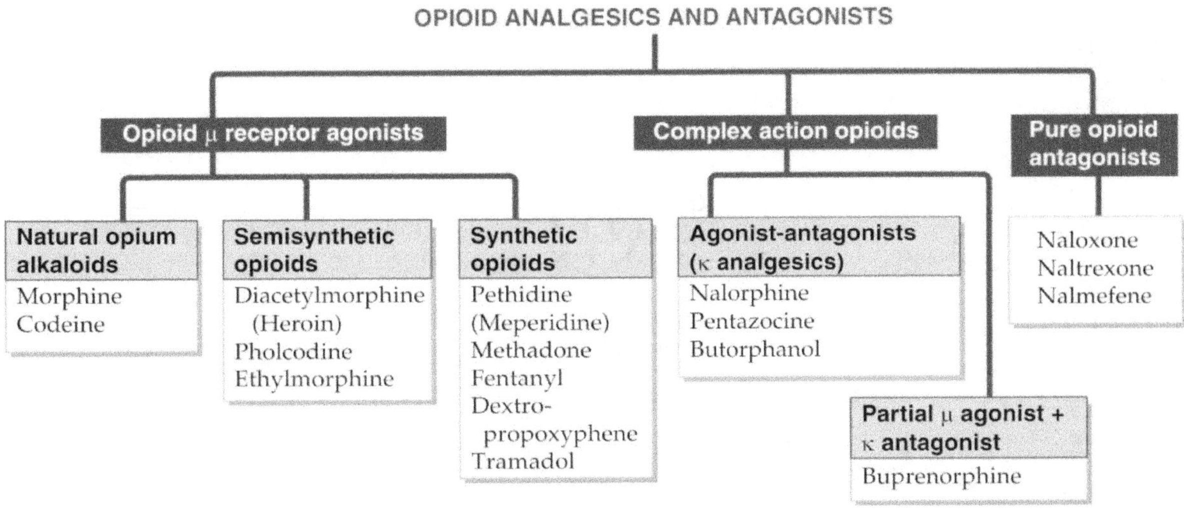


***SAR of Morphine***

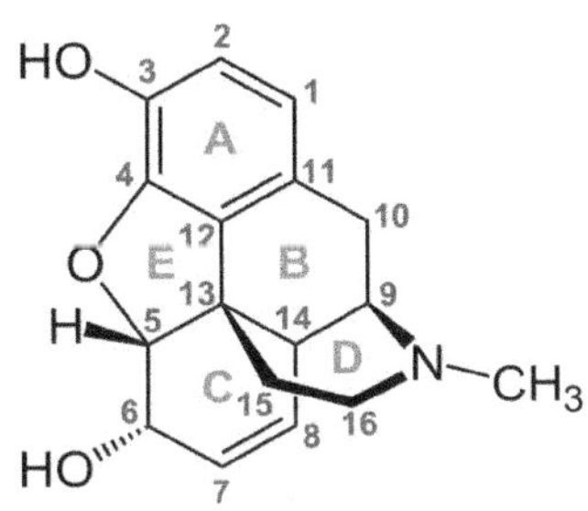


(i) Morphine has 5 Chiral centers. Only the Levo (-) rotatory isomer is active

(ii) The OH group in the phenolic ring and basic Nitrogen is needed for activity and seen in all potent μ agonist. Activity can be preserved or enhanced by removing other rings changing -OH to just –H or -OCH3 lowers activity as seen with codeine.

(iii) The Nitrogen is mostly tertiary with a methyl substitution in morphine. The size of substituent on Nitrogen dictates potency and agonist or antagonist activity.

  (a) Increasing size from methyl (ie 1 C) to 3 or 5 carbon (especially with double bonds or

  (b) small cyclic/aromatic rings) results in antagonist activity

  (c) Still larger substitution restores agonist activity in more potent form

  - If R = 3-5 carbons then μ antagonist effect (more valid if presence of double bond or Small carbocyclic ring)
  - If R = > 5 carbon (in chain or ring) then increased μ agonist effect

(iv) Reduction of 7, 8 double bond increases activity.

(v) Inclusion of Hydroxyl group at 14 increases activity.

(vi) Removal of Hydroxyl at 6 increases activity

(vii) Oxidation of Hydroxyl to keto group at 6 increases activity, if there is also reduction of 7,8 double bond eg hydrocodone

(viii) Acetylation of Hydroxyl at 6 increases activity

(ix) Removal of the ether linkage produces compounds called morphinans that has increases activity

### OPIOD Analgesics Structures

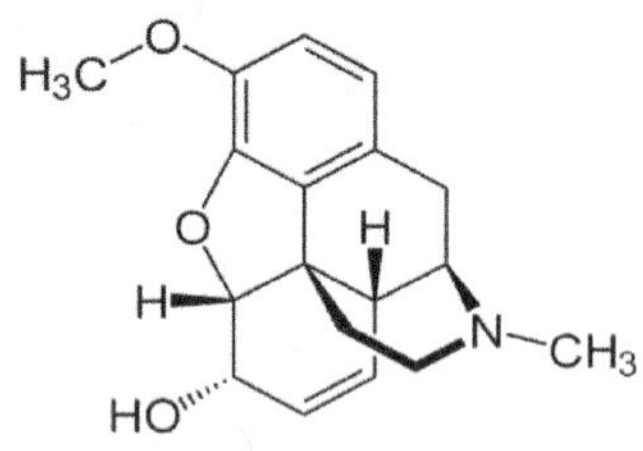

**Codiene**

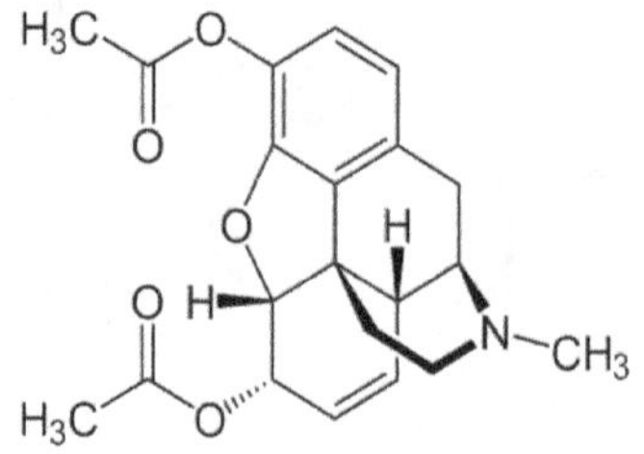

**Heroine**

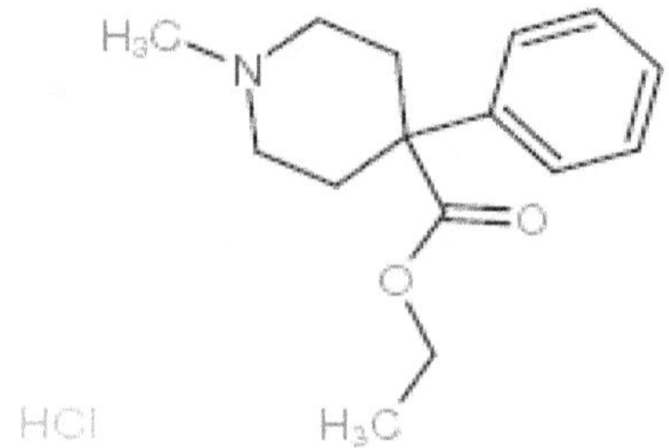

**Meperidine**

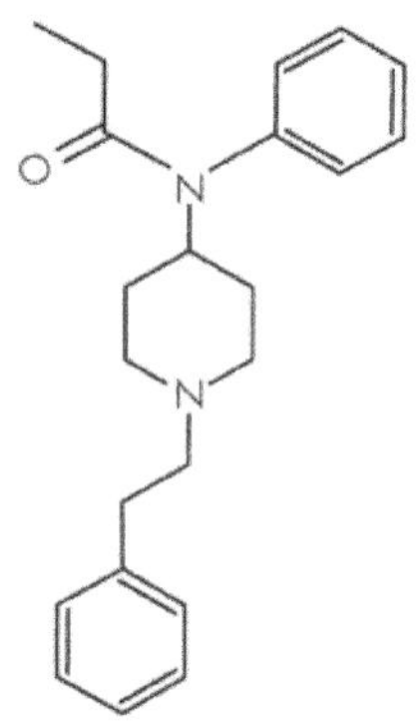

**Fentanyl**

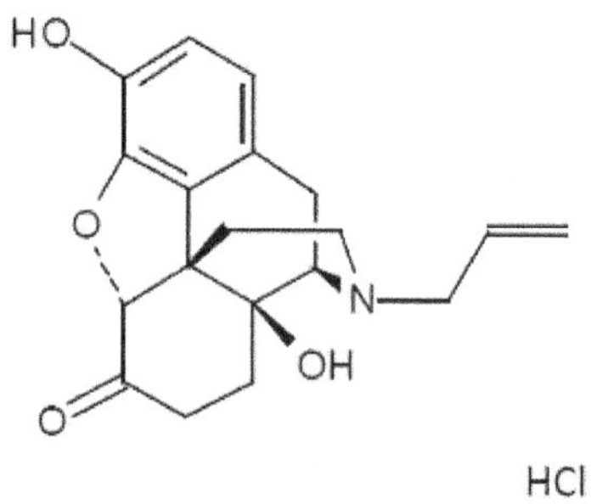

**Buprenorphine**

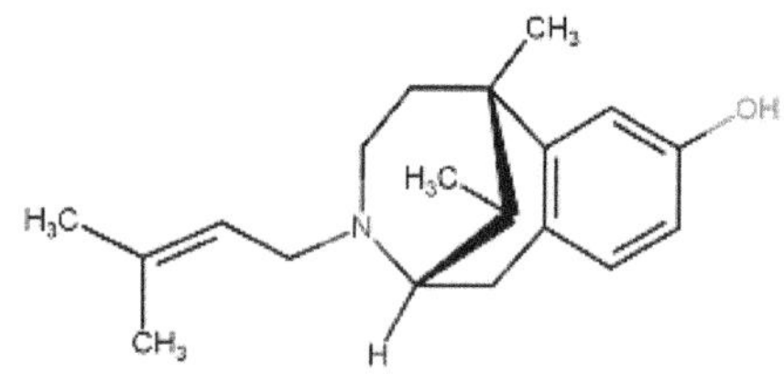

**Pentazocine**

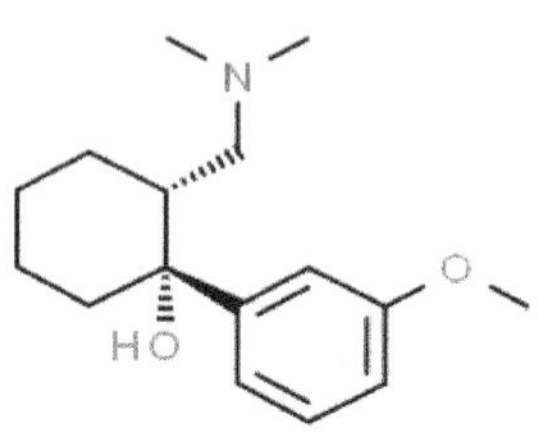

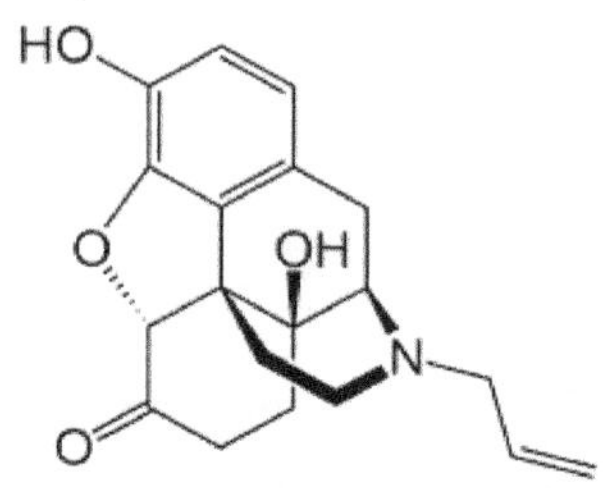

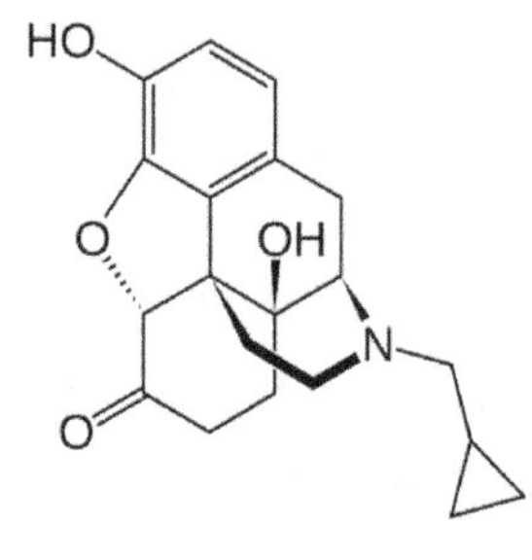

## 2.4 Antimicrobial Drugs

Drugs in this class differ from all others in that they are designed to inhibit/kill the infecting organism and to have no/minimal effect on the recipient. This type of therapy is generally called ***chemotherapy*** which has come to mean 'treatment of systemic infections with specific drugs that selectively suppress the infecting microorganism without significantly affecting the host.' The basis of selective microbial toxicity is the action of the drug on a component of the microbe (e.g. bacterial cell wall) or metabolic processes (e.g. folate synthesis) that is not found in the host, or high affinity for certain microbial biomolecules (e.g. trimethoprim for bacterial di hydrofolate reductase). Due to analogy between the malignant cell and the pathogenic microbes, treatment of neoplastic diseases with drugs is also called **'chemotherapy'**.

## Antibacterial Drugs

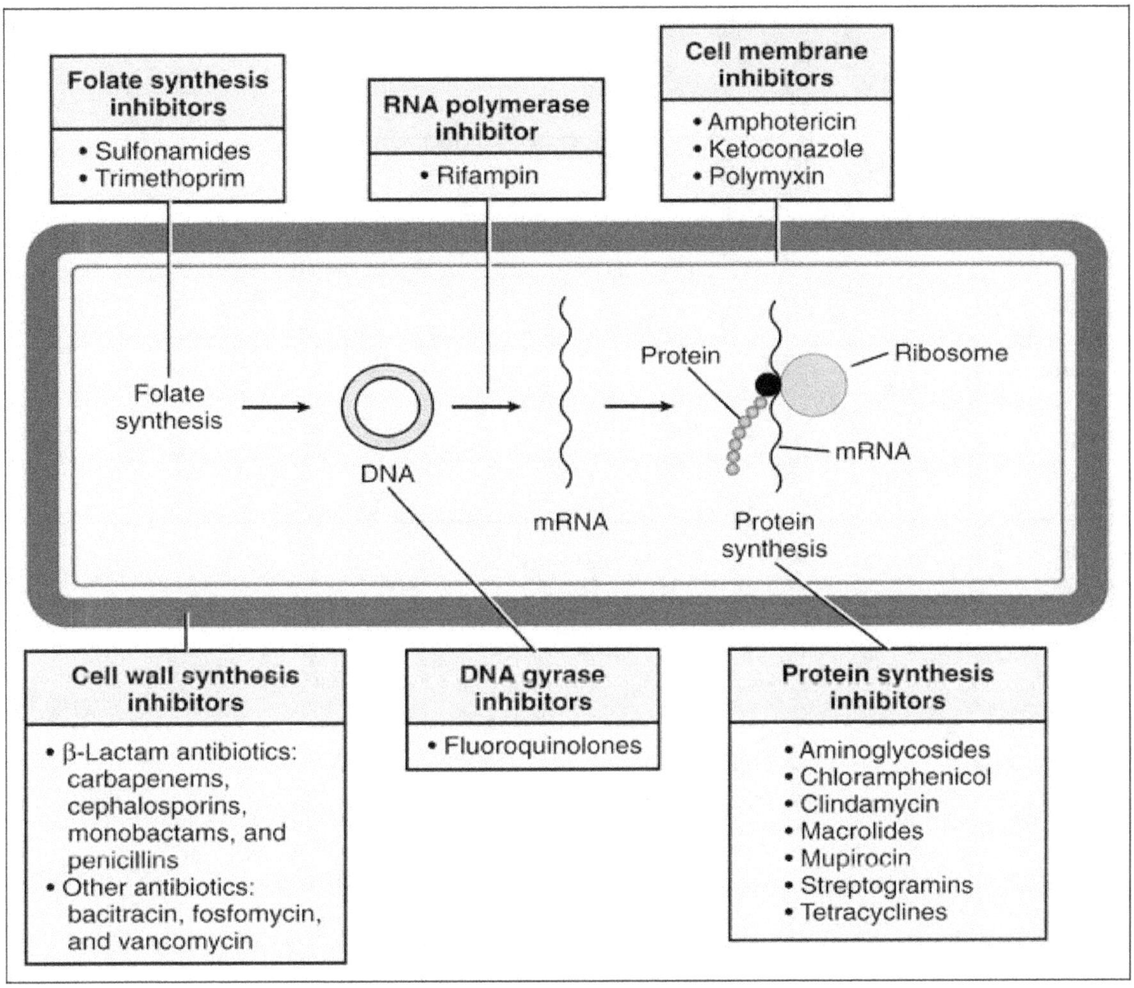


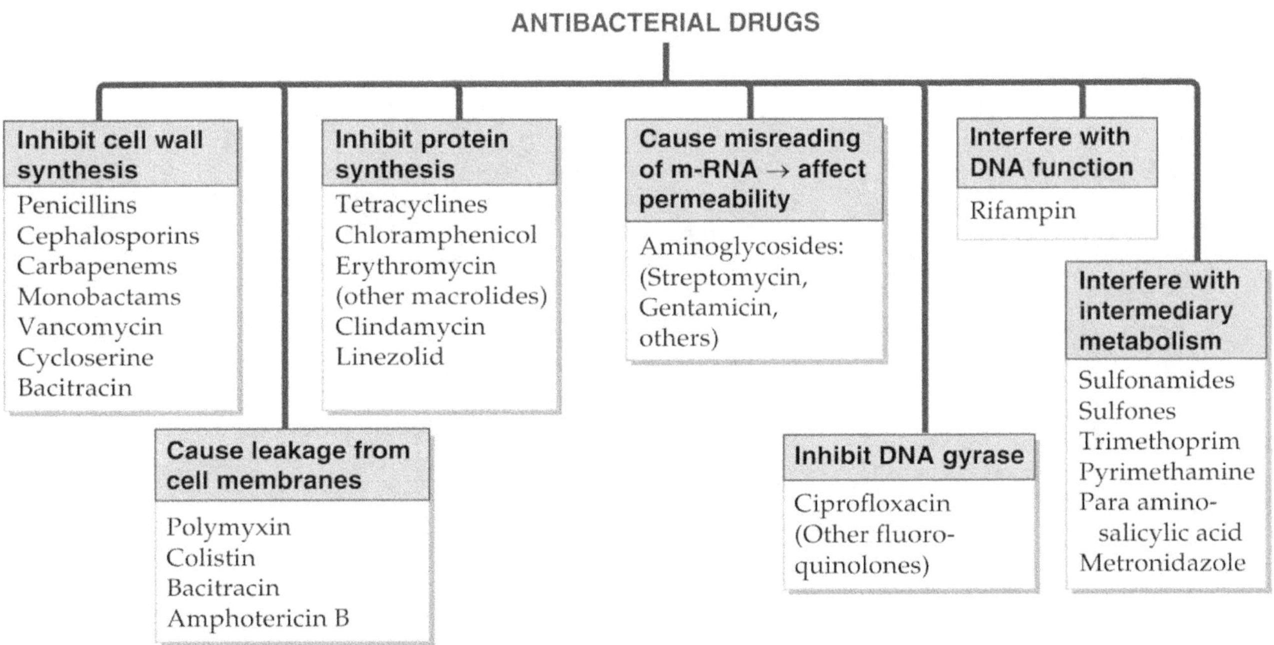

| | |
|---|---|
| Penicilline | 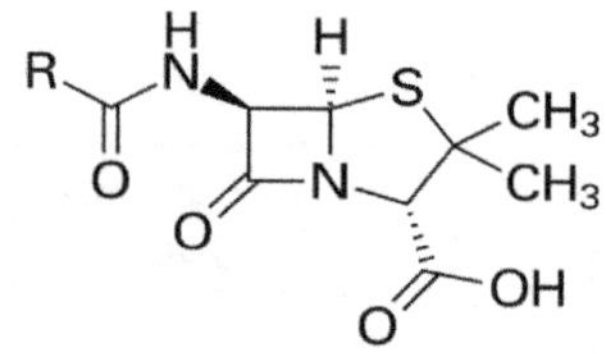 |
| Cephalosporin | 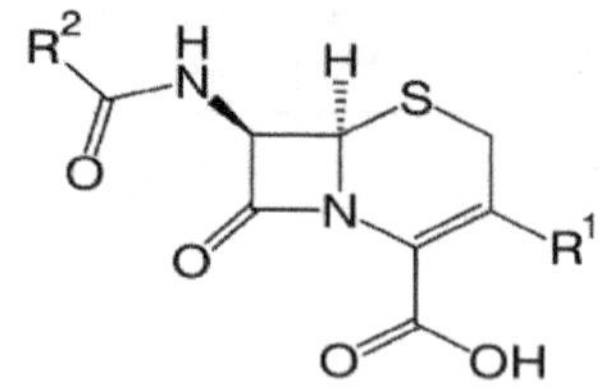 |
| Carbapenem | 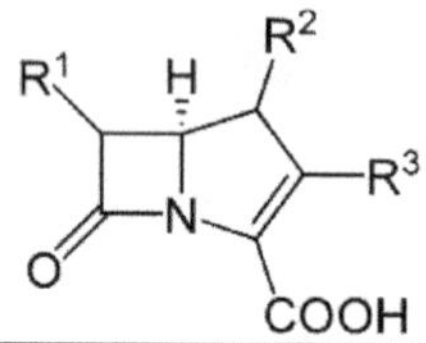 |
| Polymyxin | 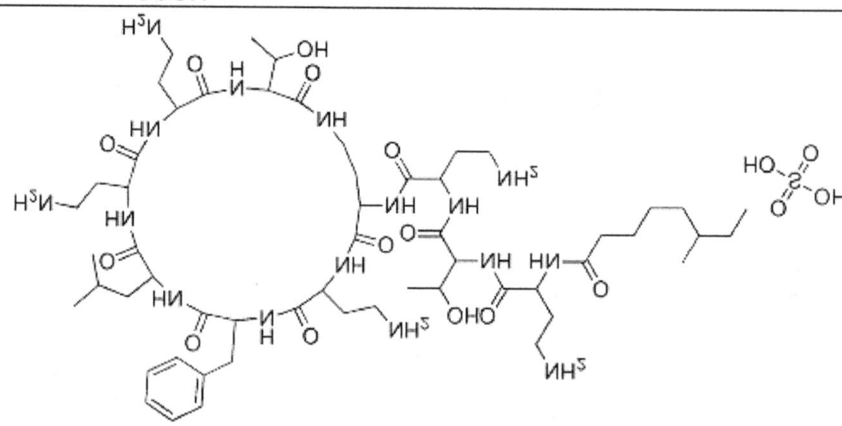 |
| Colistin | 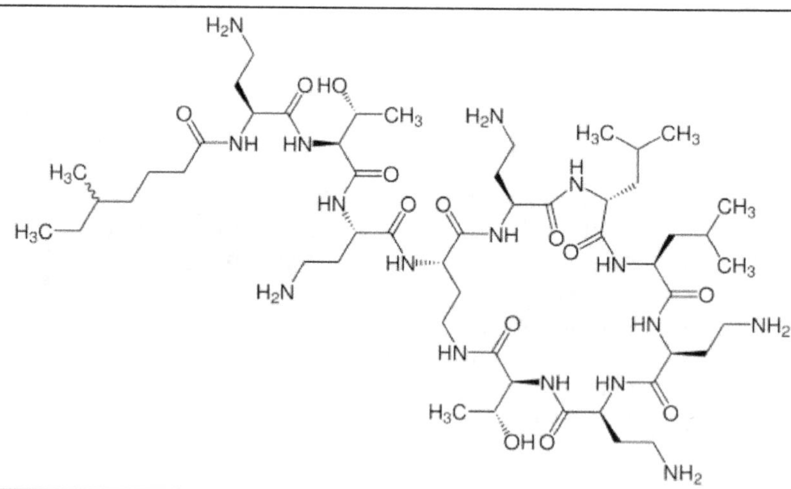 |

**Table** *Contd...*

| | |
|---|---|
| Amphotericin B | 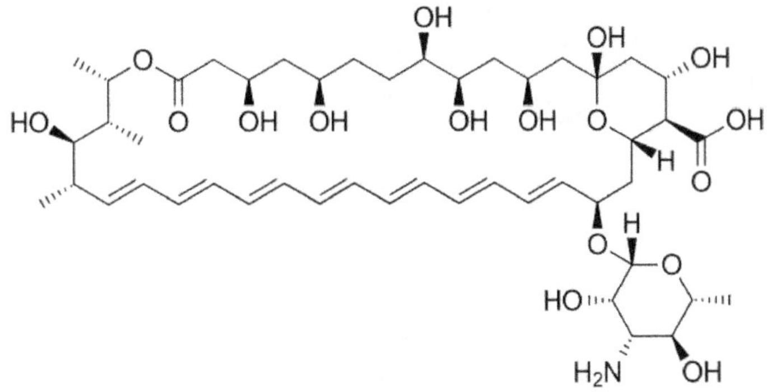 |
| Tetracycline | 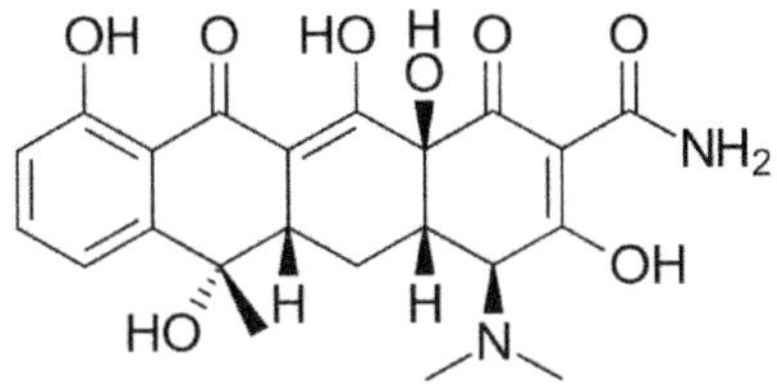 |
| Erythromycin | 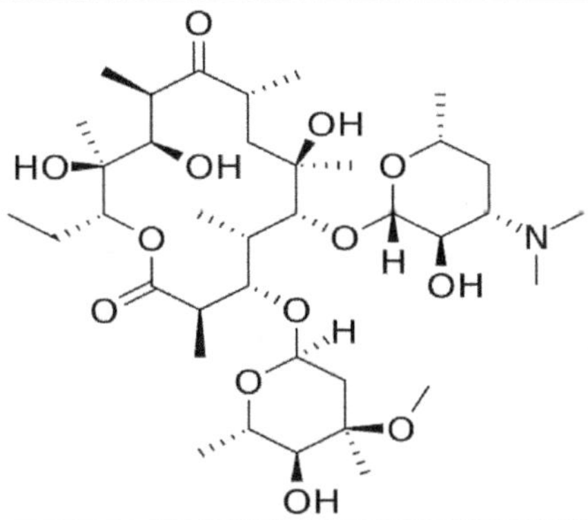 |
| Aminoglycoside | 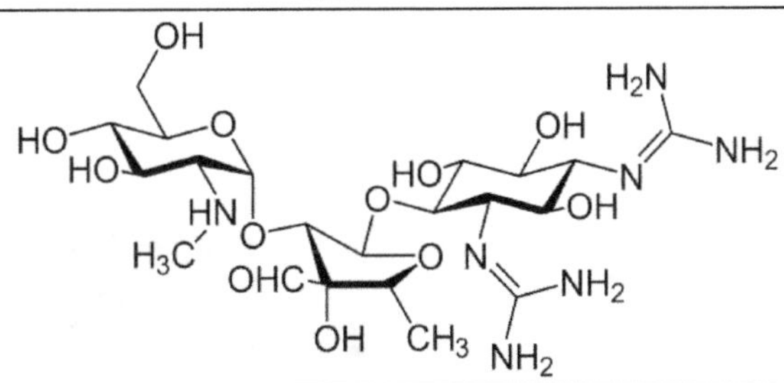 |
| Ciprofloxacin | 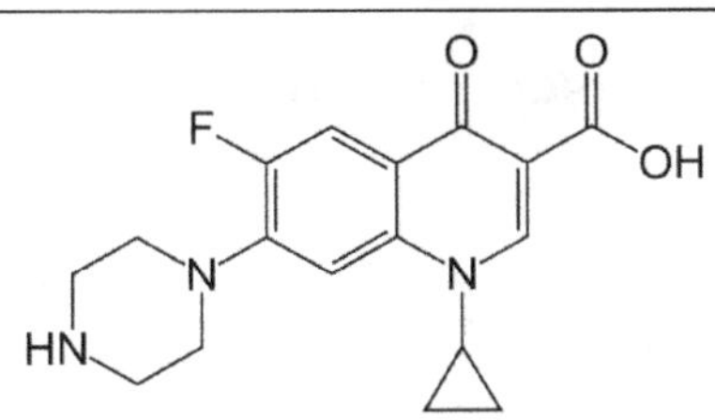 |

**Table** *Contd...*

| | |
|---|---|
| Rifampicin | 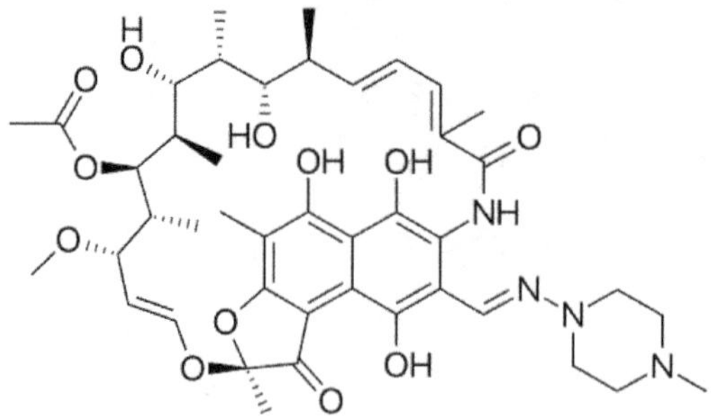 |
| Sulfonamide | 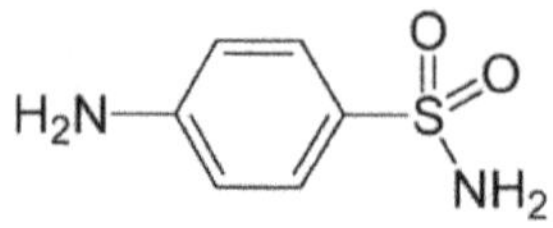 |
| Metronidazole | 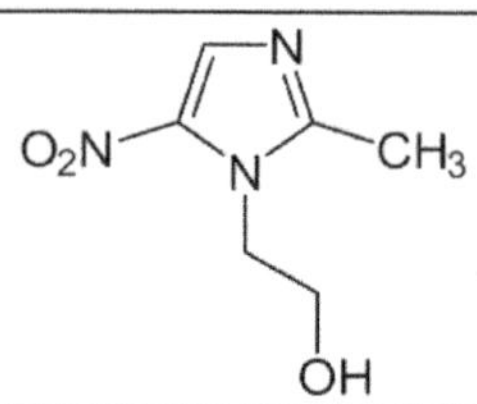 |

### SULFONAMIDES

- **Short acting**
  - Sulfadiazine
- **Intermediate acting**
  - Sulfamethoxazole
- **Long acting**
  - Sulfadoxine
  - Sulfamethopyrazine
- **Special purpose**
  - Sulfacetamide sod.
  - Sulfasalazine
  - Silver sulfadiazine
  - Mafenide

### QUINOLONE ANTIMICROBIALS

- **Nonfluorinated quinolone**
  - Nalidixic acid
- **Fluoroquinolones**
  - **First generation**
    - Norfloxacin
    - Ciprofloxacin
    - Ofloxacin
    - Pefloxacin
  - **Second generation**
    - Levofloxacin
    - Moxifloxacin
    - Gemifloxacin
    - Prulifloxacin
    - Lomefloxacin
    - Sparfloxacin

| | |
|---|---|
| Sulfadiazine | 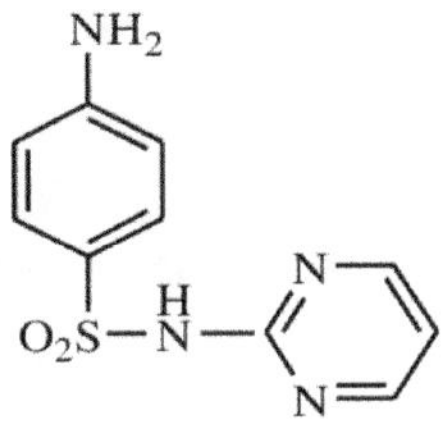 |
| Sulfamethoxazole | 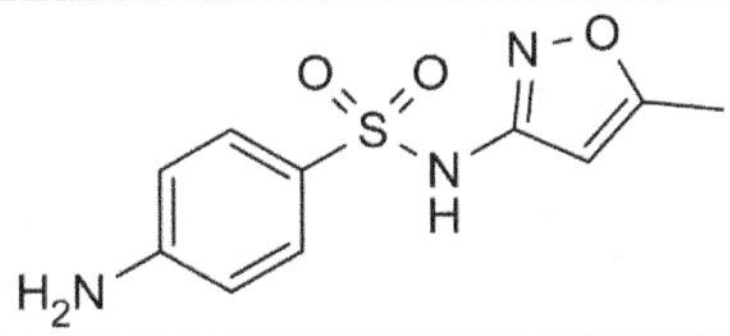 |
| Sulfadoxine | 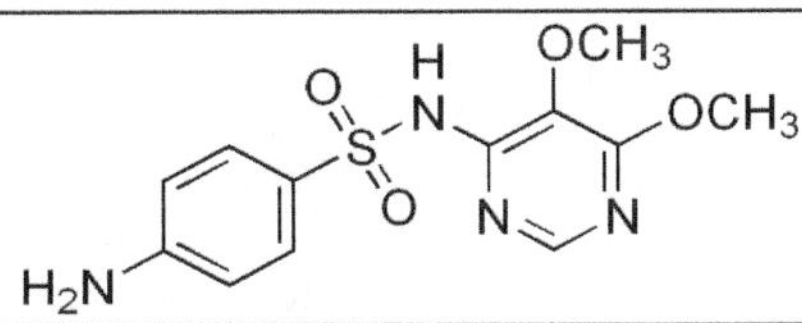 |
| Sulfasalazine | 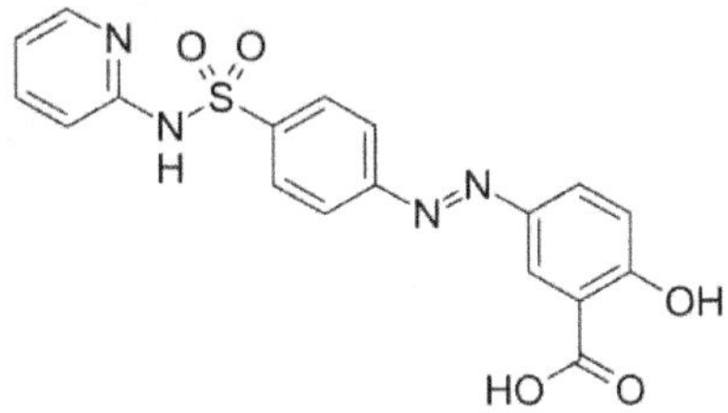 |
| Mafenide | 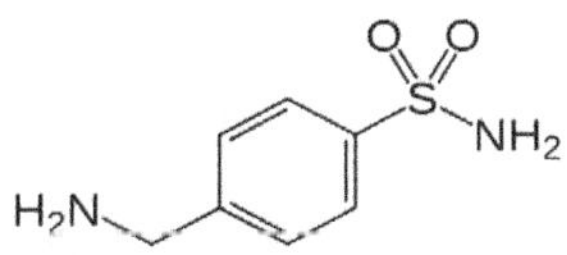 |
| Nalidixic acid | 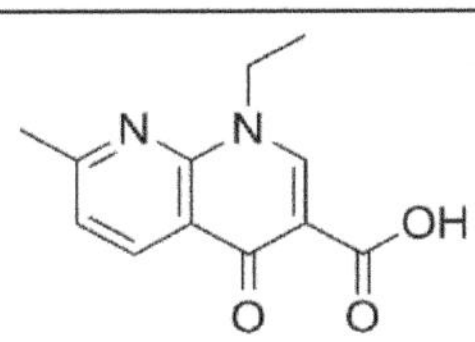 |
| Norfloxacin | 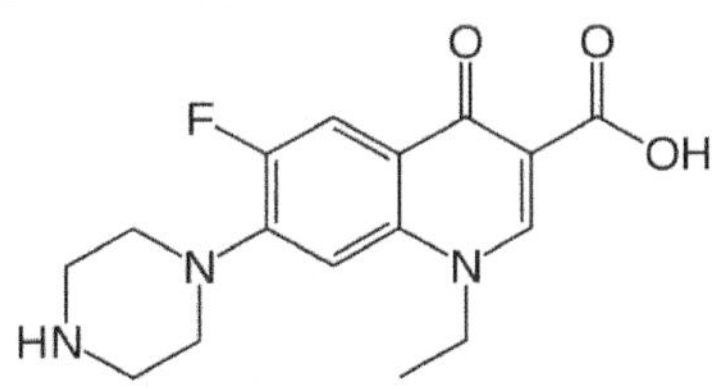 |
| Levofloxacin | 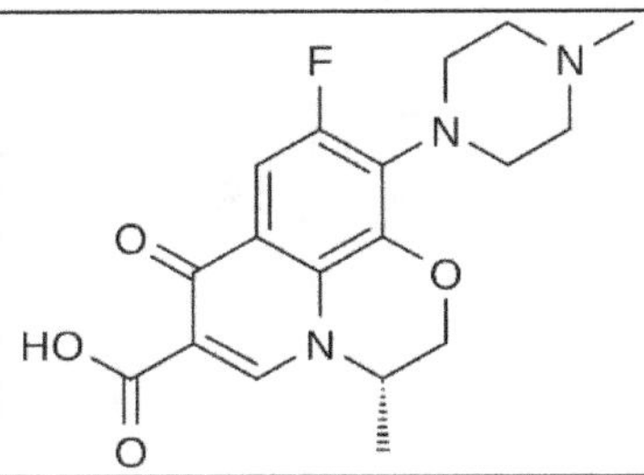 |

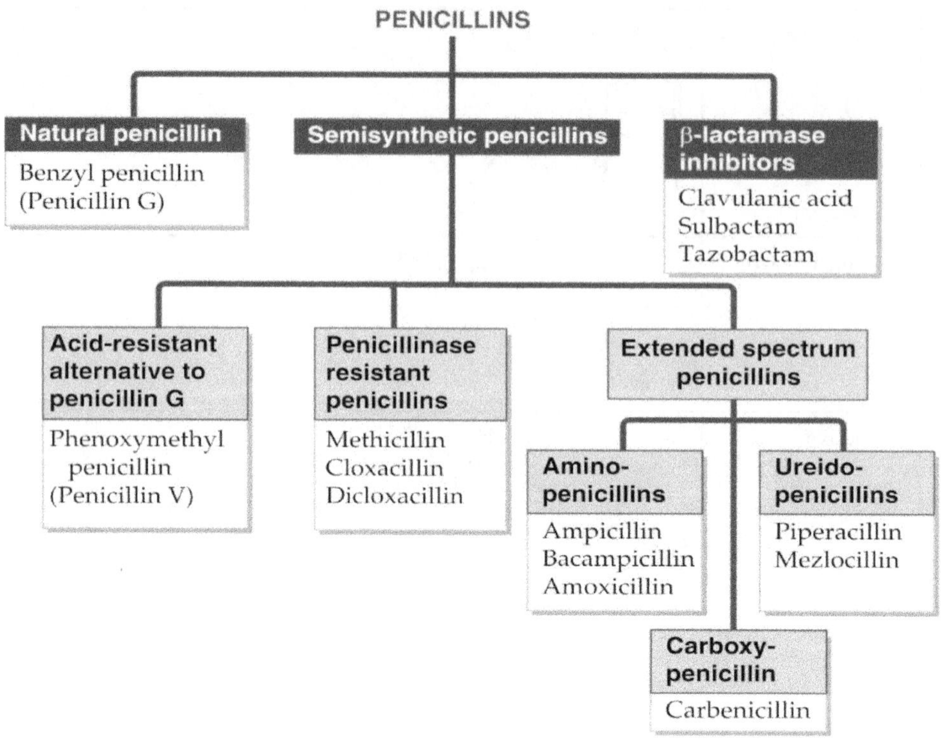


| Penicillin-G | 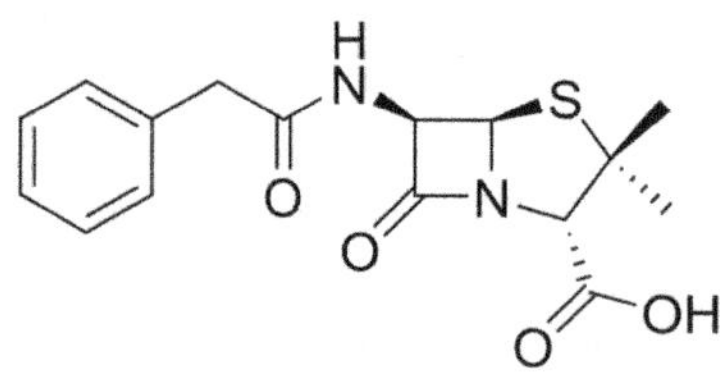 |
|---|---|
| Phenoxymethylpenicillin | 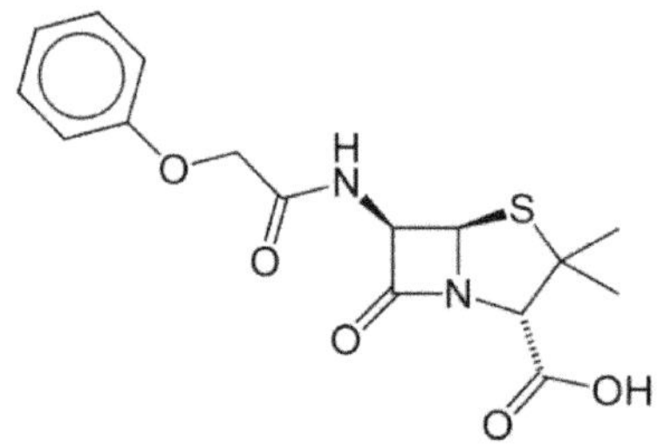 |
| Cloxacillin | 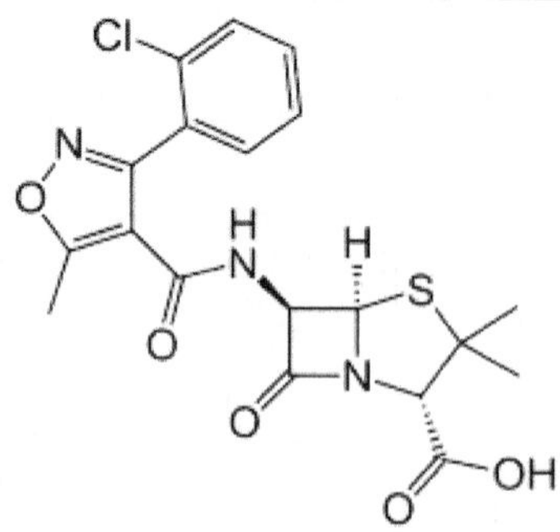 |

**Table** *Contd...*

| | |
|---|---|
| Saulbactum | 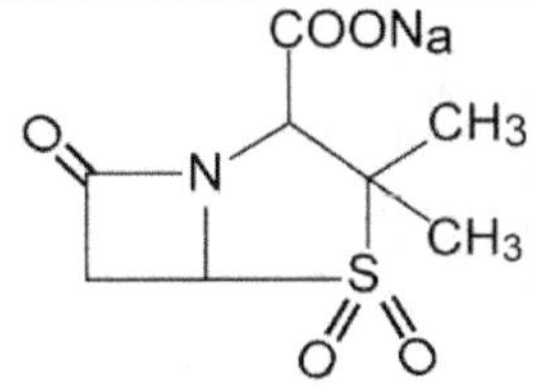 |
| Ampicillin | 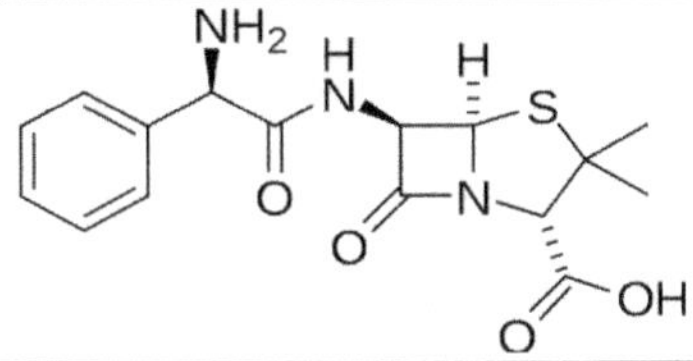 |
| Carbenicillin | 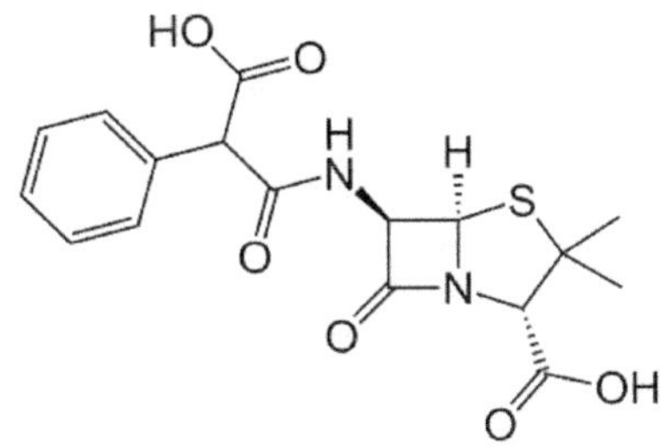 |

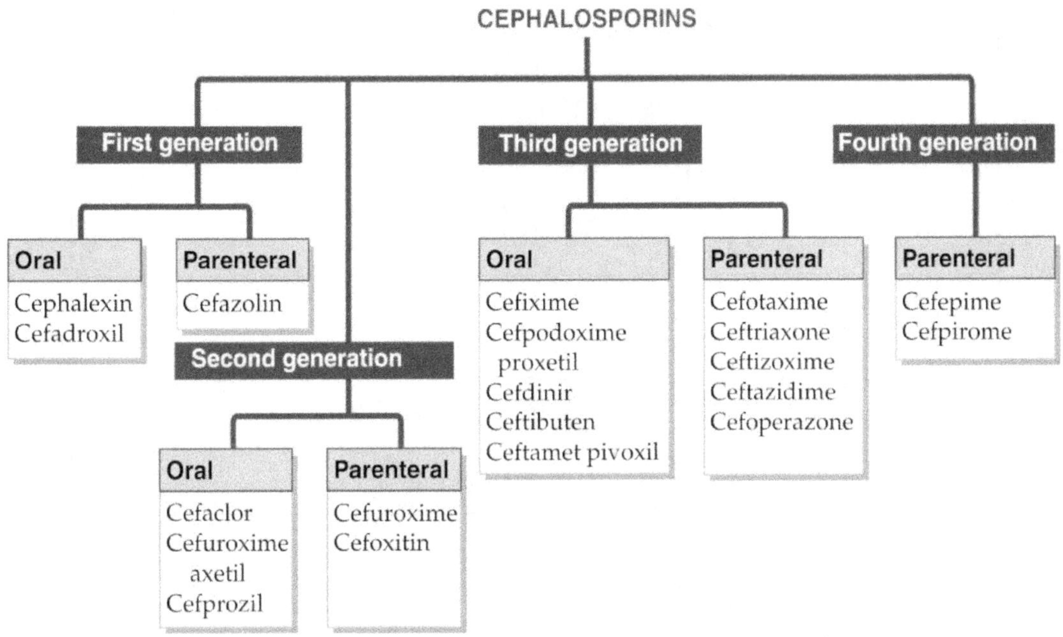


| | |
|---|---|
| Cefalexin | 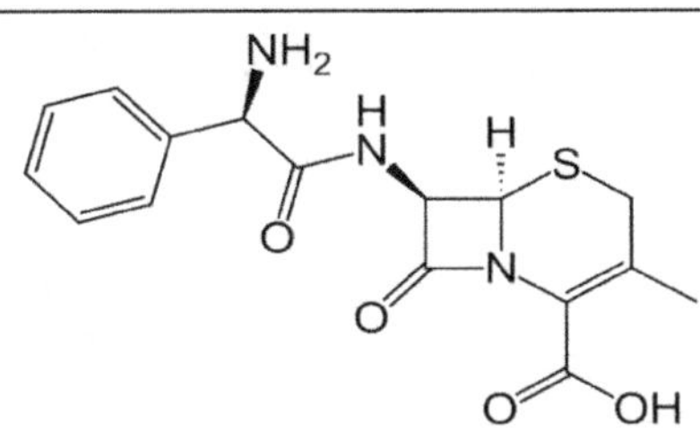 |

**Table** *Contd...*

| | |
|---|---|
| Cefezoline | 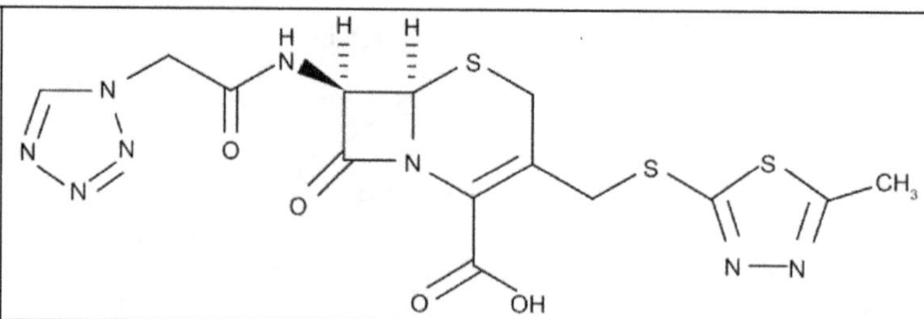 |
| Cefaclor | 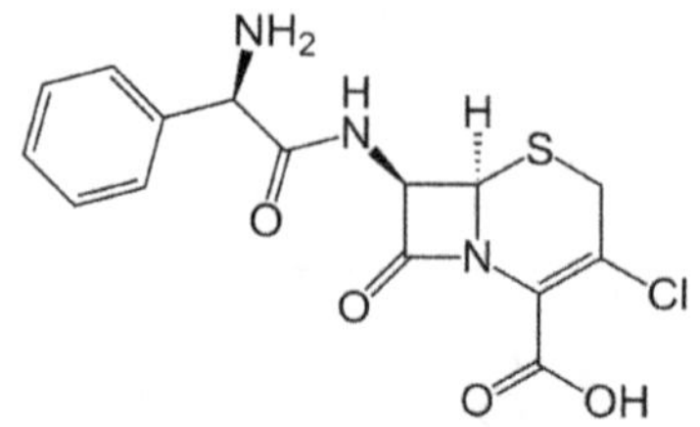 |
| Cefoxitin | 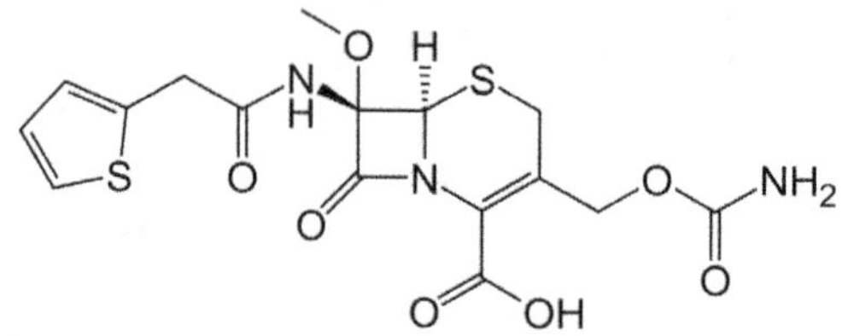 |
| Cefixime | 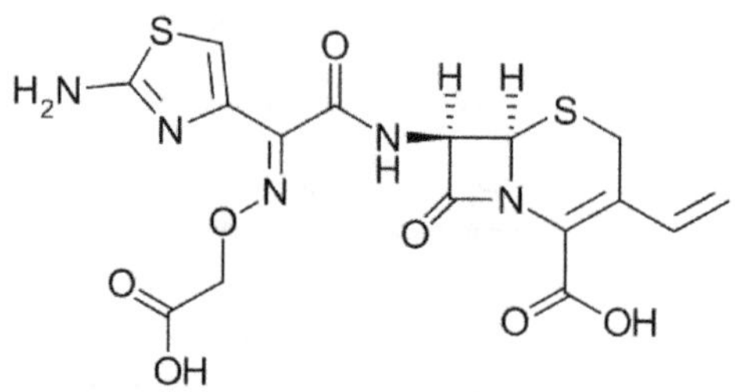 |
| Cefdinir | 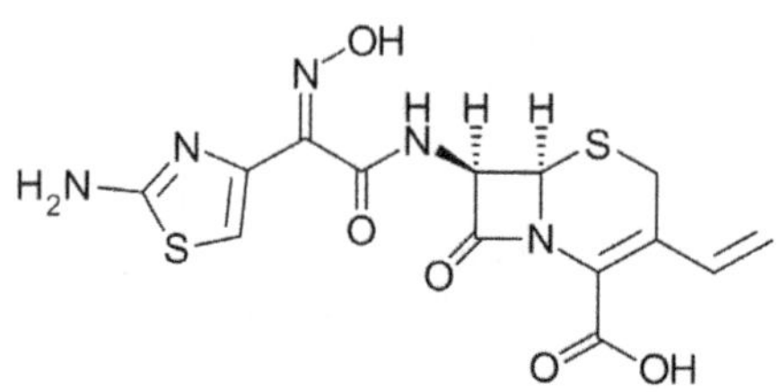 |
| Cefotaxime | 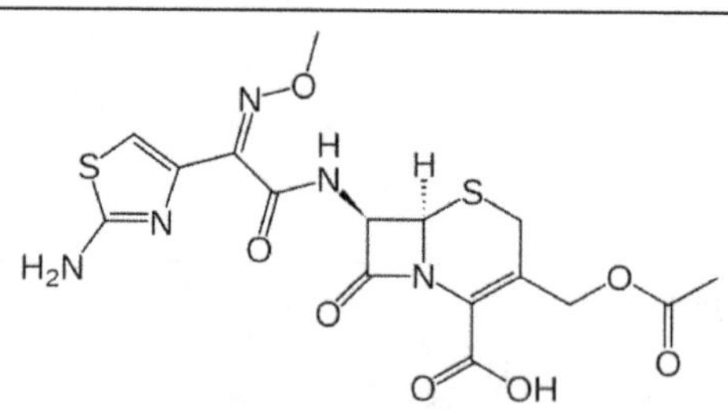 |
| Cefepime | 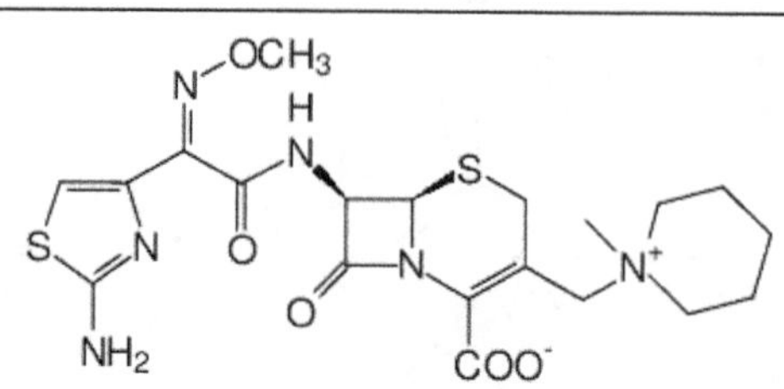 |

**ANTITUBERCULAR DRUGS**

- **First line drugs**
  - Isoniazid
  - Rifampin
  - Pyrazinamide
  - Ethambutol
  - Streptomycin
- **Second line drugs**
  - **Fluoroquinolones**
    - Ofloxacin
    - Levofloxacin
    - Moxifloxacin
    - Ciprofloxacin
  - **Other oral drugs**
    - Ethionamide
    - Prothionamide
    - Cycloserine
    - Terizidone
    - Paraamino-salicylic acid (PAS)
    - Rifabutin
    - Thiacetazone
  - **Injectable drugs**
    - Kanamycin
    - Amikacin
    - Capreomycin

| | |
|---|---|
| Isoniazid | 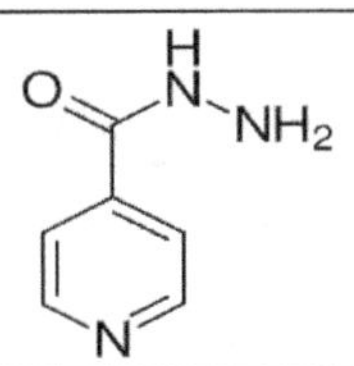 |
| Ethambutol | 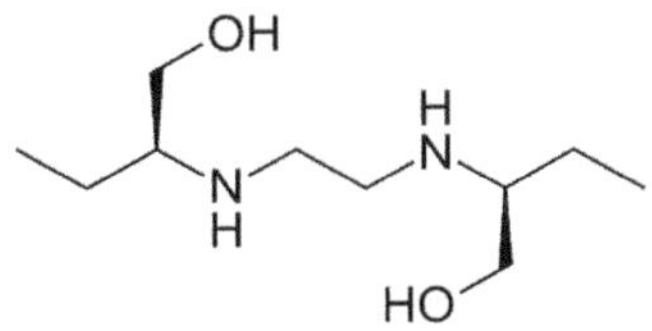 |
| Rifampicin | 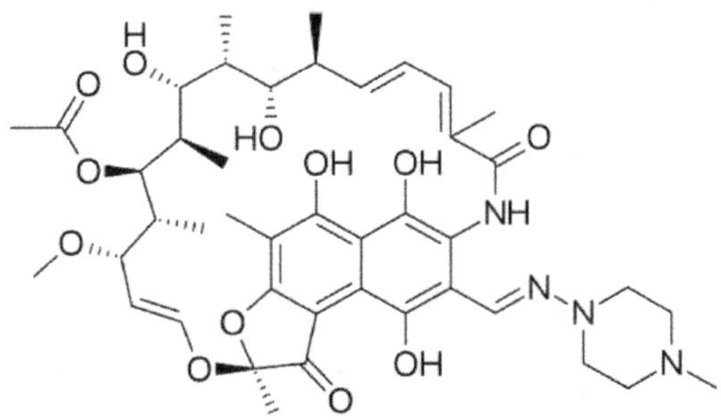 |
| Oflaxacine | 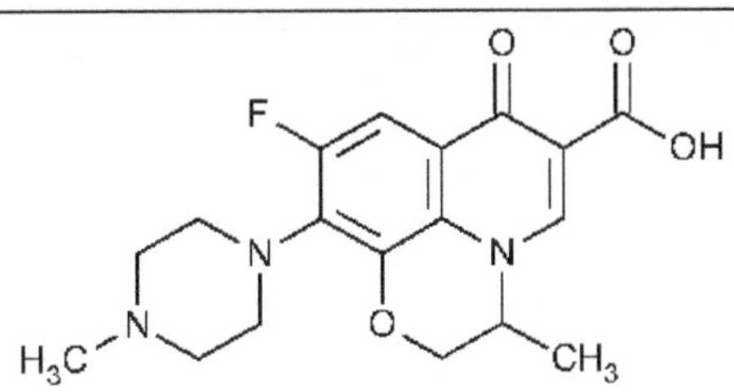 |
| Ciprofloxacin | 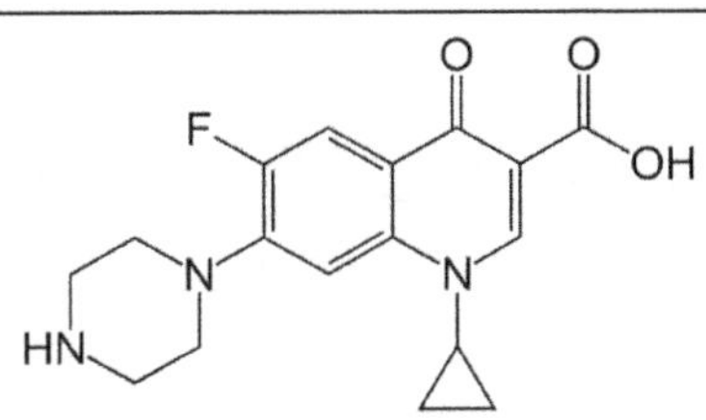 |

**Table** *Contd...*

| | |
|---|---|
| Rifabutin | 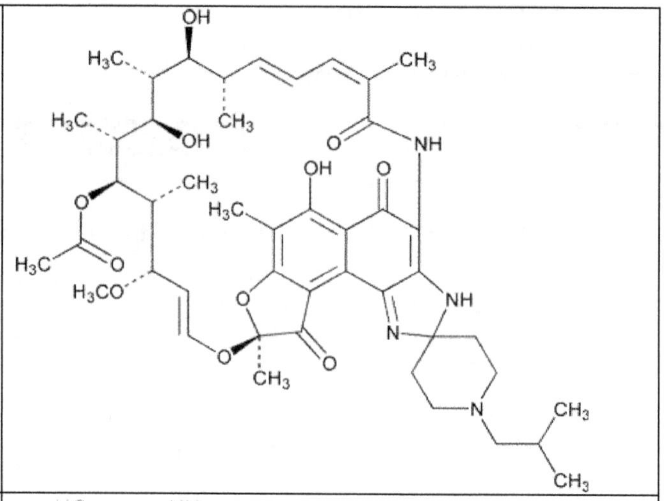 |
| Amikacin | 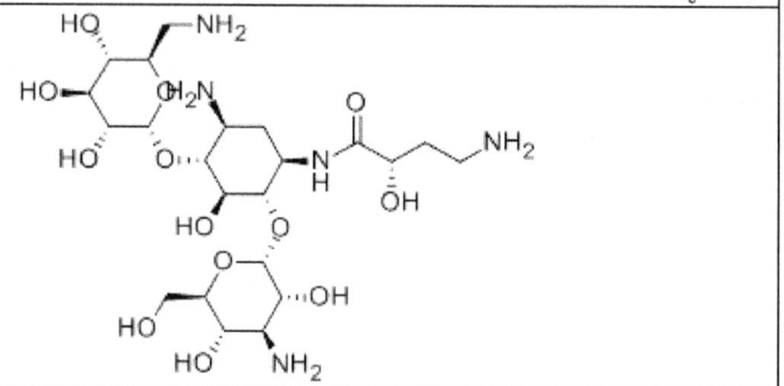 |
| Kanamycin | 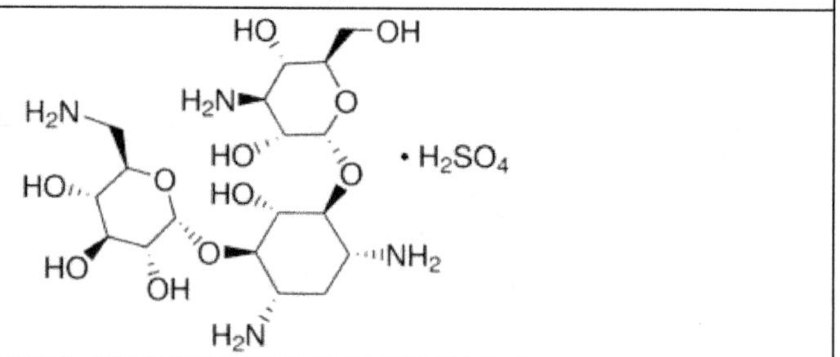 |

ANTIFUNGAL DRUGS

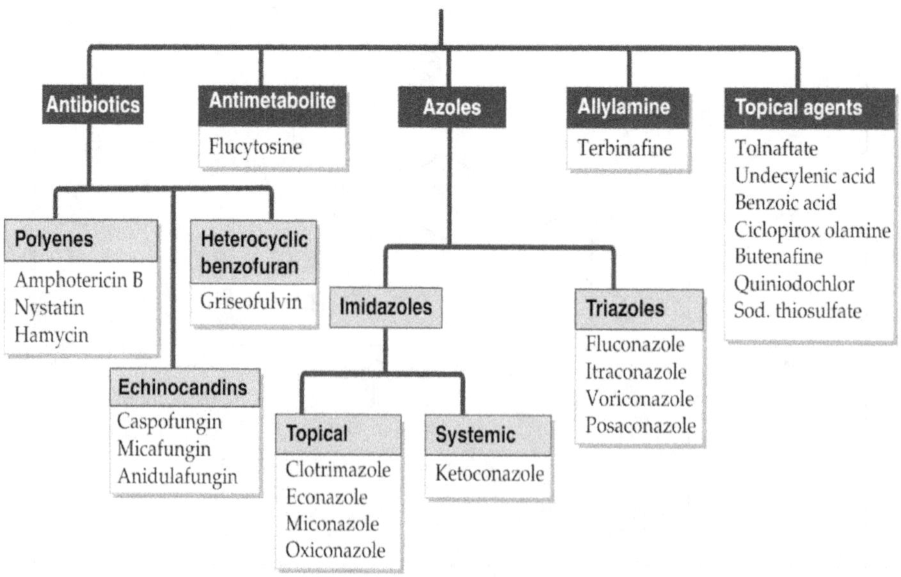

| | |
|---|---|
| Nystatin | 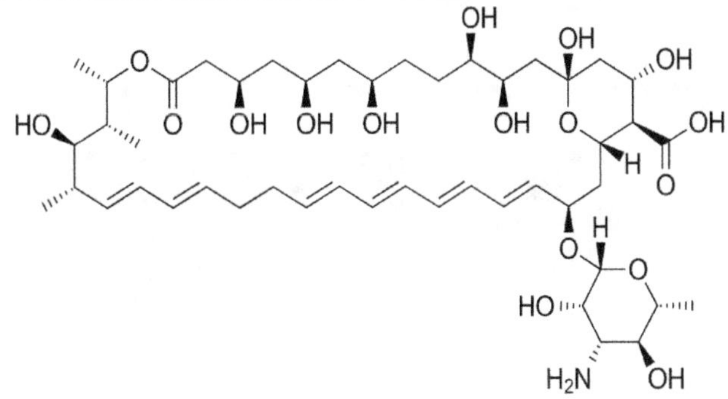 |
| Griseofulvin | 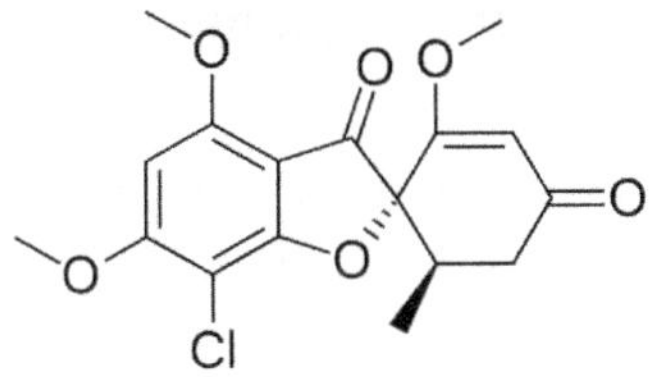 |
| Flucytocin | 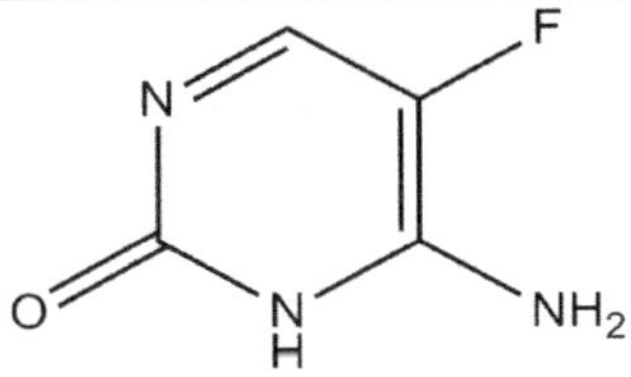 |
| Clotrimazole | 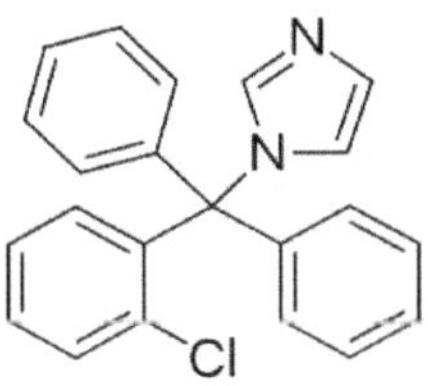 |
| Ketoconazole | 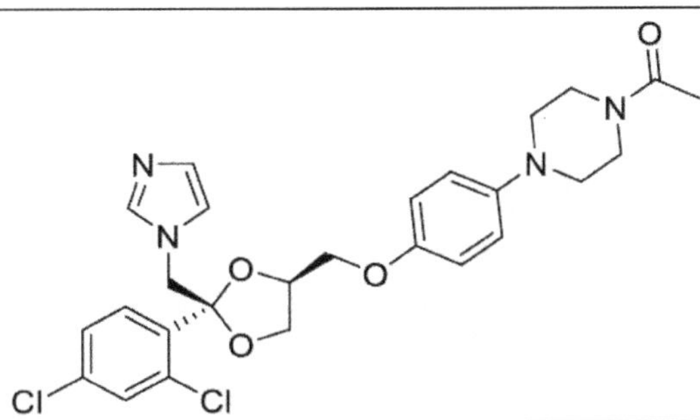 |
| Fluconazole | 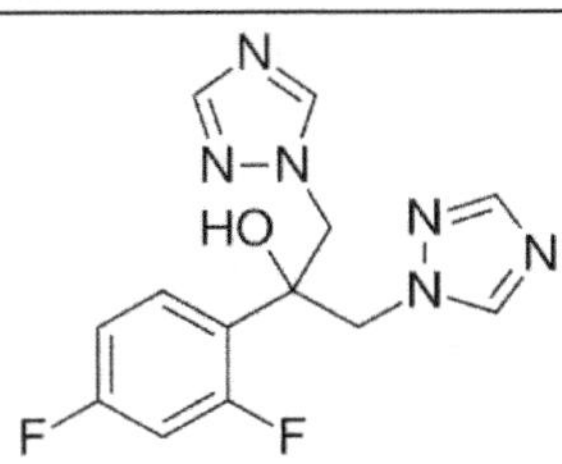 |
| Benzoic acid | 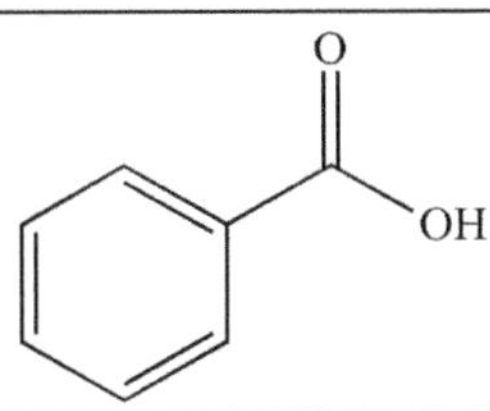 |

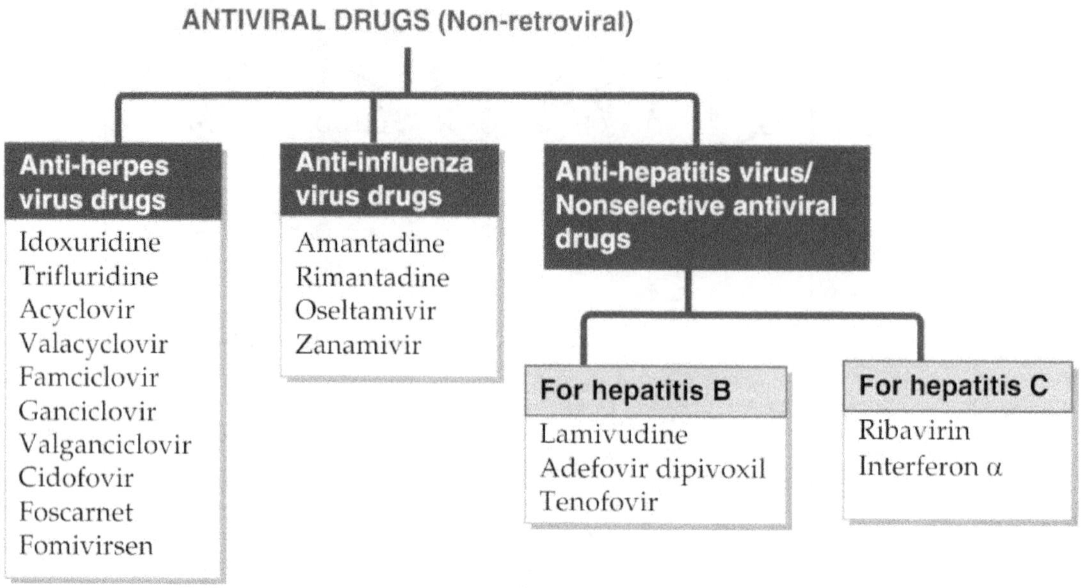


| | |
|---|---|
| Acyclovir | 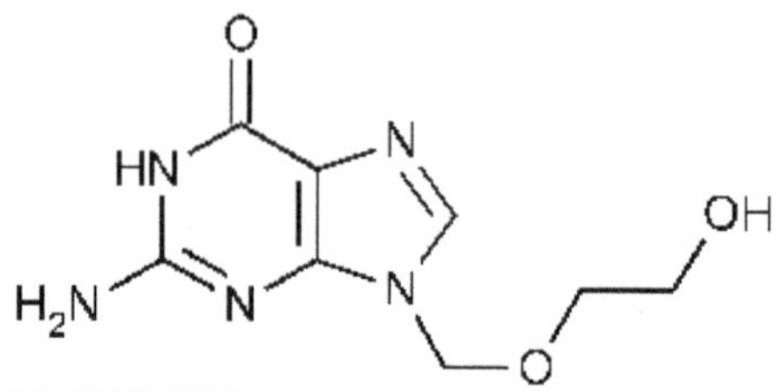 |
| Idoxuridine | 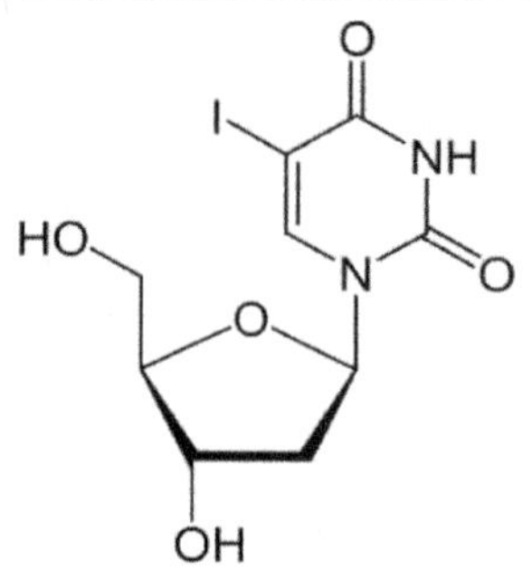 |
| Ganciclovir | 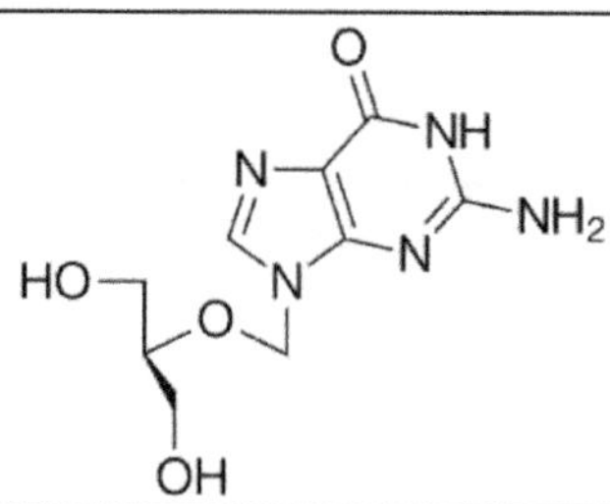 |
| Amantadine | 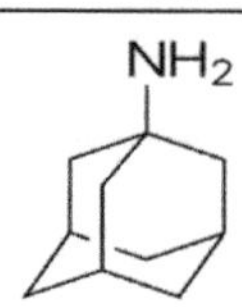 |

**Table** *Contd...*

| | |
|---|---|
| Rimantadine | 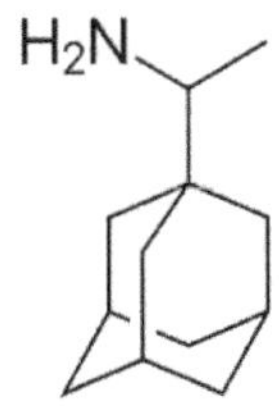 |
| Lamivudine | 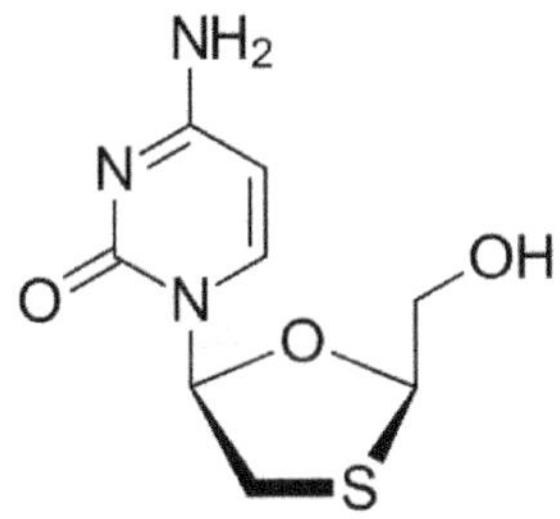 |
| Ribavirin | 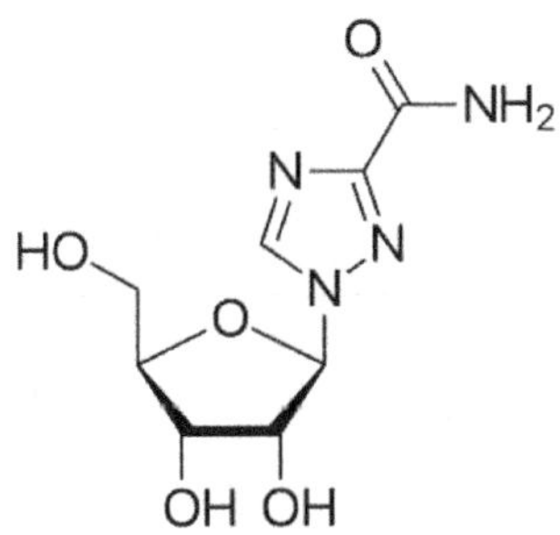 |

## ANTIRETROVIRUS DRUGS

**Nucleoside reverse transcriptase inhibitors (NRTIs)**
- Zidovudine
- Didanosine
- Stavudine
- Lamivudine
- Abacavir
- Emtricitabine
- Tenofovir

**Non-nucleoside reverse transcriptase inhibitors (NNRTIs)**
- Nevirapine
- Efavirenz
- Delavirdine

**Protease inhibitors (PIs)**
- Ritonavir
- Atazanavir
- Indinavir
- Nelfinavir
- Saquinavir
- Amprenavir
- Lopinavir

**Entry inhibitor**
- Enfuvirtide

**CCR-5 receptor inhibitor**
- Maraviroc

**Integrase inhibitor**
- Raltegravir

| Zidovudine | 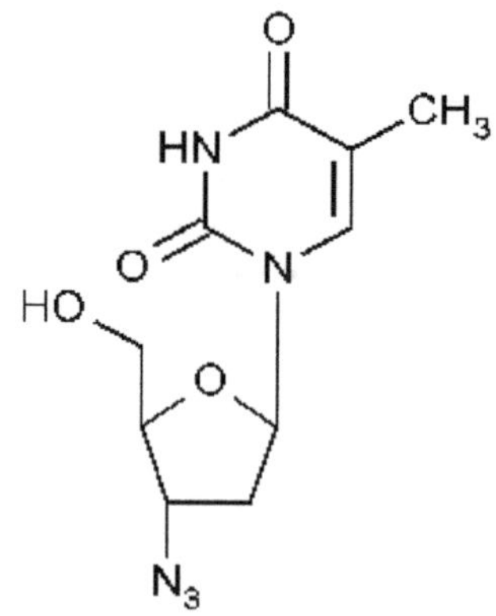 |
|---|---|
| Efavirenz | 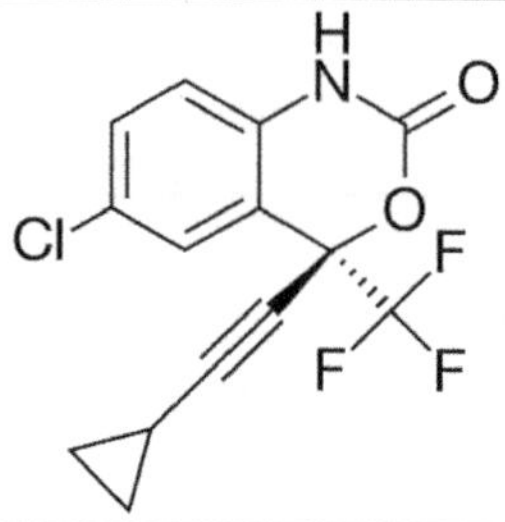 |
| Ritonavir | 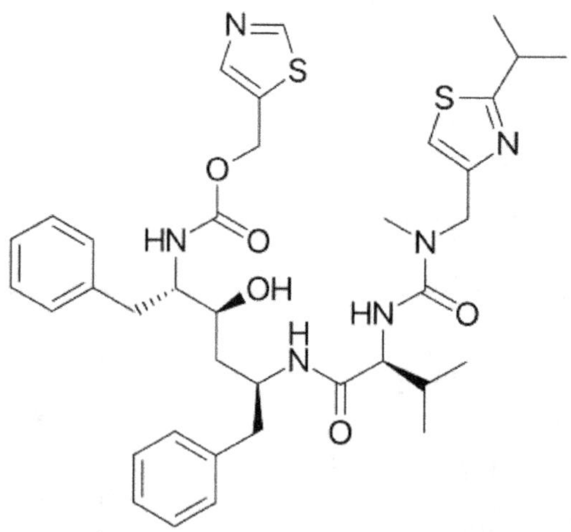 |
| Raltegravir | 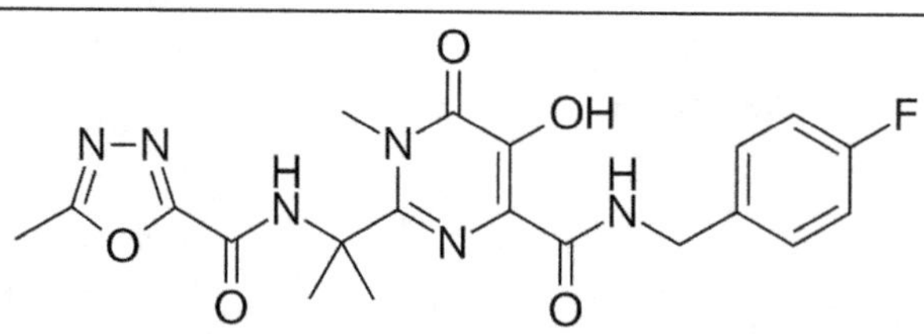 |
| Maraviroc | 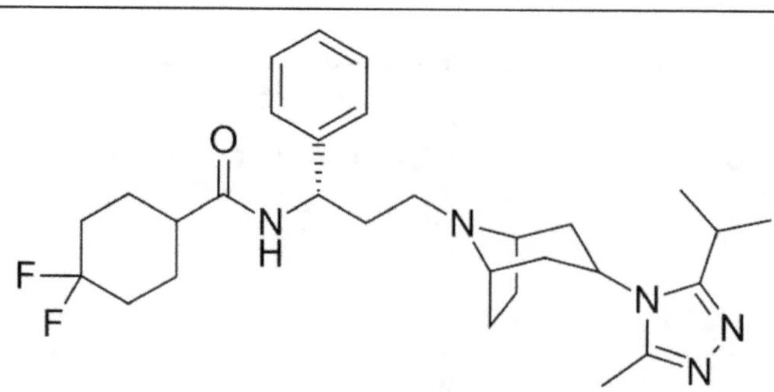 |

**Table** *Contd...*

| Saquinavir | 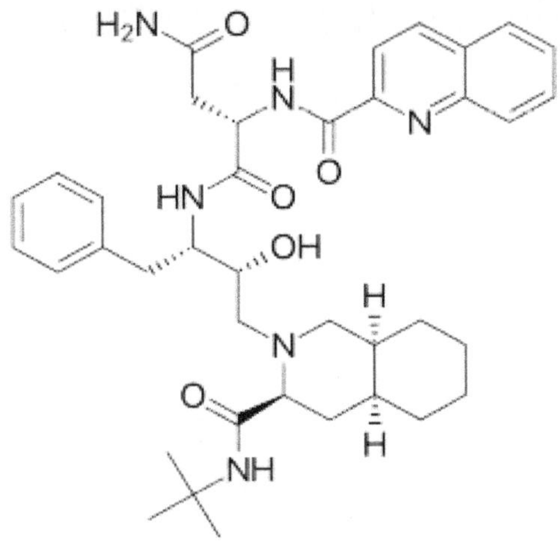 |
| --- | --- |

## 2.5 Autacoids and Related Drugs

**Antihistaminic Drugs**

Histamine: a chemical messenger mostly generated in mast cells

- Mediates a wide range of cellular responses
- Allergic and inflammatory reactions
- Gastric acid secretion
- Neurotransmission in parts of the brain.
    - ✓ Histamine is present in practically all tissues, with significant amounts in the lungs, skin, blood vessels, and GI tract
    - ✓ Found at high concentration in mast cells and basophils
    - ✓ As neurotransmitter in the brain.
    - ✓ Also occurs as a component of venoms and in secretions from insect sting

**Histamine Synthesis, Storage and Release**

Histamine is formed by the decarboxylation of histidine by histidine decarboxylase In mast cells, histamine is stored in granules If histamine is not stored, it is rapidly inactivated by the enzyme amine oxidase.

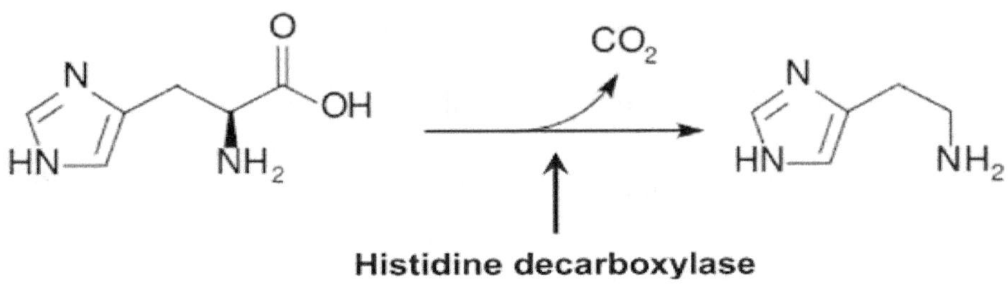


***Release of histamine***

- ➢ Most often, histamine is just one of several chemical mediators released in response to stimuli
- ➢ The stimuli for release of histamine from tissues may include destruction of cells as a result of cold, toxins from organisms, venoms from insects and spiders, and trauma
- ➢ Allergies and anaphylaxis can also trigger significant release of histamine.

# Histamine: Storage and Release

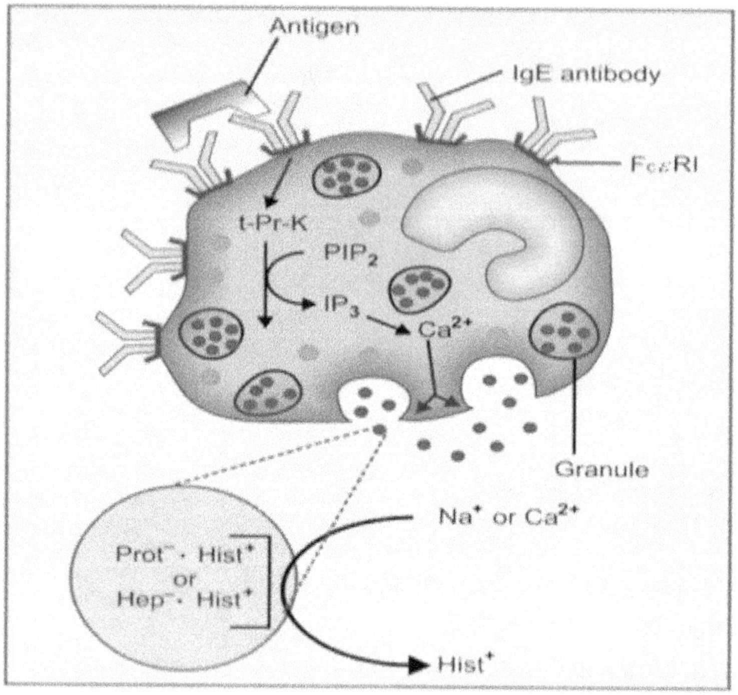


**Classification**

HISTAMINERGIC AGONISTS

| Nonselective agonists ($H_1 + H_2 + H_3$) | Selective $H_1$ agonists | Selective $H_2$ agonists | Selective $H_3$ agonists |
|---|---|---|---|
| Histamine | 2-Methyl histamine | Dimaprit | (R) α-Methylhistamine |
| Betahistine | 2-Pyridyl ethylamine | Impromidine | Imetit |
| | 2-Thizolyl ethylamine | | |

$H_1$ ANTAGONISTS
(Conventional antihistaminics)

| Highly sedative | Moderately sedative | Mildly sedative | Second generation (nonsedating) antihistaminics |
|---|---|---|---|
| Diphenhydramine | Pheniramine | Chlorpheniramine | Fexofenadine |
| Dimenhydrinate | Cyproheptadine | Dexchlorpheniramine | Loratadine |
| Promethazine | Meclozine | Triprolidine | Desloratadine |
| Hydroxyzine | Cinnarizine | Clemastine | Cetirizine |
| | | | Levocetirizine |
| | | | Azelastine |
| | | | Mizolastine |
| | | | Ebastine |

**Mechanism of Action**

- Released in response to certain stimuli and binds to various types of histamine receptors (H1, H2, H3, and H4)
- H1 and H2 receptors are widely expressed and are the targets of clinically useful drugs
- H1 receptors are important in producing smooth muscle contraction and increasing capillary permeability
- Histamine promotes vasodilation of small blood vessels by causing the vascular endothelium to release nitric oxide
- Can enhance secretion of proinflammatory cytokines in several cell types and in local tissues
- H1 receptors mediate many pathological processes, including allergic rhinitis, atopic dermatitis, conjunctivitis, urticaria, bronchoconstriction, asthma, and anaphylaxis
- Histamine stimulates the parietal cells in the stomach, causing an increase in acid secretion via the activation of H2 receptors.
- Histamine causes contraction of airway smooth muscle, stimulation of secretions, dilation and increased permeability of the capillaries, and stimulation of sensory nerve endings
- If the release of histamine is slow enough to permit its inactivation before it enters the bloodstream, a local allergic reaction results
- If histamine release is too fast for inactivation, a full-blown anaphylactic reaction occurs.

The H1-receptor blockers can be divided into first and second generation drugs.

- First generation drugs
    - Penetrate the CNS and cause sedation
    - Interact with other receptors, producing a variety of unwanted adverse effects
- Second-generation agents
    - Specific for peripheral H1 receptors
    - Do not penetrate the BBB causing less CNS depression than the first generation drug
    - Desloratadine, fexofenadine and loratadine show the least sedation
    - Cetirizine and levocetirizine are partially sedating.

The action of all the H1-receptor blockers is qualitatively similar

- Block the receptor-mediated response of a target tissue
- Much more effective in preventing symptoms than reversing them
- Have additional effects due to binding to cholinergic, adrenergic, or serotonin receptors
- Cyproheptadine also acts as a serotonin antagonist on the appetite center, sometimes used off label as an appetite stimulant and in treating anorgasmy associated SSRIs
- Antihistamines such as azelastine and ketotifen also have mast cell–stabilizing effects

**Adverse Effects**

- Sedation: (First-generation H1 antihistamines)
- Diphenhydramine may cause paradoxical hyperactivity in young children
- Fatigue, dizziness, lack of coordination, and tremors
- First-generation antihistamines exert anticholinergic effects, Dryness, blurred vision and retention of urine
- The most common adverse reaction associated with second-generation antihistamines is headache
- Topical Diphenhydramine can cause hypersensitivity such as contact dermatitis when applied to the skin.

## Prostaglandins

Prostaglandins and related compounds are produced in minute quantities by almost all tissues.

- They generally act locally on the tissues in which they are synthesized
- They are rapidly metabolized to inactive products at their sites of action.
- The prostaglandins do not circulate in the blood in significant concentrations.

**Classification**

PROSTAGLANDINS (PGs)

| Natural PGs | Prostaglandin analogues |
|---|---|
| Dinoprostone ($PGE_2$) | Carboprost (15-methyl $PGF_{2\alpha}$) |
| Gemeprost | Misoprostol (methyl $PGE_1$ ester) |
| Dinoprost ($PGF_{2\alpha}$) | Latanoprost ($PGE_2$ analogue) |
| Alprostadil ($PGE_1$) | Travoprost |
| Prostacyclin ($PGI_2$) (Epoprostenol) | Bimatoprost |

***Synthesis of Proglandins***

Arachidonic acid is the primary precursor of the prostaglandins

- Free arachidonic acid is released from tissue phospholipids by the action of phospholipase A2
- There are two major pathways arise from arachidonic acid, the cyclooxygenase and the lipoxygenase pathways.

1. **Cyclooxygenase pathway:**
   - All eicosanoids with ring structures (that is, the prostaglandins, thromboxanes, and prostacyclins) are synthesized via the cyclooxygenase pathway.
   - Two related forms of the cyclooxygenase enzymes have been described.
   - Cyclooxygenase-1 (COX-1) is responsible for the physiologic production of prostanoids,
   - Cyclooxygenase-2 (COX-2) causes the production of prostanoids that occurs in sites of chronic disease and inflammation.
   - COX-1 is enzyme regulates normal cellular processes for example
     1. gastric cytoprotection i.e. decrease level of HCL
     2. vascular homeostasis,
     3. platelet aggregation
     4. Contraction of uterus
     5. Regulation of blood flow to kidney
2. **Lipoxygenase pathway:**
   - Alternatively, several lipoxygenases can act on arachidonic acid to form leukotrienes.
   - Leukotrience cause bronchoconstriction.
   - Antileukotriene drugs, such as zileuton, zafirlukast, and montelukast, are treatment options for asthma

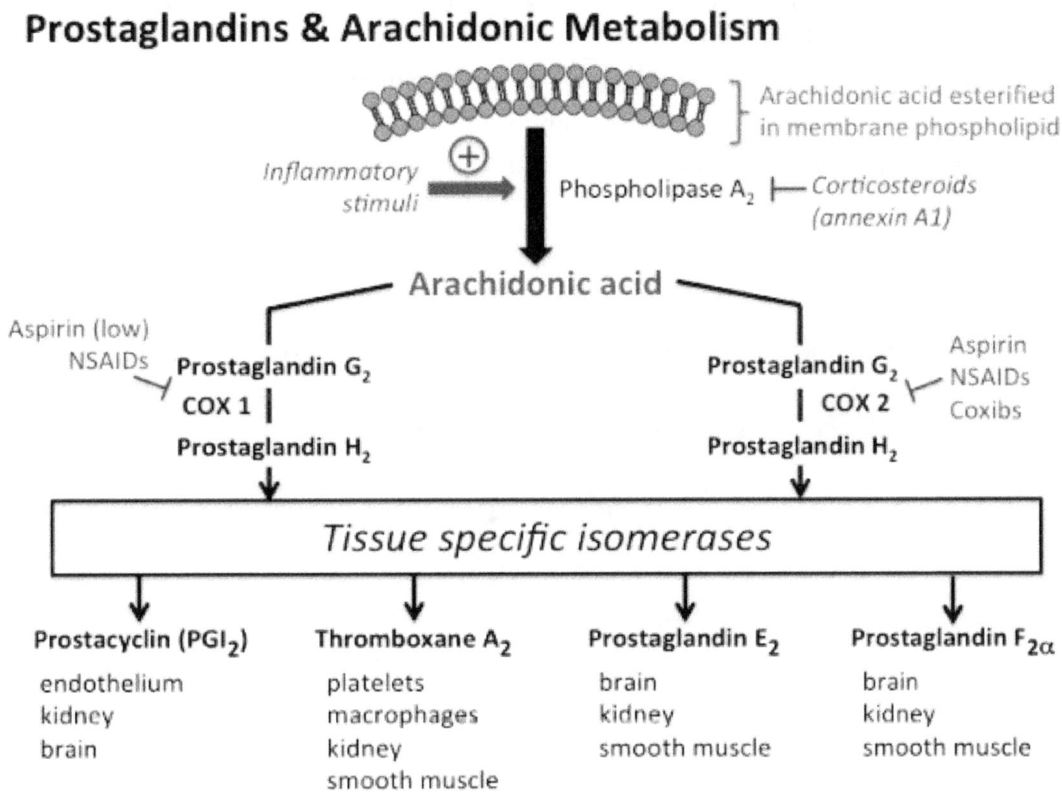


***Therapeutic uses of prostaglandins***

1. **Alprostadil**
   - Alprostadil is a PGE1 analogue.
   - Therapeutically, alprostadil can be used to treat erectile dysfunction
   - ductus arteriosus open in neonates with congenital heart conditions until surgery is possible
2. **Lubiprostone**
   - Lubiprostone is a PGE1 derivative
   - treatment of chronic idiopathic constipation, opioid-induced constipation
   - Therapeutic uses of prostaglandins
3. **Misoprostol**
   - Misoprostol is a PGE1 analog,
   - Used to protect the mucosal lining of the stomach during chronic NSAID treatment.
   - There is a combination product containing diclofenac and misoprostol.
   - Misoprostol is also used off-label in obstetric settings for labor induction

**Non Steroidal Anti Inflammatory Drugs (NSAIDs)**

NSAIDs- Drug with analgesic (without impairing consciousness), antipyretic, and anti inflammatory effects.

***Mechanism of Action***

- NSAIDs block the COX enzymes, reduce prostaglandins, inflammation, pain, and fever are reduced.
- COX-1 produced prostaglandins that support platelets and protect the stomach.

- Reduced prostaglandins that protect the stomach and support blood clotting, so NSAIDs can cause ulcers in the stomach and promote bleeding.
- Cyclooxygenase (COX) is found bound to the endoplasmic reticulum. It exists in 3 isoforms:
  - ✓ COX-1 (constitutive) acts in physiological conditions.
  - ✓ COX-2 (inducible) is induced in inflammatory cells by pathological stimulus.
  - ✓ COX-3 (in brain).

**NSAIDs**

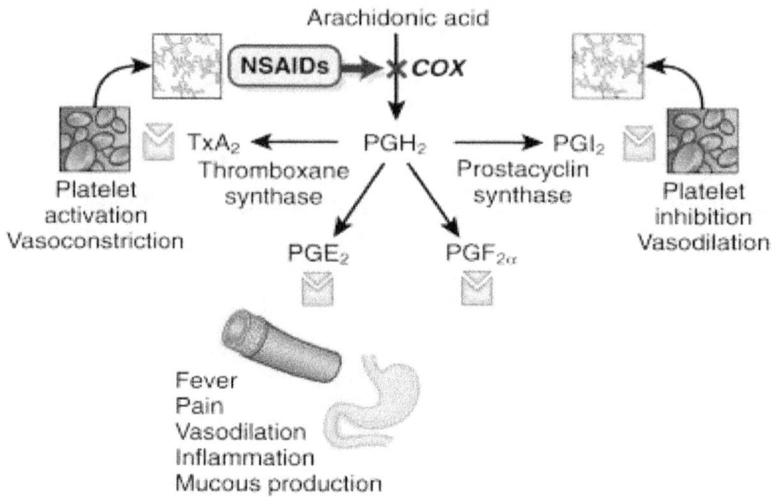


**Classification**

NONSTEROIDAL ANTIINFLAMMATORY DRUGS/ANTIPYRETIC-ANALGESICS

- **Preferential COX-2 inhibitors**: Nimesulide, Diclofenac, Aceclofenac, Meloxicam, Etodolac
- **Selective COX-2 inhibitors**: Celecoxib, Etoricoxib, Parecoxib
- **Analgesic-antipyretics with poor antiinflammatory action**
  - **Para aminophenol derivative**: Paracetamol (Acetaminophen)
  - **Pyrazolone derivatives**: Metamizol (Dipyrone), Propiphenazone
  - **Benzoxazocine derivative**: Nefopam
- **Nonselective COX inhibitors**
  - **Salicylates**: Aspirin
  - **Propionic acid derivatives**: Ibuprofen, Naproxen, Ketoprofen, Flurbiprofen
  - **Fenamate**: Mephenamic acid
  - **Enolic acid derivatives**: Piroxicam, Tenoxicam
  - **Acetic acid derivatives**: Ketorolac, Indomethacin, Nabumetone
  - **Pyrazolone derivatives**: Phenylbutazone, Oxyphenbutazone

***Side effects of NSAIDs***

*Gastrointestinal*

- ✓ Direct irritation : acidic molecules
- ✓ Indirect irritation: inhibit COX-1, reduce protective prostaglandins

- ✓ nausea, vomiting, dyspepsia, gastric ulcer/bleeding, diarrhea
- ✓ Duration of therapy, dose

*Cardiovascular*

- ✓ 80% increase risk with newer COX-2 and high dose traditional NSAID
- ✓ Heart failure risk

*Renal*

- ✓ Decrease prostaglandins→ constriction of afferent arteriole → decreased renal perfusion →alter renal function
- ✓ salt and fluid retension, hypertension
- ✓ Caution: NSAID with ACE inhibitor, diuretic
- ✓ Rare: ARF, ATN, nephrotic syn.

*Other*

- ✓ Allergy: shortness of breath
- ✓ Asthma: a higher risk for serious allergic reaction with a serious allergy to one NSAID are likely to have similar reaction to a different NSAID
- ✓ photosensitivity

## 2.6 Hormones and Related Drugs

### Antidiabetic Agents

**Diabetes mellitus (DM)** It is a metabolic disorder characterized by hyperglycaemia, glycosuria, hyperlipidaemia, negative nitrogen balance and sometimes ketonaemia. A widespread pathological change is thickening of capillary basement membrane, increase in vessel wall matrix and cellular proliferation resulting in vascular complications like lumen narrowing, early atherosclerosis, sclerosis of glomerular capillaries, retinopathy, neuropathy and peripheral vascular insufficiency.

ORAL ANTIDIABETIC DRUGS

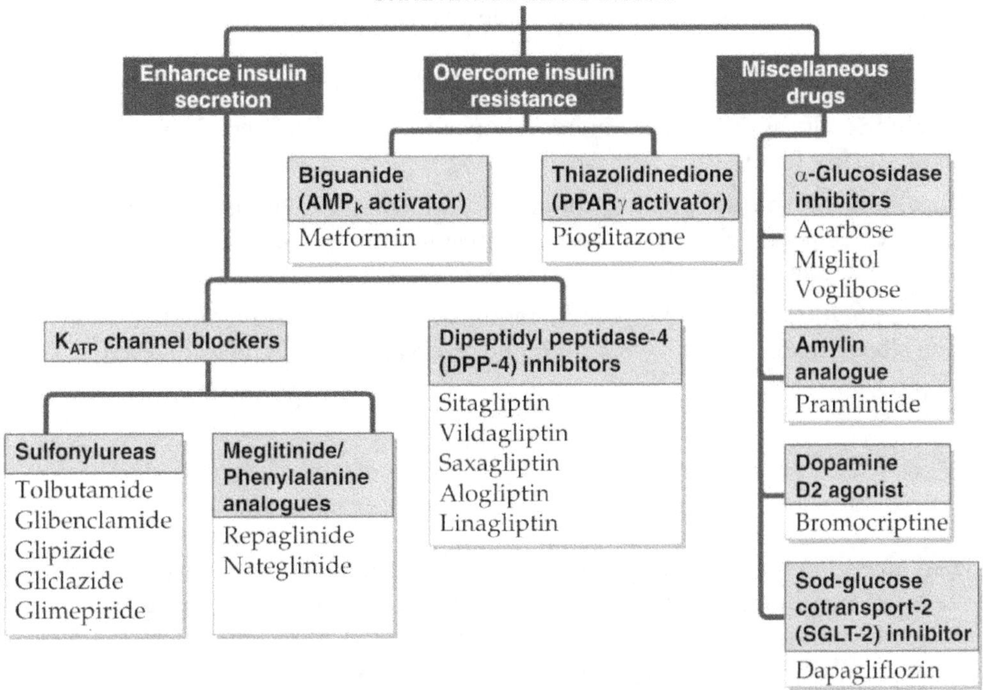

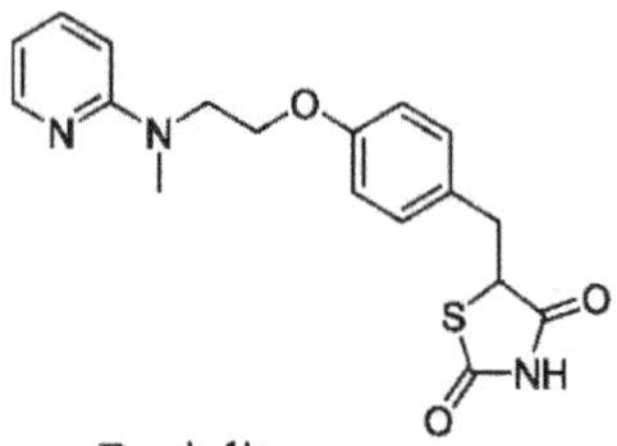
Rosiglitazone

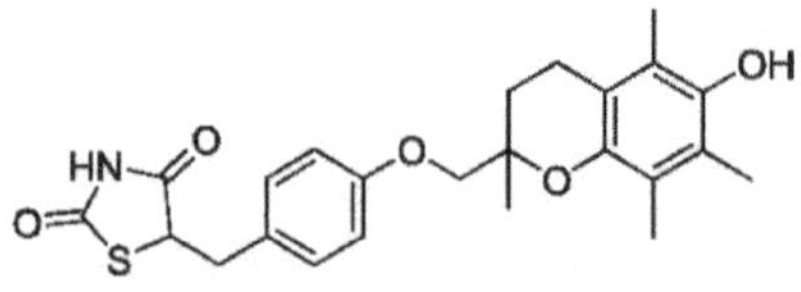
Troglitazone

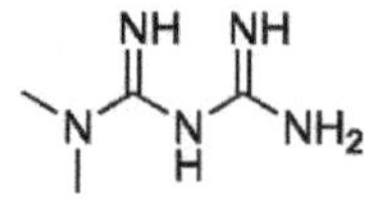
Metformin

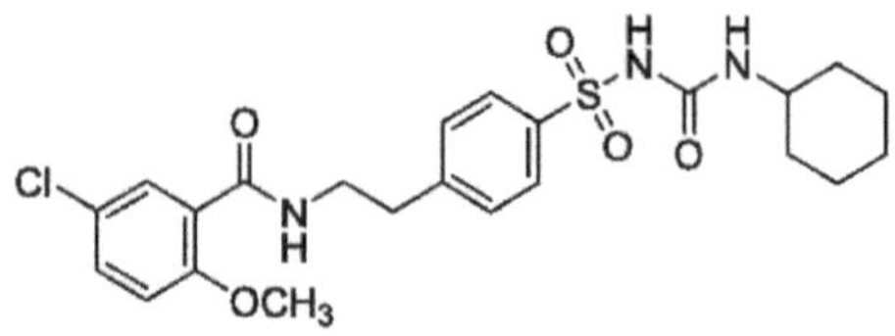
Glibenclamide

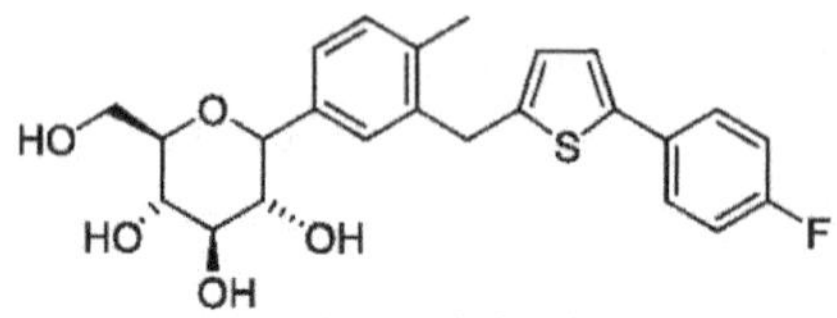
Canagliflozin

**Mechanism of Action**

- **Sulfonylureas** bind to adenosine triphosphate-sensitive potassium channel (K-ATP channel) in the beta cells of the pancreas. This leads to the inhibition of those channels and alters the resting membrane potential of the cell, causing an influx of calcium and the stimulation of insulin secretion.
- **Meglitinides** exerts its effects via different pancreatic beta cell receptors, but they act similarly by regulating adenosine triphosphate-sensitive potassium channels in pancreatic beta cells, thereby causing an increase in insulin secretion.
- **Metformin** increases hepatic adenosine monophosphate-activated protein kinase activity thus reducing hepatic gluconeogenesis and lipogenesis as well as increasing insulin-mediated uptake of glucose in muscles.
- **Thiazolidinediones** bind to peroxisome proliferator-activated receptor gamma to increase peripheral uptake of glucose and decrease hepatic glucose production.
- **Alpha-glucosidase inhibitors** competitively inhibit alpha-glucosidase enzymes in the intestine that digest the dietary starch thus inhibiting the polysaccharide reabsorption as well as the metabolism of sucrose to glucose and fructose.
- **DPP-4 inhibitors** inhibit the enzyme dipeptidyl peptidase 4 (DPP- 4) and prolong the action of glucagon-like peptide. This inhibits glucagon release, increases insulin secretion, and decreases gastric emptying thus decreasing blood glucose levels.
- **SGLT2 inhibitors** inhibit sodium-glucose cotransporter 2 (SGLT-2) in proximal tubules of renal glomeruli, causing inhibition of 90% glucose reabsorption and resulting in glycosuria in people with diabetes which in turn lowers the plasma glucose levels.
- **Cycloset,** a sympatholytic dopamine D2 receptor agonist, will reset the hypothalamic circadian rhythm which might have been altered by obesity. This results in the reversal of insulin resistance and the decrease in glucose production.

## 2.7 Gastrointestinal Drugs

### Antiulcer Drugs

Gastric and duodenal ulcers are breaks in the gastric and duodenal mucosa. Both gastric and duodenal ulcers relate to the corrosive action of pepsin and hydrochloric acid on the mucosa of the upper gastrointestinal tract. Ulcers generally range between 3 mm and several centimeters in diameter. Peptic ulcer can be diagnosed either by direct visualization using an **endoscope** or by using **contrast radiography.**

Causes of peptic ulcers are:

- Congenital hyperacidity.
- Mental strain and emotional stress that make the nervous system stimulate the excessive production of gastric acid.
- Undesirable eating habits, irregular meals or overeating.
- Smoking and excessive alcohol are direct causes of increased morbidity.
- Drugs such as aspirin and painkillers for rheumatism irritate and damage gastric mucosa.

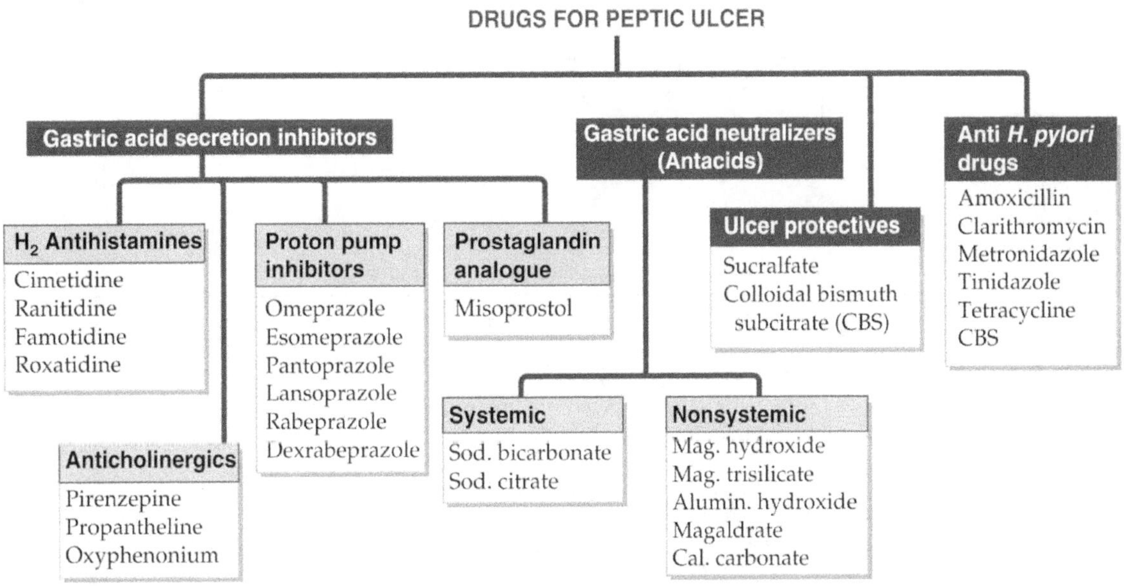


**Mechanism of action**

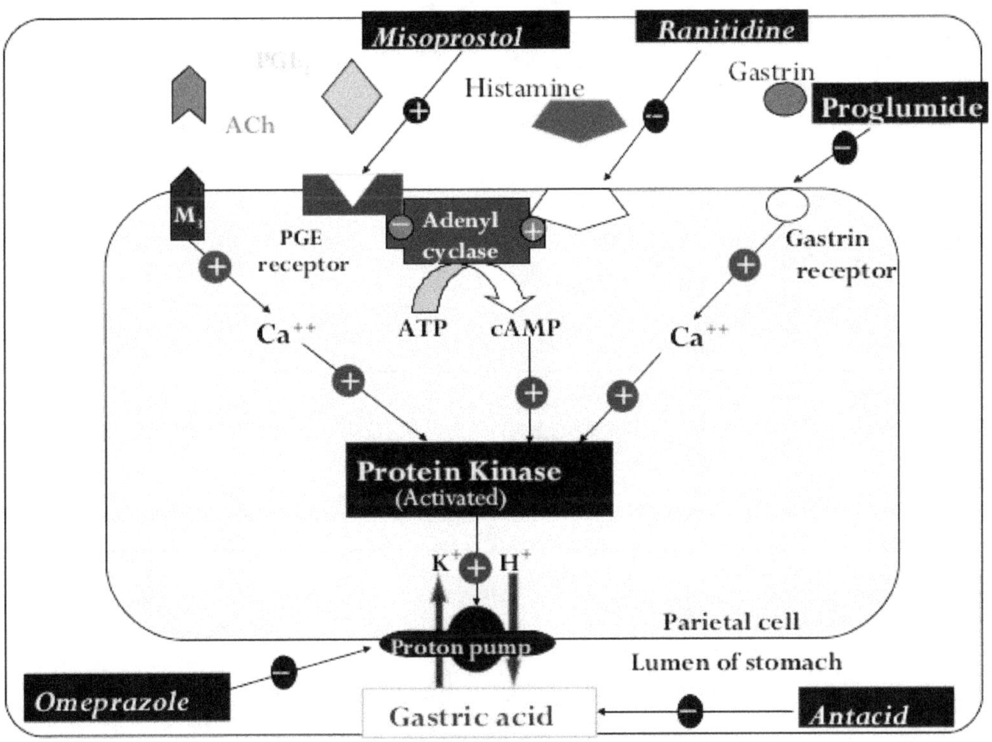

| | |
|---|---|
| Cimetidine | 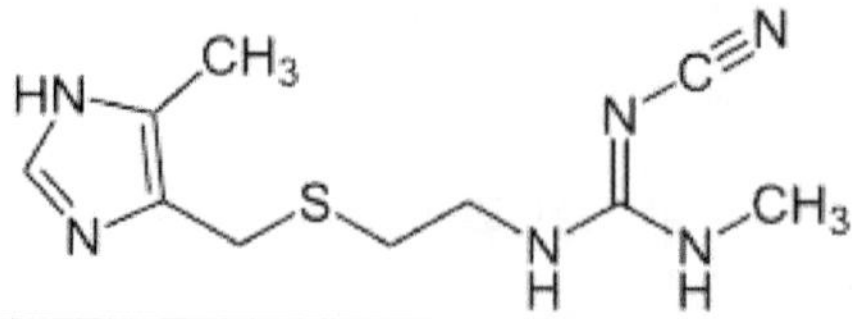 |
| Ranitidine | 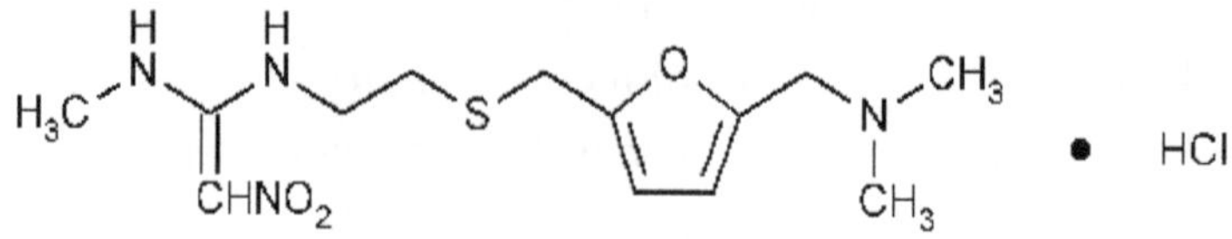 |
| Omeprazole | 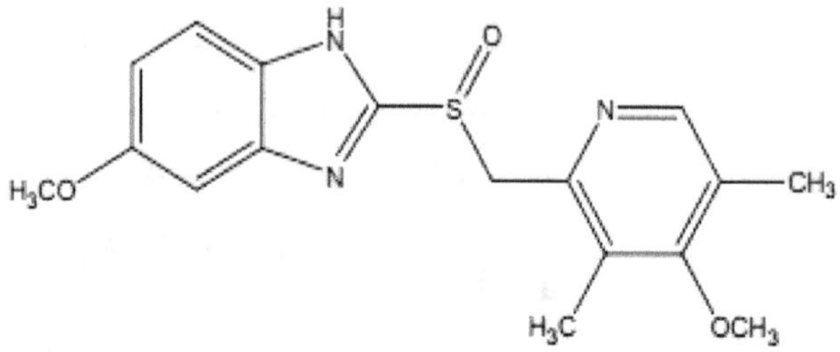 |
| Pentorazole | 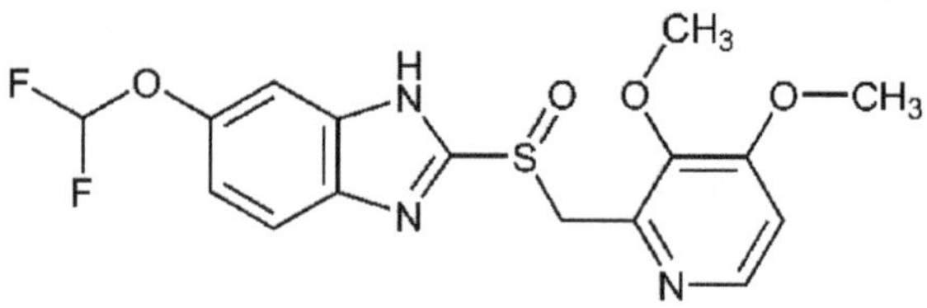 |
| Famotidine | 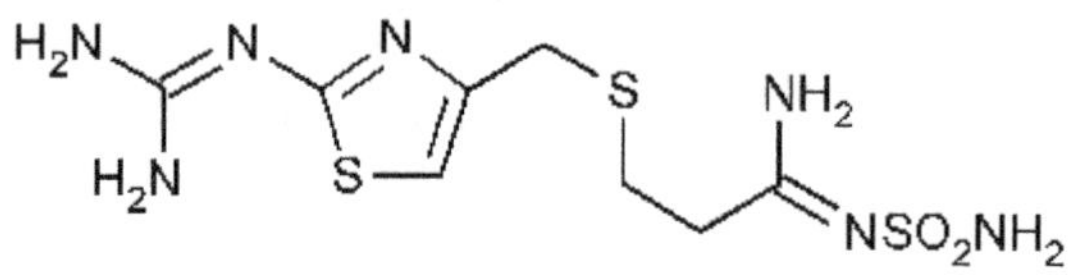 |
| Roxatidine | 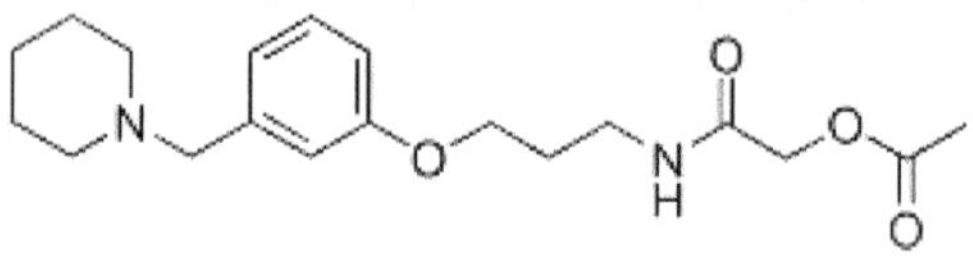 HCl |
| Lansoprazole | 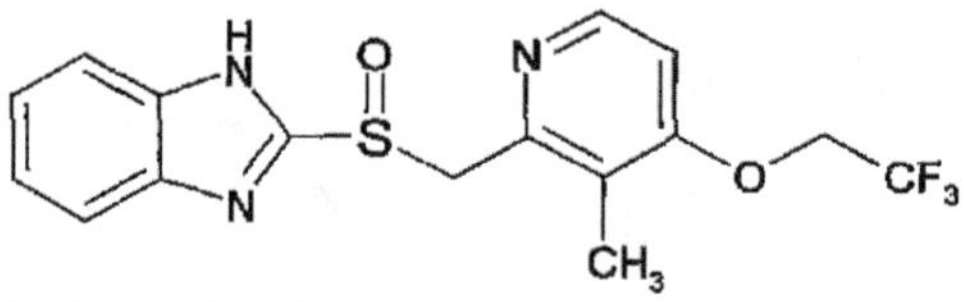 |
| Misoprostol | 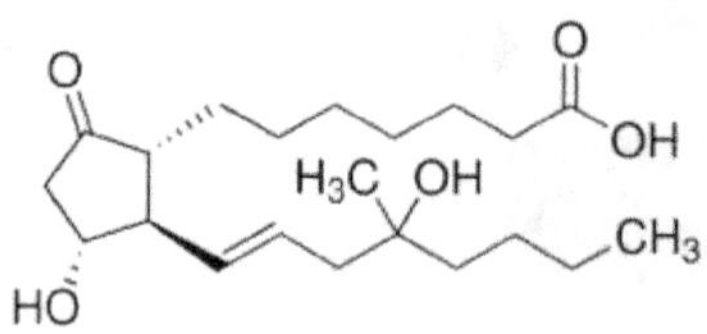 |

# Pharmacology MCQs

1. Tick the substance which changes the activity of an effector element but doesn't belong to second messengers:
   (a) cAMP (b) cGMP
   (c) G–protein (d) Calcium ions
2. What kind of substances can't permeate membranes by passive diffusion?
   (a) Lipid-soluble
   (b) Non-ionized substances
   (c) Hydrophobic substances
   (d) Hydrophilic substances
3. Pick out the appropriate alimentary route of administration when passage of drugs through liver is minimized:
   (a) Oral (b) Transdermal
   (c) Rectal (d) Intraduodenal
4. Half life (t ½) doesn't depend on:
   (a) Biotransformation
   (b) Time of drug absorption
   (c) Concentration of a drug in plasma
   (d) Rate of drug elimination
5. What term is used to describe a decrease in responsiveness to a drug which develops in a few minutes?
   (a) Refractoriness (b) Cumulative effect
   (c) Tolerance (d) Tachyphylaxis
6. Which one of the following groups is responsible for the potency and the toxicity of local anesthetics?
   (a) Ionizable group
   (b) Intermediate chain
   (c) Lipophylic group
   (d) All of the above
7. Indicate the drug, which has greater potency of the local anesthetic action:
   (a) Lidocaine (b) Bupivacaine
   (c) Procaine (d) Mepivacaine
8. Ionizable group is responsible for:
   (a) The potency and the toxicity
   (b) The duration of action
   (c) The ability to diffuse to the site of action
   (d) All of the above
9. Indicate the local anesthetic, which is used for spinal anesthesia:
   (a) Tetracaine (b) Cocaine
   (c) Dibucaine (d) Bupivacaine
10. Which of the following local anesthetics is called a universal anesthetic?
    (a) Procaine (b) Ropivacaine
    (c) Lidocaine (d) Bupivacaine
11. Most serious toxic reaction to local anesthetics is:
    (a) Seizures
    (b) Cardiovascular collapse
    (c) Respiratory failure
    (d) All of the above
12. Bethanechol has all of the following properties EXCEPT:
    (a) It is extremely resistant to hydrolysis
    (b) Purely muscarinic in its action
    (c) It is used for abdominal urinary bladder distention
    (d) It exerts both nicotinic and muscarinic effects
13. Which of the following cholinomimetics is commonly used in the treatment of glaucoma?
    (a) Pilocarpine (b) Lobeline
    (c) Acethylcholine (d) Neostigmine
14. Which of the following drugs is used for acute toxic effects of organophosphate cholinesterase inhibitors?
    (a) Atropine (b) Pilocarpine
    (c) Pralidoxime (d) Edrophonium

15. Atropine is frequently used prior to administration of inhalant anesthetics to reduce:
    (a) Muscle tone
    (b) Secretions
    (c) Nausea and vomiting
    (d) All of the above
16. Atropine is now rarely used for the treatment of peptic ulcer because of:
    (a) Slow gastric empting and prolongation of the exposure of the ulcer bed to acid
    (b) Low efficiency and necessity of large doses
    (c) Adverse effects
    (d) All of the above
17. Which of the following antimuscarinic drugs is a selective M1 blocker?
    (a) Atropine (b) Scopolamine
    (c) Pirenzepine (d) Homatropine
18. Which of the following drugs is useful in the treatment of Parkinson's disease?
    (a) Benztropine (b) Edrophonium
    (c) Succinylcholine (d) Hexamethonium
19. Which of the following drugs has "double-acetylcholine" structure?
    (a) Rocuronium (b) Carbachol
    (c) Atracurium (d) Succylcholine
20. Direct effects on the heart are determined largely by:
    (a) Alfa1 receptor (b) Alfa2 receptor
    (c) Beta1 receptor (d) Beta2 receptor
21. Which of the following effects is related to direct beta1-adrenoreceptor stimulation?
    (a) Bronchodilation (b) Vasodilatation
    (c) Tachycardia (d) Bradycardia
22. Which of the following agents is a beta2–selective antagonist?
    (a) Tolazolin (b) Pindolol
    (c) Ergotamin (d) Butoxamine
23. Beta-receptor antagonists cause:
    (a) Stimulation of lipolysis
    (b) Stimulation of gluconeogenesis
    (c) Inhibition of glycogenolysis
    (d) Stimulation of insulin secretion
24. Indicate a beta receptor antagonist, which has very long duration of action:
    (a) Metoprolol (b) Propranolol
    (c) Nadolol (d) Pindolol
25. Which of the following drugs has both alfa1-selective and beta-blocking effects?
    (a) Labetalol (b) Betaxolol
    (c) Propranolol (d) Timolol
26. Select a hypnotic drug, which is a benzodiazepine derivative:
    (a) Zolpidem (b) Flurazepam
    (c) Secobarbital (d) Phenobarbitone
27. Hepatic microsomal drug-metabolizing enzyme induction leads to:
    (a) Barbiturate tolerance
    (b) Cumulative effects
    (c) Development of physical dependence
    (d) "hangover" effects
28. Which of the following agents inhibits hepatic metabolism of hypnotics?
    (a) Flumasenil (b) Cimetidin
    (c) Phenytoin (d) Theophylline
29. Which of the following hypnotic agents is a positive allosteric modulator of GABAA receptor function?
    (a) Zaleplon (b) Flurazepam
    (c) Zolpidem (d) All of the above
30. Which of the following agents blocks the chloride channel directly?
    (a) Secobarbital (b) Flumazenil
    (c) Zaleplon (d) Picrotoxin
31. The antiseizure drug, which induces hepatic microsomal enzymes, is:
    (a) Lamotrigine
    (b) Phenytoin
    (c) Valproate
    (d) None of the above
32. Which of the following antiseizure drugs is a prodrug, metabolized to phenobarbital?
    (a) Phenytoin (b) Primidone
    (c) Felbamate (d) Vigabatrin

33. Valproate is very effective against:
    (a) Absence seizures
    (b) Myoclonic seizures
    (c) Generalized tonic-clonic seizures
    (d) All of the above

34. The mechanism of valproate action is:
    (a) Facilitation glutamic acid decarboxylase, the enzyme responsible for GABA synthesis and inhibition of GABA amino transferase, the enzyme responsible for the breakdown of GABA (enhance GABA accumulation)
    (b) Inhibition of voltage sensitive Na+ channels
    (c) Inhibition of low threshold (T-type) Ca2+ channels
    (d) All of the above

35. Benzodiazepine´s uselfulness is limited by:
    (a) Tolerance
    (b) Atropine-like symptoms
    (c) Psychotic episodes
    (d) Myasthenic syndrome

36. Which of the following antiparkinsonian drugs is an antiviral agent used in the prophylaxis of influenza A2?
    (a) Selegiline (b) Sinemet
    (c) Pergolide (d) Amantadine

37. Which of the following drugs is most commonly used for causing a noxious reaction to alcohol by blocking its metabolism?
    (a) Naltrexone (b) Disulfiram
    (c) Diazepam (d) Morphine

38. The combination of disulfiram and ethanol leads to accumulation of:
    (a) Formaldehyde (b) Acetate
    (c) Formic acid (d) Acetaldehyde

39. Which of the following agents may be used as an antidote for ethylene glycol and methanol poisoning?
    (a) Disulfiram (b) Fomepizol
    (c) Naltrexone (d) Amphetamine

40. Which of the following analgesics is a phenanthrene derivative?
    (a) Fentanyl (b) Morphine
    (c) Methadone (d) Pentazocine

41. Which of the following agents is a full antagonist of opioid receptors?
    (a) Meperidine (b) Buprenorphine
    (c) Naloxone (d) Butorphanol

42. Indicate the opioid analgesic, which has 80 times analgesic potency and respiratory depressant properties of morphine, and is more effective than morphine in maintaining hemodynamic stability?
    (a) Fentanyl (b) Pentazocine
    (c) Meperidine (d) Nalmefene

43. Which of the following opioid analgesics is used in combination with droperidol in neuroleptanalgesia?
    (a) Morphine (b) Buprenorphine
    (c) Fentanyl (d) Morphine

44. Therapeutic doses of the opioid analgesics:
    (a) Decrease body temperature
    (b) Increase body temperature
    (c) Decrease body heat loss
    (d) Do not affect body temperature

45. Which of the following opioid analgesics is used in the treatment of acute pulmonary edema?
    (a) Morphine (b) Codeine
    (c) Fentanyl (d) Loperamide

46. Which of the following drugs has weak mu agonist effects and inhibitory action on norepinephrine and serotonin reuptake in the CNS?
    (a) Loperamide (b) Tramadol
    (c) Fluoxetine (d) Butorphanol

47. Which one of the following non-narcotic agents inhibits mainly cyclooxygenase (COX) in CNS?
    (a) Paracetamol (b) Ketorolac
    (c) Acetylsalicylic acid (d) Ibuprofen

48. For which of the following conditions could aspirin be used prophylactically?
    (a) Noncardiogenic pulmonary edema
    (b) Peptic ulcers
    (c) Thromboembolism
    (d) Metabolic acidosis

49. Indicate the nonopioid agent of central effect with analgesic activity:
(a) Reserpine (b) Propranolol
(c) Clopheline (d) Prazosin

50. Which of the following nonopioid agents is an antidepressant with analgesic activity?
(a) Fluoxetine (b) Moclobemide
(c) Tranylcypramine (d) Amitriptyline

51. Indicate the atypical antipsychotic drug:
(a) Haloperidol (b) Clozapine
(c) Thioridazine (d) Thiothixene

52. Which of the following antipsychotic drugs is typical?
(a) Clozapine (b) Quetiapine
(c) Haloperidol (d) Olanzapine

53. Which of the following antipsychotic drugs has high affinity for D4 and 5-HT2 receptors?
(a) Clozapine (b) Fluphenazine
(c) Thioridazine (d) Haloperidole

54. Select the agent, which is preferred in the treatment of the drug-induced form of parkinsonism:
(a) Levodopa (b) Bromocriptine
(c) Benztropine (d) Dopamine

55. Which of the following agents is the precursor of dopamine?
(a) Bromocriptine (b) Levodopa
(c) Selegiline (d) Amantadine

56. Indicate the antipsychotic drug having a muscarinic-cholinergic blocking activity:
(a) Chlorpromazine (b) Clorprothixene
(c) Risperidone (d) Haloperidol

57. Which of the following antipsychotic agents is used in combination with an opioid drug fentanyl in neuroleptanalgesia?
(a) Haloperidol (b) Droperidol
(c) Chlorpromazine (d) Clozapine

58. Lithium carbonate is useful in the treatment of:
(a) Petit mal seizures
(b) Bipolar disorder
(c) Neurosis
(d) Trigeminal neuralgia

59. Block of which type of Monoamine Oxydase might be more selective for depression?
(a) MAO-A
(b) MAO-B
(c) Both MAO-A and MAO-B
(d) MAO-C

60. Which of the following benzodiazepines has the shortest duration of action?
(a) Triazolam (b) Clorazepate
(c) Prazepam (d) Clordiazepoxide

61. Indicate the anesthetic, which is used intravenously:
(a) Propofol (b) Halothane
(c) Desflurane (d) Nitrous oxide

62. Most of drugs are antacids EXCEPT:
(a) Misoprostol (b) Maalox
(c) Mylanta (d) Almagel

63. Indicate an antiemetic agent which is related to neuroleptics:
(a) Metoclopramide (b) Nabilone
(c) Tropisetron (d) Prochlorperazine

64. Indicate the drug belonging to antagonists of heparin:
(a) Aspirin (b) Dicumarol
(c) Dalteparin (d) Protamine sulfate

65. Aglycone is essential for:
(a) Plasma protein binding
(b) Half-life
(c) Cardiotonic action
(d) Metabolism

66. This drug prolongs repolarization:
(a) Flecainide (b) Sotalol
(c) Lidocaine (d) Verapamil

67. This drug is used intravenously to terminate supraventricular tachycardias:
(a) Nifedipine
(b) Verapamil
(c) Both of the above
(d) None of the above

68. Which of the following nitrates and nitrite drugs are long-acting?
   (a) Nitroglycerin, sublingual
   (b) Isosorbide dinitrate, sublingual (Isordil, Sorbitrate)
   (c) Amyl nitrite, inhalant (Aspirols, Vaporole)
   (d) Sustac

69. Which of the following antianginal agents is a calcium channel blocker?
   (a) Nitroglycerin (b) Dipyridamole
   (c) Minoxidil (d) Nifedipine

70. Which of the following antianginal agents is a myotropic coronary dilator:
   (a) Dipyridamole (b) Validol
   (c) Atenolol (d) Alinidine

71. Which of the following antianginal agents refers to reflex coronary dilators:
   (a) Dipyridamole (b) Validol
   (c) Atenolol (d) Alinidine

72. Which of the following antianginal agents is a potassium channel opener:
   (a) Dipyridamole (b) Validol
   (c) Atenolol (d) Minoxidil

73. This drug is a directly acting vasodilator:
   (a) Labetalol (b) Clonidine
   (c) Enalapril (d) Nifedipine

74. Tick the positive inotropic drug of non-glycoside structure:
   (a) Digitoxin (b) Digoxin
   (c) Dobutamine (d) Strophanthin

75. Tick the drug influencing the blood flow which is related to antiplatelet agents:
   (a) Heparin (b) Aspirin
   (c) Pyracetam (d) Tanakan

76. Indicate the nootropic agent useful in disorders of brain circulation:
   (a) Aspirin (b) Pyracetam
   (c) Warfarin (d) All the above

77. Vasopressin possesses the following:
   (a) Antidiuretic property
   (b) Vasodilatation property
   (c) Release of a thyroid hormone into the plasma
   (d) Diuretic property

78. Radioiodines (I131 and I132) is suitable for:
   (a) Elderly patients (over 45 years)
   (b) Pregnant women
   (c) Nursing mothers
   (d) Younger patients

79. Which of the following nitrates and nitrite drugs are long-acting?
   (a) Nitroglycerin, sublingual
   (b) Isosorbide dinitrate, sublingual (Isordil, Sorbitrate)
   (c) Amyl nitrite, inhalant (Aspirols, Vaporole)
   (d) Sustac

80. Duration of nitroglycerin action (sublingual) is:
   (a) 10-30 minutes (b) 6-8 hours
   (c) 3-5 minutes (d) 1.5-2 hours

81. Side effect of nitrates and nitrite drugs are, EXCEPT:
   (a) Orthostatic hypotension, tachycardia
   (b) GI disturbance
   (c) Throbbing headache
   (d) Tolerance

82. A ganglioblocking drug for hypertension treatment is:
   (a) Hydralazine (b) Tubocurarine
   (c) Trimethaphan (d) Metoprolol

83. This drug is a directly acting vasodilator:
   (a) Labetalol (b) Clonidine
   (c) Enalapril (d) Nifedipine

84. Choose the vasodilator which releases NO:
   (a) Nifedipine
   (b) Hydralazine
   (c) Minoxidil
   (d) Sodium nitroprusside

85. Diabetic coma is treated by the administration of:
   (a) Lente insulin
   (b) Glucose
   (c) Crystalline insulin
   (d) Oral anti-diabetic drugs.

86. The action of insulin is potentiated by:
    (a) Sulphonylureas
    (b) Glucagon
    (c) Biguanides
    (d) None of the above

87. Serious side effects of glucocorticoids include the following:
    (a) Adrenal suppression
    (b) Insomnia, behavioral changes (primarily hypomania)
    (c) Rounding, puffiness, fat deposition and plethora alter the appearance of the face – moon faces
    (d) All of the above

88. Which of the following drugs is a thromboxane A2 receptor (TXA2) antagonist?
    (a) Sulotroban
    (b) Zileuton (Zyflo)
    (c) Zafirleukast (Accolate)
    (d) Diclofenac

89. Which category of histamine H1 antagonists is recognized for as second-generation antihistamines?
    (a) Alkylamines (propylamines); i.e. Brompheniramine
    (b) Piperidines; i.e. Loratadine, Fexofenadine
    (c) Ethylenediamines; i.e. Suprastine
    (d) Phenothiazines; i.e. Promethazine

90. Which of histamine H1 antagonists is noted for the ulcerogenic effect?
    (a) Diazoline (b) Loratadine
    (c) Suprastine (d) Dimedrol

91. Side effect of first-generation histamine H1 antagonists is:
    (a) Aplastic anemia
    (b) Vomiting, tinnitus, decreased hearing
    (c) Sedation
    (d) Gastric ulcers and upper gastrointestinal bleeding

92. Mechanism of action of cyclosporine A is:
    (a) Complement-mediated cytolysis of T lymphocytes
    (b) ADCC towards T lymphocytes
    (c) Inhibits calcineurin
    (d) Compete for Fc receptors with autoantibodies

93. Class of sirolimus (rapamycin) is:
    (a) Immunoglobulins
    (b) Interferons
    (c) Immunosuppressive agents
    (d) Monoclonal antibodies

94. Which of the following vitamins is given along with isoniazide in treatment of tuberculosis?
    (a) Nicotinic acid (b) Riboflavin
    (c) Pyridoxine (d) Ascorbic acid

95. This drug binds bile acids in the GI tract:
    (a) Cholestyramine (Questran)
    (b) Nicotinic acid (niacin)
    (c) Gemfibrozil (Loprol)
    (d) Probucol (Lorelco)

96. The drug can cause ototoxicity:
    (a) Acetazolamide (Diamox)
    (b) Furosemide (Lasix)
    (c) Hydrochlorothiazide (Hydrodiuril)
    (d) Amiloride (Midamor)

97. Tick the drug belonging to glycopeptides:
    (a) Vancomycin (b) Lincomycin
    (c) Neomycin (d) Carbenicillin

98. Pick out the beta-lactamase inhibitor for co-administration with penicillins:
    (a) Clavulanic acid (b) Sulbactam
    (c) Tazobactam (d) All of the above

99. Which of the following drugs is used for systemic and deep mycotic infections treatment:
    (a) Co-trimoxazol (b) Griseofulvin
    (c) Amphotericin B (d) Nitrofungin

100. Tick the drug, which is effective against mycobacteria only:
    (a) Isoniazid (b) Streptomycin
    (c) Rifampin (d) Kanamycin

101. Rifampin has the following unwanted effect:
    (a) Dizziness, headache
    (b) Loss of hair
    (c) Flu-like syndrome, tubular necrosis
    (d) Hepatotoxicity

102. Tick the antimalarial drug having a gametocidal effect:
(a) Mefloquine (b) Primaquine
(c) Doxycycline (d) Sulfonamides

103. Tick the drug for cestodosis (tapeworm invasion) treatment:
(a) Piperazine (b) Praziquantel
(c) Pyrantel (d) Ivermectin

104. Which one of the following drugs is prescribed for the treatment of Philadelphia chromosome positive patients with Chronic myeloid Leukemia?
(a) Pentostatin (b) Methotrexate
(c) Imatinib (d) L-Asparaginase

105. Which of the following monoclonal antibodies is prescribed for patients with non-Hodgkin's Lymphoma?
(a) Infliximab (b) Abciximab
(c) Gemtuzumab (d) Rituximab

106. Identify the drug which is NOT used in the treatment of malaria caused by *Plasmodium falciparum* :
(a) Artemisinin (b) Primaquine
(c) Quinine (d) Mefloquine

107. Which one of the following drugs does NOT act through G-Protein coupled receptors?
(a) Epinephrine (b) Insulin
(c) Dopamine (d) TSH

108. Which one of the following drugs is most effective in preventing transmission of HIV virus from the mother to the foetus?
(d) Lamivudine (b) Zidovudine
(c) Indinavir (d) Ribavirin

109. Improvement of memory in Alzheimer's disease is brought about by drugs which increase transmission in
(a) cholinergic receptors
(b) dopaminergic receptors
(c) GABAergic receptors
(d) adrenergic receptors

110. Which of the following non-opioid analgesics is a prodrug?
(a) Piroxicam (b) Celecoxib
(c) Nabumetone (d) Ketorolac

111. Which one of the following drugs is NOT a typical anti-psychotic agent?
(a) Chlorpromazine (b) Haloperidol
(c) Risperidone (d) Flupentixol

112. Which one of the followings is a plasminogen activator?
(a) Tranexamic acid
(b) Streptokinase
(c) Aminocaproic acid
(d) None of the above

113. Myasthenia gravis is diagnosed with improved neuromuscular function by using
(a) Donepezil (b) Edrophonium
(c) Atropine (d) Pancuronium

114. Which one of the following drugs specifically inhibits calcineurin in the activated T lymphocytes?
(a) Daclizumab (b) Prednisone
(c) Sirolimus (d) Tacrolimus

115. The chemical behaviour of morphine alkaloid is
(a) acidic (b) Basic
(c) neutral (d) amphoteric

116. Which one of the followings is used as a mood stabilizer for bipolar disorder and also in certain epileptic convulsions?
(a) Phenytoin (b) Lithium
(c) Sodium valproate (d) Fluoxetine

117. The given antibiotic is an example of ansamycins:
(a) Roxythromycin (b) Adriamycin
(c) Aureomycin (d) Rifamycin

118. The effects observed following systemic administration of levodopa in the treatment of Parkinsonism have been attributed to its catabolism to dopamine. Carbidopa, can markedly increase the proportion of levodopa that crosses the blood brain barrier by
(a) increasing penetration of levodopa through BBB by complexation with it
(b) decreasing peripheral metabolism of levodopa
(c) decreasing metabolism of levodopa in the CNS
(d) decreasing clearance of levodopa from the CNS

119. Aminotransferases usually require the following for their activity :
   (a) Niacinamide (b) Vitamin B12
   (c) Pyridoxal phosphate (d) Thiamine

120. Measurement of inulin renal clearance is a measure for
   (a) Effective renal blood flow
   (b) Renal drug excretion rate
   (c) Active renal secretion
   (d) Glomerular filtration rate

121. Select the correc: combination of drugs for the treatment of patients suffering from Hepatitis C:
   (a) Interferon with Ribavirin
   (b) Interferon with Zidovudine
   (c) Interferon with Stavudine
   (d) Interferon with Lamivudine

122. Aliskiren acts by
   (a) inhibiting the conversion of Angiotensin I to II
   (b) inhibiting the release of rennin
   (c) inhibiting the binding of Angiotensin II to the receptor
   (d) inhibiting the action of aldosterone

123. Digitalis toxicity is enhanced by co-administration of
   (a) Potassium (b) Quinidine
   (c) Diuretics (d) Antacids

124. Which one of the following drugs is withdrawn from the market due to *torsade de pointes?*
   (a) Chlorpromazine (b) Astemizole
   (c) Haloperidol (d) Domperidone

125. Ganciclovir is mainly used for the treatment of infection caused by
   (a) Cytomegalovirus
   (b) Candida albicans
   (c) Herpes zoster virus
   (d) Hepatitis B virus

126. Identify the one rational combination which has clinical benefit:
   (a) Norfloxacin – Metronidazole
   (b) Alprazolam - Paracetamol
   (c) Cisapride – Omeprazole
   (d) Amoxycillin - Clavulanic acid

127. Stevens Johnson sjmdrome is the most common adverse effect associated with one of the following category of drugs :
   (a) Sulphonamides (b) Macrolides
   (c) Penicillins (d) Tetracyclines

128. Nicotinic action of acetylcholine is blocked by the drug
   (a) Atropine (b) Carvedilol
   (c) Neostigmine (d) d-Tubocurarine

129. Selective serotonin reuptake inhibitor is
   (a) Imipramine (b) Iproniazide
   (c) Fluoxetin (d) Naphazoline

130. Cyclophosphamide as anticancer agent acts as
   (a) alkylating agent before metabolism
   (b) alkylating agent after metabolism
   (c) phosphorylating agent after metabolism
   (d) DNA intercalating agent

131. Streptomycin can NOT be given orally for treatment of tuberculosis because
   (a) it gets degraded in the GIT
   (b) it causes severe diarrhoea
   (c) it causes metallic taste in the mouth
   (d) it is not absorbed from the GIT

132. Many xenobiotics are oxidized by cytochrome P450 in order to
   (a) increase their biological activity
   (b) increase their disposition in lipophilic compartments of the body
   (c) increase their aqueous solubility
   (d) all of the above

133. Rabies vaccine (living) is prepared using
   (a) Sheep blood (b) Mice lymph
   (c) Horse plasma (d) Fertile eggs

134. Geriatric population should be included in the following Phase of clinical trials
   (a) Phase I (b) Phase II
   (c) Phase III (d) Phase

# Answer Key Pharmacology

1. c
2. d
3. c
4. b
5. d
6. c
7. b
8. c
9. a
10. c
11. d
12. d
13. a
14. c
15. b
16. d
17. c
18. a
19. d
20. c
21. c
22. d
23. c
24. c
25. a
26. b
27. a
28. b
29. d
30. d
31. b
32. b
33. d
34. d
35. a
36. d
37. b
38. d
39. b
40. b
41. c
42. a
43. c
44. a
45. a
46. b
47. a
48. c
49. c
50. d
51. b
52. c
53. a
54. c
55. b
56. a
57. b
58. b
59. a
60. a
61. a
62. a
63. d
64. d
65. c
66. b
67. b
68. d
69. d
70. a
71. b
72. d
73. d
74. c
75. b
76. b
77. a
78. a
79. d
80. a
81. b
82. c
83. d
84. d
85. c
86. c
87. d
88. a
89. b
90. a
91. c
92. c
93. c
94. c
95. a
96. b
97. a
98. d
99. c
100. a

101. a
102. c
103. b
104. b
105. c
106. b
107. b
108. b
109. a
110. c
111. c
112. b
113. b
114. d
115. b
116. c
117. d
118. b
119. c
120. d
121. b
122. b
123. b&c
124. b
125. a&c
126. d
127. a
128. d
129. c
130. b
131. d
132. d
133. d
134. b

# Pharmaceutical Chemistry MCQs

1. Which of the following is an accurate description of the phospholipid bilayer in cell membranes?
   (a) It is made up of two layers of phospholipid polymers
   (b) It is made up of two layers of phospholipid molecules with the tails pointing away from each other.
   (c) It is made up of two layers of phospholipid molecules with the tails lying parallel to each other.
   (d) It is made up of two layers of phospholipid molecules with the tails interacting with each other.
2. Which of the following statements is true regarding the phospholipid bilayer in cell membranes?
   (a) Water and ions are unable to cross the bilayer due to the charges present in the head groups.
   (b) Water and ions are unable to cross the bilayer due the hydrophobic tails of the phospholipid molecules.
   (c) Water and ions are encouraged to cross the bilayer by interacting with the charges present in the head groups.
   (d) The molecules in the bilayer are fluid, and so the cell membrane is porous allowing the passage of ions and water across the cell membrane.
3. Which of the following statements is true
   (a) Drugs and drug targets generally have similar molecular weights.
   (b) Drugs are generally smaller than drug targets.
   (c) Drugs are generally larger than drug targets.
   (d) There is no general rule regarding the relative size of drugs and their targets.
4. What is meant by a binding site?
   (a) The area of a macromolecular target that is occupied by a drug when it binds.
   (b) The portion of the drug to which a drug target binds.
   (c) The functional groups used by a drug in binding to a drug target.
   (d) The bonds involved in binding a drug to its target
5. Which of the following binding interactions is likely to be the most important initial interaction when a drug enters a binding site?
   (a) van der Waals interactions
   (b) hydrogen bond
   (c) ionic
   (d) induced dipole-dipole interactions
6. Which of the following underlined atoms is likely to be the strongest hydrogen bond acceptor?
   (a) amide nitrogen (RNHCOR')
   (b) aniline nitrogen (ArNH2)
   (c) amine nitrogen (RNH2)
   (d) carboxylate oxygen (RCO 2-)
7. Which of the following underlined protons is likely to be the strongest hydrogen bond donor?
   (a) alcohol (ROH)
   (b) amine (RNH2)
   (c) phenol (ArOH)
   (d) ammonium ion (RNH3+)
8. Which of the following functional groups is most likely to participate in a dipole-dipole interaction?
   (a) Aromatic ring (b) Ketone
   (c) Alcohol (d) Alkene
9. Which of the following statements is untrue?
   (a) Desolvation is an energy expensive process that involves the removal of water from polar functional groups prior to a drug binding to its binding site.
   (b) Water molecules surrounding a hydrophobic region of a drug form an ordered layer of molecules with low entropy.

(c) Interaction between the non-polar regions of a drug and the non-polar regions of a target require the removal of an ordered water coat and represents a gain in binding energy due to increased entropy.
(d) An increase in entropy results in a greater positive value of $\Delta G$ and a greater chance of binding.

10. What term is used to indicate the ability of a cancer to invade other parts of the body and to produce secondary tumours?
(a) Carcinogenesis (b) Apoptosis
(c) Metastasis (d) Mutagenesis

11. Which molecules are involved in the anchoring of cells to an extracellular matrix?
(a) Integrins (b) Interleukins
(c) Angiostatin (d) Cyclins

12. Cyclophosphamide is commonly used in anticancer therapy. Which of the following statements is not true of the above structure?
(a) It is relatively non-toxic.
(b) It acts as a prodrug.
(c) It cannot be taken orally.
(d) The structure is metabolised to release acrolein

13. What is the term used to indicate the growth of new blood vessels?
(a) Biosynthesis (b) Angiogenesis
(c) Apoptosis (d) Metastasis

14. Which of the following inhibits angiogenesis?
(a) VEGF (b) FGF-2
(c) Angiostatin (d) Interleukin-6

15. What sort of therapy involves administration of an antibody linked to an enzyme, such that the enzyme activates a prodrug?
(a) ADAPT (b) GDAPT
(c) ADEPT (d) GDEPT

16. An isosteric replacement for carboxylic acid group is
(a) Pyrrole (b) Isoxazole
(c) Phenol (d) tetrazole

17. For glyburide, all of the following metabolic reactions are logical EXCEPT
(a) O-demethylation
(b) Aromatic oxidation
(c) Benzylic hydroxylation
(d) Amide hydrolysis

18. Ethambutol molecule has
(a) two chiral centers and 3 stereoisomers
(b) two chiral centers and 4 stereoisomers
(c) two chiral centers and 2 stereoisomers
(d) one chiral center and 2 stereoisomers

19. Amitryptyline is synthesized from the following starting material:
(a) Phthalic anhydride
(b) Terephthalic acid
(c) Phthalamic acid
(d) Phthalimide

20. The common structural feature amongst the three categories of anticonvulsant Drugs barbiturates, succinimides and hydantoins is
(a) Ureide
(b) Imidazolidinone
(c) Dihydropyrimidine
(d) Tetrahydropyrimidine

21. Chemical nomenclature of procaine is
(a) 2-Diethylaminoethyl 4-aminobenzoate
(b) N,N-Diethyl 4-aminobenzoate
(c) 4-Aminobenzamidoethyl amine
(d) 4-Amino-2-dimethylaminoethyl benzoate

22. Barbiturates with substitution at the following position possess acceptable Hypnotic activity:
(a) 1,3-Disubstitution
(b) 5,5-Disubstitution
(c) 1,5-Disubstitution
(d) 3,3-Disubstitution

23. Proton pump inhibitors like omeprazole and lansoprazole contain the following ring system :
(a) Pyrimidine (b) Benzimidazole
(c) Benzothiazole (d) Oxindole

24. Artemisinin contains the following group in its structure:
    (a) An endoperoxide
    (b) An exoperoxide
    (c) An epoxide
    (d) An acid hydrazide

25. In thiazides following substituent is essential for diuretic activity:
    (a) Chloro group at position 6
    (b) Methyl group at position 2
    (c) Sulphamoyl group at position 7
    (d) Hydrophobic group at position

26. Oxidative phosphorylation involves
    (a) Electron transport system
    (b) Substrate level phosphorylation
    (c) Reaction catalyzed by succinic thiokinase in TCA cycle
    (d) None of the above

27. The following protein/polypeptide has a quaternary structure:
    (a) cc-Chymotrypsin (b) Hemoglobin
    (c) Insulin (d) Myoglobin

28. To what extent are the three nitrogens of histamine ionised at blood pH?
    (a) all three nitrogens are fully ionised
    (b) all three nitrogens are not ionised at all
    (c) the side chain nitrogen is fully ionised and the heterocyclic nitrogens are not ionised
    (d) the side chain nitrogen and one of the heterocyclic nitrogens are fully ionized

29. Three binding regions were proposed to be present in the binding site of the H2 receptor. Which of the following statements is incorrect?
    (a) There is a binding region for the imidazole ring of histamine analogues which is common for agonists and antagonists.
    (b) There is a binding region which interacts ionically with the α-nitrogen of histamine and results in agonist activity.
    (c) There is a binding region further away from the imidazole ring that produces an antagonist effect if occupied.
    (d) The α-nitrogen of histamine can only bind to the agonist binding region while the guanyl group of Nα-guanylhistamine can only bind to the antagonist binding region.

30. The following structures show some of the important molecules leading to the discovery of burimamide (B).

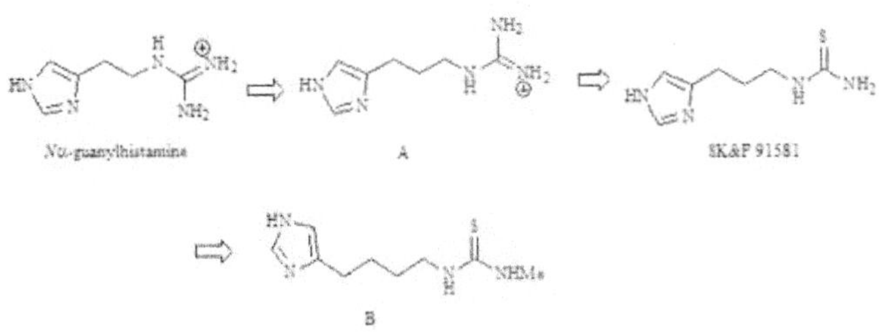


    What strategy was used in developing burimamide from SK&F 91581?
    (a) extension
    (b) chain extension
    (c) substituent variation
    (d) isosteric replacement

31. The following structures show some of the important molecules leading to the discovery of burimamide (B).

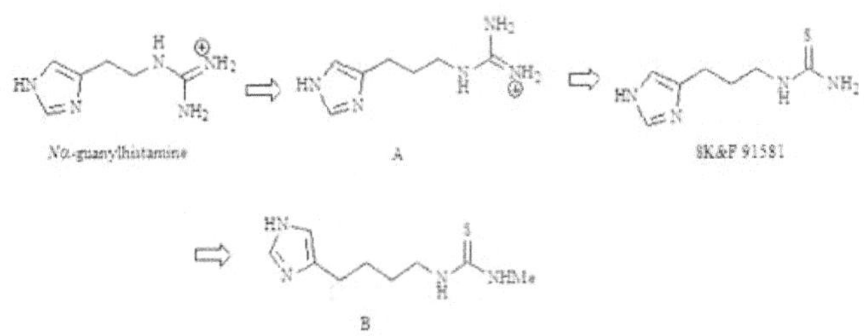


    Which of the following statements concerning burimamide is untrue?
    (a) it established the existence of H2-receptors
    (b) it was a good antagonist at H2 receptors with only weak partial agonist activity
    (c) it inhibited gastric acid release from parietal cells
    (d) it indicated that binding to the antagonist binding region involved hydrogen bonding and not ionic bonding

32. The following diagram shows development of H2-antagonists from burimamide (structure B).

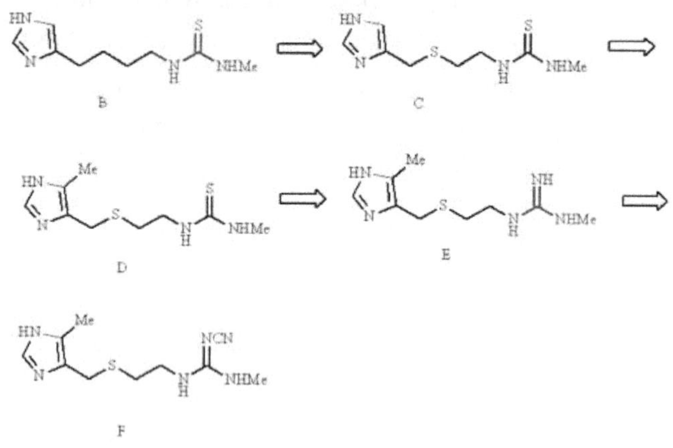

A sulphur atom was inserted into the side chain of structure C. What effect did this change have?

(a) it introduced an extra binding interaction
(b) it stabilised the molecule
(c) it increased the percentage population of the active heterocyclic tautomer
(d) it prevented ionisation of the terminal functional group

33. Once activated, the proton pump inhibitors bind to exposed amino acids in the proton pump. Which amino acid is involved?

(a) Serine (b) cysteine
(c) Lysine (d) histidine

34. Identify the correct name for the following peptide.

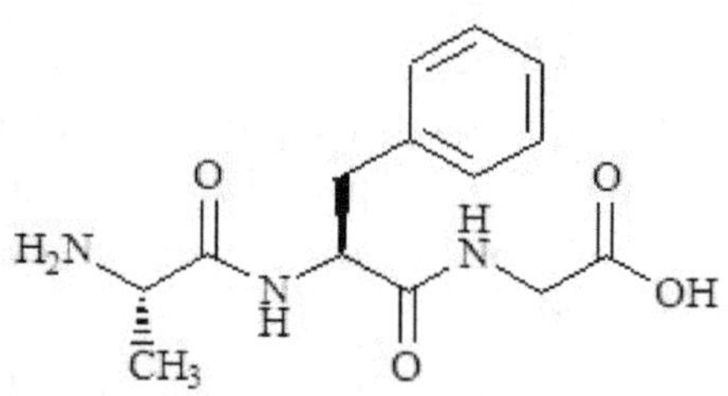

(a) L-alanyl-L-phenylalanyl-glycine
(b) glycyl-L-phenylalanyl-L-alanine
(c) L-phenylalanyl-L-alanyl-glycine
(d) L-alanyl-glycyl-L-phenylalanine

35. Which of the following single letter codes represents the structure below?

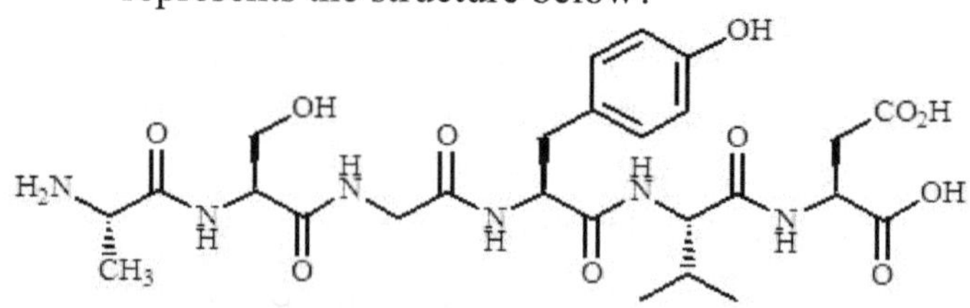

(a) DVYGSA (b) ASGYVD
(c) EVFGSA (d) ASGFVE

36. Which of the following statements is true about a peptide bond (RCONHR')?

(a) It is non planar.
(b) It is capable of forming a hydrogen bond.
(c) The cis configuration is favoured over the trans configuration.
(d) Single bond rotation is permitted between nitrogen and the carbonyl group.

37. Identify the strongest form of intermolecular bonding that could be formed involving the residue of the amino acid valine.

(a) ionic bond
(b) hydrogen bond
(c) van der Waals interactions
(d) none of the above

38. Identify which of the following terms refers to the order in which amino acids are linked together in a protein.

(a) primary structure
(b) secondary structure
(c) tertiary structure
(d) quaternary structure

39. The following antibiotic structure is an intercalating agent. What role does the ionic group serve in making this molecule an effective intercalating agent?

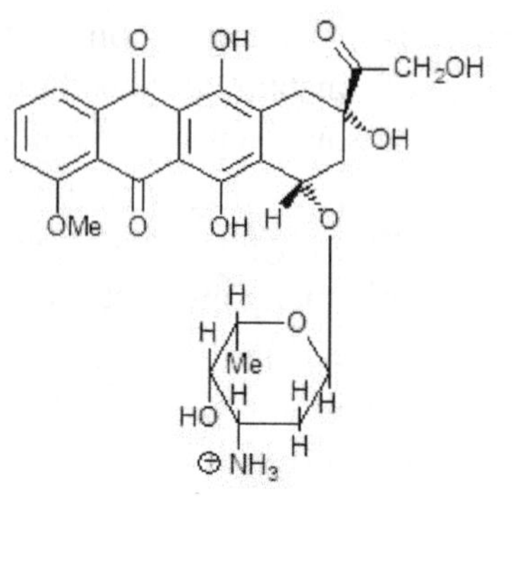

(a) It increases water solubility allowing high dose levels to be used.
(b) It interacts with charged phosphate groups in DNA to stabilise intercalation.
(c) It acts as a strong hydrogen bond donor with nucleic acid bases to stabilise intercalation.
(d) It only becomes protonated when it enters cells and so becomes trapped within the cell leading to high concentrations of drug.

40. Which term best describes the mechanism of action for fluoroquinolones?
(a) Alkylating agent
(b) Antisense agent
(c) Chain cutter
(d) Topoisomerase poison

41. The following antibacterial agent was used in the Second World War.

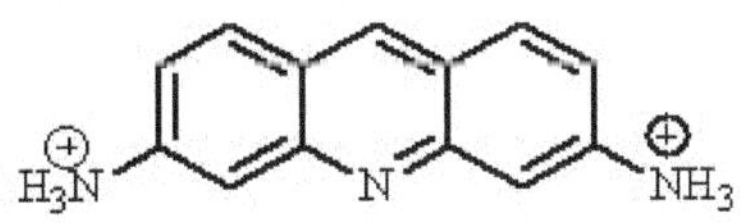

What is the name of the structure?
(a) Erythromycin (b) Proflavine
(c) Chloramphenicol (d) Rifampicin

42. The following antibacterial agent was used in the Second World War.

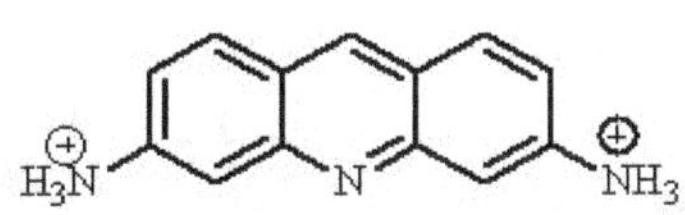

Which of the following terms best describes its mechanism of action?
(a) Alkylating agent (b) Chain cutter
(c) Antisense agent (d) Intercalating agent

43. The following structure is a synthetic antibacterial agent called ciprofloxacin.

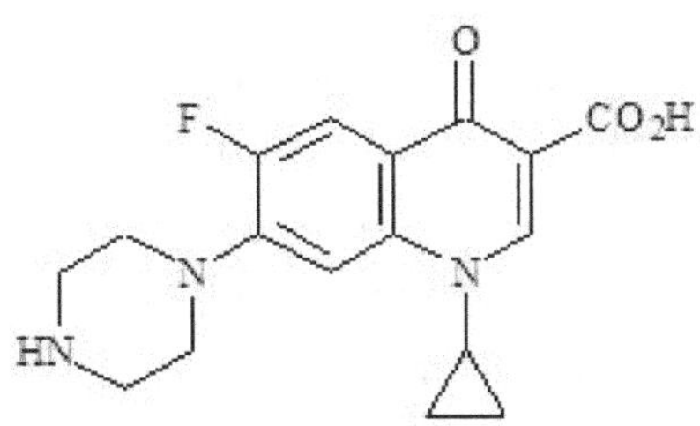

What is its mechanism of action?
(a) Topoisomerase poison
(b) Metallating agent
(c) Chain terminator
(d) Antisense agent

44. The following anticancer agent is called busulfan.

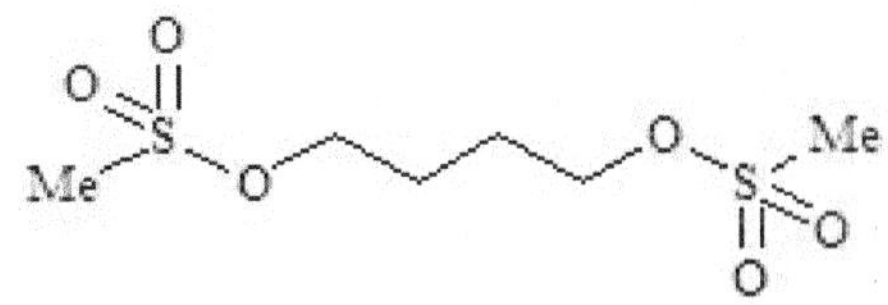

What is the drug's mode of action?
(a) Metallating agent (b) Intercalator
(c) Chain terminator (d) Alkylating agent

45. What is the mode of action of the anticancer agent calicheamicin γ1?
(a) Alkylating agent
(b) Chain cutting agent
(c) Antisense agent
(d) Intercalating agent

46. The following structure is used in the treatment of brain tumours.

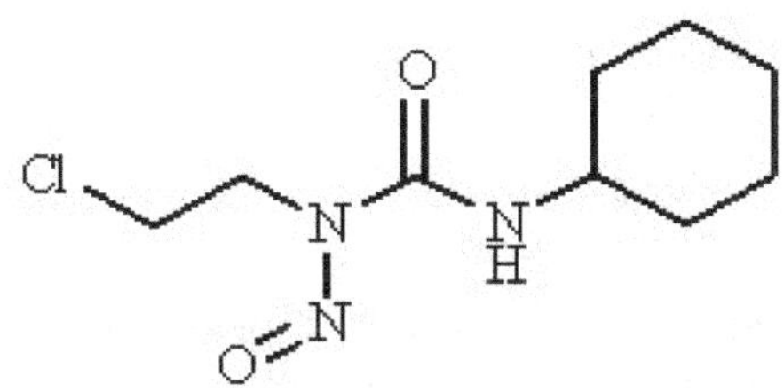

What is the structure called?
(a) Carmustine
(b) Lomustine
(c) Streptozotocin
(d) Cyclophosphamide

47. The following agent is used for the treatment of testicular and ovarian cancers.

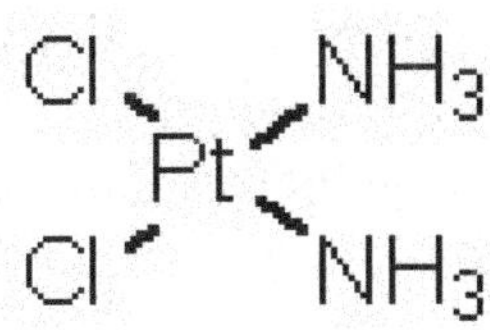

Which of the following statements is untrue regarding the above structure?

(a) The chlorine groups are displaced before the drug becomes active.
(b) Intrastrand cross linking of DNA results from the action of the agent.
(c) Base pairing between adenine and thymine is disrupted by the agent.
(d) The compound acts as a metallating agent.

48. The following general structure is representative of sulphonamides. Which of the following statements is true for active sulphonamides?

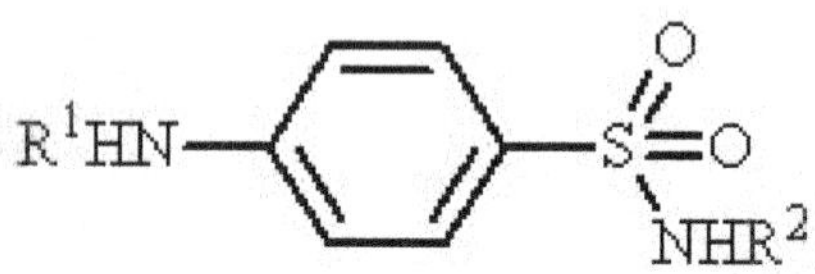


(a) R1 can be H or an alkyl group
(b) R2 must be hydrogen
(c) The aromatic ring is essential
(d) The sulphonamide functional group can be replaced with an ester

49. Which of the following statements is true regarding the properties of benzylpenicillin?

(a) It is a bacteriostatic agent.
(b) It is active over a wide range of bacterial species.
(c) It is resistant to β-lactamases.
(d) Certain individuals may have an allergic response to it.

50. What crucial feature of a penicillin is involved in its mechanism of action?

(a) Carboxylic acid (b) β-lactam ring
(c) Acyl side chain (d) Thiazolidine ring

51. What reaction is catalysed by a β-lactamase enzyme?

(a) The final cross-linking reaction to form the bacterial cell wall
(b) The hydrolysis of the acyl side chain from penicillin structures
(c) The hydrolysis of the four-membered ring present in penicillins
(d) The biosynthesis of the penicillin structure from the amino acids valine and cysteine

52. Which of the following statements is accurate in explaining why Gram negative bacteria are generally more resistant to penicillins than Gram positive bacteria?

(a) Gram negative bacteria have a thicker cell wall
(b) Gram negative bacteria have an outer hydrophilic membrane that acts as an extra barrier
(c) Gram negative bacteria can concentrate β-lactamase enzymes in the periplasmic space
(d) Gram negative bacteria produce smaller quantities of transpeptidase enzyme

53. What role does the acetoxy group at the 3-position of cephalosporins have in enhancing antibacterial activity?

(a) It acts as a steric shield and masks enzymatic attack at the β-lactam ring.
(b) It acts as a good leaving group when the β-lactam ring is opened.
(c) It takes part in a transesterification reaction with the carboxylic acid group at position 4.
(d) It increases the reactivity of the β-lactam ring by neighbouring group participation.

54. The following structure (cefalexin) is a first generation cephalosporin. The following structure (cefalexin) is a first generation cephalosporin.

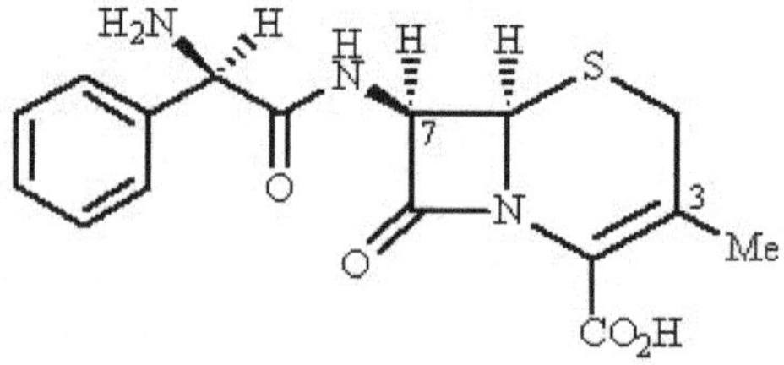


Which of the following statements is true for the methyl substituent at position 3?

(a) It is a good leaving group
(b) It is generally good for activity
(c) It is good for oral activity
(d) It acts as a steric shield

55. Morphine is an important analgesic.

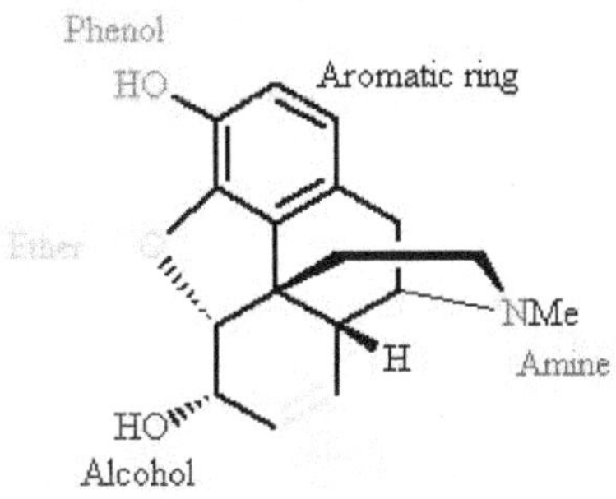

What interactions are involved in binding the phenol group to the target binding site?
(a) Ionic interactions
(b) Hydrogen bonding interactions
(c) van der Waals binding interactions
(d) The group has no binding role

56. The following structure is more active than morphine as an analgesic.

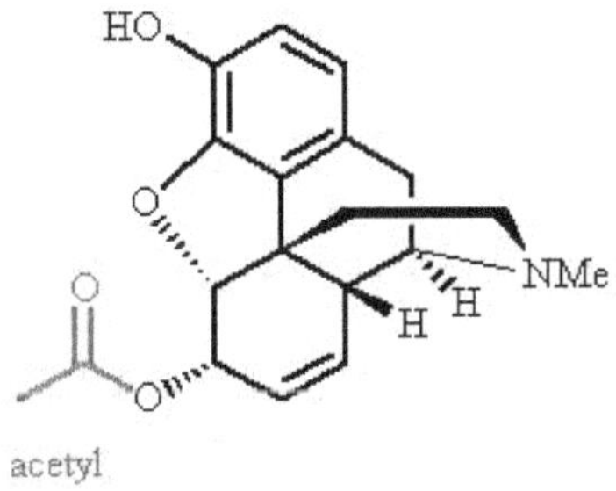

What is this structure called?
(a) 6-acetylmorphine
(b) 3-acetylmorphine
(c) heterocodeine
(d) heteromorphine

57. Propose the likely analgesic activity of 3-acetylmorphine relative to diamorphine and 6-acetylmorphine.
(a) 3-acetylmorphine should be more active than 6-acetylmorphine and diamorphine.
(b) 3-acetylmorphine should be less active than 6-acetylmorphine and diamorphine.
(c) 3-acetylmorphine should be more active than 6-acetylmorphine and less active than diamorphine.
(d) 3-acetylmorphine should be less active than 6-acetylmorphine and more active than diamorphine.

58. The following agent is used clinically as an analgesic.

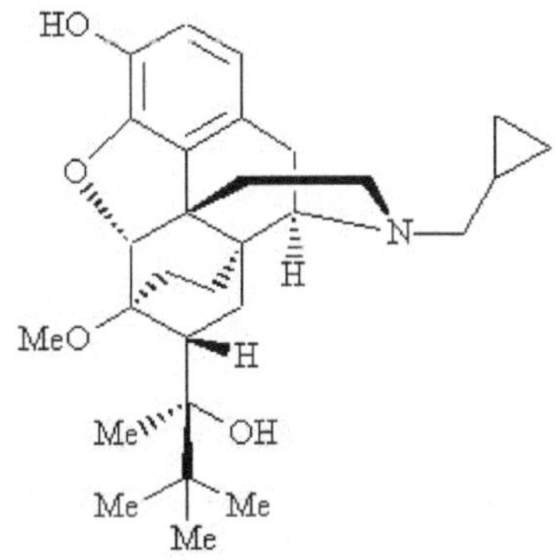

What is it called?
(a) Etorphine (b) thebaine
(c) Buprenorphine (d) diprenorphine

59. The binding site of analgesic receptors has two hydrophobic binding regions in the vicinity of the ionic binding region. One is responsible for agonist activity and the other is responsible for antagonist activity. Which of the following statements is true?
(a) The antagonist hydrophobic binding region is closer to the ionic binding region than the agonist hydrophobic binding region.
(b) The agonist hydrophobic binding region is closer to the ionic binding region than the antagonist hydrophobic binding region.
(c) The antagonist hydrophobic binding region and agonist hydrophobic bind regions are equidistant from the ionic binding region.
(d) The relative positions of the hydrophobic regions vary depending on the type of analgesic receptor concerned.

60. What type of structures are the compounds (i) - (iv)?

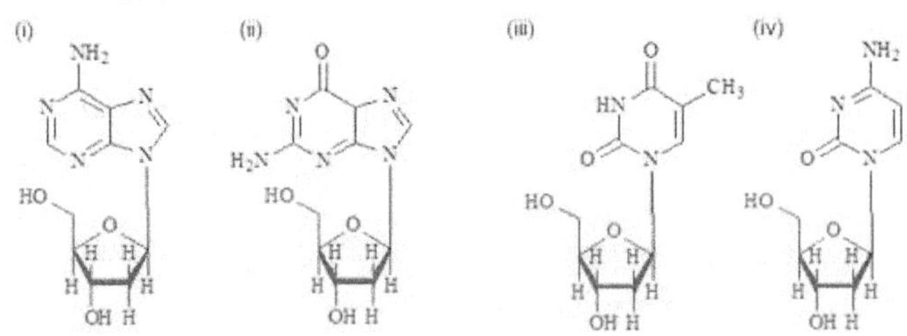

(a) nucleic acids (b) nucleotides
(c) nucleosides (d) deoxyriboses

61. To which of the following does thymine form hydrogen bonds in DNA?
    (a) Adenine (b) thymine
    (c) Cytosine (d) guanine

62. What term is used to describe the process by which DNA is copied to produce two daughter DNA molecules?
    (a) Reproduction (b) replication
    (c) Translation (d) transcription

63. What term is used to describe the process by which a segment of DNA is copied to produce a molecule of messenger RNA?
    (a) Reproduction (b) replication
    (c) Translation (d) transcription

64. Which of the following mutations is most likely to be disruptive to protein synthesis or function?
    (a) UAU to UAC (b) UAU to UUU
    (c) UAU to UAA (d) UAU to CAU

65. Which of the following strategies will increase the polarity and water solubility of a drug?
    (a) Removing polar functional groups
    (b) Adding extra alkyl groups
    (c) Replacing an aromatic ring with a nitrogen containing heterocyclic ring
    (d) Replacing an alkyl group with a larger alkyl group

66. Losartin was developed from structure (I) as an antihypertensive agent by replacing a carboxylic acid group with a tetrazole ring. Which of the following statements is incorrect?

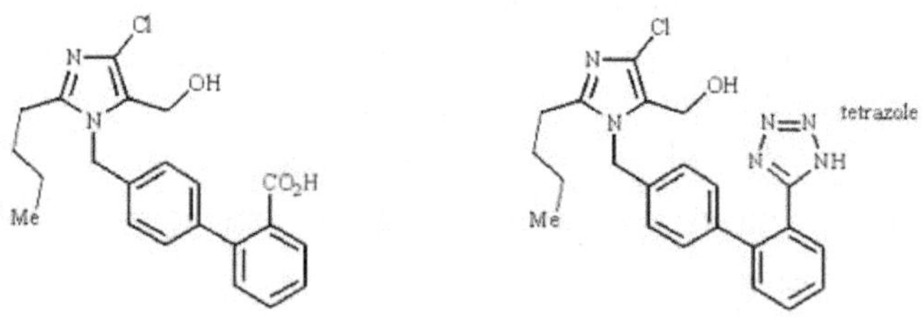


(I) Losartan

    (a) The tetrazole ring represents a bio-isostere.
    (b) The tetrazole ring mimics a carboxylic acid in being planar.
    (c) The tetrazole ring mimics a carboxylic acid in being acidic.
    (d) The tetrazole ring is more polar than a carboxylic acid.

67. Why does chlorpropamide have a longer antibiotic activity than tolbutamide?

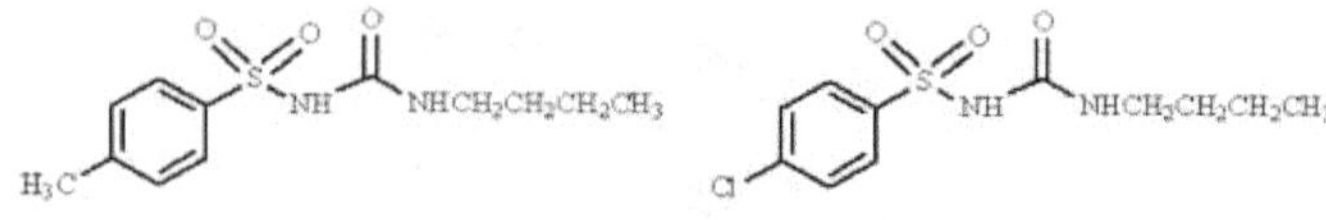

Tolbutamide Chlorpropamide

    (a) The chloro group of chlorpropamide has an electron-withdrawing effect on the aromatic ring and stabilises the molecule.
    (b) The methyl group of tolbutamide is susceptible to drug metabolism whereas the chloro substituent of chlorpropamide is not.
    (c) The urea group of tolbutamide is more susceptible to hydrolysis than the urea group of chlorpropamide.
    (d) The sulfonamide group of tolbutamide is more susceptible to hydrolysis than the sulfonamide group of chlorpropamide.

68. Carbachol is more stable than acetylcholine to hydrolysis. Which of the following statements is not true?

Carbachol Acetylcholine

    (a) The blue coloured methyl group of acetylcholine is susceptible to oxidation by cytochrome p450 enzymes.
    (b) The blue coloured nitrogen of carbachol stabilises the neighbouring carbonyl group.
    (c) Carbachol contains a urethane group while acetylcholine contains an ester group.
    (d) The blue coloured NH2 group of carbachol is a bio-isostere for the blue coloured CH3 group of acetylcholine.

69. Some drugs containing an ester group are inactive in vitro, but are active once the drug has been absorbed in vivo. What term is used for such drugs?
    (a) Postdrugs (b) predrugs
    (c) Metabolites (d) prodrugs

70. In Parkinson's disease, there is a lack of the neurotransmitter dopamine in the brain. Adding dopamine itself is not very effective for a

variety of reasons. Which of the following statements is not a valid explanation?

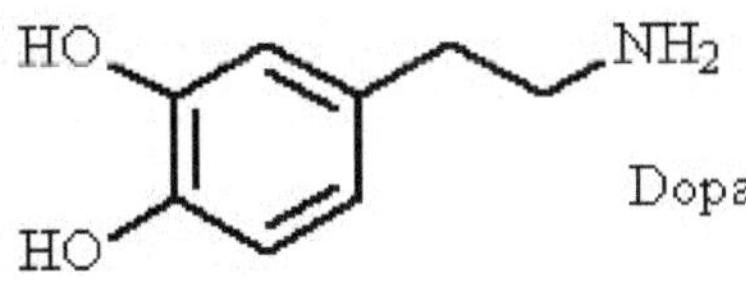


Dopamine

(a) Dopamine is too polar to cross the blood-brain barrier.
(b) Dopamine is chemically unstable.
(c) Dopamine is metabolised to inactive metabolites.
(d) Dopamine shows no selectivity between dopamine receptors in the brain and peripheral dopamine receptors.

71. Candoxatril is an ester prodrug for candoxatrilat which inhibits protease enzymes. Which of the following statements is incorrect?

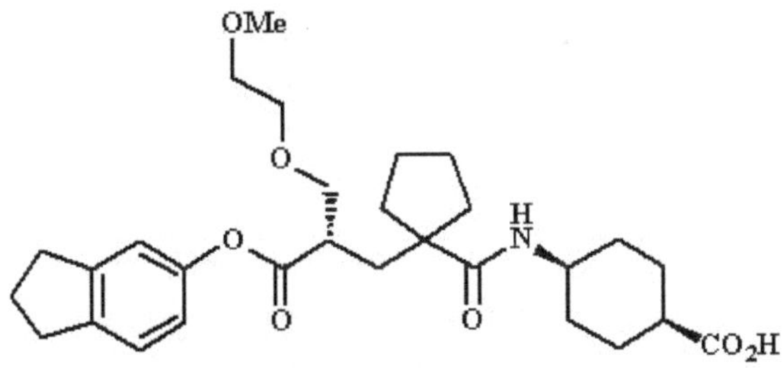


Candoxatril

(a) Hydrolysis of the ester reveals a carboxylic acid group on candoxatrilat.
(b) The parent drug can be administered orally, whereas the ester prodrug cannot.
(c) The bicyclic leaving group is non-toxic.
(d) The bicyclic system is electron with-drawing and speeds up the rate of ester hydrolysis.

72. Some peptides and proteins have been used as drugs. Which of the following statements is untrue?
(a) Protein drugs suffer a disadvantage in that they could produce an immune response.
(b) Peptides and proteins generally show poor bioavailability.
(c) Peptide drugs are susceptible to peptidase enzymes.
(d) Peptide drugs are susceptible to metabolic enzymes but not to digestive enzymes.

73. Which species of the following is used to bombard with the sample for which mass spectroscopy has been performed?
(a) Alpha particles (b) Neutrons
(c) Electrons (d) Protons

74. What are the main criteria on which mass spectrometer used for?
(a) Composition in sample
(b) Relative mass of atoms
(c) Concentration of elements in the sample
(d) Properties of sample

75. Which of the following statement is false for mass spectroscopy?
(a) Mass spectroscopy is used to identify unknown compounds within a sample, and to elucidate the structure and chemical properties of different molecules
(b) Particle are characterized by their mass to charge ratios (m/z) and relative abundances
(c) This technique basically studies the effect of ionizing energy on molecules
(d) This technique can be used on all state of matter

76. The ultraviolet spectrum of benzonitrile shows a primary absorption band at 224 nm. If a solution of benzonitrile in water, with a concentration of 1x 10-4 molar, is examined at a wavelength of 224 nm, the absorbance is determined to be 1.30. The cell length is 1 cm.

What is the molar absorptivity of this absorption band?
(a) $2.3 \times 104$ (b) $3.3 \times 104$
(c) $1.3 \times 104$ (d) $4.3 \times 104$

77. What is the correct order of $\lambda$max for n–> $\pi^*$ transition for the following three compounds?
(a) RCOOH > RCOOR' > RCONH2
(b) RCOOH = RCOOR' = RCONH2
(c) RCOOH = RCOOR' < RCONH2
(d) RCOOH = RCOOR' > RCONH2

78. What is the correct order of $\lambda$max for n –> $\pi^*$ transition for the R-CN, R-NO2, and R-N=N-R?
(a) R-CN < R-NO2 < R-N=N-R
(b) R-CN = R-NO2 = R-N=N-R
(c) R-CN > R-NO2 > R-N=N-R
(d) R-CN > R-NO2 < R-N=N-R

79. Which of the following main component of mass spectroscopy deal with resolving the ions into their characteristics mass components according to their mass-to-charge ratio?
    (a) Ion Source
    (b) Analyzer
    (c) Detector System
    (d) Analyzer tube
80. Which is the mildest reducing agent which reduces only carbonyl group in presence of nitro, carboxyl, double bond and ester groups?
    (a) LiAIH4 (b) Na-NH3
    (c) NaBH4 (d) H2-Ni
81. Alcohol on refluxing with Cr2O7 gives:
    (a) Ester (b) Aldehyde
    (c) Sugar (d) Carboxylic acid
82. What is the relation between wave number of IR absorption and the reduced mass?
    (a) Wave number is directly proportional to reduced mass
    (b) Wave number is inversely proportional to reduced mass
    (c) Wave number is independent of the reduced mass
    (d) Wave number is directly proportional to square of reduced mass
83. A compound C8 H6 decolorizes Br2 in CCl4 and gives a white precipitate with Tollen's reagent. It has sharp band at 3300 cm-l and weak bands at 3085, 2110 cm-l. What is this compound?
    (a) Phenyl acetylene (b) Phenyl propylene
    (c) Phenyl ethylene (d) Octene
84. Why ketenes absorb in IR at a very high frequency (2150 cm-1)?
    (a) The inner C is sp hybridized
    (b) The more s character in a bond, the stronger it is
    (c) Inner C is sp2 hybridized
    (d) Inner C is sp3 hybridized
85. Which compound having molecular formula C5H10 shows absorption at 1380 cm-1?
    (a) 2-Methyl-1-butene
    (b) Cyclopentane
    (c) Pentyne
    (d) Methylcyclobutane
86. Why in the IR spectrum of Benzoyl chloride, a weak band near 1750 cm-1 is formed?
    (a) Inductive effect
    (b) Fermi resonance between C = O band and first overtone
    (c) Conjugation effect
    (d) Hyperconjugation effect
87. Since the nuclei in a polyatomic molecule do not always vibrate in a simple harmonic manner, there arises which of the following situation?
    (a) Harmonicity
    (b) Anharmonicity in molecular vibrations
    (c) Fundamental frequencies
    (d) Infrared
88. What is the relation between restoring force, f to the displacement q in Hooke's law?
    (a) f = -kq (b) f = kq
    (c) f = kq2 (d) f = -kq2
89. The intensity of an absorption band is always proportional to which of the following factor?
    (a) Atomic population
    (b) Molecular population of the initial state
    (c) Molecular population of the final state
    (d) Temperature
90. For HCI, = 1.63 x 10-27 kg, the observed frequency = 2890 or v = 8.67 x 1013 Hz. What is the force constant K?
    (a) 4.83 m dyn Å-1 (b) 8.43 dynes cm-1
    (c) 483 μm-1 (d) 4.83 dyn Å-1
91. How many Hertz does 1 ppm correspond to for an PMR spectrometer operating at a radio frequency of 60 MHz and 100 MHz?
    (a) 6 Hz, 10 Hz (b) 60 Hz, 100 Hz
    (c) 100 Hz, 60 Hz (d) 10Hz, 100Hz
92. The distance between the centers of the peaks of doublet is called as?
    (a) Coupling constant
    (b) Spin constant
    (c) Spin-spin coupling
    (d) Chemical shift

93. $H_2$, $CH_4$, $C_2H_6$ and $C_6H_6$ exhibit which PMR spectra?
(a) Singlet (b) Doublet
(c) Triplet (d) Quintet

94. The 1H NMR spectrum of $CH_3OCHClCH_2Cl$ will exhibit ________
(a) A three proton doublet. One proton singlet and a two proton doublet
(b) A three proton singlet. One proton singlet and a two proton doublet
(c) A three proton singlet. One proton triplet and a two proton doublet
(d) A three proton triplet. One proton triplet and a two proton triplet

95. Location of M1 Receptor is:
(a) Autonomic Ganglia
(b) Heart
(c) Smooth Muscle
(d) All of the above

96. Bioisosteres are similar in which parameter:
(a) Physical (b) Chemical
(c) Biological (d) Both (a) and (b)

97. Solubility of drug in a particular solvent depends on:
(a) Chemical structure (b) Particle size
(c) Crystal formation (d) All of the above

98. What is the protein content of cytochrome P450
(a) Heme protein CYP450
(b) NADPH- CYP450 reductase
(c) NADH- CYP450 reductase
(d) Both (b) and (c)

99. Which of the following is not Phase I metabolic reaction
(a) Reduction of ketone
(b) Conjugation of alcohol
(c) Monoamine oxidase
(d) Ester hydrolysis

100. All muscarinic receptors are:
(a) Ligand Gated ion channels
(b) G- protein coupled receptor
(c) Enzyme linked receptors
(d) Nuclear receptor

101. The amino acid precursor for the catecholamine is
(a) Serine (b) Phenylalanine
(c) Tyrosine (d) Choline

102. The alpha methyl substitution on the ethylene bridge of Acetylcholine shows increase in:
(a) Muscarinic activity
(b) Nicotinic activity
(c) Both of the above
(d) None of the above

103. Dicyclomine belong to which of the following category?
(a) Antiparkinsonian
(b) Vasicoselective
(c) Antisecretory-antispasmodic-Quaternary Compounds
(d) Antisecretory-antispasmodic-Tertiary amine

104. Tolazoline is
(a) Alpha 1 selective
(b) Alpha 2 selective
(c) Both Alpha 1 and Alpha2 selective
(d) None of the above

105. Naturally occurring Noradrenaline is rapidly metabolized by:
(a) COMT
(b) MAO
(c) Cholinesterases
(d) None of the above

106. Barbiturates act by:
(a) Increasing GABA inhibition
(b) By binding to A1 receptor
(c) Through GPCR
(d) All of the above

107. Antipsycotic drugs are also called:
(a) CNS depressant
(b) CNS Stimulant
(c) Neuroleptics
(d) Antidepressant

108. Which of the following is a D2 blocker?
(a) Clozapine
(b) Loxapine Succinate
(c) Haloperidol
(d) Prochlorperazine Maleate

109. Hydantoin is:
    (a) Imidazolidine-2, 2- dione
    (b) Imidazolidine-2, 4- dione
    (c) Imidazolidine-2, 5- dione
    (d) Imidazolidine-2, 3- dione

110. Which of the following is selective NMDA receptor antagonist?
    (a) Ketamine (b) Thiopental
    (c) Diazepam (d) Methohexital

111. Which of the following is the drug of choice in cardiac surgery for anesthesia?
    (a) Enflurane (b) Isoflurane
    (c) Halothane (d) Thiopentone

112. Which one is not an Opioid receptor?
    (a) Mu (b) Kappa
    (c) Delta (d) Gamma

113. Aspirin is a:
    (a) p-amino phenol derivative
    (b) Salicylic acid Derivative
    (c) Anthranilic acid derivative
    (d) Oxicam Derivative

114. Which one the following is a selective COX-2 Inhibitor?
    (a) Etorcoxib (b) Piroxicam
    (c) Miloxicam (d) Diflunisal

115. When considering electrophillic substitution, aromatic substitution the halides are
    (a) Ortho / Para directing and deactivatin
    (b) Ortho / Para directing and activating
    (c) Meta directing and deactivating
    (d) Meta directing and activating

116. Sulponation of Phenol at room temperature gives
    (a) p-isomer
    (b) o-isomer
    (c) Both a and b
    (d) None of the above

117. Phenol is better bronsted acid than cyclohexenol because
    (a) I is a better proton donor
    (b) The cyclohexyl group is an electron donating group by induction which stabilizes the anion formed in the reaction
    (c) Phenol is able to stabilize the anion formed in the reaction by the resonance
    (d) None of the above

118. When chloride is present at meta position in benzene nucleus of aromatic acid shows
    (a) Electron donating resonance effect
    (b) Electron withdrawing inductive effect
    (c) Both a and b
    (d) None of the above

119. The specific gravity of lipid is
    (a) 0.2 (b) 0.8
    (b) 1.0 (d) 1.5

120. Rancidity of lipids containing food is due to
    (a) Hydrogenation of unsaturated fatty acids
    (b) Reduction of fatty acids
    (c) Oxidation of fatty acids
    (d) Dehydrogenation of saturated fatty acids

121. Dietary fats are transported by
    (a) Chylomicrons (b) Liposomes
    (c) Lipid globules (d) Oil droplets

122. Which of the following is important in testing the purity of butter and ghee?
    (a) R. M. value
    (b) Saponification value
    (c) Iodine value
    (d) Acetyl value

123. An aromatic molecule will have
    (a) Have $(4n + 2)$ $\pi$ electrons
    (b) Be cyclic
    (c) Be planar
    (d) All of the above

124. Benzene act as
    (a) Nucleophile
    (b) Electrophile
    (c) Both a and b
    (d) None of the above

125. 1- Nitronaphthalene on reduction yields
    (a) 1- Naphthylamine
    (b) 2- Naphthylamine
    (c) 1- Naphthol
    (d) 2- Naphthol

126. Upon ozonolysis, phenanthrene gives,
   (a) Phenanthroquinone
   (b) Diphenic acid
   (c) Phenanthric acid
   (d) Diphenylaldehyde

127. Cyclopropane when reacted with bromine it gives
   (a) 1,2-dibromopropane
   (b) 1,3-dibromopropane
   (c) 1,4-dibromopropane
   (d) 1,1-dibromopropane

128. Which of the following cycloalkanes has lowest heat of combustion?
   (a) Cyclopropane
   (b) Cyclopentane
   (c) Cyclohexane
   (d) Cycloheptane

129. Anthracene undergoes electrophillic substitution reactions mainly at
   (a) C-1 (b) C-2
   (c) C-9 (d) C-4

130. Which of the following cycloalkanes has the more strain energy?
   (a) Cyclobutane (b) Cyclopentane
   (c) Cyclohexane (d) Cyclopropane

131. The boat conformation has how many eclipsing H-H interactions?
   (a) 1 (b) 2
   (c) 4 (d) 6

132. Resonance energy for Naphthalene is
   (a) 88 kcal/mole (b) 36 kcal/mole
   (c) 47 kcal/mole (d) 61 kcal/mole

133. PAHs stand for
   (a) Polyaromatic Hydrocarbons
   (b) Polyaromatic halides
   (c) Polyamines as Histamines
   (d) None of these

134. PAHs are
   (a) Polar
   (b) Non-Polar
   (c) Both a and b
   (d) None of these

135. The diazonium salts are reaction product of reaction of nitrous acid with
   (a) primary aliphatic amines
   (b) primary aromatic amines
   (c) secondary aliphatic amines
   (d) secondary aromatic amines

136. Phenol is used
   (a) in alcoholic beverages
   (b) as anaesthetics
   (c) in antiseptics
   (d) as moth repellant

137. C-C Bond Length in benzene is
   (a) greater than C-C bond length in ethane
   (b) shorter than C-C bond length in ethylene
   (c) same as that of C-C bond length in ethylene
   (d) intermediate between C-C bond length in ethane and C-C bond length in ethylene

138. The term "Hygroscopic" means:
   (a) Loss of water of crystallization
   (b) To absorb moisture
   (c) To absorb toxins
   (d) Soapy to touch

139. Which of the following is not an electrolyte used in replacement therapy :
   (a) Sodium chloride
   (b) Potassium chloride
   (c) Calcium gluconate
   (d) Sodium fluoride

140. Physiological antidotes act by:
   (a) Absorption of the poison
   (b) Changing the chemical nature of poison
   (c) Producing the effect opposite to that of poison
   (d) By countering the effect of poison

141. The one instrument from following not used for measurement of radioactivity is
   (a) Proportional counter
   (b) G.M. Counter
   (c) Ionization chamber
   (d) Conductivity meter

142. Sodium chloride equivalent method is used to adjust tonicity of which of the following Solutions?
   (a) Isotonic (b) Hypertonic
   (c) Hypotonic (d) Saturated

143. What is the pH range of blood?
   (a) 6.2-6.3 (b) 9.1-9.2
   (c) 4.2-4.3 (d) 7.4-7.5

144. Which one of the following is a major intracellular cation?
   (a) Iron (b) Potassium
   (c) Calcium (d) Magnesium

145. Astringents act by-
   (a) Lipid precipitant
   (b) Bacterial inhibition
   (c) Protein precipitant
   (d) Enzymatic catalysis

146. According to Lewis concept, acids are those which:
   (a) accepts a lone pair of electron
   (b) gives H+ ions on dissolution in non-aqueous solution
   (c) OH- ions on dissolution in aqueous solution
   (d) donates a lone pair of electron

147. Common name of sodium hydroxide is:
   (a) Slaked Lime (b) Spirit of salt
   (c) Caustic Soda (d) Quick Lime

148. Function of granulated zinc in limit test of arsenic is:
   (a) Reduction by absorption of H2 gas
   (b) Slow and prolonged evolution of nascent H2 gas
   (c) Faster evolution of nascent H2 gas
   (d) Oxidation by absorption of H2 gas

149. Fluoride inhibits carries formation by-
   (a) Downwards acid solubility of enamel
   (b) Bacterial inhibition
   (c) Both a and b
   (d) None of the above

150. Antidote in cyanide poisoning is-
   (a) Ethanol
   (b) Atropine
   (c) Desferioxamine
   (d) Sodium thiosulphate

151. Radioactive decay is-
   (a) 1st order reaction
   (b) 2nd order reaction
   (c) 3rd order reaction
   (d) Zero order reaction

152. Which buffer is used for maintaining acid-base balance balance in the blood :
   (a) Carbonic acid-bicarbonate ion
   (b) Acetic acid and sodium acetate
   (c) Ammonium hydroxide-ammonium chloride
   (d) Formic acid-sodium formate

153. Emetics act by:
   (a) By increasing the amount of fluid
   (b) By stimulation of the chemoreceptor trigger zone
   (c) By decreasing the viscosity of the bronchial secretion
   (d) None of these

154. Physiological antidotes acts by:
   (a) Absorption of the poison
   (b) Changing the chemical nature of poison
   (c) Producing the effect opposite to that of poison
   (d) By countering the effect of poison

155. Productive cough produces
   (a) Mucus (b) Vomiting
   (c) Amalgam (d) None of these

156. Alpha rays consist of stream of –
   (a) H+ (b) He2+
   (c) Only electron (d) Only neutron

# Answer Key Pharmaceutical Chemistry

1. d
2. b
3. b
4. a
5. b
6. d
7. d
8. b
9. d
10. c
11. a
12. c
13. b
14. c
15. c
16. d
17. b
18. b
19. b
20. a
21. a
22. b
23. b
24. a
25. c
26. a
27. b
28. c
29. d
30. b
31. b
32. c
33. b
34. a
35. b
36. b
37. a
38. b
39. d
40. b
41. d
42. a
43. d
44. b
45. b
46. c
47. c
48. d
49. b
50. c
51. c
52. b
53. c
54. b
55. a
56. b
57. b
58. c
59. a
60. c
61. a
62. b
63. d
64. c
65. c
66. d
67. b
68. a
69. d
70. b
71. b
72. d
73. c
74. b
75. d
76. c
77. b
78. a
79. b
80. c
81. d
82. b
83. a
84. c
85. b
86. b
87. a
88. a
89. b
90. a
91. b
92. a
93. a
94. c
95. a
96. d
97. d
98. a
99. b
100. b
101. b
102. b
103. d
104. c
105. a
106. a
107. c
108. d
109. b
110. a
111. b
112. d
113. b
114. a
115. a
116. b
117. c
118. d
119. b
120. c

121. a
122. a
123. d
124. a
125. c
126. d
127. b
128. c
129. c
130. d
131. c
132. a
133. a
134. b
135. b
136. c
137. d
138. b
139. d
140. c
141. d
142. a
143. d
144. b
145. **c**
146. a
147. b
148. b
149. c
150. d
151. a
152. a
153. b
154. c
155. a
156. b

# Chapter 3

# Pharmacognosy

## Pharmacognosy

### 3.1 Volatile Oils and Terpenoids

- **Terpenes:** Hydrocarbon $(C_5H_8)n$
- **Terpenoids:** Hydrocarbon with oxygenated derivatives. Terpnes and terpenoids are found in all found in all volatile oils or essential oils.
- **Etherenal oil:** Evaporate when exposed to air at ordinary temperature.
- **Extraction of volatile oils:**
  - ➢ **Hydro-distillation:** Water distillation, Steam distillation.
  - ➢ **Enfleurage:** fresh flower petals spread on fatty material Fatty layer saturated with volatile principle which is extracted with lipid solvent.
  - ➢ **Ecuelle:** Oil cells ruptured mechanically using pointed projection by twisting raw material in clockwise direction.
- **Classification of Volatile oils:**
  1. **Alcohol volatile oils** – Rose oil, Peppermint, Cardamom, Coriander, Sandalwood, Orange flowers.
  2. **Aldehyde volatile oils**-Lemon Peel, Citronella, Lemon grass, Bitter almond, Cinnamon, Orange peel.
  3. **Ester volatile oils**- Lavender, Musterd, Gaultheria.
  4. **hydrocarbon volatile oils** -Turpentine, Black pepper.
  5. **Ketone volatile oils** –Caraway, Civet oil, Musk, Spermint, Buchu, Camphor.
  6. **Oxide volatile oils** -Chenopodium, Eucalyptus.
  7. **Phenolic ether volatile oils** -Anise, Fennel, Nutmeg.
  8. **Phenol volatile oils**-Clove, Creosate, Thyme
- **General Chemical test for volatile oils:**
  - Drug part (usually thin section) - alc. $sol^n$ of sudan III - Red colour globules indicators of presence of volatile.
  - Drug part (thin section)- drop of tincture alkane- Red colour indicators of presence of volatile oil.

- **Classification of Terpenoids:**

  1. Hemiterpene or isoprene $(C_5H_8)$ : Not occur in nature
  2. Monoterpenes or terpenes $(C_5H_8)_2$
  3. Sesquiterpenes $(C_5H_8)_3$
  4. Diterpenes $(C_5H_8)_4$
  5. Triterpenes $(C_5H_8)_6$
  6. Tetraterpenes or carotenoids $(C_5H_8)_8$
  7. Pentaterpenes $(C_5H_8)_{10}$
  8. Polyterpenes or rubber $(C_5H_8)n$

- **Volatile oils containing Terpenoids**

  1. Peppermint oil: Menthol
  2. Fennel oil: Anethol
  3. Sandalwood : Santalol
  4. Clove oil: Eugenol
  5. Citronella oil: Geraniol, Citronellal, Farnesol
  6. Caraway oil: Carvone, Limonene
  7. Geranium oil: Geraniol
  8. Ginger oil: Zingiberone
  9. Eucalyptus oil: Cineole

- Monoterpenoids derived from geranyl pyrophosphate
- Sesquiterpnoids derived from farnesyl pyrophosphate
- Diterpenoids derived from geranyl pyrophosphate

**Table** Detail description about volatile oils and terpenoids

| Synonym | Biological name | Part Used | Family | Chemical Constituents | Uses | Miscellaneous |
|---|---|---|---|---|---|---|
| *aloids : Biosynthesis from tryptophan* | | | | | | |
| | Claviceps purpurea | Fungal sclerotium in ovary of rye plant; secale cereale | Fungus: Clavicipitaceae Rye : Graminae | *Derivatives of Lysergic acid, Levo form is active while dextro form is inactive. Ergometrine – water soluble Ergotamine, ergosine, ergocriptine, ergocornine – water insoluble Pigments: ergosterol, fungisterol* | *Oxytocic, Prevent postpartum haemorrhage, used in treatment of migraine* | Chemical Test: 1. Ergot + Van-Urk's reagent (p-dimethylamino-benzaldehyde) blue colour. 2. Ergot + solvent ether + H2S filtrate + NaHCO3 soln red colour in aq. soln 3. Ergometrinein water blue fluorescence Ergotamine + glacial acetic acid + ethyl acetate mix. + H2SO4 blue colour with re tinge + FeCl3 blue colour. |
| **e** | Catharanthus roseus | Whole Plant | Apocynaceae | Vincristine. Vinblastine – indole part (catharanthine) dihydroindole part (Vindoline) Ajmalicine | Anticancer – in treatment of hodkin's disease and leukaemia | Microscopy: Unicellular covering trichomes. Cruciferous (anisosytic) stoma Ca. Oxalate crystals – absent. |
| **a, a otachand, dha** | Rauwolfia serpentine | Roots and Rhizome | Apocynaceae | Reserpine, Rescinnamine ajamaline, ajamalicine, yohimbine, serpentine, syrosingopine | Hypotensive transquilliser | Microscopy: Presence of Ca. oxalate crystals. Chemical Test: 1. Freshly fractured surface + Conc $HNO_3$ red colour to medullary ray 2. Reserpine + vanilline in acetic acid red colour. |

**Table** *Conta*

| me / Synonym | Biological name | Part Used | Family | Chemical Constituents | Uses | Miscellaneous |
|---|---|---|---|---|---|---|
| **-vomica, w fig, en strychni** | Stryachnos Nux-vomica | Dried ripe Seeds | Loganiaceae | Strychnine, brucine, vomicine, α –colubrine, psudostrychnine, Glycoside: Loganin, chlorogenic acid | CNS stimulant, Bitter stomachic Brucine is 4 time bitter than strachnine<br><br>Adulterants :<br>1. S. nuxblanda<br>2. S. potatorum – it contain diaboline | Microscopy: Unicellular lignified covering tricho<br>Ca oxalate crystal – abse<br>Chemical test:<br>1. T.S. of Drug + ammo vanadate + H2SO4 p colour due to strychn endospermic cells<br>2. T.S. of Drug + Conc. HNO3 yellow colour brucine in endosperm |
| **sostigma, abar beans, eal bean** | Physostigma venonosum | Seeds | Loganiaceae | Physostigmine (Eserine) present in cotyledons, on contact with air oxidised to rubeserine (red compound) Physovenine, eseramine, geneserine, hysovenine, calabatine, calabasine | Cholinergic, ophthalmic in glaucoma. | -- |
| uinoline alkaloids | | | | | | |
| **ac** | Cephaelis ipecacuahana, Cephaelis acuminata | Roots and rhizomes | Rubiaceae | Emetine, Cephaeline, psychotrine, o-methyl psychotrine, emetamine, emetine :cephaline (4:1) in rioipecac, (1:1) in panama ipecac, (2.5:1) in johor ipecac Cephaeline emetine by methylation. | Antiamoebic, emetin, expectorant, Antiprotozoal | Microscopy :<br>Roots: presence of starch (15 micron) and acicular cal. oxalate.<br>Rhizomes: starch grain ( micron)<br>Chemical test:<br>1. 2.5 g of drug + 20 ml HCl + 5 ml H2O Filtrate + 0.5g pot. ch Yellow changes to re standing due to emeti<br>2. Emetine + H2SO4 + acid bright green col |

**Table (**

| Synonym | Biological name | Part Used | Family | Chemical Constituents | Uses | Miscellaneous |
|---|---|---|---|---|---|---|
| rrowroot | Chondrodentron tomentosum, strychnos castelnaea, S. toxifera | Most of plants | Loganiaceae and Menisperm aceae | d-tubocurarine (bisbenzylisoquinoline moiety), curine, curarine, tometocurine, chondrocurine, | Skeletal muscle relaxant, used in diagnosis of myasthenia gravis | Chemical test:<br>1. d-tubocurarine + $FeCl_3$=Gr colour.<br>2. d-tubocurarine + mercuric nitrate soln =cherry red co |
| | Papaver somniferum | Latex from capsules | Papaveraceae | Morphine, Codein, Narcotine, papaverine salt of meconic acid Protopine, hydrocotarnine – minor alkaloids | Narcotic analgesic, Morphine produces respiratory depression and constipation. Stimulates CTZ causes nausea and vomiting. | Chemical test:<br>1. General test for meconic ac Opium + $H_2O$ + $FeCl_3$ red purple<br>2. Morphine + $HNO_3$ orange colour. (Codein doesn't respond to $HNO_3$)<br>3. Morphine + Pot. ferricyani $FeCl_3$ bluish green colour (Codein doesn't respond to test)<br>4. Papaverine in HCl + Pot. ferricyanide lemon yellow colour |
| | Berberis aristata | Roots and rhizomes | Berberidaceae | berberine | Astringent in inflammation of mucous membranes | -- |
| s, golden ow root | Hydrastis canadensis | Roots and rhizomes | Berberidaceae | berberine, hydrastine | To control uterine - haemorrhage | -- |
| fusion of pyrrolidine + piperidine) alkaloids | | | | | | |
| | Datura metel | Leaves and Flowering tops | Solanaceae | Scopalamine (hyoscine), l-hyoscyamine (scopoline), Atropine (less quantity) hyoscine :ester of tropic acid and scopine | Anticholinergic, in duodenal ulcers, CNS depressant, treatment of asthma and cough | Microscopy:<br>Anisocytic or cruciferous stomata present both glandular and covering trichomes presen<br>Chemical test:<br>Hyoscine + silver nitrate soln yellowish white ppt soluble in ammonia and insoluble in nitri acid. |

**Table** *Cont*

| me / Synonym | Biological name | Part Used | Family | Chemical Constituents | Uses | Miscellaneous |
|---|---|---|---|---|---|---|
| **adonna lly night leaves** | Atropa belladonna, A acuminata | Leaves and flowering tops | Solanaceae | l-hyoscyamine, its racemic form Atropine, belladonine, scopoletin, hyoscine | Anticholinergic, antispasmodic, antidotes for opium and chloral hydrate poisoning. | Microscopy: anisocytic stomata, unise multicellular covering tri also presence of uniseria unicellular glandular tric Adulterants: Phytolacca americana, solanum nigrum, ailanthu glandulosa. |
| **syamus, bane** | Hyosyamus niger | Dried leaves and flowering tops | Solanaceae | l-hyoscyamine, atropine and Hyoscine (less amount), l-hyoscyamine : ester of tropic acid and tropine | Anticholinergic, antispasmodic, relive spam of urinary tract and sedative. | Microscopy: leaf is dorsiventral, Glandular trichomes, anis stomata, prismatic or clus crystal of ca. oxalate. |
| **monium orn apple es)** | Datura Stramonium | Dried Leaves and flowering tops | Solanaceae | l-hyoscyamine, Hyoscine, Atropine (small quantity) | Anticholinergic, Mydriatics, control motion sickness, treatment of asthma | Microscopy: Cluster or prism of ca. oxalate crystals. Multicellular conical uniseriate covering tricho fewer glandular trichome Anisocytic stomata on lo epidermis Adulterants: Xanthium strumarium, so nigrum (no ca. oxalate) |
| **a** | Erythroxylon coca, Erythroxylon truxillense | Dried Leaves | Erythroxylaceae | Cocaine (methyl benzyol ecgonine), Cinnamyl-cocaine (methyl cinnamoyl ecgonine), α-truxilline (methyl α-truxilline ecgonine), tropocaine, benzoyltropane, benzoylecgonine Cinnamyl cocaine + methyl alcohol + cinnamic acid | Local aneasthetics | Microscopy: Isobilateral leaves, paracy stomata, No trichomes Chemical test: Cocaine + $H_2SO_4$ + H2C characteristic of methyl benzoate. |

**Table** *C*

| Synonym | Biological name | Part Used | Family | Chemical Constituents | Uses | Miscellaneous |
|---|---|---|---|---|---|---|
| | Duboisia myoporoides | Dried Leaves | Solanaceae | Scopalamine and atropine, nor-hyoscyamine, tigloidine, valproate, tiglyoxytropine | Anticholinergic, antidotes for pilocarpine, physostigmine | Chemical test: Atropine + HCl + gold chloride lemon yellow ppt. |
| alkaloids | | | | | | |
| | Cinchona ledgeriana; Cinchona succirubra; Cinchona officinalis | Dried Roots and stem bark | Rubiaceae | Imp: Quinine, quinidine, cinchonine, cinchonidine<br>Other: quinicine, cinchonicin, hydroquinine,hydrocinchonidine.<br>quinine, and quinidine are isomer to each other.<br>cinchonine, cinchonidine are isomer to each other.<br>phlobatannins –cinchotannic acid.<br>Glycosides: quinovin. | Antimalerial, bitter tonic<br>Quinidine – used as cardiac depressant (in treatment of arrhythmia and tachycardia, atrial fibrillation) | Microscopy:<br>Idiobalst of ca. oxalate – special characteristic.<br>Chemical test:<br>1. Quinine crystals shows blue fluorescence in UV light.<br>2. Drug + glacial acetic acid purple vapours<br>3. Thalleoquine test: Drug + bromine water + ammonia emerald green colour.<br>4. Quinidine + silver nitrate white ppt soluble in $HNO_3$ |
| heca, ee | Camptotheca acuminata | Dried stem wood | Nyssaceae | Camptothecin, 10-hydroxy Camptothecin, 10-methoxy Camptothecin, | Anti-tumour – by inhibition of topoisomerase I.<br>It also inhibit DNA replication of herpes and adenovirus. | Camptothecin – yellow needle shaped crystals. |
| lkaloids | | | | | | |
| bacco, veed | Lobelia nicotianefolia | Leaves and tops | Campanulaceae | Lobeline<br>lobelidine, lonelanine, isolobelanine, lobelanidine, | Respiratory Stimulant, in treatment of asthma. cough and pain receptors are stimulated by lobeline | Chemical test:<br>1. Lobeline + H2SO4 + formaldehyde red colour.<br>2. Lobeline Δ acetophenone recognise by smell. |

**Table** *Co*

| ame / Synonym | Biological name | Part Used | Family | Chemical Constituents | Uses | Miscellaneous |
|---|---|---|---|---|---|---|
| **ca, betel nut** | Areca catechu | Dried seeds | Palmae | Arecoline, Arecaidine, guvacine (tetrahydro-nicotinic acid), guvacoline | Respiratory Stimulant, Arecoline is para-sympathomimetic<br>Also used as anthelmentic only in veterinary practice and not used as human medicine. | - |
| dazole alkaloids | | | | | | |
| **orandi, ocarpus** | Pilocarpus jaborandi | Leaves | Rutaceae | Pilocarpine, iso-pilocarpine, Pilocarpidine Pilosine, isopilosine. Volatile oil – limonene, α-pinene, sabinene | Cholinergic (Opthalmic), Used in treatment of glaucoma | Chemical test: Pilocarpine + dil. H2SO + benzene + pot. chroma layer (bluish violet) and layer (yellow colour) |
| nazoline alkaloids | | | | | | |
| **aka adulsa, labar Nut** | Adhathod vasica | Dried and fresh leaves | Acanthaceae | Vasicine, Vasicinone | Antitussive, expectorant | Microscopy: Caryophyllaceous or dic stomata, both covering a glandular trichomes |
| ne alkaloids | | | | | | |
| **oa seeds** | Theobroma cocoa | Dried seeds | Sterculiaceae | Theobromine, Caffeine, cocoa butter | Diuretics, cocoa butter used in suppository preparation | -- |
| **, Camellia thea** | Thea sinesis | dried leaves and leaf buds | Theaceae | Caffeine, Theobromine, Theophylline colour of tea due to gallotannic acid<br>enzymatic mixture called – thease | CNS Stimulant and diuretics | -- |
| **fee** | Coffea arabica | Dried seeds | Rubiaceae | Caffeine, trigonelline smell of coffee due to volatile oil – caffeol | Stimulant, to counter effect overdosage of CNS depressant | Chemical test:<br>1. Murexide colour reac caffeine + HCl + pot. heated to dryness + v dil. ammonia purple ;colour lost on addn o<br>2. Caffeine + tannic acid ppt. |

**Table**

| Synonym | Biological name | Part Used | Family | Chemical Constituents | Uses | Miscellaneous |
|---|---|---|---|---|---|---|
| alkaloids | | | | | | |
| **a,** | Veratrum album, V. viride | Dried rhizomes and roots | Liliaceae | Germicidine, protoveratrine A and B | Hypotensive, cardicac depressant | -- |
| **ndha herry** | Withenia somnifera | Dried roots and stem bases | Solanaceae | Withanine, Somaniferine, somnine, withananine, tropine, psudotropine, glycoside – Sitoindocide VII and VIII<br>Leave - withanolide D – withaferin, withaferine A | Sedative, antirhumatic, hypotensive, immune-modulatory, sitoindoside – anti-stress activity. | -- |
| | Holarrhena antidysenterica, H. pubescens | Dried stem bark | Apocynaceae | Conessine (Kurchicine), norconessine, isoconessine, dioxyconessine | Antiamoebic | Microscopy: Prismatic ca. oxalate crystal present. |
| **kaloids (Proto-alkaloids)** | | | | | | |
| **, ng** | Ephedra gerardiana, E. equisetina, E. Sinica | Dried young stems | Ephedraceae | Ephedrine, nor- ephedrine, n-methyl ephedrine, psudo ephedrine-(alkaloidal amines) | Sympathomimetic, antiasthmatic, treatment of hay fever | Microscopy: Sunken stomata, Cluster crysta Ca. oxalate. Chemical test: Ephedrine +H2O + dil HCl + copper sulphate + NaOH viole colour + ether organic layer (purple) aq. layer (blue colour) |
| **od,** | Aconitum nepellus | Dried Roots | Ranunculaceae | Aconitine, neopelline, napelline, neoline<br>1. Aconite hydrolysis Benzoyl aconine + Acetic acid<br>2. Benzoyl aconine hydrolysis aconine + benzoic acid | In treatment of rheumatism and sciatica, used externally only highly poisonous | -- |
| **m, eeds, crocus** | Cholchicum autumnale, C. luteum | Dried seed and corn | Liliaceae | Colchicine, demecolcine<br>Colchicine – pale yellow crystals | In treatment of gout, induction of polyploidy | 1. Colchicine + 70% $H_2SO_4$ yellow colour<br>2. Colchicine + FeCl3 red col |
| **Glory lily** | Glorisa superb | dried roots and rhizomes and tubers | Liliaceae | Colchicine | In treatment of gout and inflammation, cancer. | -- |

**Table** *Con*

| ne / Synonym | Biological name | Part Used | Family | Chemical Constituents | Uses | Miscellaneo |
|---|---|---|---|---|---|---|
| oterpenoids | | | | | | |
| **phor oil, mosa oil** | Cinnamomum camphora | Wood | Lauraceae | Camphor, safrole, acetaldehyde, eugenol, d-pinene, eucalyptol, Phellandrene and cineole. natural camphor : Dextro form Synthetic Camphor: Racemic form | Rubefacient, counter- irritant, | Chemical Test: Solution of Vanillin sulphuric acid + Dr Red, violet, and fina (note: Synthetic cam detected by this test) |
| **nopodium American mseed oil, opodium, noposan** | Chenophodium ambrosioides | Fresh Flowering and fruiting | Chenopodiaceae | 70 -80% Ascaridole – unsaturated terpene peroxide, 20% p-cymene, myrcene, 1-limonene, Camphor | Anthelmintic – round warm, hook warm, dwarf tape warm, no action on large tape warm | Chemical Test: 1 ml of oil heated wi of porcelain golden y liquid. |
| **alyptus oil,** | Eucalyptus globulus | Fresh leaves | Myrtaceae | Cineole – Eucalyptol (80%), Pinene, camphene | Counter-irritant, antiseptic, expectorant | - |
| **anium oil** | Pelargonium graveolens | Fresh leaves | Geraniaceae | β – citranellol, geraniol (6070%), gerynyl acetate, citranellyl acetate | Flavouring agent | - |
| **on-grass Melissa oil** | Cymbopogan flexuousus, Cymbopogan citrates | Leaves and aerial part | Graminae | Citral – aldehyde (75%), methylheptenol, nerol, citronellal, dipentene and geraniol | Flavouring agent, Citral β ionine Synthesis of Vit. A | - |
| **pentine oil, m terbinthae** | Pinus roxburghii, Pinus longifolia, pinus palustris | Oleo-resin | Pinaceae | α – pinene (20-30%), β – pinene (5-10%), Camphene, β – phellandrene, δ-3-carene, limonene | Counter-irritant, rubefacient, chronic bronchitis, | - |
| **permint oil, tha oil** | Mentha piperita | Fresh flowering tops | Labiatae | l-menthol, Menthone, menthofuran (dirty smell - resinification), jasmone (pleasant smell), methyl isovalerate, l-limonene, isopulegone, cineole, pinene | Carminative, stimulant, flavouring agent, $Ca^{++}$ channel blocking activity – spasmolytic and smooth muscle relaxant Azulene – anti-inflammatory and antiulcer activity | - |

**Table**

| ynonym | Biological name | Part Used | Family | Chemical Constituents | Uses | Miscellaneous |
|---|---|---|---|---|---|---|
| enoids | Mentha spicata, Mentha viridis Mentha cardiana | Leaves and flowe-ring tops | Labiatae | 50% l-carvone, linalool, pinene, cineole,phellandrene | Carminative, flavour – toothpaste, mouthwashes, chewing gums | - |
| | Carum carvi | dried ripe fruits | Umbelliferae | 45-65% carvone limonene,dihydrocarvone, Carvacrol | Aromatic, | - |
| m | Elettaria cardamomum | dried ripe fruits | Zingiberaceae | 2-8 % cineole, terpineol, borneol, terpinene | Aromatic, Carminative, Flavouring agent | Adulterants: Big cardamom (4cm length x 1 cm diameter). Korarima cardamom (4x2 do not show presence of ru (present in genuine drug) |
| er | Coriandrum sativum | dried ripe fruits | Umbelliferae | Volatile oil – 90% D-linalool (Coriandrol), coriandryl acetate, L-borneol, geraniol, pinene Leaves – Vitamin A | Purgative, Aromatic, Carminative, Flavouring agent | Microscopy: Prism of $Ca^{++}$ Oxalate Adulterants: Bombay coriander fruit |
| ermum , Carum | Trychispermum ammi | dried ripe fruits | Umbelliferae | 35-60% thymol (flavour and taste), 50-60% p-cymene, 30-35% terpinene | Antispasmodic, carminatives, bronchitis | - |
| | Anethum graveolens | dried ripe fruits | Umbelliferae | Carvone – aromatic liquid dihydrocarvone, D-linonene, phellandrene | Aromatic, Carminative, Flavouring agent | - |
| Fructus m | foeniculum vulgare | dried ripe fruits | Umelliferae | Ketone, fenchone (20%) – clourless pungent liquid, phenolic ether anethone (50%) – sweet in taste and odour. | Aromatic, Carminative, expectorant | Microscopy: Presence of anomocytic stomata, Rosette crystal of $Ca^{+2}$ oxalate |
| eel, nonis | Citrus limonis | ripe fruits | Rutaceae | Volatile oil – Limonene (90%), citral (4%), Other: hesperidin, Pectin | Carminative, stimulant, Flavouring agent | - |

**Table** *Contd.*

| me / Synonym | Biological name | Part Used | Family | Chemical Constituents | Uses | Miscellaneo |
|---|---|---|---|---|---|---|
| **er orange** | Citrus aurantium | Pericarp of ripe fruit | Rutaceae | Volatile oil – Limonene (90%), Other: hesperidin, iso-hesperidin, Vit C, pectin Bitter principle: aurantiamarin (glycoside) Aldehyde: Citral and citronellal | Stomachic, aromatic, carminative | - |
| **meg, Nux chata** | Myristica fragrans | Dried kernels of seeds | Myristicaceae | Volatile oil – Myristicin, elimicin, saffrole, fatty acids – myristic acid, palmitic acid, oleic acid. Myristicin – poisonous and narcotic effect | Carminative, stimulant, aromatic | Mace: arillius od see myristica. It contain amylodextin give re with iodine Use as c carminative |
| **sia namon, nese amon** | Cinnamomum cassia | Dried stem bark | Lauraceae | Cassia oil: Volatile oil (brown) – 85% cinnamic aldehyde | Carminative, stimulant, aromatic, flavouring agent | - |
| **namon, Kalmi hini, Ceylon amon** | Cinnamomum zeylanicum, C. verum | Dried inner bark of shoots | Lauraceae | Volatile oil, pholbatannins, mannitol Volatile oil – cinnamaldehyde, eugenol, benzaldehyde, cuminaldehyde | Stomachic, Carminative, flavouring agent, antiseptic | Chemical test: Volatile oil + $FeCl_3$ Pale green colour (cinnamic acid – bro colour, eugenol – bl cassia oil shows only colour as it doesn't c eugenol |
| **manasi, d,** | Nardostachys Jatamanasi | Dried rhizomes | Velerianaceae | Jatamansic acid Ketones: Jatamansone, nardostachone Bitter principle: alcohol and its isovaleric esters | Sedative, antispasmodic, diuretics, emmenagogue, stomachic, epilepsy, hysteria | Chemical test: 80% alc. extract blui fluroscence in UV li |

**Table** *C*

| ynonym | Biological name | Part Used | Family | Chemical Constituents | Uses | Miscellaneous |
|---|---|---|---|---|---|---|
| alanga, inger | Alpinia officinarum | Dried rhizomes | Zingiberaceae | Volatile oil – Methyl cinnamate, cineaole, camphor, pinene Glanagol, galangin – yellow crystalline anti-inflammatory – sorghumol, bochmerd | Carminative, stimulant, aromatic, antibacterial, anti-rhumatism | - |
|  | Allium sativum | Bulb | Liliaceae | Volatile oil – Alliin, Allicin Alliinallicin by enzyme allinlyase | Carminative, aphrodisiac, expectorant, stimulant | - |
| cred ly basil | Ocimum sanctum | Fresh and dried leaves | Labitae | 70% eugenol, carvacrol caryophyllin, Vit C. | antibacterial and insecticidal, stimulant, spasmolytics, immuno-modulatory agents | - |
| , let | Viola odorata | Dried aerial part | Violaceae | Leaves : Essential oil, glycoside – methyl salicylate – expectorant alkaloid – odoratine Flowers: violin, rutin, cyanin | Expectorant, diaphoretic, antipyretic, antibacterial, violin is an emetic | - |
| achari, inger lily | Hedychium spicatum | Dried rhizomes | Zingiberaceae | Volatile oil – paramethoxycinnamic acid (68%), cineole, limonene, 8-caryophyllene | Stomachic, stimulant, carminative, tonic, flavouring agent | - |
| pper | Piper nigrum | unripe fruit | Piperaceae | Alkaloid – piperine Volatile oil – l-phellandrene and Caryophyllene | Carminative, stimulant, aromatic, stomachic | - |
| tiver, | Vetiveria Zizanioids | Root | Graminae | 45-60% Alcohol – vetivenol, vetiverol 8-35 % of Ketone – α & β vetivones | Carminative, stimulant, aromatic, stomachic | - |
| y oil | Rosmarinus officinalis | Fresh flowering top | Labitae | Volatile oil – 10-15 % borneol, 2.5-3% bornyl acetate, camphor 45% terpenes | Carminative, stimulant rubefacient, flavouring agent | - |

**Table** *Cont*

| ne / Synonym | Biological name | Part Used | Family | Chemical Constituents | Uses | Miscellaneo |
|---|---|---|---|---|---|---|
| se, Aniseed | Pimpinella anisum | dried ripe fruits | Umbelliferae | Volatile oil – 90% Anethol, Methyl chavicol, Anisaldehyde | Carminative, stimulant, expectorant | - |
| nmin | Cumminum cyminum | dried ripe fruits | Umbelliferae | 30-50% cumminaldehyde, α & β-pinene, phellandrene, hydrocuminine | Carminative, stimulant, diarrhoea, dyspepsia | - |
| ry, Apium | Apium graveolens | dried ripe fruits | Umbelliferae | Celery – strong aromatic flvour, D-limonene (60%), sandanoic acid, d-selinine (10%) | Carminative, stimulant, nervine sedative and tonic | - |
| ender oil | Lavandula officinalis | Fresh flowering top | Labitae | 30-40% Linalyl acetate, linalool, pinene, geraniol, cineol | Carminative, flavouring agent , aromatic. | - |
| ltheria oil, la oil, et birch oil, f ergreen, berry oil | Gaultheria procumbens | Leaves | Ericaceae | 98% methyl salicylate. Gaultherin (glycoside) hydrolysis by gaultherase methyl salicylate Enanthic alcohol – characteristic odour | Anti-rhumatism, counter irritant | Chemical test: 5 ml oil + vanillin so 2 ml of alcohol bloo colour. |
| of palmarosa ha oil anium oil, | Cymbopoaganm martini | Leaves | Graminae | Rosha oil – 85-90% geraniol, citronellal dipenetene, linaloolm terpenes | Used in perfumery, cosmetics and soap. insect repellent, anti-rhumatism | - |
| of zitronella | Cymbopogan nordus | Fresh leaves | Graminae | 40-60% geraniol, citronellal | Perfume in soap, in mosquito repellent cream, flavouring agent | - |
| k, kasturi, chus | Moschus moschiferus | Dried secretion from perpetual follicles of musk dear | Cervidae | Dark brown volatile oil – muskone (Ketonic sub.) Cholesterin, albuminoids | used in perfumery due to its strong odorous property for long time | - |

**Table (**

| ynonym | Biological name | Part Used | Family | Chemical Constituents | Uses | Miscellaneous |
|---|---|---|---|---|---|---|
| eth | Secretion from scent glands from external reproductive organs from male and female of civet cat Viverra zibetha | Viverra | Viverridae | Civetone, civetol | perfumery, flavouring agent | - |
| n, | Castor faber | dried perpetial follicles of beaver | Castoridae | Crystalline comp- castorin resin (80%) | flavouring agent | - |
| | Thymus vulgaris | Dried Leaves and flowering top | Labiatae, (Lamiaceae) | Volatile oil – thymol, carvacrol, terpineol flavonoids, caffeic acid, labiatic acid | Expectorant, antispasmodic, carminative, antifungal anthelmintic | |
| , worm onica | Artemisia cina, A. brevifolia, A. maritma | Flower-heads | Compositae | Santonin, artemisin (crystalline sub.) cineole, pinene Santonin – sesquiterpene lactone | Santonica used as anthelmintic, for round warm, hook warm, tape warm | |
| iin | Artemisia annua | Whole plant-Herb | Compositae | Artemisinin - sesquiterpene lactone | Antimalarial effect for schizonticidal activity, Artemether and artsunate are derivatives of artemisinin | |
| il | Atermisia pallens | Flowering herbs | Compositae | davanone, artemone, davana furans – responsible for aroma | perfumery, flavouring agent | |
| s bane, | Arnica montana | Flowering herbs | Compositae | Volatile oil – 4-hydroxythymodimethyl ether Helenanolides (sesquiterpene lactone) – helenalin, epoxyhelanlin arnifolin, arnicin, arnidiol, feradiol flavonoids – apigenin, quercetin kaempferol | Counter irritant, cosmetics and hair shampoo. helenaline and its derivatives – antihyperlipidemic, antitumor, anthelmintic, antifungal activity. | - |

**Table** *Cont*

| me / Synonym | Biological name | Part Used | Family | Chemical Constituents | Uses | Miscellaneo |
|---|---|---|---|---|---|---|
| of sandal d | Santalum album | Heart-wood | Santalaceae | Sesquiterpene alcohol – α & β santalol, santalal, santalone | Symptomatic relief for dysurea, diminishes the frequency of marked in the tuberculosis of bladder | - |
| ve | Eugenia Caryophyllus | Dried flower buds | Myrtaceae | Volatile oil – eugenol (70-90%), Tannins – gallotannic acid | Dental analgesic, carminative, flavouring agent | Dental analgesic, ca flavouring agent |
| s | Humulus Dried lupulus | Dried female flowers-Strobiles | Cannabinaceae | Phluroglucinol derivative – humulone, cohumulone. Volatile oil – myrcene, limonene, pinene | Sedative and spasmolytic | - |
| ssurea, costus, h | Saussuurea Lappa | Dried root | Compositae | Volatile oil – costuslactone, dihydrolactone, alkaloid – saussurine | in treatment of bronchial asthma, expectorant, powerful insecticide, anti-rheumatism | - |
| rus, bach, , Sweet flag | Acorus calamus | Dried rhizomes | Araceae | Volatile oil – asaraldehyde, asarone, eugenol bitter principle - acorine | Carminative, bitter stimulant, vermifuge insect repellent Asarone – sedative and tranquillising property | - |
| eb, abchini | Piper cubeba | Unripe fruit | Piperaceae | Volatile oil – dipentene, cadinene | Stimulant, aromatic, urinary antiseptic, in treatment of cough | Chemical test: drug + $H_2SO_4$ purple |
| erian | Velariana wallichii | Dried rhizomes | Velerianaceae | alkaloids – chatinine, valerine Volatile oil – borneol formate, borneol isovelerianate sesquiterpnes – Valepotriates, valtrate | Antispasmodic, CNS depressant action, tranquillising activity | |
| erfew, summer y, Featherfoil | Tanacetum parthenicum | dried leaves or fresh leaves and aerial part | Asteraceae or Compositae | chrysanthemin A and B, parthenolide | In treatment of migraine, vertigo, arthritis, fever and menstrual disorder. | |
| us, Yew, spatra | genus – Taxus T. baccata, T. cuspidate, T. brevifolia, T. Canadensis | | taxaceae | Taxol, cephalomannine, 10-deacetyl baccatin | In treatment of refractory ovarian cancer, lung cancer, gastric and cervical cancer. | |

Table

| ynonym | Biological name | Part Used | Family | Chemical Constituents | Uses | Miscellaneous |
|---|---|---|---|---|---|---|
| ii | Coleus Forkoshlii, Plectranthus barbalus | Roots | labiatae (lamiaceae) | diterpene – forskolin (coleonol) coleonol B, C and E | Vasodilator, cardiostimulant effect. Forskolin inhibit platelet aggregation. reduces intraocular pressure, useful in glaucoma | |
| is | Physter catodon | Intestinal tract of sperm whale | Physeteridae | Triterepene alcohol – ambrein, epicoprostanol, coprostanone | perfumery, flavouring agents | |
| | Bixa orellana | Dried seeds | Bixaceae | 70-80% bixin of total pigment – yellow colour Isobixin, trans-bixin | Colouring agent | |
| affron, ron, | Crocus sativus | Stigmas and upper parts of styles | Iridaceae | Crocin, Crocetin, Bitter – Picrocrocin Protocrocin – carotenoid glycoside | Colouring and flavouring agents, antispasmodic, emmenagogue, and stimulant | Adulterant – Carthamus tinctorius (Safflower) |

**Table** Volatile oils and terpenoids containing drug and their chemical structure of their therapeutic constitutes

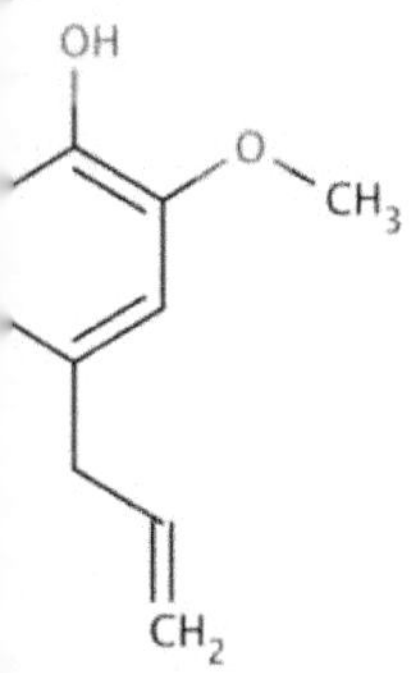

**Eugenol**

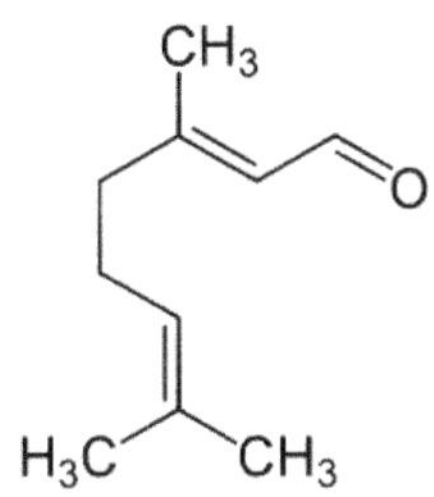

**Geranial**

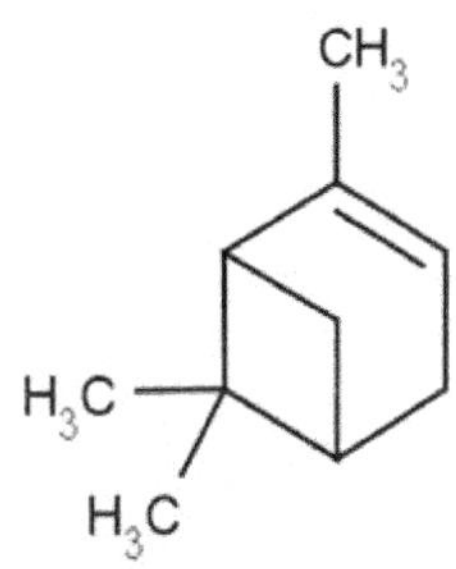

**Alpha- pinene**

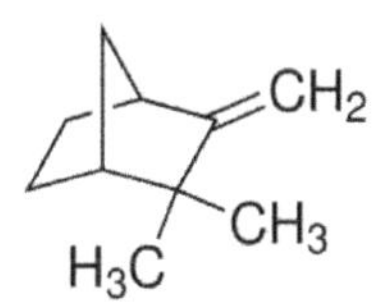

**Camphene**

**Table** *Ca*

| | | | |
|---|---|---|---|
| 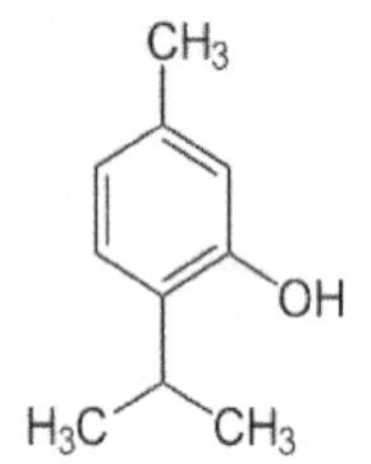 **Thymol** | 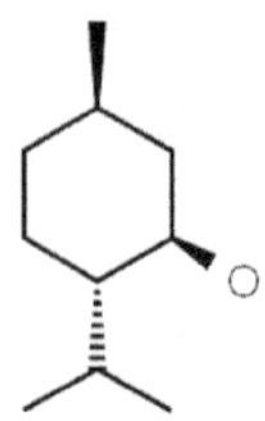 **Menthol** | 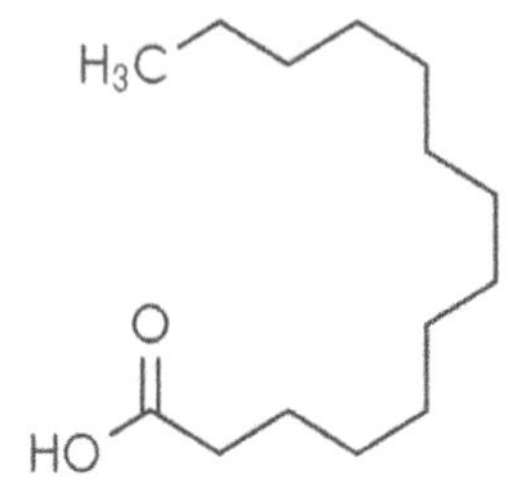 **Myriticin** | 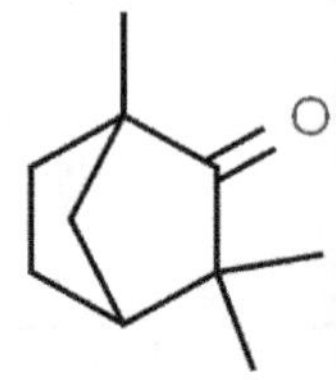 **Fenchone** |
| 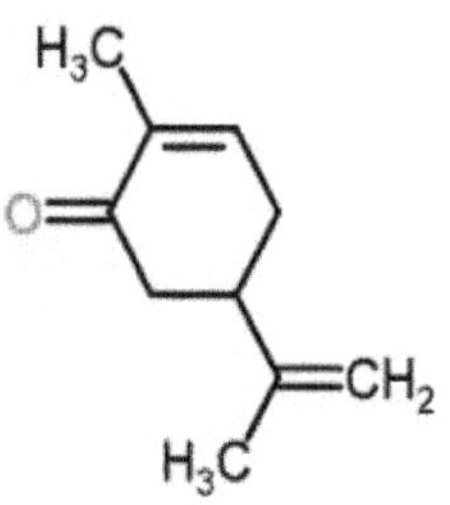 **Carvone** | 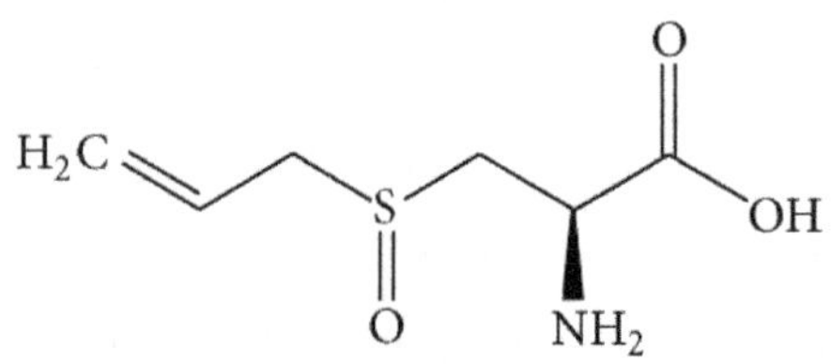 **Alliin** | 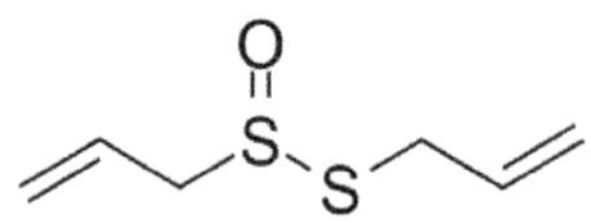 **Allicin** | 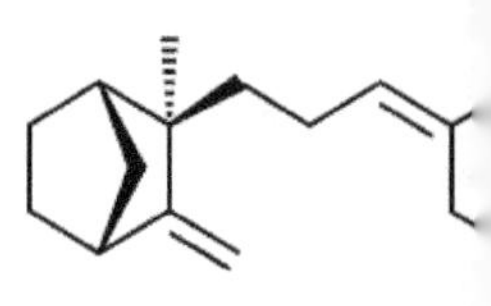 **Santalol** |
| 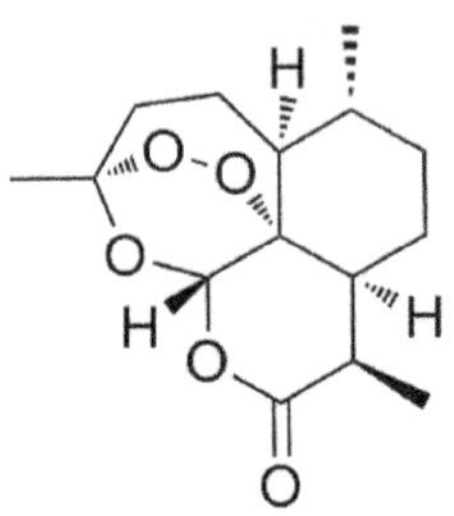 **Artemisinin** | 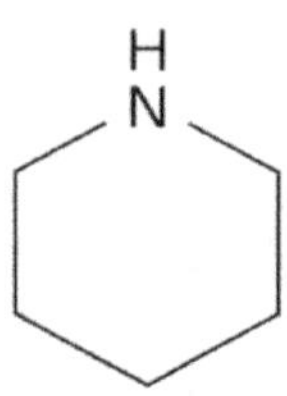 **Piperine** | 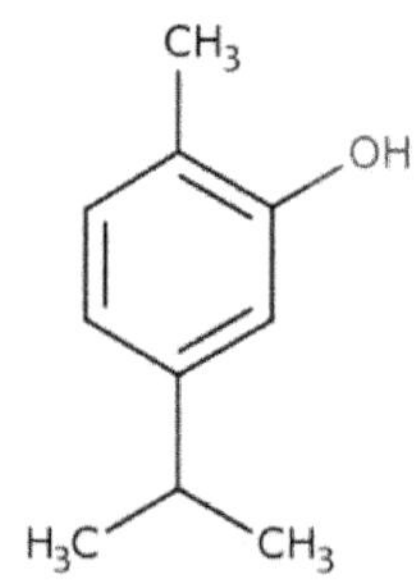 **Carvacrol** | 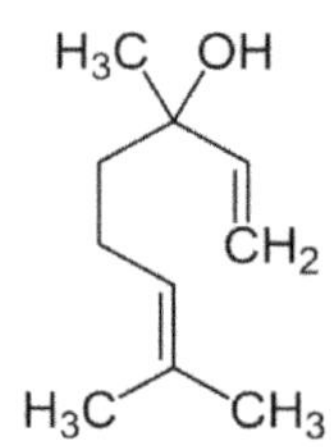 **Linalool** |

**Table**

| 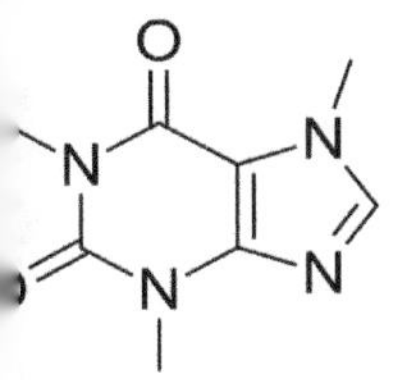 Caffeine | 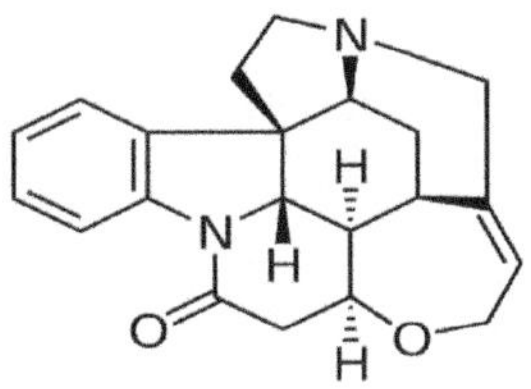 Strychnine | 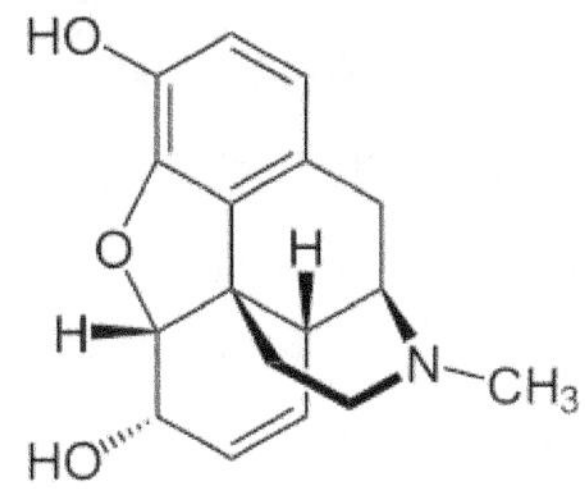 Morphine | 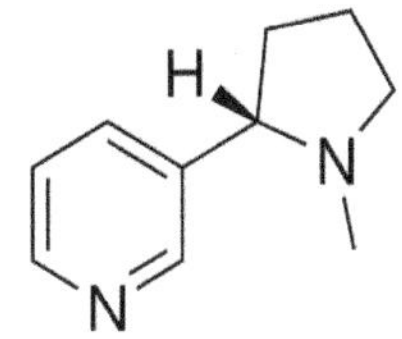 Nicotine |
|---|---|---|---|
| 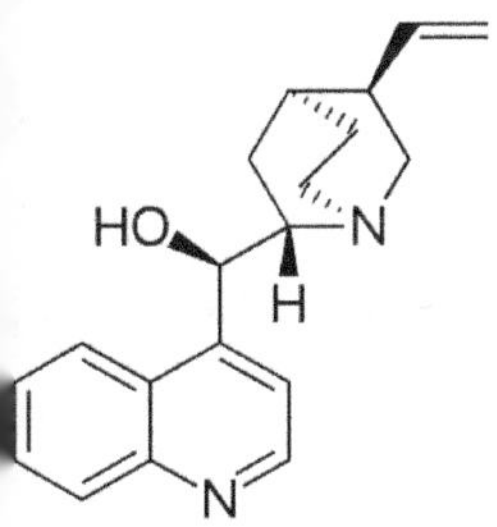 Quinine | 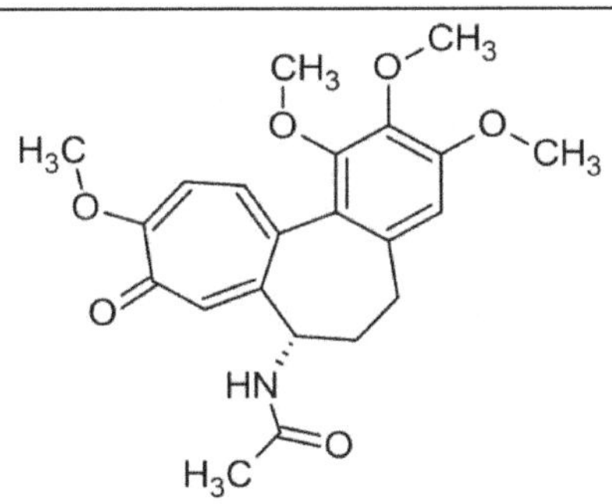 Colchicine | 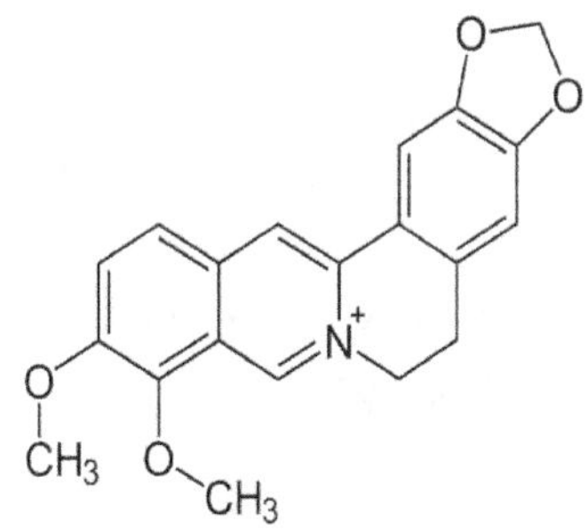 Berberine | 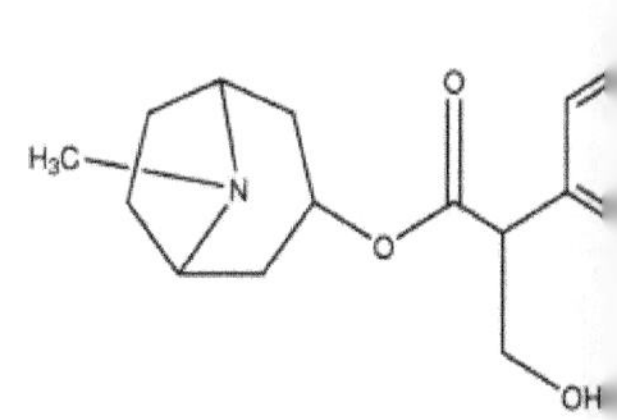 Hyoscyamine |

## Glycosides

- A glycoside is any molecule in which a sugar group is bonded through its anomeric carbon to another group via glycosidic bond.
- A glycosidic bond is a certain type of chemical bond that joins a sugar molecule to another molecule.
- Glycoside = Glycone + Aglycone
- Linkage between "Glycone" and "Aglycone" called glycosidic linkage.
- Classification of glycoside based on either glycosidic linkage or chemical nature of aglycone part-
  - ❖ Based on glycosidic linkage:
    1. C- glycosides : Cascara, aloin (aloe), flavones
    2. O- glycosides : Senna, Rhubarb
    3. S- glycosides : Isothiocynate glycoside like Sinigrin (Black mustard)
    4. N- glycosides : Nucleosides
  - ❖ Based on Chemical Nature:
    1. Anthracene glycosides

       Senna, Aloe, Rhubarb, Cascara, Hypericum, Cochineal
    2. Sterols or Cardiac glycosides

       Digitalis, Thevetia, Adonis, Indian squill, Red Squill, Stropanthus, Ouabain, Oleander, Black hellebore
    3. Saponin glycosides

       Dioscora, Safed musali, Liquorice, Shatavari, Brahmi, Ginseng, Momardica, Senega, Quillaia, Gokharu
    4. Cynogenetic and cyanophoric glycosides

       Bitter almond, Wild cherry bark
    5. Isothiocyanate glycosides

       Black mustard
    6. Flavonol glycosides

       Silymarin, Gingko, Buck wheat, Citrus
    7. Coumarin glycosides

       Tonka bean, Ammi, Psoralea, Cantharides, Mylabris
    8. Aldehyde glycosides

       Vanilla pods
    9. Phenol glycosides

       Bearberry
    10. Steroidal Glyco-alkaloids

        Solanum
    11. Glycosidal bitter and miscellaneous glycosides

        Gentian, Picrorrhiza, Chirata, Quassia, Kalmegh, Gymnema, Henna

❖ Structure of Glycosides- Theses are composed of two structural features
  - The sugar (Glycone)
  - The non sugar (Aglycone)

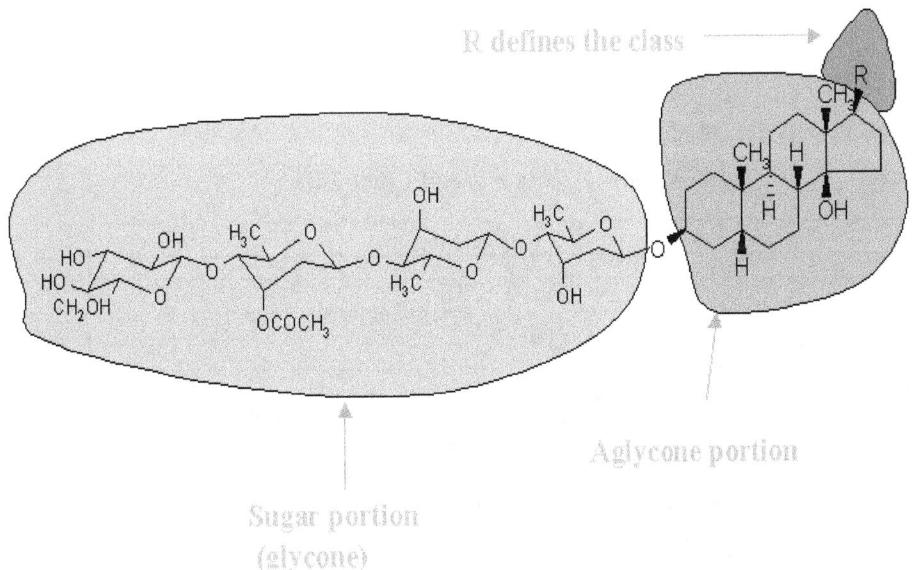


**Fig.** Structure of Glycosides

**Table** Chemical test for specific glycosides

| Glycoside | Test | Procedure | Observation |
|---|---|---|---|
| uinone glycoside | **Borntrager's test** | Cover test tube containing moist drug sample with filter paper moistened with dilute NaOH solution. Place it in water bath for several minute. Expose paper to UV light | Rose pink to red color in the amm yellow green |
| | **Modified Borntrager's test** | Boil drug with H2SO4 and aq. FeCl3 solution (5%), filter, add dichloromethane or CHCl3 to filtrate. To the lower layer (CH2Cl2 or CHCl3 layer) shake with dilute ammonia. | Rose pink to red color in the amm |
| glycoside | **Kedde's test** | Dried chloroform extract of drug + Alcohol (90%) + 2 % 3,5 dinitro benzoic acid in 90 % alcohol + 20 % NaOH Solution | Bluish to Purple color |
| | **Keller-Killiani test (Test for deoxy sugar)** | Alcoholic extract of drug + H2O+ Lead acetate solution, Filtrate + CHCl3. Dried CHCl3 extract of drug + Glacial acetic acid containing trace amount of FeCl3+ concentrated Sulphuric acid by the side of test tube. | Reddish brown layer changes to B colour (Digitoxose) |
| | **Raymond's test** | Test solution + Dinitrobenzene in hot methanolic alkali | Violet color |
| | **Legal's test** | Test solution + Pyridine + Alkaline sodium nitroprusside solution | Blood red color |
| | **Baljet's test** | Test solution + Picric acid or Sodium picrate | Yellow to Orange color |
| in e | **Fluorescence test** | Cover test tube containing moist drug sample with filter paper moistened with dilute NaOH solution. Place it in water bath for several minute. Expose paper to UV light. | Paper shows yellow green Fluorescence |
| netic e | Sodium Picrate test | Drug in the flask moisten with few drops of water + Dilute H2SO4, Suspend sodium picrate treated filter paper | HCN turn the paper to brick red formation of sodium isopurpurate. |
| | Cuprocyanate test | Dip strip of paper in guaiacum resin and moisten with dilute copper sulphate and expose to it freshly cut surface of the crude drug | Paper turns to blue with prussic ac |
| e | Froth test | Shake solution of drug in water | Stable froth (foam) formed |
| | Haemolysis test | Mix solution of Saponin (prepared in 1% normal saline) and blood and centrifuge | Red supernatant compared with control tube |

**Table** Detail description about glycoside

| ym | Biological name | Part Used | Family | Chemical Constituents | Uses | Key points |
|---|---|---|---|---|---|---|
| a, | Cassia Angustifolia | Dried leaflets | Leguminosae | Sennoside A and B (sterioisomers to each other)<br>Aglycone part – in Sennoside A (dextro-rotatory) Sennoside B (meso form)<br>Nepthalene glycoside – Tinnevallin and 6-hydroxy musizin glycoside | Purgative<br>griping effect due to resin or emodin content | • **Presence of cluster-** crystals of ca+2 oxala<br>• **Vein-islet no** -19.5 to<br>• **Stomatal index** -17-1 |
| | Cassia Acutifolia | Dried leaflets | Leguminosae | Sennoside A and B | Purgative | • **Vein-islet no**-25 to 2<br>• **Stomatal index**- 11.4 |
| , | Aloe barbadensis | Dried Leaves | Liliaceae | Aloin - Barbaloin, Aloe- emodin C-10 glycoside, isobarbaloin, β-barbaloin. | Purgative | **Adulterants**:<br>Natal aloe - resemble to it contain natalion –wea purgative action. |
| ini | Rheum Palmatum, Rheum emodi Rheum webbianum | Dried Bark | Polygonaceae | Rhein,<br>glucorhein – anthraquinones with carboxyl group. aloe-emodin, emodine, chrysophanol – anthraquinones without carboxyl group<br>Palmidine A,B and C-Heterodiantrones<br>Asringent – due to gallic acid, catechin and epicatechin. | Purgative | - |
| d | Rhamanus purshiana | Dried Bark | Rhamnaceae | Cascarosides A, B, C, and D, barbaloin, chrysaloin | Mild Purgative, emetics | **Microscopy**: Shows pre prism of Ca. oxalate cry |
| | Coccus cacti | Female insect enclosing young larvae | Coccidae | Carminic acid - 10 %<br>(Prismatic crystals) | Colouring agent | - |
| | Digitalis lanata, Digitalis purpurea | Dried Leaves | Scrophulariaceae | Digitoxin, Lanatoside, A,B and C, Digoxin<br>Purpurea glycoside A, digitonin, gitonin | Cardiotonic | **Microscopy:** anomocyti stomata, Glandular trich Collapsed covering trich |

**Table** *Co*

| Synonym | Biological name | Part Used | Family | Chemical Constituents | Uses | Key p |
|---|---|---|---|---|---|---|
| | Thevetia nerifolia | Seeds | Apocynaceae | Thevetin – mix of thevatin A and cereberoside (thevetin B) | Cardiotonic | - |
| t's eye) | Adonis vemalis | Over-ground portion | Renunculaceae | Adoniotoxin | Cardiotonic | - |
| | Nerium oleander | Leaves | Apocynaceae | Oleandrin | In cardiac insuffciency | - |
| thus | Strophanthus Kombe | Dried ripe seeds | Apocynaceae | {K- strophanthin – K-strophanthoside, K-strophanthoside β cymarin, cymarol} on hydrolysis Strophanthidin | Cardiotonic | |
| anthin) | Strophanthus gratus | Dried Seeds | Apocynaceae | Ouabain | Cardiotonic, poisonous sub | - |
| llebore | Helleborus niger | Dried Roots and rhizomes | Renunculaceae | Hellebrin | Cardiac Stimulant | - |
| uill, j, Sea la | Urginia Indica | dried bulbs | Liliaceae | Scillaren A and B | Cardiotonic | **Microscopy:** Rap oxalate crystals. |
| Squill, ill | Urginia maritima | dried scaly leaves and bulbs | Liliaceae | Cardicac glycosides: bufadienolide type Scillaren A and B | Cardiotonic, emesis in chronic bronchitis | - |
| l | Urginia maritima | Leaves of bulbs | Liliaceae | Scilliroside, scillirubroside | Rat poison | Red colour due to pigment |
| (Yam), sm root | Dioscorea deltoidea, D. composita | Dried Tubers | Dioscoreaceae | Diosgenin (Steroidal Sapogenin) its glycosides – smilagenin, epismilagenin, Yamogenin | Synthesis of medicinal steroids, General Tonic | |
| , mulethi | Glycyrrhiza glabra | Dried Roots and Stolon | Leguminosae | Glycyrrhizin (Glycyrrhizic acid) – Triterpnoid saponin, on hydrolysis yield 18-β-glycyrrhetic acid.<br>Flavonoids : isoliquiritin – antigastric effect, antispasmodic | Expectorant Treatment of peptic ulcer<br>Glycyrrhizic acid -minero-corticoid activity | **Microscopy:** cork of Ca oxalate cryst |
| sali | Chlorophytum borovillianum | Tuberous roots | Liliaceae | Hicogenin | General Tonic | - |
| i | Bacopa moniera | Fresh Leaves and Stems | Scrophulariaceae | Saponin: Bacosides A and B<br>Alkaloid: Brahmine, herpestine | Nervine tonic, in treatment of asthma, anti-cancer activity | - |

Ta

| ym | Biological name | Part Used | Family | Chemical Constituents | Uses | Key points |
|---|---|---|---|---|---|---|
| , | Various species of panax like Panax ginseng, Panax japonica, P. notaginseng | Dried Roots | Araliaceae | Ginsenosides and panaxosides (Triterpnoid saponin), oleanolic acid, Panaxadiol, panaxatriol | Adaptogen, Tonic and stimulant, immune-modulatory activity | - |
| ure | Tribalus Terrestris | Dried ripe Fruits | Zygophyllaceae | Steroidal sapogenins – diosgenin, gitogenin,chlorogenin Alkaloids – Harmine, harman | Diureticm aphrodisiac, and in gout. | - |
| | Brassica nigra | Dried ripe Seeds | Cruciferae | Sinigrin | Counter irritant, Rubefacient (externally) emetics (internally) | - |
| | Citrus | Unripe fruits | Rutaceae | Hesperidin | In capillary fragility | - |
| | Dipteryx odorata | Dried Seeds | Leguminosae | Coumarin – lactone of cis-o-caumarinic acid | Flavouring agent | |
| la | Vanilla planifolia | Unripe fruits | Orchidaceae | vanillin (4-hydroxy 3-methoxybenzaldehyde) Gluco-vanillin | Flavouring agent | - |
| | Aritostaphylos uvaursi | Dried leaves | Ericaceae | Arbutin, methyl arbutin, quercetin, ursone | Diuretics in urethritis | - |
| | Solanum Khasianum | Dried Berries | Solanaceae | Solasodine glycoalkaloid - solakhasianin | Steroidal synthesis | - |
| an | Lawsonia innermis | Fresh and dried leaves | Lythraceae | Lawson degradation of product of hennoside A, B, and C. | Antifungal and antibacterial | - |
| | Andrographis paniculata | Leaves and Shoots | Acanthaceae | bitter principle – andrographolide – bicyclic diterpenoid lactone, Kalmeghin | Bitter tonic, anthelmintic, in treatment of dysentery and dyspepsia., hepato-protective drug | |
| | Picrasma excelsa | Dried Stem Wood | Simarubaceae | Amaroid compounds – Quassin, Picrasmin (isoquassin), neoquassin | Bitter Stomachic, Anthelmentics, insecticidal activity | **Microscopy: Biseriate or multiseria medulary rays** |

**Table** Glycoside containing drug and their chemical structure of their therapeutic constitutes

| Example | Chemical Structure |
|---|---|
| **ALOE**<br>Aloin<br>Aloe-emodin<br>aloesin | 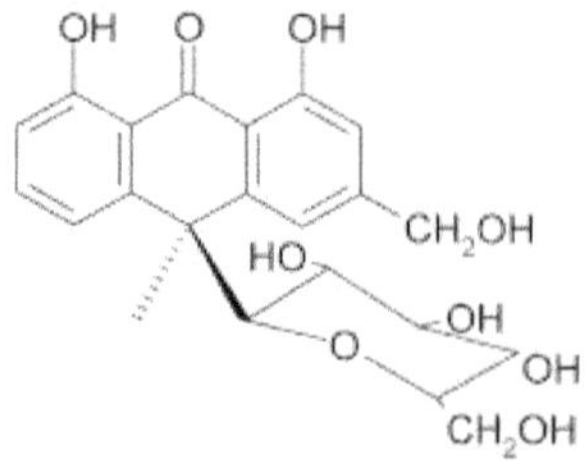<br>Aloin<br>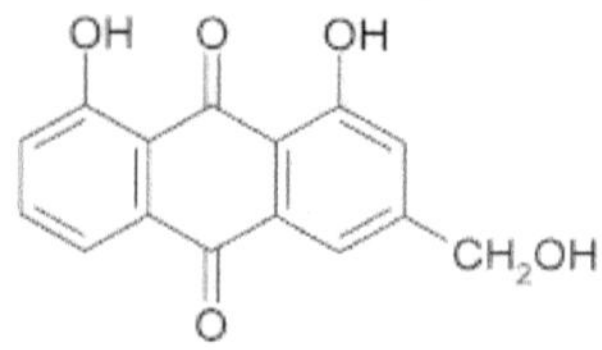<br>Aloe-emodin<br>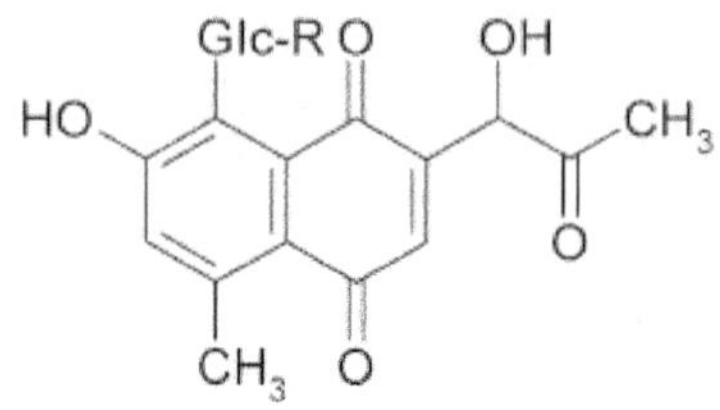<br>Aloesin |
| **SENNA**<br>Sennoside-A<br>Sennoside-B | 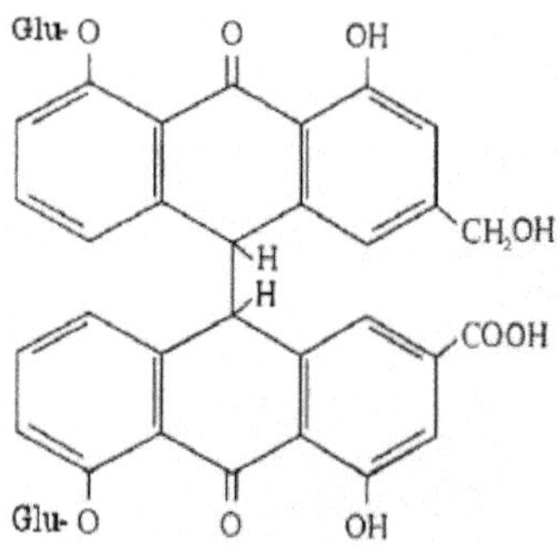<br>**Sennoside A**<br>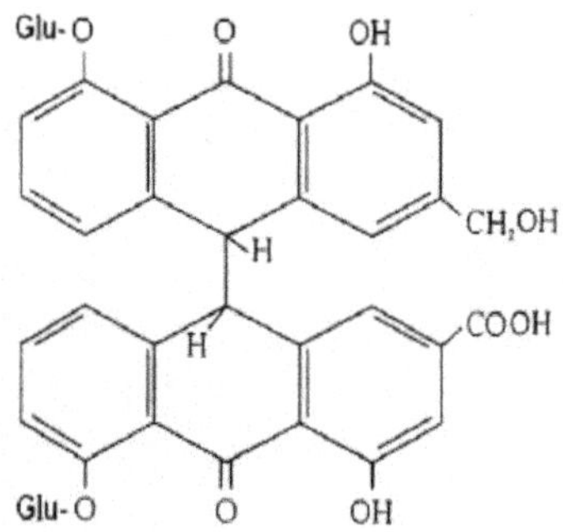<br>**Sennoside B** |
| **Rhubarb**<br>Rhein<br>Chrysophanol<br>Aloe-emodin<br>Emodin | 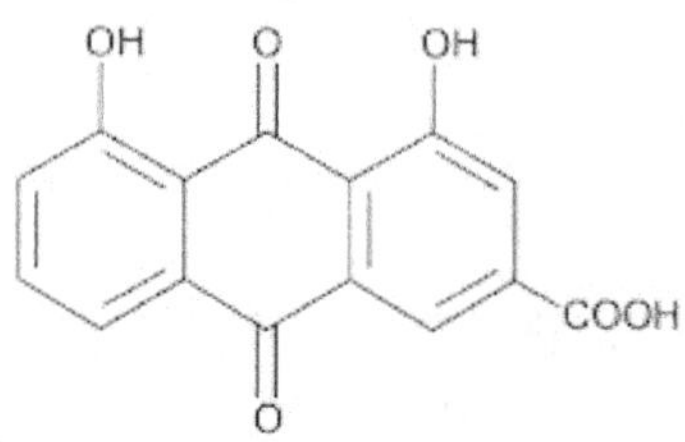<br>Rhein<br>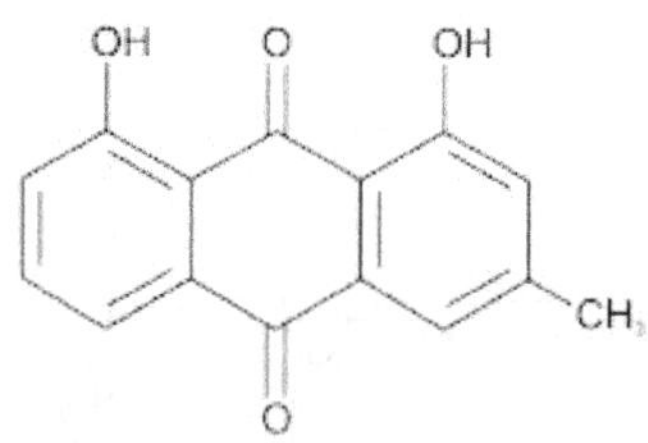<br>Chrysophanol<br>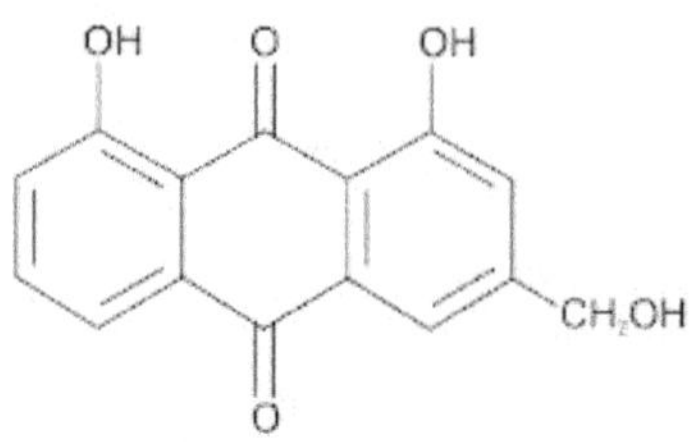<br>Aloe-emodin<br>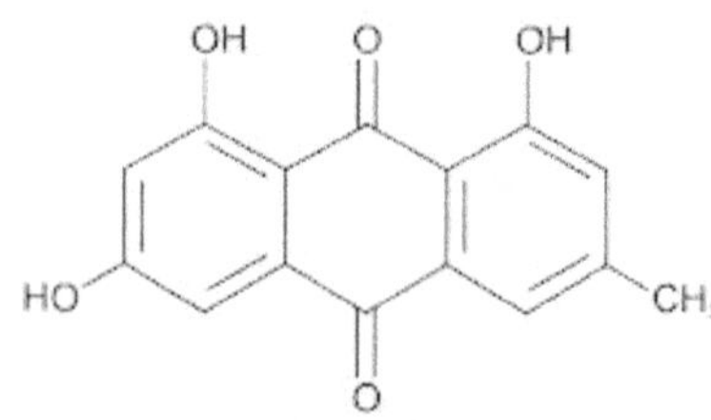<br>Emodin |

**Table** *Contd...*

| Example | Chemical Structure |
|---|---|
| **Cascara**<br>Cascaroside A<br>Cascaroside B<br>Cascaroside C<br>Cascaroside D | 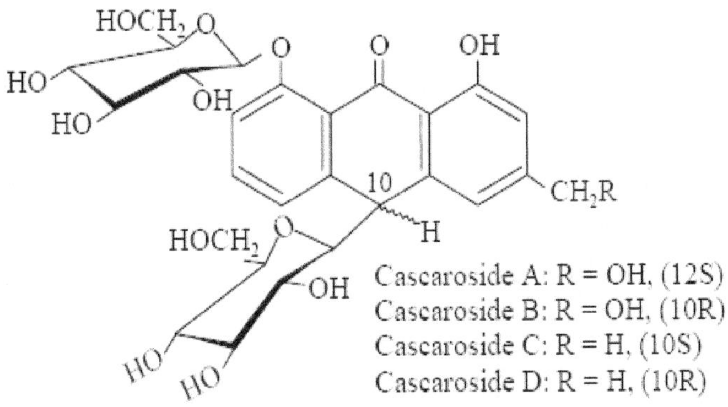<br><br>Cascarosides |
| **Digitalis purpurea**<br>Digoxin<br>Digitoxin<br>Ouabain<br>Digoxigenin | 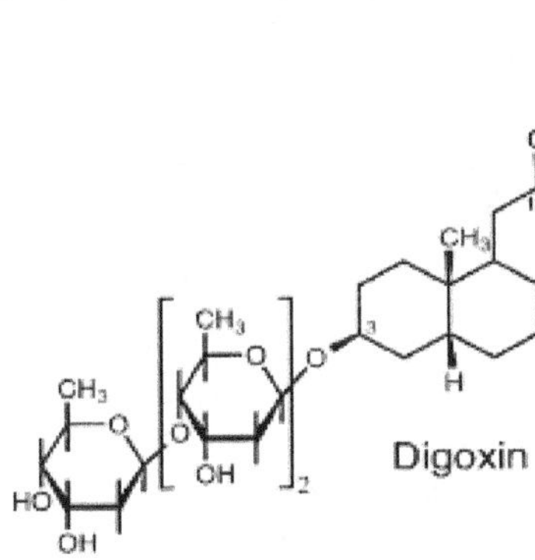 Digoxin 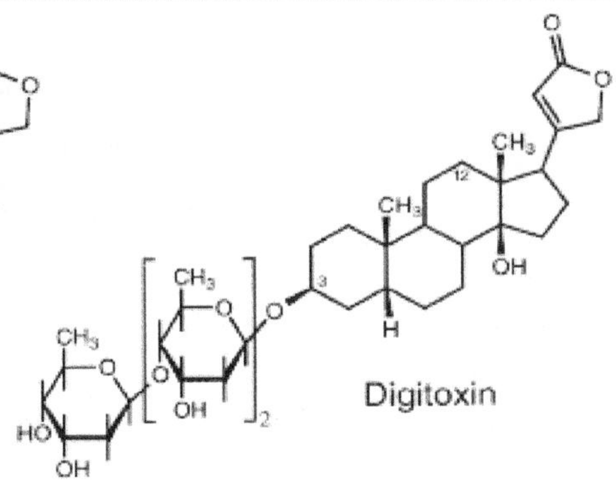 Digitoxin 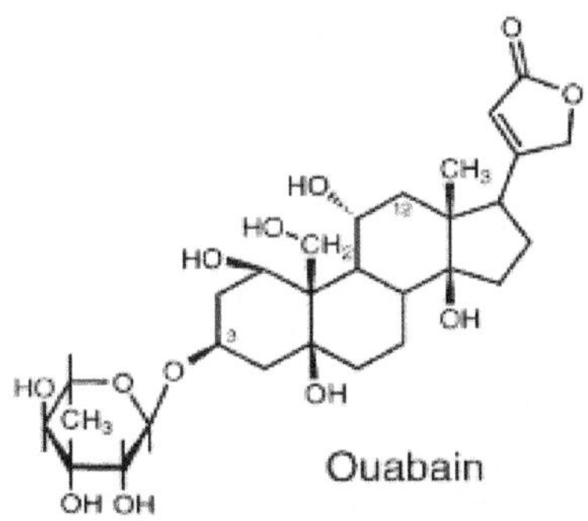 Ouabain 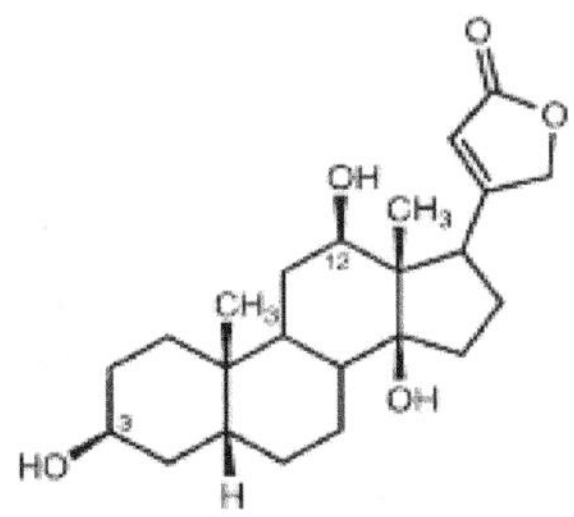 Digoxigenin |
| **Liquorice**<br>Glycyrrhetinic Acid<br>Glycyrrhizin | 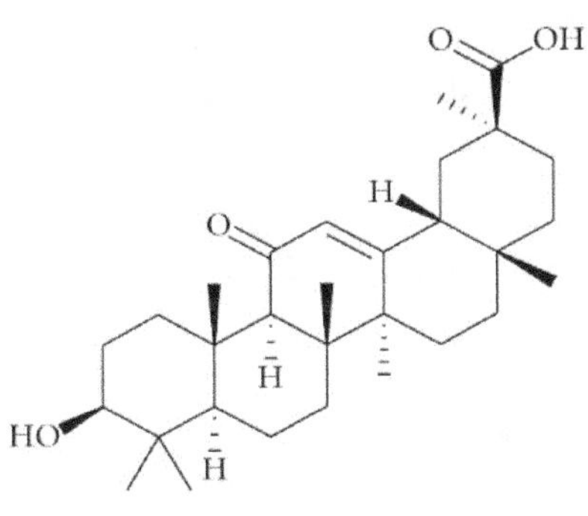 Glycyrrhetinic acid $C_{30}H_{46}O_4$ 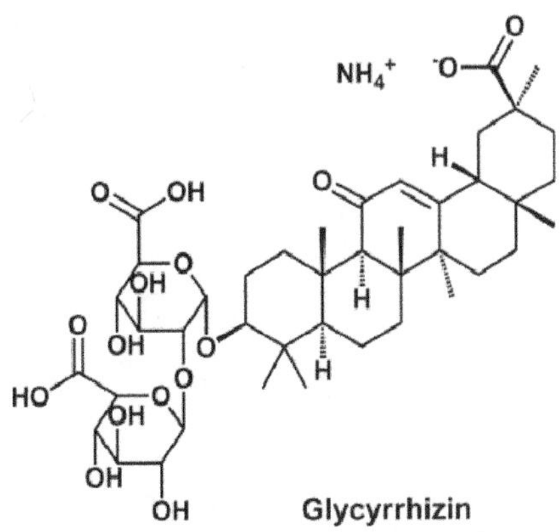 Glycyrrhizin |

**Table** *Contd...*

<table>
<tr><th>Example</th><th>Chemical Structure</th></tr>
<tr><td>Asparagus<br>Adscendin A<br>Adscendin B<br>Asparanin A<br>Asparanin B<br>Asparanin C<br>Asparanin D</td><td>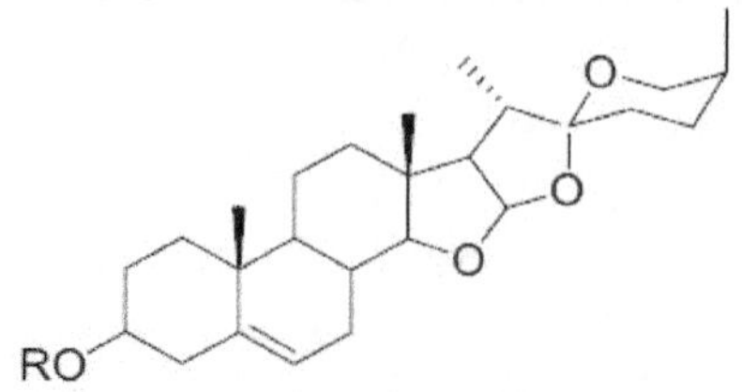<br>R= Glu(6-1), Adscendin A<br>R=Glu[(4-1)Rha](6-1)Rha, Adscendin B<br>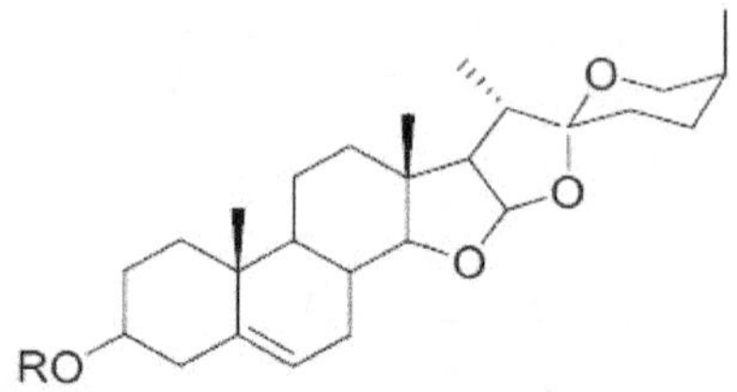<br>R= Glu(2-1)Glu, Asparanin A<br>R=Glu[(2-1)Glu](4-1)Rha, Asparanin B<br>R=Glu[(4-1)Ara](6-1)Rha, Asparanin C<br>R=Glu[(2-1)Rha](4-1)Ara, Curillin G<br>R=Glu[(2-1)Glu](4-1)Ara, Curillin H</td></tr>
<tr><td>Fenugreek<br>Rhaponticin<br>Desoxyrhaponticin<br>rhapontigenin</td><td>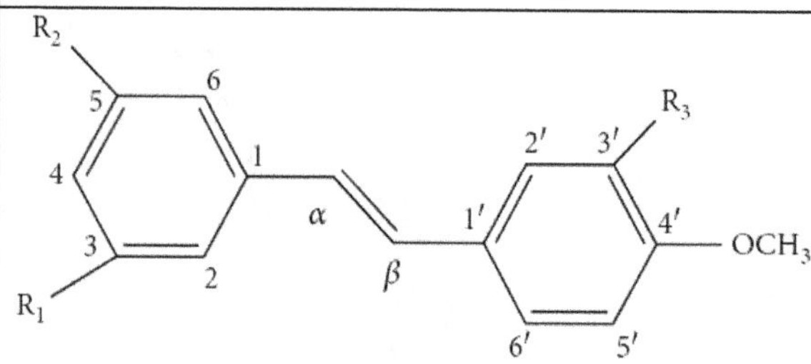
<table>
<tr><th></th><th>$R_1$</th><th>$R_2$</th><th>$R_3$</th></tr>
<tr><td>Rhaponticin</td><td>Glc</td><td>OH</td><td>OH</td></tr>
<tr><td>Desoxyrhaponticin</td><td>Glc</td><td>OH</td><td>H</td></tr>
<tr><td>Rhapontigenin</td><td>OH</td><td>OH</td><td>OH</td></tr>
</table></td></tr>
<tr><td>Ginseng<br>Ginsenoside</td><td>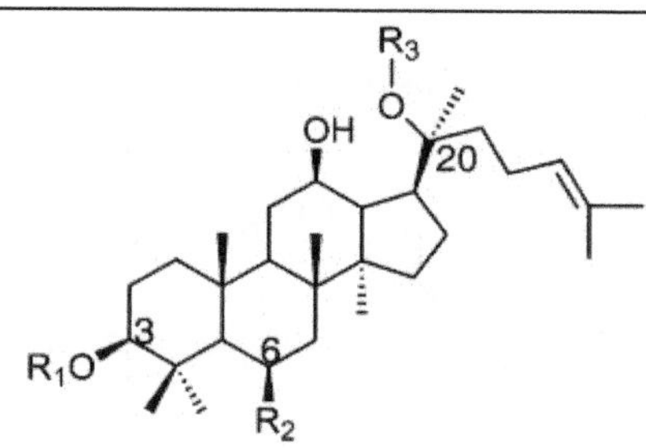
<table>
<tr><th>Ginsenoside</th><th>$R_1$</th><th>$R_2$</th><th>$R_3$</th></tr>
<tr><td>Protopanaxatriol</td><td></td><td></td><td></td></tr>
<tr><td>$Rg_1$</td><td>H</td><td>-O-glc</td><td>glc</td></tr>
<tr><td>$Rg_2$</td><td>H</td><td>-O-glc(2-1)rha</td><td>H</td></tr>
<tr><td>Re</td><td>H</td><td>-O-glc(2-1)rha</td><td>glc</td></tr>
<tr><td>Rf</td><td>H</td><td>-O-glc(2-1)glc</td><td>H</td></tr>
<tr><td>$Rh_1$</td><td>H</td><td>-O-glc</td><td>H</td></tr>
<tr><td>F1</td><td>H</td><td>-OH</td><td>glc</td></tr>
</table></td></tr>
</table>

**Table** *Contd...*

| Example | Chemical Structure |
|---|---|
| | *Protopanaxadiol*<br>**Rb₁** *glc*(2-1)*glc* H *glc*(6-1)*glc*<br>**Rb₂** *glc*(2-1)*glc* H *glc*(6-1)*ara*(p)<br>**Rg₃** *glc*(2-1)*glc* H H<br>**Rh₂** *glc* H H<br>**Rc** *glc*(2-1)*glc* H *glc*(6-1)*ara*(f)<br>**Rd** *glc*(2-1)*glc* H *glc*<br>**Ra** *glc*(2-1)*glc* H *glc*(6-1)*glc*<br>**F2** *glc* H glc |
| **Kalmegh**<br>Andrographolide<br>Andrographiside | 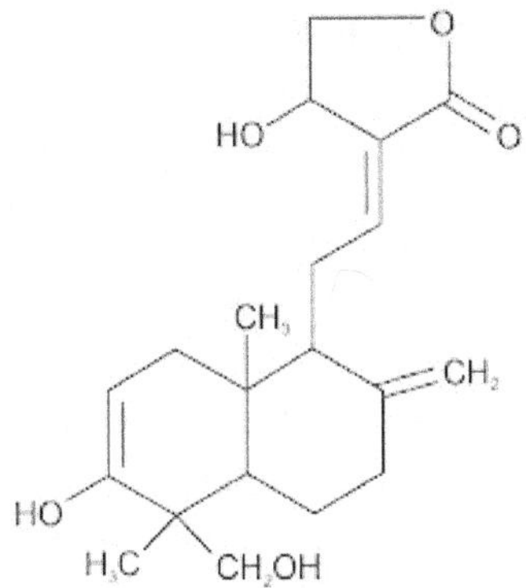  Andrographolide 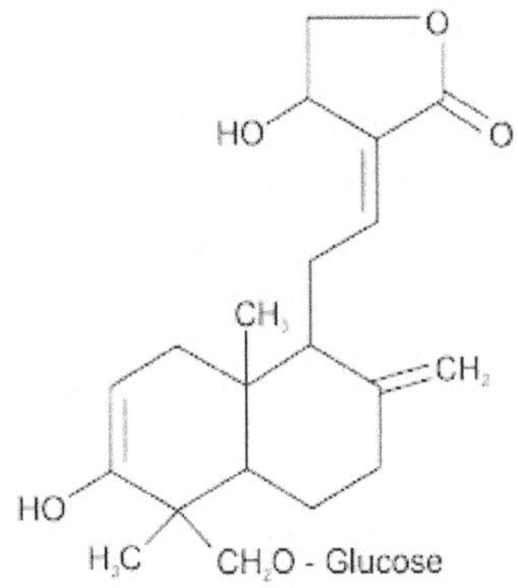  Andrographiside |
| **Vanilla pods**<br>Vanillin | 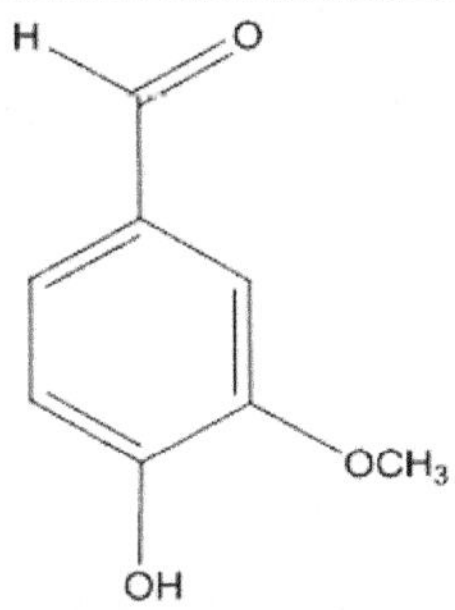  **Vanillin** |

# Pharmacognosy MCQs

1. The meaning of ''pharmakon'' is......
   (a) Knowledge (b) Science
   (c) Drug (d) Application
2. Exogenous factor for cultivation is
   (a) Transport (b) Fertilizers
   (c) Soil nation (d) Chemical
3. Embryo culture is Carried out in 1904 by
   (a) Hannig (b) Kolte
   (c) Robbins (d) Haberlandt
4. The plant which is directly used in allopathic medicine system is
   (a) Aconite (b) Digitalis
   (c) Senna (d) Kurchi
5. Bast fibers are separated from stem by
   (a) Peeling (b) Mulching
   (c) Cutting (d) Retting
6. The meaning of ''gnosis'' is
   (a) Knowledge (b) Science
   (c) Drug (d) Herbal
7. Endogenous factor for cultivation is
   (a) Transport (b) Fertilizers
   (c) Soil nature (d) Chemical race
8. Scientist ''went'' first discovered plant hormone
   (a) NAA (b) IBA
   (c) IAA (d) Kinetin
9. ''veda'' stands for
   (a) Life (b) Knowledge
   (c) Soul (d) Mind
10. Dietary fibers are used in
    (a) Laxative (b) Astringent
    (c) Antioxidant (d) Anti-tussive
11. The father of pharmacognosy is
    (a) Schmidt (b) Crr.A. Seydler
    (c) Charaka (d) Shen Nung
12. During rainy season alkaloid content in Datura is
    (a) Less (b) More
    (c) Same (d) Varies
13. Prof. Whit was first developed plant tissue culture medium for
    (a) Callus of leaves
    (b) Meristem cells of tomato
    (c) Callus of carrot
    (d) Meristem cell of tobacco
14. ''Pitta'' is belongs to
    (a) Panchabhuta (b) Kapha
    (c) Dshas (d) Vedas
15. Pulping process is used to remove
    (a) Mineral (b) Lignin
    (c) Cellulose (d) None
16. The name pharmacognosy coined in the year
    (a) 1811 (b) 1851
    (c) 1815 (d) 1814
17. Optimum temperature for propagation
    (a) 25-35° C (b) 18-28° C
    (c) 30-35°C (d) 10-20 °C
18. The process by which meristem cells converted into more cells are known
    (a) Differentiation
    (b) De-differentiation
    (c) Re-differentiation
    (d) Plasticity
19. ''kabam'' means
    (a) Old age (b) Childhood
    (c) Adult (d) None of these
20. ''Asbestos'' is an example of
    (a) Animal fiber (b) Wood fiber
    (c) Mineral fiber (d) Synthetic fiber

21. Extraction of chemical constituent from plant was first carried out from
    (a) Pikaso (b) Charaka
    (c) Galen (d) Sushrutha
22. Pythium spinosum is
    (a) Fungal pest (b) Viral pest
    (c) Bacterial pest (d) Insect
23. Regeneration capacity of plant cells are
    (a) Plasticity
    (b) Totipotency
    (c) Micropropagation
    (d) Differentiaton
24. Metals that are used in siddha system
    (a) Mercury and Gold
    (b) Mercury and Sulfur
    (c) Sulfur and gold
    (d) Gold and Copper
25. Millon's reagent reacts with animal fibre to give………. Precipitate
    (a) Violet (b) Yellow
    (c) Red (d) White
26. Anatomical atlas of crude drugs was published in the year
    (a) 1856 (b) 1815
    (c) 1862 (d) 1865
27. Bordeaux mixture is …….
    (a) Insecticide (b) Rodenticide
    (c) Herbicide (d) Fungicide
28. Synthetic seed is known as
    (a) Encapsulation of somatic seeds
    (b) Encapsulation of somatic embryos
    (c) Encapsulation of stem
    (d) Encapsulation of anthers
29. One of the four humours is
    (a) Phlegm (b) White bile
    (c) Hawa (d) Water
30. Cotton fibres are separated from seeds from
    (a) Retting (b) Plucking
    (c) Peeling (d) Ginning
31. First binomial classification of plants given by
    (a) Bentham
    (b) Hooker
    (c) Bentham and Hooker
    (d) Car Linnaeus
32. Soil pH required for available phosphorus in plant is
    (a) 5 to 8 (b) 6 to 7.5
    (c) 7 to 8 (d) 2 to 4
33. The process of formation of unorganized tissues from organized tissues is known as
    (a) Organogenesis
    (b) Re-differentiation
    (c) De-differentiation
    (d) Differentiation
34. Which one is not belongings to unani treatment
    (a) Naum-o-Yaqzah
    (b) Hawa
    (c) Harkat-o-sakoon nfsaniah
    (d) Harkat-wo-Mashroob
35. Hemp contains
    (a) High cellulose and low protein
    (b) High cellulose and low lignin
    (c) High lignin and low cellulose
    (d) High lignin and protein
36. The creator of science of genetics of plant is
    (a) Gregor mendel (b) Galen
    (c) Hooker (d) Bentham
37. Harvesting time for aerial parts of plants is
    (a) 9 to 10 am (b) 1 to 3 pm
    (c) 4 to 5 pm (d) 4 to 5 am
38. Embryo culture help in
    (a) Production of Orchids
    (b) Increasing germination of seeds
    (c) Prevent seed dormancy
    (d) Increasing breeding cycle
39. As per homeopathy medicine system, potency indicates with the symbol
    (a) C (b) P
    (c) X (d) M
40. Aflatoxin is produced from
    (a) Aspergillus versicolor
    (b) A.purpurea
    (c) A.flavus
    (d) A.purpurea

41. The father of medicine is
    (a) Theophrastus (b) Aristotle
    (c) Hippocrates (d) Charaka
42. Temperature required for root harvesting is
    (a) Above 25◦C (b) Below 23◦C
    (c) Below 35◦C (d) Above 25◦C
43. Rapid clonal multiplication is possible through
    (a) Anther culture
    (b) Seed culture
    (c) Prostoplast culture
    (d) Meristem culture
44. As per Chinese medicine system, five element are known as
    (a) Yin and yang (b) Yin and yu
    (c) Xing Wu (d) Wu Xing
45. Fabric is prepared by
    (a) Chitin (b) Biose
    (c) Hemicelluloses (d) None of these
46. Nutraceutical was first coined by
    (a) Stephen DeFelice (b) Drexler
    (c) Elder (d) Norio taniguchi
47. Small seed are harvested with
    (a) Digger (b) Forks
    (c) Seed stripper (d) Hand plucking
48. BOD incubator is
    (a) Biological oxygen demand
    (b) Bio fuel oxygen demand
    (c) Basic oxygen demand
    (d) Biological oxygen depositor
49. Example of dextrorotatory alkaloid is
    (a) Caffeine (b) Papaverine
    (c) Coniine (d) Nicotine
50. The regent mixture of copper acetate and acetic acid is known as
    (a) Benedict's reagent
    (b) Barfoed reagent
    (c) Bial's reagent
    (d) Selwanoff's reagent
51. Biomarke of withania ssomnifera is
    (a) Withanin (b) Withanolide
    (c) Withanolide-D (d) Withaferin
52. Flower are packed in
    (a) Plastic bag (b) Crates
    (c) Small bag (d) Hand plucking
53. Purple pigmentation of callus indicates
    (a) More phenolic
    (b) More flavonoids
    (c) More anthocyanin
    (d) More quinines
54. Orange colour alkaloid is
    (a) Colchicines (b) Betanin
    (c) Nicotine (d) Betanidine
55. Composition of Bial's reagent is
    (a) Orcinol, HCL and $FeCL_3$
    (b) Resorcinol , HCL
    (c) Sodium citrate , sodium carbonate
    (d) Sodium citrate, $CuSO_4$
56. The plant is having multiple stems and shorter height is known as
    (a) Herb (b) Shrub
    (c) Creeper (d) Tree
57. Enzymatic action is required for drying of drug like
    (a) Nux vomica (b) Digitalis
    (c) Cocoa seed (d) Liquorice
58. The colour of dead single cell in fluorescent diacetate is
    (a) Red (b) Blue
    (c) Pink (d) Unstain
59. Volatile liquid alkaloid is
    (a) Colchicines (b) Betanin
    (c) Nicotine (d) quinine
60. Red colour red algae is due to
    (a) Mucilage (b) Phycoerythrin
    (c) Gelidium (d) All of these
61. Eugenol is the plant constituent
    (a) Amla (b) Hibiscus
    (c) Senna (d) Clove
62. Acacia is dried under
    (a) Shade (b) Sun light
    (c) Vacuum (d) Tray dryer

63. Protoplast cell are
    (a) Cell with cell wall
    (b) Cells with cell membrane without cell wall
    (c) Cell with cell wall without cell membrane
    (d) Hybrid cell

64. Source of quinine is
    (a) Root (b) Bark
    (c) Leaves (d) Stem

65. Bassorin is insoluble in
    (a) Water
    (b) Alcohol
    (c) Water and alcohol
    (d) None of these

66. Cochineal product is procured from
    (a) Male insect
    (b) Female insect
    (c) Male and female insect
    (d) None of these

67. Aloe is store in
    (a) Vacuum
    (b) Gunny bag
    (c) Goat skin
    (d) Plastic scaled cover

68. Agrobacterium is required for culture of
    (a) Protoplast (b) Hair root
    (c) Anther (d) Seed

69. Composition of mayer's reagent is
    (a) Pot-bismuth iodide
    (b) Iodine pot iodide
    (c) Pot- mercuric iodide
    (d) Mercuric iodide

70. The major amino acid present in honey is
    (a) Leucine (b) Proline
    (c) Aspartic acid (d) Glycine

71. Cocoa butter is adulterated with
    (a) Paraffin (b) Lime stone
    (c) Lard (d) Kokum butter

72. Plant materials are extracted by using slow flow of solvent, is known as
    (a) Maceration (b) Decoction
    (c) Percolation (d) infusion

73. Biotransformation is possible through
    (a) protoplast culture
    (b) immobilized cell culture
    (c) organ culture
    (d) micropropagation

74. Alkaloid forms white colour precipitate when react with
    (a) Picrolonic acid (b) Sulphuric acid
    (c) Mercuric iodide (d) Hager's reagent

75. ''Aniline chloride test '' is performed to detect adulteration of honey with
    (a) Inverted sugar
    (b) Cane sugar
    (c) Glucose
    (d) Commercial sugar

76. Anomocytic stomata present in
    (a) Datura (b) Digitalis
    (c) Senna (d) peppermint

77. soxhlet apparatus in an example of
    (a) Digestion
    (b) Percolation
    (c) Continuous Hot Extraction
    (d) Maceration

78. HEPA filter remove particle size of
    (a) 0.03μM (b) 0.3 μM
    (c) 0.003 μM (d) 3 μM

79. One of the reagent used in Vitali Morin Test is
    (a) Sulphuric acid
    (b) Chloroform
    (c) Amino benzaldehyde
    (d) KOH

80. Chemoprotein is an example of
    (a) Simple protein
    (b) Derived protein
    (c) Conjugation protein
    (d) None of these

81. Lignified tarichome is present in
    (a) Belladonna (b) Digitalis
    (c) Nux vomica (d) Tea

82. Cytokinins are used for
    (a) Root formation
    (b) Shoot formation
    (c) Root inhibition
    (d) Shoot inhibition

83. Example of sterilants is
    (a) 2% NaCl
    (b) 2% sodium hypochlorite
    (c) 1% sodium sulphate
    (d) 2% sodium sulphate

84. Sodium molybdate in concentrated sulphuric acid is known as
    (a) Rosequin reagent (b) Van Urk's reagnt
    (c) Froehd's test (d) None

85. Light colour getatine is obtained by bleaching in
    (a) $H_2S$ (b) $H_2O_2$
    (c) $SO_2$ (d) Lead acetate

86. Hydathodes are present in
    (a) Vasaka (b) Piper betel
    (c) Cannabis (d) coffee

87. Stringolactones are derived from
    (a) Fatty acid
    (b) Carotenoids
    (c) Smoke of burning plant
    (d) Steroidal compound

88. Cereal anther culture is suitable in
    (a) N-6 medium (b) Nitsch's medium
    (c) B-5 medium (d) MS medium

89. Solvent that is not use for separation of aglycone
    (a) Chloroform (b) Acetone
    (c) Ether (d) Pet. Ether

90. Moisture content in gelatin is
    (a) 17% (b) 6%
    (c) 16% (d) 7%

91. Rosette type calcium oxalate crystal is present in
    (a) Cinnamon (b) Ipecac
    (c) Arjuna (d) Cinchona

92. Removal of stamen from female flowering plant is known as
    (a) Bagging (b) Emasculation
    (c) Tagging (d) Crossing

93. Medium pH is optimum for tissue culture is
    (a) 4.5 (b) 7.0
    (c) 5-6 (d) 6-8

94. Example of flavones glycoside
    (a) Luteolin (b) Catechin
    (c) Querrcetin (d) Naringenin

95. Phosphate group present in alpha casein is
    (a) 10-15 (b) 8-10
    (c) 6-8 (d) 3-7

96. Haemolytic activity is carried out for
    (a) Cardiac glycoside
    (b) Saponin glycoside
    (c) Cyanogenetic glycoside
    (d) Flavonoids

97. Farmers right act in
    (a) 2001 (b) 2004
    (c) 2000 (d) 1970

98. Live attenuated vaccine is
    (a) Typhoid (b) Oral polio
    (c) Plague (d) Rabies

99. Gallic acid is found in
    (a) Eucalyptus (b) Rhubarb
    (c) Myrobalan (d) None of these

100. Proenzyme of pepsin is
    (a) Kymopepsin (b) Kimopepsin
    (c) Sarapepsinogen (d) Pepsinogen

101. The volatile oils are the complex mixture of……
    (a) Mono- and sesquiterpenes as well as phenyl-propane derivatives.
    (b) Mono- and diterpene alcohols and ethers.
    (c) sesquiterpenes and other aromatic compounds.
    (d) monoterpene acids and lactones.
    (e) monoterpene ethers and aldehydes.

102. Sesquiterpenes are formed of............in the plants.
    (a) farnezyl-pyrophosphate
    (b) stress compounds
    (c) colouring material
    (d) degraded products of triterpenes
    (e) pathological products

103. What are known as balsams?
   (a) resins dissolved in volatile oil
   (b) a mixture of volatile oils with sesquiterpenes
   (c) resins dissolved in water
   (d) polysaccharide mixed with volatile oil
   (e) juice evaporated to dryness

104. Saponin containing drugs are used as..........
   (a) Laxative.
   (b) Bitter Tonic.
   (c) Expectorant.
   (d) Emetic.
   (e) Pain Killer.

105. Alkaloids are naturally occurring compounds which contain ............in their molecules.
   (a) One or more N atom(s)
   (b) Two heterocyclic rings
   (c) One C15 side chain on the benzene ring
   (d) One or more N atom(s) originated from amino acids
   (e) One or more O atoms besides the S atoms

106. How to extract the alkaloids in mineral salt form from plant?
   (a) Heating with organic solvent.
   (b) Boiling with ammonium-hydroxide and water.
   (c) Shaking with water containing mineral acid.
   (d) Boiling with water and lead acetate.
   (e) Warming with mineral acid in organic solvent.

107. The volatile oils consist of a mixture of.........
   (a) Oxygen free mono- and diterpenes.
   (b) Aliphatic and cyclic mono- and triterpenes.
   (c) Aliphatic and cyclic mono- and sesquiterpenes and phenyl-propane derivatives.
   (d) Highly oxygenated mono- and diterpenes.
   (e) Oxygen free di- and monoterpenes

108. The iridoids are:
   (a) Constituents of volatile oils.
   (b) Starting unit of the tannin biogenesis.
   (c) Precursor of biosynthesis of saponins.
   (d) Precursors of the biogenesis of certain alkaloids.
   (e) Constituents of fixed oils.

109. What do you do for getting alkaloids in basis form from the plant material?
   (a) Adding some ammonium-hydroxide and water to the pulverised drug.
   (b) Making an extract by mineral acid and organic solvent.
   (c) Making an extract with some basis and organic solvent.
   (d) Adding to the powdered drug some mineral acid and water.
   (e) Making an extract with organic solvent and warm it.

110. Morphin is separable from its side alkaloids because:
   (a) Morphine has a piperidine ring.
   (b) Morphine has two methoxy groups.
   (c) Morphine has phenolic hydroxyl group while the side alkaloids have none.
   (d) Morphine has no phenolic hydroxyl group while the side alkaloid has it.
   (e) Morphine and its side alkaloids are inseparable.

111. Which is the right reagent for the detection of rancidity?
   (a) Concentrated nitric acid
   (b) Phloroglucinol dissolved in diluted hcl
   (c) Antimony-iii-chloride
   (d) Concentrated sulphuric acid
   (e) Phloroglucinol dissolved in ether and concentrated hcl

112. 5 Choose the right skeleton for Cinchona alkaloids.
   (a) Cevan
   (b) Tropane
   (c) Isoquinoline
   (d) Rubanol
   (e) Dammarane

113. 5. Choose the right reagent for alkaloids.
   (a) 2,4-dinitrophenylhydrazine
   (b) Iron-iii-chloride
   (c) Antimony-iii-chloride
   (d) Potassium-tetraiodomercurate
   (e) Phloroglucinol in concentrated hydrochloric acid

114. How could be prepared a mucilage extract starting from Linseed?
   (a) After grinding some water is added to the seed and warm it.
   (b) The seed is covered with water without grinding and warming.
   (c) After grinding some alcohol is added to the seed.
   (d) Without grinding some alcohol is added to the seed.
   (e) After grinding it is covered with water without warming.

115. 6 Ergot is the......................of the fungus Claviceps purpurea.
   (a) Vegetative form
   (b) Dried sclerotium
   (c) Ascospore
   (d) Conidiospore
   (e) Philamentous Hyphae

116. What is the difference between the chemical structure of cotton and starch?
   (a) Cotton consists of lines α-glucose molecules while the starch has branched β-glucose residue.
   (b) Cotton consists of unbranched β-glucose molecules the starch has also unbranched α- and β-glucose molecules.
   (c) Cotton is built up of glucose residues united by 1,4-β-D-glucose links, starch has branched and linear chains of 1,4-α-,and 1,6-α-D-glucose residue.
   (d) Both consist of branched and linear 1,2-β-D-glucose residues.

117. The haemolytic index shows:
   (a) The di- and sesquiterpene content of the volatile oils..
   (b) The saponin content of the drugs.
   (c) The steroid content of the drugs.
   (d) The aliphatic monoterpene content of the drugs.
   (e) The tannin content of the drugs

118. Which is the right structure for the flavonoids of Silybum marianum?
   (a) Dimer flavan-3,4-diol
   (b) Monomer flavon-3-ol
   (c) Flavanolignan
   (d) Simple flavanonol-glycoside
   (e) Isoflavanon-diglycoside

119. Cocaine is used as...................in the officinal medicine.
   (a) Narcotic
   (b) Emetic
   (c) Sedative
   (d) local anaesthetic
   (e) Cough suppressant

120. Choose the right test for identification of anthraquinones.
   (a) Marquis test
   (b) Froehde test
   (c) Liebermann-Burchard test
   (d) Borntraeger test
   (e) Murexid test

121. How to detect the procyanidins?
   (a) On heating with diluted NaOH procyanidines show green colour.
   (b) Procyanidins give yellow colour on concentrated nitric acid.
   (c) On heating with a mixture of cc. HCl and N BuOH procyanidines show red colour.
   (d) On heating with resorcinol procyanidins give bluish violet colour.
   (e) Procyanidins give orange precipitate on Kedde reagent.

122. The anthraquinone content of the drugs tested by ...........................
   (a) Warming with glacial acetic acid giving red precipitate.
   (b) Shaking the extract made by organic solvent with diluted ammonium-hydroxide the water phase gives red or orange colour.
   (c) Extracting with water and precipitate with lead acetate showing blue colour.
   (d) Making a water extract which shows green colour on sulphuric acid.
   (e) Making organic solvent extract which shows yellow precipitate on heating with dil. Hcl and chlorine.

123. What is the right method for making assay for volatile oil content of drugs?
(a) Water-damp distillation
(b) Extraction of light petrol
(c) Distillation by marcusson's method
(d) Determination of loss on drying
(e) Determination of alcohol extract

124. Which is the right test for the cardioactive glycosides of Foxglove leaf?
(a) Murexide
(b) Liebermann- Burchard
(c) EP
(d) 2,4-dinitro-phenylhydrazine
(e) Keller-Kiliani

125. Which of the following compounds makes model for the synthesis of methyl- psoralens?
(a) Chinine (b) Ephedrine
(c) Tubocurarin (d) Xanthotoxin
(e) Cocaine

126. How to take a sample of plant drug material according to the prescription of pharmacopoeia?
(a) 1000g of drug is taken off the upper part of the container.
(b) 100 or 200g drug has to be taken the side of the container.
(c) The number of sample depends on the number of container (N) or square root of N (at higher N). The samples has to be taken from different parts of container and the amount of the sample must be sufficient for the further analysis.
(d) Depends on the number of the container and volume of the sample.
(e) The amount and number of the sample are determined on the basis of the water content of the drug.

127. Choose the right shape for the maize starch.
(a) Oval
(b) Rounded
(c) Pentagon with a "v" form fission in the middle of the grain
(d) Triangular
(e) Dumb-bell shaped

128. Why can't use for medical purpose Rheum raponticum instead of Rheum palmatum?
(a) Because the emodin content of Rheum raponticum is too much.
(b) Because the rhein content of the Rheum raponticum is too low.
(c) Because the chrysophanol content of Rheum palmatum is higher than in case of Rheum raponticum.
(d) Because the Rheum raponticum contains a stilben derivative which has undesirable hormon activity.
(e) Because the R. raponticum has gallic acid and the amount of other tannins are too low.

129. Which of the following compounds transforms to chamazulen on Waterdamp distillation?
(a) Lavandulol (b) Farnezol
(c) Matricine (d) Gossypol
(e) Parthenolid

130. Which compound makes model for the synthesis of petidin?
(a) Psoralen (b) Cocaine
(c) Hyoscyamine (d) Morphin
(e) Physostigmine

131. Which of the following drug(s) contain(s) citric acid in a large amount?
(a) Bearberry leaf
(b) Elder flower
(c) Herniariae herba
(d) Tamarindi fructus
(e) Violae odoratae radix

132. How to get fixed oil for medical purpose?
(a) By extraction with a cold organic solvent
(b) By warm expression
(c) By extraction with cold water
(d) By cold expression
(e) By cooking with water

133. The cake of ricinus seed left after expression is unfit for use as a cattle food since it contains an extremely poisonous toxin known as ................
(a) Ricinin (b) Ricine
(c) Taxol (d) Sinigrine
(e) Lotaustralin

134. Which of the following alkaloids derived from lysine?
    (a) Emetin
    (b) Chelidonin
    (c) Cinchonidin
    (d) Brucin
    (e) obelin

135. Which of the following drugs contains inulin?
    (a) Cichoriae radix
    (b) Comfrey root
    (c) Plantain shoot
    (d) Foenigraeci semen
    (e) Tanaceti herba

136. Hasis (hashish) consists ........ of Cannabis sativa.
    (a) Gum of the male flowers
    (b) Resin of the female flowers
    (c) Gum of the male and female flowers
    (d) Pressed juice of the leaves
    (e) Latex of the tops

137. What is Opium?
    (a) Latex exudate of the unriped incised capsules after air dried.
    (b) Dried wateric extract of the riped capsules.
    (c) Dried alcoholic extract of the unriped capsules.
    (d) Concentrated alcoholic extract of the poppy straw.
    (e) Wateric extract of the riped seeds.

138. The common base skeleton of physiologically active ergoline alkaloids is:
    (a) Isolysergic acid.
    (b) Clavorubine.
    (c) Lysergic acid.
    (d) 2-phenylbenzopyrane.
    (e) Elimoclavine.

139. Codeine is:
    (a) Monomethyl ether of morphine.
    (b) Amide of apomorphine.
    (c) Acetyl derivative of morphine.
    (d) Dimethyl ether of papaverine.
    (e) Diethyl ether of morphine.

140. Skeleton of the B-type procyanidines is:
    (a) flavan-3-ol.
    (b) flavan-4-on.
    (c) lignan.
    (d) flavanolignan.
    (e) flavanonol.

141. Select the method prescribed for quantitative determination of anthraglycosides in Pharmacopoeia Hungarica Editio VII.:
    (a) Gravimetry.
    (b) High pressure liquid chromatography.
    (c) Spectrophotometry.
    (d) Gaschromatography.
    (e) Titrimetry.

142. Select the compound prescribed for quantitative determination on the base of complex formation in Pharmacopoeia Hungarica Editio VII.:
    (a) Bitter substance.
    (b) Flavonoid.
    (c) Alkaloid.
    (d) Saponin.
    (e) Phenolglycoside.

143. Which of the following physico-chemical characteristics is correct for mucilages?
    (a) Foaming
    (b) Specific colour
    (c) Specific gravity
    (d) Viscosity
    (e) Refractive index

144. Poppy straw is the industrial raw material of morphine production because .........
    (a) Poppy straw contains only morphine
    (b) Poppy straw does not contain other alkaloids
    (c) Poppy straw has the maximum morphine content
    (d) Poppy straw is the chiepest available raw material
    (e) Poppy straw contains morphine derivative

145. Definition of vegetable drugs in the Pharmacopoeia:
    (a) Plant part used in medicine.
    (b) Plant part containing the highest content of the bioactive/characteristic compound/s.
    (c) Dried part of the medicinal plant.
    (d) Plant part or its preparations described in the paragraphs of the pharmacopoeia.
    (e) Dried plant part used in medicine.

146. The whole in toto vegetable drugs of mild activity have to be rejected when ...
   (a) It contains any toxic foreign matter (plant parts).
   (b) It contains foreign matter (plant parts) more than prescribed in the corresponding paragraph of the pharmacopoeia.
   (c) It contains any toxic foreign matter (plant parts) which can not be separated.
   (d) It contains any foreign matter (plant parts).
   (e) It contains other parts of the plant more than prescribed in the corresponding paragraph of the pharmacopoeia.

147. A vegetable drug is considered as one of pharmacopoeial quality, when:
   (a) It meets both the general requirements of the pharmacopoeia and the requirements of the corresponding paragraph in the pharmacopoeia.
   (b) It meets the requirements of the corresponding paragraph in the pharmacopoeia.
   (c) It meets the requirements of the national standard i.
   (d) It meets the general requirements of the pharmacopoeia.
   (e) It meets both the general requirements of the pharmacopoeia and the requirements of the national standard i.

148. Which of the following statement is associated with the name of Janos KABAY?
   (a) Isolation of morphine.
   (b) Structure elucidation of morphine.
   (c) Industrial production of morphinanes from poppy straw.
   (d) Industrial production of morphinanes from opium.
   (e) Industrial production of morphinanes from unriped poppy capsules.

149. Which of the following statement is associated with the name of Miklos BEKESSY?
   (a) Production of essential oils by steam distillation.
   (b) Industrial production of poppy alkaloids.
   (c) Cultivation of ergot.
   (d) Isolation of morphine.
   (e) Production of ergot alkaloids by fermentation.

150. 50. Whose name of the followings is associated with the discovery of morphine?
   (a) Caventou (b) Serturner
   (c) Stoll (d) Pelletier
   (e) Scheele

151. Select the method used for the fixed vegetable oil-preparation of pharmacopoeial quality:
   (a) Solvent extraction.
   (b) Expression.
   (c) Cold-expression.
   (d) Steam distillation.
   (e) Expression and solvent extraction.

152. Quality control of medicinal plants is carried out by authority in Hungary:
   (a) National Pharmaceutical Institute.
   (b) Any institute for quality control.
   (c) Herbaria (National Medicinal Plant Trading Company).
   (d) Hungarian Bureau of Standards.
   (e) Research Institute for Medicinal Plants.

153. Which of the following vegetable drugs has the highest caffeine content?
   (a) Mate folium (b) Theae folium
   (c) Guarana (d) Coffeae semen
   (e) Colae semen

154. Which of the following cannabinoids is narcotic?
   (a) Cannabichromene
   (b) Tetrahydrocannabinol
   (c) Cannabigerol
   (d) Cannabinol
   (e) Cannabidiol

155. Select the vegetable drug which has the highest alkaloid content!
   (a) Chinae succirubrae cortex
   (b) Stramonii folium
   (c) Ipecacuanhae radix
   (d) Strychni semen
   (e) Belladonnae radix

156. Which of the following constituents is not present in Aetheroleum chamomillae?
(a) Chamazulene
(b) Matricin
(c) Spatulenol
(d) A-bisabolol
(e) En-in-dicycloethers

157. Which of the following constituents is not present in Chamomillae anthodium?
(a) Chamazulene
(b) Matricin
(c) Spatulenol
(d) A-bisabolol
(e) En-in-dicycloethers

158. Which of the followings is true for inulin?
(a) Arabin
(b) Pectin
(c) Galaktane
(d) Mannan
(e) Fructosane

159. Number of vegetable drugs which are not subject to restriction in Hungary?
(a) Less than 50
(b) Between 50 and 100
(c) Between 100 and 300
(d) Between 300 and 500
(e) More than 500

160. Which of the followings is correct for the molecular mass of tannins?
(a) Less than 200
(b) Between 200 and 500
(c) Between 500 and 1000
(d) Between 1000 and 3000
(e) More than 3000

161. Which of the following vegetable drugs is carminative?
(a) Frangulae cortex
(b) Centaurii herba
(c) Silybi mariani fructus
(d) Foeniculi fructus
(e) Graminis rhizoma

162. Which of the following vegetable drugs contains ajoene?
(a) Valerianae radix
(b) Agrimoniae herba
(c) Echinaceae radix
(d) Ginseng radix
(e) Allii sativi bulbus

163. Which of the following plant constituents can be characterized by reversible complexation with proteins?
(a) Alkaloids
(b) Saponins
(c) Tannins
(d) Mucilages
(e) Anthraglycosides

164. Morphine content in Opium is:
(a) Less than 0.5 %.
(b) Between 0.5 and 1.0 %.
(c) Between 1.0 and 5 %.
(d) Between 5 and 10 %.
(e) Between 10 and 15 %.

165. Which of the following vegetable drugs contains aucubin?
(a) Marrubii herba
(b) Agrimoniae herba
(c) Valerianae rhizoma and radix
(d) Plantaginis folium
(e) Cyani flos

166. Which of the following vegetable drugs is in the category of amara aromatica?
(a) Absinthii herba
(b) Cardui benedicti herba
(c) Gentianae radix
(d) Trifolii fibrini folium
(e) Centaurii herba

167. Hide powder is used in the traditional method of tannin quantitation because ...
(a) Hide powder gives a colour reaction with tannin.
(b) Hide powder reacts with polyphenols.
(c) Hide powder reduces tannins.
(d) Hide powder oxidizes polyphenols.
(e) Hide powder reacts with tannins.

168. What type of compound is arbutin used in urological infections?
(a) Flavonoid glycoside
(b) Phenolic glycoside
(c) Furanocoumarin
(d) Iridoid glycoside
(e) Gallotannin

169. How can you extract tertiary alkaloids in the form of salts?
   (a) Extracting with organic solvent like chloroform.
   (b) Boiling with aqueous ammonia.
   (c) Extracting with organic solvent containing alkaline solution.
   (d) Extracting with organic solvent containing acidic solution.
   (e) Extracting with an acidic aqueous solution.

170. Ginseng saponins are of the ............... series
   (a) Lupine
   (b) Ursane
   (c) Abietane
   (d) Oleanane
   (e) Dammarane

171. Choose the right compound for the following structure:
   (a) Podophyllotoxin
   (b) Taxifolin
   (c) Silybin
   (d) Hyperoside
   (e) Silychrystine

# Answer Key Pharmacognosy

1. c
2. b
3. a
4. b
5. d
6. a
7. a
8. c
9. b
10. a
11. b
12. a
13. b
14. c
15. b
16. c
17. b
18. a
19. a
20. c
21. c
22. a
23. b
24. b
25. c
26. d
27. d
28. b
29. a
30. d
31. d
32. b
33. c
34. d
35. b
36. a
37. c
38. c
39. c
40. c
41. c
42. c
43. d
44. d
45. b
46. a
47. c
48. a
49. c
50. b
51. c
52. b
53. c
54. d
55. a
56. b
57. c
58. a
59. c
60. b
61. d
62. b
63. b
64. b
65. a
66. b
67. c
68. b
69. c
70. b
71. a
72. c
73. b
74. c
75. d
76. b
77. c
78. b
79. d
80. c
81. c
82. b
83. b
84. c
85. c
86. b
87. b
88. a
89. b
90. c
91. c
92. b
93. c
94. a
95. b
96. b
97. b
98. b
99. b
100. d
101. a
102. a
103. a
104. c
105. d
106. c
107. c
108. d
109. c
110. c
111. e
112. d
113. d
114. b
115. b
116. c
117. b
118. c
119. d
120. d
121. c
122. b
123. a
124. e
125. d
126. c
127. c
128. d
129. c

| | | | | | |
|---|---|---|---|---|---|
| 130. | d | 144. | d | 158. | e |
| 131. | d | 145. | d | 159. | c |
| 132. | d | 146. | c | 160. | d |
| 133. | b | 147. | a | 161. | d |
| 134. | e | 148. | c | 162. | e |
| 135. | a | 149. | c | 163. | c |
| 136. | b | 150. | b | 164. | e |
| 137. | a | 151. | c | 165. | d |
| 138. | c | 152. | e | 166. | a |
| 139. | a | 153. | b | 167. | e |
| 140. | a | 154. | b | 168. | b |
| 141. | c | 155. | a | 169. | e |
| 142. | b | 156. | b | 170. | e |
| 143. | d | 157. | a | 171. | c |

# Chapter 4

# Pharmaceutical Jurisprudence

## Pharmaceutical Jurisprudence

### 4.1 Pharmaceutical Legislation

#### Introduction

- Law intends for regulation and control of various aspects of life.
- These aspects might be social, economic and political.
- Pharmaceutical legislation is a mixed legislation, which overlapping covers both social and economic aspects.

#### Objective

- To ensure that the patients receive drugs of required quality, tested and evaluated for safety as well as efficacy for their intended use.
- Pharmaceutical legislation is associated with the health of the society.

#### Origin

- In 1811 first chemist shop opened by Mr. Bathgate, who came to India with East India company in Calcutta.
- In 1910 they have started manufacture of tincture and spirits.
- In 1821 another firm, Smith Stanistreet and co. started apothecary shop and started manufacturing in 1918.
- In 1901 Bengal Chemical and Pharmaceutical works, a small factory was started in calcutta by Acharya P.C. Ray
- In 1903 Prof. T. K. Gajjar opens small factory at Parel for the development of Pharmaceutical units and Alembic chemical works Ltd. at Baroda

#### Drug Enquiry Committee

- Appointed by Indian Govt. in 1931
- Committee chairman was Lt. Col. R. N. Chopra
- Also called as DEC or Chopra committee
- The committee was asked to make enquiries in the said matter and then to make recommendations for smooth control of manufacture, import, distribution and sale of drugs in the interest of public health.

RECOMMENDATION of DEC - 90 recommendations with report was submitted by the committee. Important Recommendations:

- Formation of Central Pharmacy Council and State pharmacy council which would look after the education and training of professionals. Councils would maintain the register containing names and addresses of the registered pharmacist.
- Creation of drug control machinery (Departments) at the center and branches in all states.
- Establishment of a well-equipped Central Drug Laboratory (CDL) with competent staff and experts for an efficient and speedy working of Drug Control Department. Small laboratories would work under its guidance

## Scope

- Drug bill was introduced in 1940 in legislative assembly, and Drug Bill 1940 was passed, which came to force in 1947. since then drug act was amended many times and at present it covers the provisions related to Drugs, Cosmetics, Ayurveda, including Unani and Homeopathic medicines.
- The present Drug and Cosmetic Act is an improved version of the Drug Act, 1940. The main objective of this act was to regulate the import, manufacture, distribution and sale of drugs and cosmetics in India.
- The Central Government made several rules entitled the Drug and Cosmetic Rules 1945. These act and rules were amended from time to time.
- The Pharmacy act 1948 was passed with the main objective to regulate the profession of Pharmacy in India.
- In 1954 the Drug and Magic Remedies Act was passed with the main aim to control certain types of advertisements related to drug and to prohibit certain types of advertisements related to magic remedies.
- Medicinal and Toilet Preparations (Excise duty) Act, 1955 was passed providing for the levy and collection of duties of excise on medicinal and toilet preparations containing alcohol, opium Indian hemp or other narcotic drugs.
- Central government implemented Drug Price Control order 1987.
- In 1985 the Narcotic and Psychotropic Substance Act, was passed. The main objective of this act was to consolidate and amend the laws relating to narcotic drugs and Psychotropic substance.
- Other acts included were:-
    - Prevention of food Adulteration act, 1954 and rules.
    - The Industries (Development and Regulations) Act, 1951.
    - The Industrial Employment (Standing order) Act 1946 and rules.
    - Industrial Dispute Act, 1947.
    - Factory Act, 1948.
    - The Indian Patent and Design Act 1970.
    - The Trade and Merchandise Mark, 1958.
    - The Epidemic Disease Act, 1897.
    - Shops and Establishment acts of respective states.

## Bhore Committee

- October 1943---Health Survey and Development Committee – by Government of India.
- Chairman----Sir Joseph Bhore.
- COMMITTEE RECOMMENDATIONS-

- Establishment of an All India Pharmaceutical Council and provincial Pharmaceutical Council
- Strengthening of profession standards of pharmacists
- Maintaining disciplinary control
- Starting of revised courses of study
- Setting up of Central Drug Laboratory
- Rigid enforcement of the Drug and Cosmetics Act, 1940

### Bhatia Committee

- ➢ Government of India in 1953---Appointed
- ➢ Pharmaceutical Enquiry Committee
- ➢ Chairman---Major-general S.L.Bhatia
- ➢ Made a comprehensive enquiry into the working of pharmaceutical industry.
- ➢ In June 1954, 212 recommendations have been implemented.

### Mudaliar Committee

- ➢ In 1959, Healthy Survey and Planning Committee appointed
- ➢ Chairman- DR.A. LAKSHMANSWAMY MUDALIAR
- ➢ Recommended the inclusion of indigenous systems of medicine under the purview of the Drugs Act.

### Hathi Committee

- ➢ Important milestone in pharmaceutical legislation history is Hathi Committee
- ➢ Chairman- JAISUKH LAL HATHI
- ➢ This committee covered all the aspects of Licensing, price control, imports, role of foreign sector quality control.

### The Pharmacy Council of India

The Pharmacy Council of India consists of the following:

- ✓ Six members, among whom at least one teacher of pharmaceutical chemistry, pharmacy. Pharmacology and pharmacology elected by the University Grants Commission.
- ✓ Six members, four of whom are persons possessing a degree or diploma in and practicing pharmacy or pharmaceutical chemistry, nominated by the Central Government.
- ✓ One member elected from amongst themselves by the members of the medical Council of India.
- ✓ The Director General of Health Services or an authorized person by him.
- ✓ The Drugs Controller of India or an authorized person by him,
- ✓ The Director of Central Drugs Laboratory,
- ✓ A representative of the University Grants Commission,
- ✓ A representative of the All India Council for Technical Education.
- ✓ One member to represent each state elected from each state council and who is a Registered Pharmacist
- ✓ One member to represent each state nominated by the State Government who is a Registered Pharmacist
- ✓ One member to represent each Union territory, nominated by the Union territory
- ✓ Council, being eligible for registration under section 31 of the Act

## State Pharmacy Councils

The State Pharmacy Council consists of the following

- Six members, elected from amongst themselves by registered pharmacists,
- Five members, of whom three are persons possessing a prescribed degree or diploma in pharmacy or
- Pharmaceutical chemistry or registered pharmacist, nominated by State Government.
- One member, elected from amongst themselves by the members of each Medical
- Council or the Council of Medical Registration of the State,
- The chief administrative medical officer of the State or his authorised person,
- The officer-in-charge of drugs control organisation of the State or his authorised person,
- The Government Analyst.

## Joint State Councils

A Joint State Council consists of the following:

- Not less than three and not more than five members elected amongst themselves by the registered pharmacists of each of the participating States,
- Not less than three but not more than four members nominated by each participating State Government.
- One member elected from amongst themselves by the members of each Medical Council or the Council of Medical Registration of each participating State,
- The chief administrative medical officer of each participating State or his authorized person,
- The officer in-charge of drugs control organisation of each participating State or his authorised person.
- The Government Analyst of each participating State.

## Registration of Pharmacists

The register shall include the following particulars, namely:

- The full name and residential address of the registered person;
- The date of his first admission to the register;
- His qualifications for registration;
- His professional address, and if he is employed by any person, the name of
- such person;
- Such further particulars as may be prescribed.

Preparation of first register-

- For the purpose of preparing the first register, the State Government shall by notification in the Official Gazette constitute a Registration Tribunal consisting of three persons, and shall also appoint a Registrar who shall act as Secretary of the Registration Tribunal.
- The State Government shall, by the same or a like notification, appoint a date on or before which applications for registration, which shall be accompanied by the prescribed fee, shall be made to the Registration Tribunal.
- The Registration Tribunal shall examine every application received on or before the appointed date, and if it is satisfied that the applicant is qualified for registration under section 31, shall direct the entry of the name of the applicant on the register.
- The first register so prepared shall thereafter be published in such manner as the State Government may direct, and any person aggrieved by a decision of the Registration Tribunal expressed or implied in

the register as so published may, within sixty days from the date of such publication, appeal to an authority appointed by the State Government in this behalf by notification in the Official Gazette.

- The Registrar shall amend the register in accordance with the decisions of the authority appointed under sub-section (4) and shall thereupon issue to every person whose name is entered in the register a certificate of registration in the prescribed form **The name of the registered pharmacist can be removed from the register by the Executive Committee, if it is found that,**
- His name has been entered by error or on account of misrepresentation or suppression of material fact, or
- He has been convicted of any offence or has been guilty of any infamous conduct in any professional respect; or
- A person employed by him for the purposes of his business of pharmacy or employed to work under him in connection with any business of pharmacy has been convicted of any such of offence or has been guilty of any such infamous conduct as would, if such person were a registered pharmacist, render him liable to have his name removed from the register.

## 4.2 Drug and Cosmetic ACT 1940 (Rules 1945)

The Drugs and Cosmetics Act, 1940 is an Act of the Parliament of India which regulates the import, manufacture and distribution of drugs in India. The primary objective of the act is to ensure that the drugs and cosmetics sold in India are safe, effective and conform to state quality standards. The related Drugs and Cosmetics Rules, 1945 contains provisions for classification of drugs under given schedules and there are guidelines for the storage, sale, display and prescription of each schedule. Amendments; The Act has been amended several times.

The following are a list of amending acts:

1. The Drugs (Amendment) Act, 1955 (11 of 1955).
2. The Drugs (Amendment) Act, 1960 (35 of 1960).
3. The Drugs (Amendment) Act, 1962 (21 of 1962).
4. The Drugs and Cosmetics (Amendment) Act, 1964 (13 0f 1964).
5. The Drugs and Cosmetics (Amendment) Act, 1972 (19 of 1972).
6. The Drugs and Cosmetics (Amendment) Act, 1982 (68 of 1982).
7. The Drugs and Cosmetics (Amendment) Act, 1986
8. The Drugs and Cosmetics (Amendment) Act, 1995 (71 of 1995)

**Table** Sale Drug (from for license)

| S. No. | Category | Wholesale | Retail |
|---|---|---|---|
| 1 | Drug other than those specified C,$C_1$ and X | 20 B | 20 |
| 2 | Other than schedule C and $C_1$ (motor vehicle) | 20 BB | - |
| 3 | Drug specified in schedule C, $C_1$ and excluding in X | 21 B | 21 |
| 4 | Drug specified in schedule C and $C_1$ (motor vehicle) | 21 BB | - |
| 5 | Schedule X Drug | 20 G | 20 F |

**Restricted Licenses:**

- Drug specified in C,$C_1$ and X – 20 A
- Drug specified in C and $C_1$ not X – 21 A
- No Licence for schedule X.

**Specific Requirement for Plant and Equipment**

[II Schedule M]

| | |
|---|---|
| 1. External Preparation: - | 30sq. – Basic Install |
| | 10 sq. – ancillary are |
| 2. Oral Liquid Preparation: - | 30sq. – Basic Install |
| | 10 sq. – ancillary are |
| 3. Table Preparation: - | 60sq. – Basic Install |
| | 20 sq. – ancillary are |
| 4. Powder Preparation: - | 30sq. – Basic Install |

## Schedules to the Rules

**Schedules to the rules**

| TYPE | CONTENT |
|---|---|
| "A" | Performa for **forms no. 1 to 50**( Application, issue, renewal, etc.) |
| "B" | **Rates of fee** for test or analysis by CDL or Govt. analysts |
| "C" | List of **Biological and special products (Injectable)** applicable to special provisions.<br>Ex. Sera, Vaccines, Penicillin.....etc |
| "$C_1$" | List of Biological and special products **(nonparenteral)** applicable to special provisions.<br>Ex. Digitalis, Hormones , Ergot |
| "D" | List of drugs that are **exempted** from provisions of **import** |
| "$E_1$" | List of poisonous substances under the **Ayurvedic , Siddha and Unani systems** |
| "F" | Provisions applicable to **blood bank** |

**Schedules to the rules**

| TYPE | CONTENT |
|---|---|
| "$F_1$" | Special provision applicable to biological and special products, e.g. Bacterial and viral vaccines, sera from living animals, bacterial origin diagnostic agents |
| "$F_2$" | Standards for **surgical dressings** |
| "$F_3$" | Standards for **umbilical tapes** |
| "FF" | Standards for **ophthalmic preparations** |
| "G" | List of substances required **to be used under medical supervision** and labelled accordingly Ex. Metformin, Anti Histaminic, ...etc. |
| "H" | List of substances **(prescription)** that should be sold by retail only on prescriptions of **R.M.P.** Ex. Atenolol, Lorazepam, Dapson ...etc. |

## Schedules to the rules

| TYPE | CONTENT |
|---|---|
| "J" | List of **diseases and ailments** that drug should **not claim to cure**<br>Ex. Cancer, AIDS, Cataract, Diabetes…etc |
| "K" | List of drugs that are **exempted** from certain provisions regarding **manufacture** |
| "M" | Requirements of manufacturing premises, **GMP requirements** of factory premises, plants and equipments |
| "$M_1$" | Requirements of factory premises for manufacture of **Homeopathic medicines** |
| "$M_2$" | Requirements of factory premises for manufacture of **cosmetics** |
| "$M_3$" | Requirements of factory premises for manufacture of **medical devices** |
| "N" | List of **equipment to run a Pharmacy** |
| "O" | Standards for **disinfectant fluids** Ex… Phenol, H2O2, alcohol…. |

## Schedules to the rules

| TYPE | CONTENT |
|---|---|
| "P" | **Life period(expiry)** of drugs Ex. Insulin Inj. – 24 months |
| "Q" | **Coal tar colors** permitted to be used in cosmetics Ex. Caramel, TiO2, Toney red….. |
| "R" | Standards for **mechanical contraceptives** |
| "$R_1$" | Standards for **medical devices** |
| "S" | Standards for **cosmetics** |
| "T" | Requirements (GMP) of factory premises for **Ayurvedic, Siddha, Unani** drugs |
| "U" | Manufacturing and analytical records of **drugs** |

47

## Schedules to the rules

| TYPE | CONTENT |
|---|---|
| "$U_1$" | Manufacturing and analytical records of **cosmetics** |
| "V" | Standards for **patent or proprietary medicines** |
| "W" | List of drugs marketed under generic names- **Omitted** |
| "X" | List of **narcotic** drugs and **psychotropic** substances<br>EX. Opium, Morphine, Barbital…… |
| "Y" | Requirement and guidelines on **clinical trials** for import and manufacture of new drugs |

48

### Administrative Bodies

The central Government and State Government establish:

**A. Advisory:**

(i) Drugs Technical Advisory Board.
(ii) Drugs Consultative Committee.

**B. Analytical:**

(i) The Central Drug Laboratory.
(ii) Drugs Control Laboratory in States.
(iii) Government Analyst.

**C. Executive:**

(i) Licensing Authority
(ii) Drug Inspector.
(iii) Customs Collector.

## 4.3 The Pharmacy ACT, 1948

### Introduction

In India there was no restriction to practise the profession of pharmacy. One could practise this profession as any other profession. Persons, having no knowledge and having no education in pharmacy or pharmaceutical chemistry or pharmacology, were engaged in this profession. Hundreds of cases were brought to the notice of the Government wherein the compounding, mixing, or dispensing of medicines was being done by persons who were not adequately educated in this line. The system was causing great harm to the health of people by wrong compounding, mixing or dispensing. It was found necessary to enact a law for the regulation of the profession and practice of pharmacy. To achieve this goal the Pharmacy Bill, 1947 was introduced in the Legislature which was later referred to the Select Committee.

**List of Amending Acts and Adaptation Orders**

1. The Adaptation of Laws Order, 1950
2. The Adaptation of Laws (No.3) Order, 1956.
3. The Pharmacy (Amendment) Act, 1959 (24 of 1959).
4. The Pharmacy (Amendment) Act, 1976 (70 of 1976).
5. The Pharmacy (Amendment) Act, 1982 (22 of 1982).
6. The Delegated Legislation Provisions (Amendment) Act, 1985 (4 of 1986).

### Statement of Objects and Reasons

PHARMACY ACT -1948 desirable that, as in most other countries, only persons who have attained a minimum standard of professional education should be permitted to practise the Profession of Pharmacy. It is accordingly proposed to establish a Central Council of Pharmacy, which will prescribe the minimum standards of education and approve courses of study and examinations for Pharmacists, and Provincial Pharmacy Councils, which will be responsible for the maintenance of provincial registers of qualified pharmacists. It is further proposed to empower Provincial Governments to prohibit the dispensing of medicine on the prescription of a medical practitioner otherwise than by, or under the direct and personal supervision of, a registered pharmacist.

### Pharmacy Council of India

**The Pharmacy Council of India Consists of the Following:**

(i) Six members, among whom at least one teacher of pharmaceutical chemistry, pharmacy. Pharmacology and pharmacology elected by the University Grants Commission.

(ii) Six members, four of whom are persons possessing a degree or diploma in and practicing pharmacy or pharmaceutical chemistry, nominated by the Central Government.

(iii) One member elected from amongst themselves by the members of the Medical Council of India

(iv) The Director General of Health Services or an authorized person by him.

(v) The Drugs Controller of India or an authorized person by him,

(vi) The Director of Central Drugs Laboratory,

(vii) A representative of the University Grants Commission,

(viii) A representative of the All India Council for Technical Education

(ix) One member to represent each state elected from each state council and who is a registered pharmacist,

(x) One member to represent each state nominated by the State Government who is a registered pharmacist.'

(xi) One member to represent each Union territory, nominated by the Union territory Council, being eligible for registration under section 31 of the Act,

## 4.4 Narcotic and Psychotropic Substance Act and Rules

### Introduction

The statutory control over narcotic drugs was being exercised under The Opium Act, 1852, The Opium Act, 1878 and The Dangerous Drugs Act, 1930. The provisions of these enactments were found to be inadequate because of the passage of time and developments in the field of illicit drug traffic and drug abuse at national and interactional level. To consolidate and to amend the existing laws relating to narcotic drugs a comprehensive legislation was considered to be necessary. Accordingly the Narcotic Drugs and Psychotropic Substances Bill was introduced in the Parliament.

### Objective

1. To consolidate and amend the existing low related NP drugs.
2. To make stringent provisions.
3. Enhance penalties for offences.
4. To make provision for manufacturing and cultivation and processing of NP drug.

### History

- Before 1857 there is no legal rules regarding (NDPS ACT) opium derivatives.
- Frist time in 1857 opium act was introduced.
- It is further amended in opium act 1878.
- India participate in second international opium conference at Geneva in 1925 for connection related to dangerous drug.
- Dangerous drug act was introduced in 1930.
- Central opium rules are come in 1934.
- Further dangerous drug act was amended in 1957.
- Central manufactured drug rules are come in force in 1962.

- Narcotic and psychotropic act was passed inparliament in 16 September 1985 by president "CUIANI ZAIL SINGH"and bill was introduced it loksabha in 23 Aug. 1985.
- Both are come in force as (narcotic and psychotic substance act and rules in 14 November 1985)
- It was amended two time in 1988 and 2001
- Narcotic control bureall was setup in 1986.

### Reasons

The starter control over narcotic drugs is exercised in India through a number of Central and State enactments. The principal Central Acts, namelp the Opium Act, 1857, the Opium Act, 1878 and the Dangerous Drugs Act, 1930 were enacted a.long time ago. With the passage of time and the developments in the field of illicit drug haffic and drug abuse at national and international level, many deficiencies in the existing laws have come to notice, some of which are indicated below: (i) The scheme of penalties under the present Acts is not sufficiently deterrent to meet the challenge of well organized gangs of smugglers. The Dangerous Drugs Act, 1930 provides for a maximum term of imprisonment of 3 years with or without fine and 4 years imprisonment with or without fine for repeat offences. Further, no minimum punishment is prescribed in the present laws, as a result of which drug traffickers have been sometimes let off by the courts with nominal punishment. The country has for the last few years been increasingly facing the problem of transit traffic of drugs coming mainly from some of our neighboring countries and destined mainly to Western countries. (ii) The existing- Central laws do not provide for investing the officers of a number of important Central enforcement agencies like Narcotics, Customs, Central Excise, etc.,

## 4.5 Drug (Price Control) Order DPCO (6 JUN 1995)

In exercise of the powers conferred by section 3 of the Essential Commodities Act, 1955 (10 of 1955), the Central Government hereby makes the following Order, namely:-

1. Short title and commencement:
   - This Order may be called the Drugs (Prices Control) Order, 1995
   - It shall come into force on the date of its publication in the Official Gazette.

### History

In 1966, parliament members felt that manufacturers charging high rate on drugs. to control on high drug rates, DPCO 1966 was passed under section 3 of Essential Commodities Act 1955.

↓

DPCO 1966 replaced by DPCO 1970.

↓

In 1974, Hathi committee was formed and submitted it's reports in 1975.

↓

DPCO 1970 Replaced By DPCO 1979.

↓

DPCO 1979 Replaced By DPCO 1987.

↓

DPCO 1987 Replaced By DPCO 1995.

↓

Finally DPCO 1995 Replaced By DPCO 15th may 2013.

↓

Indian government releases DPCO 2013, expanding price controls to **652 drugs**.

**Schedule – 1 ORDER**

- According DPCO act 1995 bulk drug to (essential drug list) – contain 74 drug.
- But according to DPCO act 2013 it contain 652 bulk drug.

**Schedule – 2 ORDER**

Forms for approval or revision of price.

Form 1 - application for fixation revision of price

Form 2 - information related with price of non-schedule bulk drug.

Form 3 - application for approval revision of scheduled formulation.

Form 4- application for approval revision for price of scheduled formulation imported in finished form.

Form 5 - form of price list.

Form 6 - yearly information of turnover and allocation of sales and expenses.

**Schedule – 3 ORDER**

DPCO ACT 1955 -It specifies maximum pre – tax return on sales turnover of manufacturer importer of formulation a b c categories.

(a) Category - large unit turnover -rs.6 carod per annum.
(b) Category - medium size unit turnover– rs.1 crore to 6 carodperannum.
(c) Category - other unit – turnover less than rs. 1 crores perannum

### Calculation of Retail Price of Formulation:

Formula for calculation-

$$R.P. = (M.C. + C.C. + P.M. + P.C.) \times (1 + MAPE/100) + E.D.$$

Where, R.P. = retail price

M.C. = material cost

C.C. = conversion cost

P.M. = packaging material cost

P.C. = packing charges

E.D. = excise duty

MAPE = maximum allowable post manufacturing expenses

## 4.6 Drugs and Magic Remedies Act and Its Rules

### Introduction

Under competition of marketing of any product, advertising has become a part of our life. Modern age is called 'advertisement' era. It has occupied special position in our life. Media (TV, Internet) and newer method for advertisement has brought massive progress. However if drugs are advertised to general public, it may lead to self medication. Ethical advertising is never objectionable, while unethical or misuse of advertisement (for promoting sale of drugs) cause harm to the user of the advertised goods. (e.g pen or a drug for curing disease condition – lead to worse). Hence it becomes necessary that drugs be advertised only to doctors, pharmacist, nurses and other personnel of the medical profession and not directly to the public as in case of consumer goods.

Another problem in India might be selling of magic remedies such as Kavachas, mantras, talishmans etc for sexual disorders and venereal disease, which are claimed to be universal cure of any disease. Advertisement in the magazines, newspapers and on the premises of doctors, hakims or vaids claiming cure of disease. Innocent peoples are often trapped of such unsocial activity which leads waste of time, money, spoil their health and prematurely leave the world.

Recent years there has been great increase in the objectionable advertisements (sexual content and muscle improving) published in newspaper and magazine and internet. This leads to self-medication with harmful drugs which cause a great harm. To stop such practice, The Drugs and Magic Remedies Act **1954,** was passed. The act as well as rule came into force in **1st April, 1955** and amended in **1963 and 2020** and extends all over India except Jammu and Kashmir.

## Objective

- To control certain type of advertisement relating to drugs.
- To prohibit certain kind of advertisement relating to magic remedies which make false claim and are likely to misled the public.

## Definitions

**Advertisement** - Any notice, circular, label, wrapper, any announcement in orally of by means of producing transmitting sound and light.

**Drug** – any chemical substances or medicines are used for internal or external treatment of human beings or animals or used for diagnosis, cure, mitigation, treatment or prevention of disease or other than food that influence in structure or organic function of the body

**Magic remedy** – This includes a talisman (a ring or stone that bring luck), mantra, kavacha have miraculous power or in the cure, diagnosis, treatment or influencing any structure or organic function of the body.

## Prohibition of Advertisements

**(a) Certain drugs for treatment of certain diseases and disorders:**

No person shall not take part in the publication of any advertisement relating to any drug in terms which suggest-

1. Miscarriage or prevention of conception in women or
2. Maintenance or improvement of the sexual pleasure of human beings or
3. Rectification of menstrual disorder in women or
4. Diagnosis, cure, mitigation, treatment or prevention of any disease, disorder or condition specified in the Schedule J of the drug and cosmetic rules 1945.

**(b) Misleading advertisements relating to drugs:**

Any person shall not take any part in the publication of any advertisement relating to a drug if the advertisement contains any matters which-

1. directly or indirectly gives a false brand regarding the true character of the drug; or
2. makes a false claim for the drug; or

**(c) Magic remedies for treatment of certain diseases and disorders.**

Any person shall not take any part in the publication of advertisement related to any magic remedy which directly or indirectly claims to efficient for purposes of specified in section (a).

**(d) Import into, and export from, India of certain advertisements.**

Any person shall not import into, or export from, the territories to which this Act extends any documents containing an advertisement under in section a or in section b or section c, and any document containing any such advertisements shall be deemed to be goods of which the import or export has been prohibited under section 19 of the Sea Customs Act,1878.

## Exempted Advertisements

1. Any registered medical practitioner has displayed advertisement on sign board or notice his buildings showing that treatment of any disease or disorder.
2. Any matter related to the disease or disorder showing on the book or treatise.
3. Any advertisement relating to any drug sent confidentially (by posting) to the registered medical practitioner or whole seller or retail chemist and showing the specification "For the use only of registered medical practitioner or a hospital or a laboratory".
4. Any advertisement relating to a drug printed or published by the state or central govt
5. Any advertisement, labels or sets of instruction are permitted under the Drugs and Cosmetics Act and Rules.

## Advertisements Exempted Conditionally

| S. No | Class of advertisement | Condition |
|---|---|---|
| 1. | 1. Leaf let or literature on packing of Drugs'.<br>2. Drug advertisement in medical, pharmaceutical, scientific and technical journals | 1. Only such information shall be shown on advertisement that required for the guidance of registered medical practitioner. The contents of the matter as follows-<br>A. Therapeutic use of drugs<br>B. Route of administration<br>C. Dosage form<br>D. Side effects<br>E. Any precaution observed during treatment<br>2. Any claim made in the advertisement in respect of the drug shall not false or misleading |
| 2. | 1. Price lists or therapeutic indexes published by manufacturers, importers or distributers of drugs under Drugs and Cosmetics Act & Rules 1940<br>2. Medical literature distributed by medical retailers appointed by manufacturers, importers under Drugs and Cosmetics Act & Rules 1940 | 1. Only such information shall be shown on advertisement that required for the guidance of registered medical practitioner. The contents of the matter as follows<br>A. Therapeutic use of drugs<br>B. Route of administration<br>C. Dosage form<br>D. Side effects<br>E. Any precaution observed during<br>Treatment.<br>2. The distribution of such literature is confined only to the physician, hospital, dispensaries, medical and research institution, chemist and druggists under Drugs and Cosmetics Act & Rules 1940.<br>3. Any claim made in the advertisement in respect of the drug shall not false or misleading |

**Offences and Penalties:** Whoever breaks any of the provisions of this Act shall, on conviction, be punishable-offences under the act can be tried only in the court of the president magistrate or magistrates of the first class.

| Offences | Penalties (Imprisonment/fine) |
|---|---|
| 1. **First conviction** | 1. 6 months or fine or both 1 year or fine or both |
| 2. **Second conviction** | 2. As per rule |
| 3. **Offence by company-**<br>• In-charge person as well as compony (with knowledge)<br>• Guilty without knowledge | 3. Forfeiture of any document, article or thing, includes its content |

**Powers of entry, search, etc.:**

Any Gazetted Officer authorised by the State Government may, within the local limits of the area for which he/she is so authorised,

1. Enter and search at all reasonable times, with such assistants, if any, as he/she considers necessary, any place in which he has reason to believe that an offence under this Act has been or is being committed.
2. Seize any advertisement which he has reason to believe contravenes any of the provisions of this Act.
3. Where any person seizes anything under clause (b), he shall, as soon as may be, inform a Magistrate and take his orders as to the custody.

### Amendments

On February 03, 2020, the Ministry of Health and Family Welfare, Government of India, put forth a proposal to amend the Drugs and Magic Remedies (Objectionable Advertisement) Act, 1954, in view of major concerns raised on implementation and effectiveness of the same-

- The act shall be called the Drugs and Magic Remedies (Objectionable Advertisements) (Amendment) Act, 2020, and shall come into force on such date as the Central Government may, by notification in the Official Gazette, appoint.
- The new amendment, the government has substituted a clause in section 2, for clause (a) which states that " 'advertisement' means any audio or visual publicity, representation, endorsement or pronouncement made by means of light, sound, smoke, gas, print, electronic media, internet or website and includes any notice, circular, label, wrapper, invoice, banner, poster or such other documents".
- The sub clause of section 3 of Drugs and Magic Remedies (Objectionable Advertisements) Act, 1954 states that Prohibition of advertisement of certain drugs for treatment of certain diseases and disorders for "the maintenance or improvement of the capacity of human beings for sexual pleasure; or. The new amendment also includes a sub clause after sub clause 2 of section 3 which states that "after consultation with Ayurvedic, Siddha and Unani Drugs Technical Advisory Board constituted under section 33C of the Drugs and Cosmetics Act, 1940 in respect of Ayurvedic, Siddha and Unani system of medicines."\
- The draft bill has also expanded the list of diseases from 54 to 78 on which the ministry prohibits any advertisements which claim to cure "any" of the 78 diseases, disorders or conditions that it has specified. The current law identifies 'magic remedy' in the form of a talisman, mantra, kavacha or any other charm which supposedly possesses miraculous powers to diagnose, cure, mitigate, treat or prevent any disease in human beings or animals or for effect or influence in any way the structure or any organic function of the body of human beings or animals.

## 4.7 Intellectual Property Rights (IPR)

**What is Intellectual Property?**

Intellectual property (IP) refers to creations of the mind: inventions, literary and artistic works, and symbols, names, images, and designs used in commerce.

Creations of the mind- Creativity is the ability to

- Think / come up with new idea
- Design new "inventions"
- Produce "works of art"
- Solve problems in new ways, or develop a new idea based on an "original" knowledge.
- Novel or unconventional approach.

IP and IPR have evolved over centuries, it was not until the 19th century that the term intellectual property began to be used and not until the late 20th century that it became commonplace in the majority of the world.

**Intellectual Property Rights?**

Intellectual Property Rights are rights once granted allows the creator(s) or owner(s) of the intellectual property to exclude others from exploiting the same commercially for a given period of time.

**Need of intellectual Property Rights**

The intellectual property rights were essentially recognized and accepted all over the world due to some very important reasons-

- To provide an incentive to individuals for new creations
- To accord due recognition to the creators and inventors
- To ensure material reward for intellectual property
- To make available genuine and original products.

**Governing Laws in India for IPR as follows**

- Patent Act 1970
- Trade Marks Act (1958 original) 1999
- The Copyright Act 1957
- The design Act 2000

**Bodies regulating IPR**

- WIPO(World Intellectual Property Organization)
- WTO(World Trade Organization)
- GATT(General Agreement on Tariffs and Trade)

**Types of Intellectual Property**

1. Copyright
2. Trademarks
3. Geographical indication
4. Patents
5. Utility models
6. Designs

**Copyright**

**Definition:** Copyright is a federal protection from unauthorized copying or performance given to the authors of original works of authorship. The term original in the copyright law means that the work originated with the author. There is no requirement for novelty or uniqueness as there is in patent law. Copyright law protects the expression of an idea. Not the idea itself.

**Copyrightable works categories:**

1. Literary works (including computer programs);
2. Pictorial, graphic and sculptural works
3. Motion pictures and other audiovisual works.

Examples of copyrightable subject matter include: Songs, movies and books (but not their titles), labels on products.

**What Cannot Be Copyrighted:**

1. Works that have not been fixed in a tangible form of expression.
2. Titles of books or magazines
3. Ideas, themes, procedures, methods of operation, systems, processes, concepts as opposed to a written description or explanation or illustration of the same.
4. Works consisting entirely of information that is common property and containing no original authorship.

**Duration of Copyright**

- For works created on or after January 1, 1978, and works originally created before January 1, 1978 but not published or registered by that date, the duration of a copyright is the life of the author plus 70 years.

**Registration a copyright**

- By completing a simple application form, along with the appropriate fee.
- Need not send a copy of your work,
- It may appear with the same title, but if each work has been created independently, each will have its own copyright protection.

**Advantages and Disadvantages**

- Advantages: easy to obtain in short period of time for a low cost and are easily maintained.
- Disadvantages: not protect the underlying ideas or functions performed by the software.

## Trademarks

**Definition:** A trademark is any word, name, symbol, or device, or any combination of these, which identifies goods in a way to distinguish them from the goods of others.

**Purpose of trademark:**

- For quickly identify the source of a given product or service.
- Preventing from free-riding on the good reputation of others.

**Types of Marks:**

1. Fanciful - for the purpose of functioning as a mark and has no other meaning: XEROX.
2. Arbitrary- words used for the mark do not in any way describe anything about the product at all: APPLE computers
3. Suggestive - a mark which merely "suggests" but does not describe qualities or functions: GLEEM toothpaste.
4. Merely Descriptive -identifies to mind the characteristics, functions, purpose, use of a product: HOUR AFTER HOUR deodorant.

**Geographical Indication**

**Definition:** (GI) is defined as any indication that identifies a good as originating from a particular place, where a given quality, reputation or other characteristics of the good are essentially attributable to its geographical origin.

- It is the six Trade-Related Intellectual Property Rights (TRIPS) of the World Trade Organisation (WTO).
- In India the Geographical Indications of Goods (Registration and Protection) Act, 1999 (Act 48 of 1999) came into force with effect from 15 September 2003.
- **Darjeeling Tea** was the first good to be registered as a Geographical Indication good in India.
- Example of GI anstherir states: G.I STATE
    - Solapuri Chaddar-Maharashtra
    - Maysor Silk -Karnataka
    - Puneri Pagdi– Maharshtra
    - Madhubani Paintaings–Bihar

## Patents

**Definition:** A patent is a right to exclude others from making, using or selling a claimed invention.

Invention patentable if

- new (novel)
- useful
- not obvious
- pertains to patentable subject matter

**Types of patent**

1. Utility Patents: cover the useful or working features of an invention
2. Design Patents: cover the physical appearance or ornamental design of an article
3. Plant Patents: cover certain new and distinct, invented or discovered asexually reproduced plants.

**Duration of patent:** 20 yr – Utility patent and 14yr- Design patent

**Fee for filing patent:**

- The Government fee for filing a patent application in India is Rs.750/- for individuals and Rs.3,000/- for legal entities.
- No fee for 1st and 2nd year.
- Renewal fee, on yearly basis, is required to be paid for 3rd to 20th for keeping the patent in force.
- Patent lapses if renewal fee is not paid within the prescribed period.

**Utility models**

- Grant protection from 5 to 10 yrs
- Covers product not methods process material
- Granted within few months
- Fees for application and maintenance are cheaper than patents.

**Design right**

- The appearance of the whole or part of product (shape, line, colours)
- Must not be dictated by technical function.

### Organization Structure of IPR

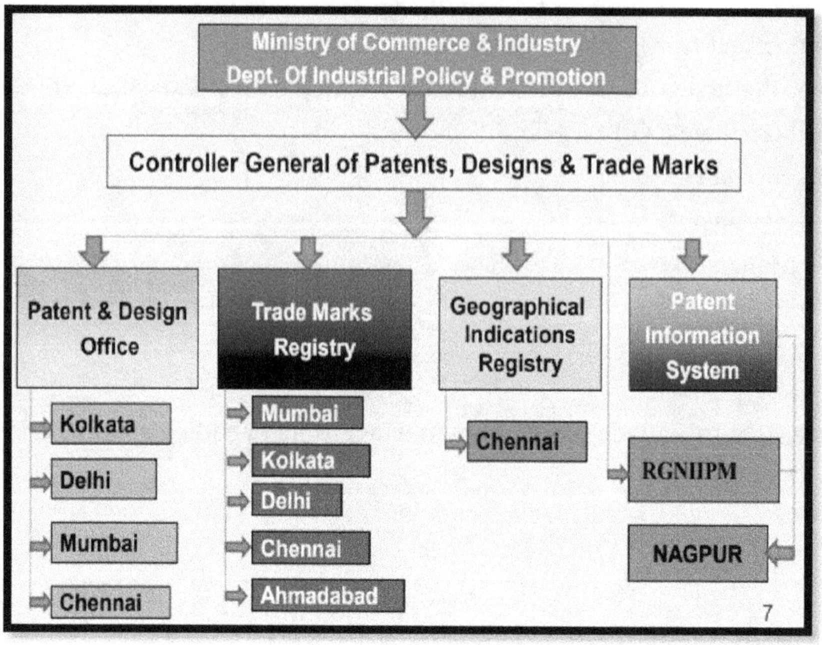


### Validity of IPR

| Sl No. | IPR | Maximum Protection | Renewal | Act/Rule |
|---|---|---|---|---|
| 1 | Patent | 20 Yrs | *Every year (mandatory) | The Patents Act,1970 Amended in 2005 |
| 2 | Trade Mark | Life long | After 10yrs | The Trade Marks Act, 1999 Amended in 2010 |
| 3 | Design | 15 Yrs | After 10 years for next 5 years | The Designs Act, 2000 & Designs (Amendment) Rules, 2014 |
| 4 | Copyright | 60 years | Not require | The Copyright Act, 1957 Amended in 2012 |
| 5 | Geographical Indication (GI) | Life long | After 10 Yrs | The Geographical Indications of Goods (Registration and Protection) Act, 1999 |

***Patents will cease and be transferred to public domain if Patents are not renewed within 6 month of expiry of concerned year by paying renewal fee.**

13

## 4.8 Prevention of Cruelty to Animals ACT

### Introduction

- In modern day research, animal are considered as important experimental subject because if their physiological similarity to human beings.

- For establishing the safety and therapeutic efficacy of drugs, experimentation on animal is usually unavoidable.
- 108 Nobel Prizes awarded for Physiology or Medicine, 96 were directly dependent on animal research. Addiction (monkeys), Alzheimer's Disease (mice), Diabetes – Type I (mice), Heart Damage (rats), HIV/AIDS (monkeys, mice) are Current examples of animal research in medicine for establishing for safety and therapeutic efficacy of drugs.
- The clinical trials under the drug and cosmetic act and rules are prepared by data generation on animal toxicology and animal pharmacology.
- This implies that the animal may be subject to injury, pain or suffering and even death. But causing unnecessary pain and injury is unethical.
- The prevention of cruelty to animal act 1960 (which repeals the act of 1890) has been enacted to prevent the infliction of unnecessary pain or suffering on animal.
- As recognition of the general awareness about animal welfare, the Breeding of and experiments on animal (control and prevention) Riles, 1998 have been recently incorporated.
- The act extends to the whole of India except the state of Jammu and Kashmir.

## Objective

1. To prevent the infliction of unnecessary pain or suffering on animals as well as to prevent to cruelty to animals.
2. Animals: this term include any living creature except human being.
3. Cruelty: it is not define under this act but it roughly means the infliction of unnecessary pain or suffering.

## Definitions

- **Animal**- Any leaving creature other than human being.
- **Domestic anima-** means any animal which is tamed or which has been or is being sufficiently tamed to serve some purpose for the use of human or which, although it neither has been nor is intended to be so tamed, is or has become in fact wholly or partly tamed.
- **Captive animal**- means any animal (not being a domestic animal) which is in capacity or confinement, whether permanent or temporary, or which is subjected to any appliance of contrivance for the purpose of hindering or preventing its escape from captivity or confinement or which is pinioned or which is or appears to be maimed.
- **Board** – Animal welfare board established under sec- 4 of the act.
- **Breeder** – Breeds animals for the purpose of transfer to the authorized institution for performing experiments.
- **Committee** – Control and supervision on animals under section 15 of the act.
- **Establishment** – Any individual, company, firm, corporation, institution except college (upto PG label) performing experiments on animals.
- **Experiment** – Use of an animal for the purpose of acquiring knowledge of a biological, psychological, ethological, physical or chemical nature.
- **Institutional Animals Ethics Committee**- A body/committee comprising a group of persons to control and supervision on experimented animals.
- **Contract Research** – Any research undertaken by an individual, company, firm, corporation or institution on behalf of a foreign individual, corporation or institution.
- **Collaborative Research** – Any research undertaken between two or more research institution without any financial consideration and is meant for advancement of scientific research and human welfare.

## Cruelty to Animals -Includes:

- Subjecting any animal **to unnecessary pain** or suffering or treatment, or
- Employing any **unfit animal** for work or labour, or
- Willfully and unreasonably administering any **injurious drug** or substance to any domestic or captive animal, or
- Keeping or confining any animal in any **cage** of insufficient size not permitting it reasonable movement, or
- **Failure to provide** any animal with sufficient food, drink or shelter by its owner, or
- Unnecessary mutilating any animal or killing any animal in an unnecessarily cruel manner.
- Treating animal cruelly is an offence punishable with fine upto Rs. 50 in the first instance and if a second offence is committed within three years of the previous offence, the fine may extend to Rs. 100, or with imprisonment up to three months, or with both.

**Institutional Animal Ethics Committee (IAEC):**

- IAEC consist of
  1. A biological scientist
  2. Two scientists from different biological dept.
  3. A veterinarian physician
  4. A scientist from animal facility of the establishment concern
  5. A scientist from outside of the institution
  6. A social person
  7. A representative of the Committee for the Purpose of Control and Supervision of Experiments on Animals (CPCSEA)
  8. A specialist (radioactive substance or deadly microorganisms) may be co-opted.
- An eight-member IAEC is constituted in every registered institute.
- All research project proposals using small animals, such as rats, mice, rabbits or guinea
- pigs, have to be approved by the IAEC before initiation.
- Every member of the IAEC has the right to question/reject of a project; unapproved
- proposals are referred to a subcommittee of experts for scrutiny and possible approval.
- The IAEC cannot approve research projects on large animals, such as dogs, cats, nonhuman
- primates, cattle, goats and sheep.

## Function of IAEC

- To review and approve research proposals involving lab animals
- To provide suggestions for modification of the proposals wherever necessary.
- To conduct periodic supervision of Institute's animal facility.
- To ascertain ethical use of animals and protection of well being of animals during and after research. When research activity is not found in accordance to CPCSEA guidelines to help adopt correct measures.
- To see that all those persons involved in animal care and research are adequately trained to handle the animals.
- To ensure that GLP guidelines are followed in animal facility to protect the researchers and all others involved in animal handling.

### Committee for the Purpose of Control and Supervision of Experiments on Animals (CPCSEA)

- Constituted by Central Government.
- Central Government nominates one of the member as chairman
- Committee has power to regulate its own procedure
- Central Government gives grants and funds to CPCSEA
- Subcommittee can be formed to execute various functions
- Committee may appoint staff members, officers and other employee.

### Duties and Powers of the Committee

To take all such measures as may be necessary to ensure that animals are not subjected to unnecessary pain or suffering before, during or after the performance of experiments on them.

- The registration of persons or institutions carrying on experiments on animals is essential;
- The reports and other information which shall be forwarded to the Committee by persons and institutions carrying on experiments or, animals.

### Objectives of the Rules made by CPCSEA

- In particular, and without prejudice to the generality of the foregoing power, rules made by the Committee shall be designed to secure the following objects, namely –
  1. In cases where experiments are performed in any institution, the responsibility therefore is placed on the person in charge of the institution. In cases where experiments are performed outside an institution by individuals responsibility therefore is placed on the person. The individual person must be technically qualified and competent.
  2. Experiments should be performed with **due care and humanity** and that as far as possible experiments involving operations are performed under the influence of some anesthetic of sufficient power to prevent the animals feeling pain.
  3. That experiment on animals are avoided wherever it is possible to do so; as for example; in medical schools, hospitals, colleges etc. if other teaching devices such as books, models, films may equally suffice.
  4. That experiment **on larger animals are avoided** when it is possible to achieve the same results by experiments upon small laboratory animals like guinea-'pigs, rabbits, frogs and rats.
  5. As far as possible, **experiments are not performed merely for the purpose of acquiring manual skill.**
  6. Animals intended for the performance of experiments are properly **looked after both before and after experiments.**
  7. **Suitable records are maintained** with respect to experiments performed on animals.
- All rules made by the Committee shall be binding on all individuals performing experiments outside institutions and on person's in-charge of institutions in which experiments are performed.

### Offences and Penalties

1. Preforming operation like Phooka or any other operation to improve lactation which injurious to health of animal is punishable with fine up to Rs. 1000/- or imprisonment up to 2 year or with both. Animal may be forfeited by the government.
2. Contravention of any order made by the committee or breach of any condition imposed by the committee is punishable with fine up to Rs. 200/-. If person has guilty of the offence and shall be punishable accordingly.

## 4.9 Medical Termination of Pregnancy ACT

### Introduction

The MTP Act, 1971 preamble states "an Act to provide for the termination of certain pregnancies by registered medical practitioners and for matters connected therewith or incidental thereto".

Short title, extent and commencement.

1. **MTP Act** may be called the Medical Termination of Pregnancy Act, **1971.**
2. Medical Termination of Pregnancy **Act**, 1971 and **Rules** thereunder **1975.**
3. It extends to the whole of India except the State of Jammu and Kashmir.
4. It shall come into force on such date as the Central Government may, by notification in the Official Gazette, appoint.

### Objectives

- Aims to improve the maternal health scenario by preventing large number of unsafe abortions and consequent high incidence of maternal mortality & morbidity.
- Legalizes abortion services
- Promotes access to safe abortion services to women
- Offers protection to medical practitioners who otherwise would be penalized under the Indian Penal Code (sections 315-316)

### Definitions

(a) "**guardian**" means a person having the care of the person of a minor.

(b) "**lunatic**" a person who is mentally ill.

(c) "**minor**" means a person who, under the provisions of the Indian Majority Act, 1875 (9 of 1875), is to be deemed not to have attained his majority.

(d) "**registered medical practitioner**" means a medical practitioner who possesses any recognised medical qualification as defined in **clause (h) of section 2 of** the Indian Medical Council Act, 1956 (102 of 1956), whose name has been entered in a State Medical Register and who has such experience or training in gynecology and obstetrics as may be prescribed by rules made under this Act.

**(e)** "**admission register**" means the register maintained under **regulation 5.**

(f) **"approved place"** means a place approved under rule 4 of the MTP Rules 1975.

(g) **"place"** means such building, tent, vehicle or vessel or hospital or clinic which is used or intended for used, for the termination of any pregnancies.

**Circumstances for termination of Pregnancy by RMP**

1. Pregnancy is not more that 12 weeks old:

   **Conditions:**

   (a) Serious injury to physical or mental health of the woman and

   (b) Child to be born would be seriously handicapped.

2. More than 12 weeks but less than 20 weeks: If pregnancy caused because of rape or as a result of failure of any contraceptive device used by any married woman or her husband for the purpose of family planning, it may presumed to constitute a grave injury to the mental health of pregnant woman. Opinion of two RMPs required for termination of pregnancy between 12 and 20 weeks

3. Woman with 18 years or more: with her written consent.
4. Woman with less than 18 years: lunatic with written consent of her guardian.

**Experience or Training**

This act prescribes the experience and training in gynecology and obstetrics for RMP who should have to terminate the pregnancy.

1. Before commencement of the act:- Should have registration in state medical register and have more than 3 years of experience and practice in mentioned field.
2. After Commencement of the act:-

**For termination up to 12 weeks:**

- A practitioner who has assisted a registered medical practitioner in performing 25 cases of MTP of which at least 5 were performed independently in a hospital established or maintained or a training institute approved for this purpose by the Government.

**For termination up to 20 weeks:**

- A practitioner who holds a post-graduate degree or diploma in Obstetrics and Gynecology.
- A practitioner who has completed six months house job in Obstetrics and Gynecology. or

1. A practitioner who has at least one-year experience in practice of Obstetrics and Gynecology at a hospital which has all facilities.

**Places for Pregnancy Termination**

- Should have approval from government.
- Termination of pregnancies may be done under safe and hygienic conditions.
- Facilities required: Operation table, instruments, anesthetics equipment, resuscitation equipment, sterilization equipment, Drugs and parenteral fluids for emergency use.

**Maintenance of admission register**

- Head of the hospital or owner of the approved place should maintain register in prescribed form of the admission of women for the termination of their pregnancies.
- Serial number should be given to each entry in the register.
- Fresh serial number need to be given in each calendar year.
- Serial number of each year should be distinguishable.
- Information should not be disclosed.

**Offences and Penalties**

- Offences Penalties Termination of pregnancy by a person who is not RMP Punishable under IPC Any person who willfully contravenes or fails to comply with the requirements of any regulations made by state govt. 1000 rupees.
- As per IPC penalties abortion practitioner- 3 years imprisonment or fine or both.
- Women- 7 years imprisonment or fine or both.
- The fetus has the right to live as per MTP ACT 1971.

## 4.10 Code of Pharmaceutical Ethics

- **Introduction** – ethics is moral principles that govern a person's behavior or the conducting of an activity. Ethics recommending concepts of right and wrong behavior. Ethics seeks to resolve questions of human morality by defining concepts such as good and evil, right and wrong, virtue and vice, justice and crime.
- **Ethics** – ethics may be defined as **"the code of moral principles"**

**Or**

**"The science of morals".**

  - **Professional ethics -** Professional ethics are principles that govern the behaviour of a person or group in a business environment. Like values, professional ethics provide rules on how a person should act towards other people and institutions in such an environment.
  - Code of pharmaceutical ethics framed by the **Pharmacy Council of India**.
  - It helps to guide the Indian pharmacist as to how he should conduct himself in relation to **himself**, his **patron** and **the general public, co-professionals, and member of the medical and other health professionals.**

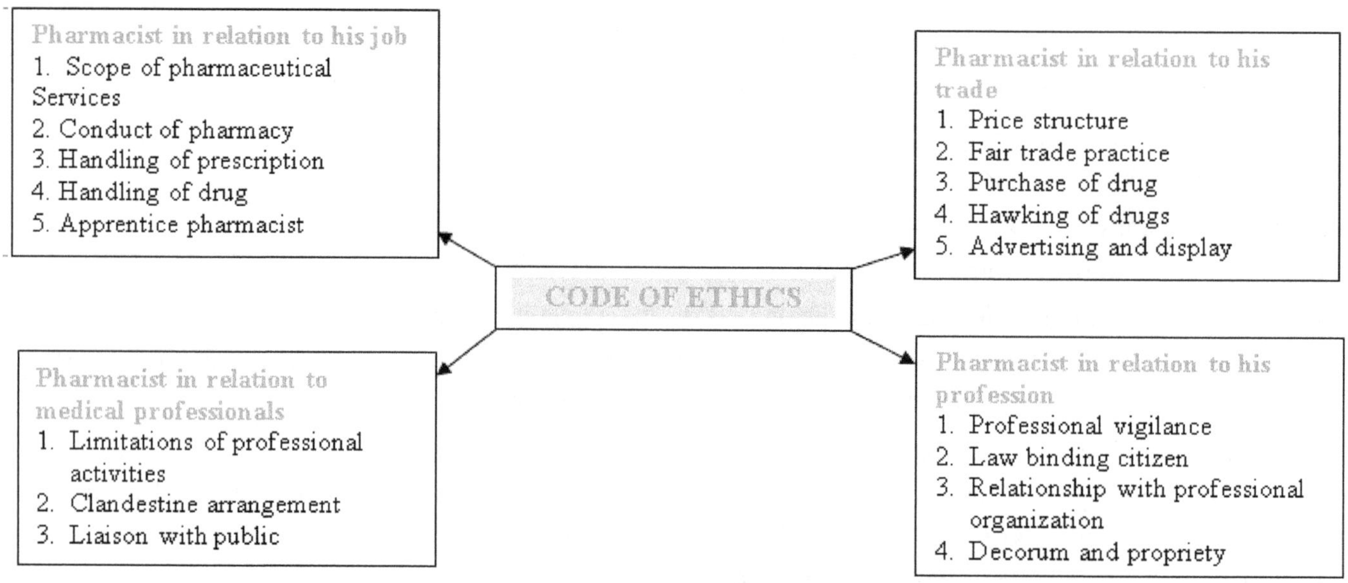

# Pharmaceutical Jurisprudence MCQs

1. The AICTE Act came into force w.e.f.
   (a) 26th March, 1988
   (b) 28th March, 1989
   (c) 28th March, 1988
   (d) 6th March, 1979.
2. The headquarters of AICTE is in
   (a) Delhi (b) Mumbai
   (c) Kolkata (d) None of these.
3. The medicinal and toilet preparation Rules were passed in
   (a) 1955 (b) 1956
   (c) 1957 (d) 1958.
4. According to MTP Act Alcohol means
   (a) 50% methyl alcohol
   (b) methyl alcohol
   (c) 50% ethyl alcohol
   (d) ethyl alcohol.
5. The pharmacy bill was introduced in
   (a) 1948 (b) 1949
   (c) 1945 (d) 1946.
6. Antiserums and toxoids are tested at
   (a) Chennai (b) Lucknow
   (c) Izatnagar (d) Delhi.
7. In case of schedule X drug, the prescription should be in
   (a) Duplicate (b) Triplicate
   (c) Only one copy (d) Five copies.
8. Licence to sell drug specified C & C1 is given in form no.
   (a) 19 (b) 18
   (c) 21 (d) 24.
9. The chairman of DTAB is
   (a) President, PCI
   (b) Drug controller of India
   (c) Union Health Minister
   (d) Director General Health Service.
10. In which year the Central Register of Pharmacist is maintained by the PCI as per as the provision of Pharmacy Act?
    (a) 1940 (b) 1948
    (c) 1976 (d) 1984.
11. The requirements and guidelines for clinical trials come under which of the following schedules?
    (a) Schedule K (b) Schedule V
    (c) Schedule Y (d) Schedule U.
12. In the Drugs and Cosmetics Act and Rules, the Schedule relating to GMP is
    (a) Schedule M (b) Schedule C
    (c) Schedule Y (d) Schedule H
13. Class 100 area is referred to
    (a) Manufacturing area
    (b) Aseptic area
    (c) Clean room
    (d) Ware house
14. Which one of the following is NOT an ex-officio member of Pharmacy Council of India?
    (a) The Director General of Health Services
    (b) The Director of Central Drugs Laboratory
    (c) The Drugs Controller General of India
    (d) The Director of Pharmacopoeia Laboratory
15. Schedule D is related to-
    (a) fees for test or analysis by central drugs laboratories or state drug laboratories
    (b) list of drugs exempted from the provision of import of drugs
    (c) standards for surgical dressings
    (d) good laboratory practice

16. The members of the D.T.A.B. hold the office for a period of-
    (a) 3 years (b) 1 years
    (c) 5 years (d) 7 years
17. Good manufacturing practices for Ayurvedic , siddha and all Unani medicines comes under
    (a) Schedule T (b) Schedule S
    (c) Schedule U (d) Schedule M
18. Form 26 A is
    (a) certificate of renewal of loan licence to manufacture for sale of drugs other than those specified in schedule X
    (b) application for the grant / renewal of a licence to manufacture for sale og Aurvedic / Siddha or Unani drugs
    (c) licence to sell, stock or exhibit or offer for sale, or distribute by wholesale drugs specified in schedule C and C(1) excluding those specified in schedule X
    (d) Memorandom to government analyst
19. Form 32A is
    (a) licence to manufacture drugs for purposes of examination, test or analysis
    (b) loan licence to manufacture cosmatics for sale or for distribution
    (c) memorandom to government analyst
    (d) form in which the inspection book shall be maintained
20. Schedule J is related to
    (a) disease and ailment (by whatever name described) which can not be treated by any drug currently available in the market
    (b) provisions applicable to the production of all sera from living animals
    (c) standards for umbilical tapes
    (d) drugs marketed under generic nameonly
21. Requirements and guidelines for permission to import and /or manufacture of new drug for sale or to undertake clinical trials comes under
    (a) Schedule Y (b) Schedule T
    (c) Schedule W (d) Schedule A
22. Application for grant/renewal of licence to manufacture blood products for sale or distribution is applied in
    (a) Form 38 (b) Form 27E
    (c) Form 28 (d) Form 32A
23. Report of test or analysis by approved institution is granted in
    (a) Form 38 (b) Form 39
    (c) Form 40 (d) Form 41
24. licence to sell, stock or exhibit or distribute by wholesale drugs specified in schedules C and C(1) excluding those specified in schedule X
    (a) 21 B (b) 20 A
    (c) 20 B (d) 22 A
25. Particulars to be shown in the manufacturing records , records of raw materials, analytical records of drugs is specified in
    (a) Schedule P (b) Schedule L
    (c) Schedule U (d) Schedule S
26. Application for the grant or renewal of a licence to manufacture for sale or for distribution of homoeopathic medicines is made in
    (a) 25 C (b) 31 A
    (c) 24 F (d) 24 C
27. The appointment of drug inspector is under act of
    (a) 51 of IPC (b) 22 of IPC
    (c) 41 of IPC (d) 21 of IPC
28. drug sample taken by drug inspector for analysis are sending to
    (a) drug controller
    (b) government analyst
    (c) chemical analyst
    (d) testing lab
29. Joint state pharmacy council is constitute under section _______pf pharmacy act
    (a) 19 (b) 20
    (c) 10 (d) 12
30. For registration of pharmacist in state, the pharmacy act provide for constitution of
    (a) registrar of state pharmacy council
    (b) registrar of co-operative society
    (c) registrar of central pharmacy council
    (d) none of the above
31. Central register of pharmacist is maintained by
    (a) central government (b) AICTE
    (c) state government (d) PCI

32. Which among given is not the common member of PCI and DTAB?
    (a) director general of health services
    (b) director of CDL, Kolkata
    (c) Drug controller of india
    (d) director of CDRL, Lucknow
33. Which of the following are functions of pharmacy council of india?
    (a) to prescribe minimum standard of education required as a pharmacist.
    (b) drafting of education regulations to be fulfilled by the institutions for the approval for imparting education in pharmacy
    (c) To provide uniform implementation of the educational standards through out the country.
    (d) All of the above
34. PCI was constituted in
    (a) 1949 (b) 1951
    (c) 1950 (d) 1955
35. A person whose name is for the time being entered in the register of the state in which he is for the time being residing or carrying on his profession or business of pharmacy is called
    (a) registered pharmacist
    (b) displaced person
    (c) repatriate
    (d) none of the above
36. executive committee may order that the name of a registered pharmacist shall be removed from the register if
    (a) his name has been enter into the register by error or on account of misrepresentation or suppression of a material fact.
    (b) he has been convicted of any offence or has been guilty of any infamous conduct in any professional respect
    (c) a person employed by him for the purposes of his business of pharmacy has been convicted of any such offence.
    (d) all of the above
37. Offences of pharmacy act include
    (a) Falsely claiming to be a registered pharmacist.
    (b) failure to surrender certificate of registration
    (c) dispensed by unregistered person
    (d) all of the above
38. The penalty fir offence " dispensing by unregistered person" are
    (a) imprisonment for a term which may extend to six months, or with fine not exceeding one thousand rupees or with both
    (b) fine up to fifty rupees
    (c) life time imprisonment
    (d) 1000 Rs fine
39. joint state pharmacy council are constituted for
    (a) 1 yr
    (b) 2 yr
    (c) 5 yr
    (d) indefinite years
40. which act provide to levy and collect excise duties on medical and toilet preparations containing alcohoal, opium, hemp or other narcotic drugs?
    (a) Poisons act
    (b) Medicinal and toilet preparation act
    (c) Pharmacy act
    (d) Drug and cosmetic act
41. The use of indian hemp plant requires specific license under which of the following act
    (a) Medicinal and toilet preparation act
    (b) Poisons act
    (c) Drug and cosmetic act
    (d) Pharmacy act
42. The premises or any part of the premises approved and licensed for the manufacture and storage of medicinal and toilet preparations containing alcohol, opium, Indian hemp and other narcotic drugs or narcotics on which duty has not been paid is known as
    (a) Bonded manufactory
    (b) Non Bonded manufactory
    (c) Spirit store
    (d) laboratory

43. which of the following statement is true for opium?
    (a) The capsules of the poppy (palaver somniferous L) whether in their original form or cut crushed or powdered and whether are not juice has been extracted there from
    (b) The spontaneously coagulated juice of such capsule which has not been submitted to any manipulations other than those necessary for packing and transport and
    (c) Any mixture , with or without neutral materials of any of the above forms of opium, and includes and derivative of opium.
    (d) All of the above
44. The manufacturing and sale in the non bonded manufactory shall be handled
    (a) Between the sunrise to sunset only on such days and times as fixed by the excise commissioner
    (b) Only on Sunday
    (c) Only on holidays
    (d) Any time
45. What is the penalty for offence “improper keeping of accounts”?
    (a) Fine upto Rs 100
    (b) Fine upto 2000
    (c) 6 month imprisonment
    (d) 6 month imprisonment with fine
46. What is the penalty for offence “disclosing any information by excise officer”?
    (a) Fine upto 100
    (b) Fine upto 1000
    (c) 6 month imprisonment
    (d) 6 month imprisonment with fine
47. Which of the following statement is correct for cannabis(hemp)
    (a) Charas, that is separated resin ,in whatever form crude or purified, obtained from the cannabis plant and also includes concentrated preparation and resin known as hashish oil or liquid hashish
    (b) Ganja, that is, the flowering or fruiting tops of the cannabis plant (excluding the seeds and leaves when not accompanied by the tops) by whatever name they may be known or designated; and
    (c) Any mixture with or without any nutral material, of any of the above farms of cannabis or any drink prepared therefrom
    (d) All of the above
48. Government opium factory situated in
    (a) Ghajipur (b) Kasauli
    (c) Lucknow (d) izatnagar
49. -------- resin is obtained from Indian hemp plant
    (a) Charas (b) Bhang
    (c) Opium (d) codeine
50. prevention of illicit traffic in narcotic and psychotropic drug act was come in
    (a) 1986 (b) 1987
    (c) 1988 (d) 1990
51. Narcotic drugs and psychotropic drug act 1985, came in effect on
    (a) 1.11.1985 (b) 14.11.1986
    (c) 14.11.1985 (d) 1.11.1986
52. As per narcotic drugs, controlled substance eans
    (a) Drug notified in central government gazzatte
    (b) Drug banned by state
    (c) Drug include in controlled price list
    (d) Drug dispensed by RMP
53. What is the penalty for offence “cultivation of opium, cannabis or coca plants without license”?
    (a) Rigorous imprisonment up to 10 years +fine up to Rs. 1 lakh
    (b) Fine 2000 Rs.
    (c) Imprisonment up to 6 month
    (d) Fine 1000 Rs.
54. Drugs and magic remedies (objectionable advertisements) act was passed in
    (a) 1954 (b) 1985
    (c) 1991 (d) 1945
55. Which act provides regulations for objectionable advertisements
    (a) Poisons act
    (b) Drug and magic remedies act
    (c) Medicinal and toilet preparation act
    (d) Pharmacy act

56. Which of the following disease is not listed in the schedule of drugs and magic remedies act 1954?
    (a) Deafness (b) Goitre
    (c) Glaucoma (d) diarrhoea

57. According to drugs and magic remedies act 1954, no person shall involve in the publication if any advertisement related to any drug for
    (a) The procurement of miscarriage in women or prevention of conception in women
    (b) The maintenance or improvement of the capacity of human being for sexual pleasure
    (c) The correction of menstrual disorder in women
    (d) All of the above

58. Magic remedies which is claimed to have miraculous powers to cure, diagnose, prevent or mitigate a disease in humans or animals include
    (a) Any talisman
    (b) Mantra
    (c) Amulet
    (d) All of the above

59. Prevention of cruelty to animals act was passed in
    (a) 1960 (b) 1985
    (c) 1945 (d) 1956

60. Which of the following is /are functions of the animal welfare board
    (a) To keep the law in force in, India for the prevention of cruelty to animals under constant study and advice the government of the amendments to be undertaken in any such law from time to time
    (b) To advice the central government on the making of rules under this act with a view to preventing unnecessary pain or suffering to animals generally, and more particularly when they are being transported from one place to another or when they are used as performing animals or when they are
    (c) to advice the govt. or any local authority or other person on improvements in the design of vehicles so as to lessen the burden on drought animals
    (d) all of the above

61. Any research undertaken by an individual, company, firm, corporation or institution on behalf of a foreign individual, company, firm, corporation or institution for any consideration is called
    (a) contract research
    (b) collaborative research
    (c) experiment
    (d) research methodology

62. The main function of CPCSEA
    (a) registration of establishment s conducting animal experimentation or breeding of animals for this purpose
    (b) permission for conducting experiments involving use of experiments,
    (c) recommendation for import of animals for use in experiments,
    (d) all of the above

63. for addition of a medicine into NLEM, 2015 which of the following criteria is to be followed
    (a) medicine to be useful in disease which is a public health problem in India
    (b) medicine have proven efficacy and safety profile based on valid scientific evidence
    (c) medicine to be comparatively cost effective
    (d) all of the above

64. For deletion of a medicine into NLEM, 2015 which of the following criteria is to be followed?
    (a) medicine has been banned in India
    (b) existence of reports of concerns on the safety profile of a medicine
    (c) the disease burden for which a medicine is indicated is no longer a national health concern
    (d) all of the above

65. what is /are the objectives of DPCO 2013
    (a) to increase the number of drugs from 74 to 652, whose prices are controlled by DPCO
    (b) to permit the firms to sell their new drugs, at or below the prices fixed by the govt.
    (c) to control the manufacturing of existing drugs, the firms can not stop their production without taking the permission
    (d) all of the above

66. The drug price control order DPCO 2013 was issued on
    (a) 15.05.2013 (b) 19.09.2013
    (c) 1.1.2013 (d) 03.03.2013
67. Government of India appointed a drug enquiry committee under the chairmanship of
    (a) Col. Ramnatha . N. chopra
    (b) Dr. A.L.Mudaliar
    (c) Jaysukhlal Hathi
    (d) M.L. Schroff
68. The main recommendation of Chopra committee is/are
    (e) to control quality ofproduction of drugs and pharmaceutical, committee establish testing laboratories in all states and a central drug laboratory to control the quality of imported drugs. the laboratory should equipped with competent staff
    (f) to provide the course for training of pharmacist and prescribe minimum qualification for the registration as the pharmacist
    (g) registration of every medicine manufacture in India or imported from outside country
    (h) all of the above
69. The recommendation of Bhore committee are
    (a) setting up central drug laboratory
    (b) establishment of all India Pharmaceutical council and provincial pharmaceutical council
    (c) starting of revised courses of study for licentiate pharmacist, pharmaceutical technologist and graduate pharmacist
    (d) all of the above
70. The Pharmacist should keep in mind the following points while dealing with his trade
    (a) price structure
    (b) fair trade practice
    (c) purchase of drugs
    (d) all of the above
71. The pharmacist should keep in mind the following points while dealing with his profession
    (a) professional vigilance
    (b) law abiding citizens
    (c) relationship with professional organisations
    (d) all of the above
72. The pharmacist should keep in mind the following points while dealing with his medical profession
    (a) limitation of professional activity
    (b) cladenstine arrangement
    (c) liaison with public
    (d) all of the above
73. A 20 week pregnancy can be terminated with the consent of
    (a) doctor holding M.B.B.S. degree
    (b) doctor holding M.D. degree
    (c) Gynaecologist
    (d) two registered medical practioner
74. A registered medical practitioner shall not be guilty of any offence under any law if any pregnancy is terminated
    (a) if the length of the pregnancy does not exceed twelve weeks
    (b) if the length of the pregnancy exceeds twelve weeks but does not exceed twenty weeks
    (c) where a pregnancy occure due to failure of any device used by any married women or her husband for the purpose of limiting the number of children
    (d) all of the above
75. Any person who wilfully contravenes or wilfully fails to comply with the requirements of any regulation under medical termination of pregnancy act shall be liable to be punished
    (a) with fine which may extend to one thousand
    (b) imprisonment of 6 months
    (c) fine of 10000Rs
    (d) both b &c
76. medical termination of pregnancy act was passed in
    (a) 1971 (b) 1965
    (c) 1947 (d) 1945

77. The officer designated by the public authorities in all administrative units or offices under it to provide information to the citizens requesting for information under the act is known
   (a) state information officer
   (b) chief information commissioner(CIC)
   (c) public information officer
   (d) assistant public information officer

78. The main objective of the right to information act is
   (a) to empower the citizens to secure access to information under the control of public authorities
   (b) promote transparency and accountability in the working of the govt.
   (c) make our democracy work for the people in real sense
   (d) all of the above

79. APIO forward application for information to
   (a) PIO
   (b) the head of the authority
   (c) first appellate authority
   (d) third party

80. RTI act 2005 mandates public information officer must providethe information as asked by the applicant
   (a) within 30 days of receipt of RTI application
   (b) within 7 days of receipt of RTI application
   (c) within 10 days of receipt of RTI application
   (d) within 90 days of receipt of RTI application

81. The definition of record under the act includes
   (a) any document , manuscript and file
   (b) any microfilm, microfiche and facsimile copy of a document
   (c) any reproduction of image embodied in such microfilm
   (d) all of the above

82. The distinctive signs that identify certain goods produced or provided by a specific person or enterprise are known as
   (a) geographical indications
   (b) trade mark
   (c) patent
   (d) copyright

83. An exclusive right granted to the applicant for an invention which is a product or a process or a new way of doing something or offers a new technical solution to a problem is known as
   (a) geographical indications
   (b) trade mark
   (c) patent
   (d) copyright

84. Patent is granted for ---------------from the filling date of the application
   (a) 20 years (b) 10 years
   (c) 1 years (d) 5 years

85. The categories of works that can be protected by copyright laws include
   (a) Novels
   (b) Films, musical compositions, and choreography
   (c) paintings, drawings, photographs and sculpture
   (d) all of the above

86. The Excise-Officer-in-charge of bonded laboratory may permit to take a sample from each batch of finished preparation free of duty up to a maximum amount of
   (a) 250 ml (b) 150 ml
   (c) 100 ml (d) 50 ml

87. As per specification given in schedule P of drugs and cosmetic act, the diphtheria toxic has expiry period of
   (a) 6 month (b) 12 month
   (c) 2 years (d) 5 years

88. The term of patent for ordinary invention from the date of patent is
   (a) 7 years (b) 14 years
   (c) 5 years (d) 10 years

89. Grant of patent, under patent act , may be opposed by a person from the date of advertisement of acceptance within a period of
   (a) 4 month (b) 8 month
   (c) 1 year (d) 2 years

90. VDRL antigen is to be tested and analysed by the
    (a) drug inspector
    (b) excise commissioner
    (c) serologist and chemical examiner
    (d) drug controller of India

91. Import of cosmetics intended for use on the eye brow or eye lash containing coaltar dyes is
    (a) Permitted (b) exempted
    (c) Prohibited (d) dutyable

92. an example of artificial color is
    (a) titanium dioxide (b) caramel
    (c) cochineal (d) curcumin

93. Chloramphenicol comes under schedule
    (a) G (b) H
    (c) W (d) P

94. A12 week pregnancy can be terminated with the consent of --------medical practitioners
    (a) Two (b) one
    (c) Three (d) five

95. drugs and chemists shops are exempted for the provision of
    (a) opening time (b) closing time
    (c) both a and b (d) lunch time

96. Section -14 of the factories act state that
    (a) effective measures should be taken by the employers to keep workrooms free from dust and flame
    (b) a factory must be fenced by safeguards of substantial construction
    (c) adequate arrangement should be made for running canteens and dispensary for employees
    (d) aseptic environment should be maintain around the manufacture process

97. price of formulation sold to retailer in case of scheduled drug as per drugs(price control)order should be
    (a) retail price minus 5%
    (b) retail price minus 10%
    (c) retail price minus 16%
    (d) retail price and 15 % local taxes

98. legal categories of drugs introduced in amendment of drugs and cosmetics act in 1982 were
    (a) 2 (b) 4
    (c) 6 (d) 10

99. 'Ganja' as per the narcotic drugs and psychotropic substance act means
    (a) flowering and fruiting tops of cannabis sativa
    (b) flowering and fruiting top, leaves and seeds of cannabis sativa
    (c) roots of cannabis sativa
    (d) all parts of cannabis sativa

100. Major amendment in drugs and cosmetic act was made in-------
    (a) 1975 (b) 1982
    (c) 1985 (d) 1986

101. import of drugs for personal use contains average doses in mg up to
    (a) 200 (b) 150
    (c) 100 (d) 50

102. patent and priority medicines can be imported to some extent in
    (a) crude conditions (b) multidose vials
    (c) bulk form (d) unit containers

103. drug retail sale licences are issued by
    (a) drugs controller of India
    (b) Union health minister
    (c) Drug controller authorities of the states

104. Names from the resister can be removed only by an order of the
    (a) PCI
    (b) registration tribunal
    (c) executive committee
    (d) Director of health

105. Example of narcotic drug is
    (a) Coca (b) opium
    (c) Charas (d) all of the above

106. Any person contravenes any condition of prevention of cruelty to animals act is punished with a fine of Rs.
    (a) 1000 (b) 1500
    (c) 3000 (d) 200

107. every year the Register of state pharmacy council is required to print the registers
(a) 1st January (b) 1st march
(c) 1st April (d) 1st june

108. establishment which have a qualified person and engage in compounding of drugs is
(a) drug store
(b) chemists and druggists
(c) pharmacy
(d) testing laboratory

109. digitalis belongs to schedule
(a) E (b) X
(c) G (d) H

110. Schedule X drug is
(a) Amphetamine (b) cyclobarbital
(c) Glutethimide (d) all of the above

111. The pharmacy council of India is also known as
(a) State pharmacy council
(b) joint pharmacy council
(c) central pharmacy council
(d) central druggist association

112. Persons from teaching professions are nominated in PCI by
(a) state government
(b) central government
(c) executive committee
(d) election

113. The secretary of PCI may also act as its
(a) Registrar (b) treasurer
(c) both a and b (d) vici- president

114. The quantities of sample taken for analysis should not be less than
(a) 10 ml (b) 20 ml
(c) 5 ml (d) 50 ml

115. A drug sample taken by the drug inspector for analysis is sent of
(a) drug controller
(b) drug inspector
(c) excise commissioner
(d) government analyst

116. from a bonded laboratory the spiritous preparations are sent to the following for the determination of the alcohol strength
(a) government analyst
(b) excise commissioner
(c) chemical examiner
(d) drug inspector

117. Biological and microbiological tests are conducted at
(a) Mumbai (b) Calcutta
(c) Chennai (d) kasauli

118. As per the drugs and cosmetic act chemist and druggist mean, premises for sale of drug which have
(a) qualified person and drugs are compounded
(b) qualified person but drugs are not compounded
(c) compounding facilities but qualified person is not needed
(d) any experience holding person who can formulate compositions

119. government opium factory is situated at
(a) Delhi (b) Mumbai
(c) Hyderabad (d) Neemuch

120. Dangerous drugs act and rules relates to the year
(a) 1948 (b) 1955
(c) 1940 (d) 1930

121. If the product has been substituted wholly or partly by another drug of substance, it is known as
(a) Spurious drug (b) Adulterated drug
(c) Misbranded drug (d) Poisonous drug

122. Drug for examination, test or analysis can be imported under a licence in form
(a) 10 (b) 11
(c) 12 (d) 13

123. Licences for the manufacture of medicinal and toilet preparation are issued by
(a) Director of health services
(b) Central govt.
(c) Excise commissioner of the states
(d) commissioner of the central excise

124. Categories of drugs introduced in the amendment of drugs and cosmetics act are
(a) Drugs specified in schedule X
(b) Drugs specified in schedule C,C(1) and X
(c) Drugs specified in schedule C and C(1) excluding those specified in schedule X
(d) all of the above

125. Schedule M (GMP) and Y were introduced in drugs and cosmetic act in
(a) 1976 (b) 1982
(c) 1988 (d) 1980

126. list of ailments and diseases that a drug should not claim to cure is given in schedule
(a) L (b) J
(c) C (d) H

127. Drugs by air can be imported into India through
(a) Ahemdabad (b) Delhi
(c) Chennai (d) all of the above

128. Opium can be exported from the part of
(a) Chennai
(b) Vishakhapatnam
(c) Mumbai
(d) none of the above

129. Example of schedule 'X' is
(a) Ciprofloxacin (b) Emetin
(c) Quinidine (d) diazepam

130. A state council may appoint a Registrar who may act as
(a) Secratary
(b) Treasurer
(c) Vice- president
(d) Executive member

131. drug samples from magistrate are sent for analysis to
(a) State drug control laboratory
(b) Pharmacy council of India
(c) Central drug laboratory
(d) Regional Research Laboratory

132. Joint state pharmacy councils are constituted for
(a) 3 years (b) 1 years
(c) 5 years (d) indefinite period

133. The front of a pharmacy shall bear an inscription
(a) Chemist
(b) Manufacturer
(c) pharmacy
(d) Chemist and druggist

134. manufacturer without bond licences are issued by
(a) excise commissioner
(b) drug inspector
(c) govt. analyst
(d) registrar

135. Condoms are tested at
(a) central toxicological research institute
(b) Indian veterinary research institute
(c) Indian pharmacopoeial laboratory
(d) Indian rosin and turpentine institute

136. The left hand top corner of the lable of schedule 'X'drugs contains symbol
(a) XRs (b) Rx
(c) RMP (d) TDS

137. list of the substances that are required to be used only under medical supervision and which are labelled accordingly are included in schedule
(a) R (b) G
(c) FF (d) C and C (1)

138. In case of schedule X drugs are prescription should be in
(a) Duplicate (b) triplicate
(c) only one copy (d) five copies

139. The tablet or capsule drugs specified in schedule X can be marketed in packing not exceeding
(a) 200 unit doses (b) 150 unit doses
(c) 100 unit doses (d) 250 unit doses

140. The education regulations are laid down by
(a) Central govt.
(b) State govt.
(c) Pharmacy council of India
(d) Ayurvedic council of India

141. Cure for blindness is an example of the following advertisement
(a) Prohibited (b) exempted
(c) Regular (d) permitted

142. All shops and establishment are required to be registered with
(a) Central govt. (b) municipality
(c) Commissioner (d) chief inspector

143. opium has been under legislative control since
(a) 1820 (b) 1857
(c) 1925 (d) 1949

144. drugs consultative committee advises
(a) Central govt. (b) (D)T.(A)(B)
(c) State govt. (d) all of the above

145. The 4th edition of Indian pharmacopoeia was published in the year
(a) 1966 (b) 1985
(c) 1996 (d) 1955

146. Standards for mechanical contraceptive are given in schedule
(a) S (b) R
(c) Q (d) T

147. Spurious drugs meaning which are
(a) imitations
(b) substitutes
(c) resemble other drugs
(d) all of the above

148. manufacturing of drugs for the purpose of act includes all the operation related to drugs concept
(a) formulating, manufacturing
(b) finishing and coating
(c) packing, labelling and sale
(d) compounding, dispensing or packing in retail business

149. medicinal hemp includes
(a) tincture of hemp
(b) powder of hemp
(c) aerial parts
(d) all parts

150. The magic remedies act was passed and enforced in the year
(a) 1954 (b) 1948
(c) 1919 (d) 1930

151. Phenobarbitone sodium belongs to
(a) Schedule X (b) Schedule R
(c) Schedule O (d) Schedule L

152. Under drugs and cosmetics act, the licences for the manufacture of drugs are issued by
(a) Drug controller of India
(b) Government of India
(c) Drug controller of the state
(d) drug inspector

153. the drugs and cosmetic act has been divided into---parts
(a) 15 (b) 16
(c) 18 (d) 24

154. list of minimum equipment for efficient running of a pharmacy is given in schedule
(a) M (b) N
(c) Q (d) R

155. Drug (price control) order came into force in the year
(a) 1970 (b) 1987
(c) 1955 (d) 1960

156. central register of pharmacists is maintained by
(a) state health ministry
(b) pharmacy council of India
(c) state pharmacy council
(d) drug controller of India

157. licences for the manufacture of medicinal and toilet preparation under bond are issued by
(a) customs collector
(b) excise commissioner of the state
(c) pharmacy council of India
(d) commissioner for central excise

158. medical termination of pregnancy act was passed in the year
(a) 1971 (b) 1980
(c) 1871 (d) 1949

159. Life period of drugs is dealt in
(a) Schedule Q (b) Schedule R
(c) Schedule P (d) Schedule T

160. Example of schedule G drugs is
(a) penicillin injection
(b) penicillin tablet
(c) sulfonal
(d) none of the above

161. Advertising of the report of a government analyst is
    (a) permitted
    (b) prohibited
    (c) some reports can be advertised
    (d) all of the above
162. The chairman of (D)T.(A)(B) is
    (a) President, PCI
    (b) Drug controller of India
    (c) Union health minister
    (d) Director general health services
163. talisman, mantras and kavachas come under
    (a) misbranded drugs
    (b) poisonous drugs
    (c) magic remedies
    (d) psychotropic drugs
164. The excise officer may permit the manufacturer to take a sample for analysis without excise duty up to a maximum of
    (a) 250 ml (b) 500 ml
    (c) 100 ml (d) 50 ml
165. government opium factory is situated at
    (a) Ghazipur (b) Lucknow
    (c) Srinagar (d) Culcutta
166. no repacking license is issued to
    (a) Schedule C drugs
    (b) Schedule G drugs
    (c) Schedule J drugs
    (d) Schedule H drugs
167. The first edition of Indian pharmacopoeia was published in the year
    (a) 1940 (b) 1985
    (c) 1955 (d) 1950
168. pharmacy council of India is reconstituted every
    (a) 6 years (b) 2 years
    (c) 3 years (d) 5 years
169. Any mixture of coca containing more than following amount of cocaine is dangerous drug
    (a) 0.01% (b) 0.05%
    (c) 0.10% (d) 0.02%
170. The poisons act was passed in the year
    (a) 1857 (b) 1919
    (c) 1948 (d) 1971
171. premises licensed for the sale of drugs which have a qualified person but where in the drugs are not compounded are called
    (a) Industry
    (b) chemist and druggist
    (c) warehouse
    (d) drugstore
172. The central drug laboratory is established at
    (a) Calcutta (b) Lucknow
    (c) Mumbai (d) Kasauli
173. The members of the (D)T.(A)(B) hold the office for a period of
    (a) 1 years (b) 3 years
    (c) 5 years (d) 7 years
174. All registers in the sale of drugs should be maintained for
    (a) 5 years (b) 4 years
    (c) 3 years (d) 2 years
175. Which of the following are prohibited to be imported
    (a) Toilet preparation
    (b) misbranded drugs
    (c) unani drugs
    (d) schedule ‘C’ and ‘G’ drugs
176. The drug bill was introduced in the year
    (a) 1930 (b) 1931
    (c) 1940 (d) 1948
177. if the manufacturing license is cancelled the loan license is
    (a) suspended
    (b) cancelled
    (c) renewed
    (d) none of the above
178. The magic remedies act was passed and enforced in the year
    (a) 1954 (b) 1944
    (c) 1919 (d) 1930

# Answer Key Pharmaceutical Jurisprudence

1. c
2. a
3. a
4. d
5. a
6. d
7. a
8. c
9. d
10. b
11. c
12. a
13. b
14. b
15. a
16. a
17. a
18. b
19. a
20. a
21. b
22. b
23. a
24. c
25. d
26. d
27. b
28. b
29. a
30. d
31. d
32. d
33. a
34. a
35. d
36. d
37. a
38. d
39. b
40. a
41. a
42. d
43. a
44. a
45. b
46. d
47. a
48. a
49. c
50. c
51. a
52. a
53. a
54. b
55. d
56. d
57. d
58. a
59. d
60. a
61. d
62. d
63. d
64. d
65. a
66. a
67. d
68. d
69. d
70. d
71. d
72. d
73. d
74. a
75. a
76. c
77. d
78. a
79. a
80. d
81. b
82. c
83. a
84. d
85. a
86. d
87. b
88. a
89. c
90. c
91. b
92. b
93. a
94. c
95. a
96. c
97. b
98. a
99. b
100. c
101. d
102. c
103. c
104. d
105. d
106. c
107. c
108. a
109. d
110. c
111. b
112. c
113. a
114. d
115. c
116. d
117. b
118. d
119. d
120. a

121. b
122. c
123. d
124. c
125. b
126. d
127. d
128. d
129. b
130. a
131. d
132. c
133. a
134. c
135. a
136. b
137. b
138. c
139. c
140. a
141. a
142. b
143. d
144. c
145. b
146. d
147. d
148. a
149. a
150. a
151. c
152. c
153. b
154. b
155. b
156. b
157. a
158. c
159. d
160. b
161. d
162. c
163. a
164. a
165. a
166. c
167. d
168. c
169. d
170. b
171. a
172. b
173. b
174. b
175. b
176. b
177. a
178. a

# Chapter 5

# Microbiology

## 5.1 General Microbiology & Identification of Bacteria

### Glossary

| | | |
|---|---|---|
| X-factor | - | Required for growth of certain Haemophilus spp. |
| Widal test | - | A slide agglutination test for typhoid or paratyphoid fever |
| Weil- Felix test | - | An agglutination test for typhus using proteus spp. |
| Wasserman antibodies | - | An antibodies against Cardiolipin |
| Warburz respirometer | - | An apparatus used to study enzyme reaction where an exchange of gases takes places |
| Voges- Proskaner | - | A test for the presence of acetylme thlycarbinol to assist in distinguishing between species of conform. |
| Vincents angina | - | An ulcerative condition of the tonsils of gums caused by a spirochete & fusio form bacillus |
| V-factor | - | Nicotinamide adenine dinucleotide required for the growth of Haemophilus spp. |
| VDRL | - | A microscopic agglutination screening test for the detection of Wassermann antibodies in the serum, of syphilitic patients |
| Ultrafiltration | - | A method for the removel of all but the very smallest particle |
| Turbidostatic | - | A device for maintaining microorganisms in continuous culture monitors cell culture, monitor cell density & regulates dilution rate to maintain cell density at a constant value |
| Transposns | - | Units of DNA which can move from on DNA molecule to other |
| Translation | - | The process in which genetic information in mRNA directs the order of assembly of specific amino acids during protein synthesis |
| Transformaiton | - | The phenomenon by which certain bacteria incorporate DNA from related strains into their genetic make up |
| Termostable | - | Relatively resistant to heat, resistant to the temperature. Of 100°C (212°F) |
| Thermohile | - | An organism that grows best at temp above 45°C |
| Thermolabile | - | Destroyed by heat at temp below 100°C (212°F) |
| Stenothermophile | - | An organism which grows at 60°C or higher & cannot grow at mesophilic temperature (true /obligate temperature) |
| RNA polymerse | - | An enzyme that synthesizes mRNA or a DNA template |
| Reverse transcriptase | - | An enzyme that synthesizes of a DNA molecule using RNA a template |

| | | |
|---|---|---|
| Resolution | - | The smallest distance by which two objects can be separated and still be visualized as separate objects |
| Repression | - | A decrease in the rate of synthesis of an enzyme specifically caused by a small molecule |
| Puterfication | - | The decomposition of proteins by micro-organism producing disagreeable odors. |
| Psychotorph | - | Organism able to grow at 0°C but which grows best at a temperature above 20°C |
| Psychotrophile | - | A cold lowing organism capable growing at 0°C or lower, organism that cannot grow above 20°C |
| Phototraph | - | Organism nutritionally independent & able to synthesize all required growth factor. |
| Photolithotroph | - | Organism obtaining energy from light uses inorganic compounds as a source of electron |
| Photoautotroph | - | organism obtaining energy from light uses carbon dioxide as its carbon sources. |
| Phosphatase list | - | A list to determine the efficiency of pasteurization of milk |
| Phenol coefficient | - | Ratio between greatest dilution of a test germicide capable of killing a test organism in 10 minute but not in 5 minute of greatest dilution of phenol giving the same result. |
| Oxidase test | - | A test for presence of cytochrome C |
| Opsonin | - | An antibody that renders microorganism susceptible to ingestion by phagocytosis |
| O-antigens | - | Polysaccharide antigens extending from G(-) ve bacteria |
| Mesophile | - | A bacterium growing best but at moderate temperature range 25- 40 °C |
| Khan test | - | A microscopic flocculation test for syphilis |
| Iosenzyme | - | Any one of group of enzyme of different structural forms that possess identical catalytic properties |
| Invetase | - | An enzyme that hydrolysis sucrose to glucose an fructose |
| Hybridoma | - | A hybrid cell resulting from the fusion of a myeloma cell with an antibody producing β lymphocytes |
| Holoenzyme | - | Apoenzyme+ coenzyme |
| Halophile | - | Organism whose growth stimulated b higher salt conc. |
| Fibrinolysin | - | A substance producedby haemolytic streptococci that can liquefy clotted blood plasma (streptokinase) |
| Fastidious organism | - | Organism difficult to isolate due to its special nutritional requirement |
| Faculitative anaerobe | - | Organism which does not require carbon dioxide or growth grows in aerobic and anaerobic condition |
| Exotoxin | - | A toxic protein excreted by a microorganism into surrounding medium |
| Exoenzyme | - | An enzyme excreted by organism into environment |
| Endotoxin | - | A heat toxin which consist of lipopolysaccharide, located in outer membrane of G-(-ve bacteria) |
| Endonuclease | - | Enzyme that exercises a damaged segment of DNA |

Coenzyme $F_{420}$ - A Flavin like coenzyme unique to methanogenic bacteria

Coenzyme M - Coenzyme unique to methanogenic bacteria involve methyl transfer reaction.

Co-factor - Metal ion which function in combination with enzyme protein

Cellulose - Cellulose to cellulobiose

Catalase - Enzyme that converts hydrogen peroxide to water & oxygen

Brophile - Organism growing under high hydrostatic pressure

Antitoxin - Antibody capable of uniting with neutralizing with specific toxin

Amylase - An enzyme that hydrolysis starch

Allosteric Enzyme - Regulatory enzyme with a binding or catalytic site for the substrate at different site.

Acid curd - Milk protein coagulated by acid

Obligatory anaerobes - Do not tolerate oxygen an die in its presence

## Identification of Bacteria

Once a bacteria has been obtained in pure culture, it has to be identified – it is performed by two methods:

(a) By study of morphology : It depends on a number of factors such as the strain studied, nature of the culture medium, temperature and time of incubation.

(b) Staining reactions: Sample stains bring out the morphology best. Differential and special stains are necessary to bring out characteristics like flagella, capsules, spores and metachromatic granules.

## Various Staining Methods in Microbiology

| | |
|---|---|
| Moller's method & Schafer fulton tech<br>Modified Ziehl-Neelse's tech. | Spore stain |
| Tliss method (Negative staining) | Capsule staining |
| Flagella | Modified Leif son's method |
| Albert stain | Diphtheria bacillus |
| Ziehl Nielson stain | Acid fast |
| Gram stain | Gram (+VE), Gram (-VE) |
| Fenlgen stain | DNA |
| Giemage stain | Rickettsia &Protoza |
| Volutin granules & metachromatic granules | Diluted methylene blue |
| Poly β-hydroxy butyrate | Nile blue |
| Glycogen | Iodine |
| Corynebacterium | Metachromatic stains, methylene blue |
| Diphtheriae | Albert's method, Neisser's stain |
| Pneumococci | India-ink |
| Spirochaetes | Giemsa, Levaditi's, fontana |
| TB, Leprosy, Nocardia | Acid fact |
| Anthrax | Sudam black |
| Trichomonas | Brillant crystal violet (1%) |

### Genetic transfer in Bacteria

There are four method of genetic transfer of material in bacteria:

(i) **Transformation:** It is a artificial process. It's brought about by treatment of the bacterial cells with J calcium chloride a temperature shock.

(ii) **Transduction:** It is transfer of DNA of one bacterial cell into another cell by "viral infection".

(iii) **Conjugation:** In this process, D.N.A transfer directly from one bacterial cell to another by a mechanism that requires cell to cell contact. In this process, plasmids are mostly transferred as a genetic element.

(iv) **Transposons:** It's a DNA sequence in which transpose blocks of genetic material back and forth between cell chromosomes an smaller replicons such as plasmids.

## Genetic Engineering

It is the method of isolating genes coding for any desired protein from micro-organism or from cells of higher form of life including man an inserting them into suitable micro-organisms.

## Bacterial Spores

Spores are resistant structures formed by bacteria as endospores, which can survive adverse condition such as heat, drying freezing radiations and action of toxic chemicals.

## Sterilisation

It is destruction or removal of all living organism including spores.

### Different types of sterilization

(i) **Tyndallisation:** Repeated steaming at 100°C of culture media (sugar solution) on each of three successive days, allowing spores to germinate and to kill subsequently.

(ii) **Autoclaving:** it is the Process for killing vegetative and spores by coagulation of protein. It is done at 121°C 15 $lbs/in^3$ pressure for 15 minutes. Eg. All material not spoiled by heat can be subjected autoclaving as, dressing, instruments (glass and metal)

(iii) **Incineration:** It is for disposal of soiled dressing, laboratory media and human tissue using oil fired hospital incinerators.

(iv) **Flaming:** It is used for sterilisation of wire loops and glassware (small) in microbiological laboratories.

- (i) **By use of chemical:** Several chemicals used for the purpose of sterilisation. As,
  - (a) **Glutraidehyde:** 1 to 2% as alkaline aqueous solutions 5 to 20 minute used for the instrument sterilisation as, cystoscope, endoscope and various dental instruments.
  - (b) **β-Propiolactone:** A liquid, which rapidely hydrolyse to hydrocrylic acid in aqueous solutions. It is used for vaccines inactivation.
  - (c) **Ethylene Oxide:** An inflammable gas used as a mixture of $CO_2$ at 50°C in a suitable chamber. Humidity must be adequate. It is used for the sterilisation of heat sensitive equipments as rubber tubing, gloves, bronchoscope, cyrtoscope, and heart-lung machine. Cutting and sharp instruments like blades, scissiors and knives.
- (ii) Vaccines are sterilised by Formalin 0.5%, heat at 60°C for 1 hour or by β-Propiolactone

## Assay of Drugs

The measure of the biological activity of drug is called its potency. Assay is the estimation of the potency of the activity principle in the unit quantity of medical preparation.

Types of Assays

There are three types of assay

(i) Chemical assay

(ii) Biological assay

(iii) Immunological assay

**(i) Chemical assay**

The potency of the achive principle in the drug preparation is determined by chemical method. The choice of chemical method, depands upon the nature of the functional group.

**(ii) Biological assay (Bioassay)**

It is the method of the estimation of concentration of the active principle in the unit weight of the drug in terms of biological response in the treated organism.

**Methods of (Bioassay)**

As bioassay involves the measurement of the concentration of the specific active ingredient present in the crude drug sample of drug.

## 5.2 Assay of Antibiotics & Vitamins

| Antibiotics | Sources | Assay |
|---|---|---|
| Amphoterician B | Streptemycesnodosus | Sacchromyces cerevisiae |
| Bacitracin | Bacukkyssybtilis | Micrococcus luteus |
| Cycloserine | Streptemycesarchidaceous | Staphylococcus aureus |
| Cephalosporin | Cephalosporiumacremonium | |
| Chlorotetracycline | Stremptycesaeurofaciens | Baciluscerus |
| Neomycin (CP) | Stremptemycesfradiae | Staphylococcus epidermidis |
| Neomycin (T) | | Klebsoiellapeneumoniae |
| Doxorubicin | Streptemycespneucitieus | |
| Griseofulvin | Pencilliumgriseofulvin | |
| Penicillin<br>Benzyl penicillin<br>Phenoxy methyl<br>Penicillin<br>Benzathin penicillin | Penicillumnotatum<br>Penicillumchrysogenum | Bacilus subtilis |
| Streptomycin | Streptemycesgriseus | Klebsoiella pneumoniae |
| Vancomycin | Streptmycesorientalis | B. subtilis |
| Lincomycin | Streptemyceslincolenecis | |
| Mrardin | Mradiauniformis | |
| Erythromycin | Streptemyceserythareus | Micrococcus leuteus |
| Polymyxin – B | Bacillus polymyxa | Bordetella bronchiseptica |
| Framicetrin (Soframycin) | Streptemycesdecaris | B. pumilus<br>B. subtilis |
| Mitomycin – C | Stremptmycescaespitosus | |
| Kanamycin – B | Streptmyceskanamyceticus | B. subtilis |

**Table** *Contd...*

| Antibiotics | Sources | Assay |
|---|---|---|
| Gentamycin | Micromonosporopurpurea | Staphylococcus epidermidis |
| Novobiocin | Streptemycesniveus | Staphylococcus epidermidis |
| Nystatin | Streptemycesnoursei | Sccharmoyces cerevisiae |
| Oxy-tetracycline | Streptemycesrimosus | Staphylococcus aureus |
| Paramonician | Streptemycesrimosus | |
| Tobramycin | Streptemycestenebrarius | Staphylococcus aureus |
| Refampicin | Streptemycesmediteerrani | B. subtilis |
| Fusidic ᾱ | Fusidiumcoccineum | |
| Chloromphenicol | Streptemycesvenzuelae | Sareinalutea |
| Clavulanic ᾱ | Streptemycescalvuligerus | |
| Tetracycline | Streptemycesaureeofaciens | Bacillus cereus,<br>Staphylococcus aureus |
| Amikacin | | Staphylococcus aureus |
| Doxycline | | Staphylococcus aureus |
| Framicetrin sulphate | | B. pumilus<br>B. subtils |
| Carbenicillin | | Pseudomonusaueriginosa |
| Ampicillin | | Micrococcus luteus |
| Cephalexin | | Staphylococcus aureus |
| Bleomycin | | Mycobacterium smegmatics |
| Candidicin | | Saccharomyces cerevisiae |
| Capreomycin | | Klebsiella pneumoniae |
| Cephalothin | | Staphylococcus aureus |
| Cephapirin | | Staphylococcus aureus |
| Cloxacillin | | Staphylococcus aureus |
| Colistimethate sodium | | Brodetellabronchiseptica |
| Colistin | | Brodetellabronchiseptica |
| Demeclocycline | | Staphylococcus aureus |
| Dihydrostreptomycin (CP) | | B. subtilis |
| Dihydrostreptomycin (T) | | Klebsiellapenumoniae |
| Gramicidin | | Entrococcushairae |
| Kanamycin | | Staphylococcus aureus |
| Methacycline | | Staphylococcus aureus |
| Nafcillin | | Staphylococcus aureus |
| Netlmicin | | Staphylococcus epidermidis |
| Nystain | | Saccharomyces cerevisiae |
| Paromomycin | | Staphylococcus epidermidis |
| Rolitetracycline | | Staphylococcus aureus |
| Spectinomycin (T) | | Klebsiella pneumoniae |
| Tylosin | | Staphylococcus aureus |

- All tetracycline's, kanamycin sulphate, cephalexin ------- Staphylococcus aureus
- Ampicillin, Bacitracin, Erythromycin, Lincomycin----------- Micrococcus luteus

### Microorganism in Vitamin Assay

| Vitamins | Organism used for assay | Temp. of incubation period | pH | Sterilization by |
|---|---|---|---|---|
| Niacin | Lactobacillus plantarum | 37°C | 6.8 | Autoclave |
| Calcium pantothanate | Lact. Plantarum | 37°C | 6.8 | Autoclave |
| Vit$B_{12}$ | Lactobacillus leichmani | 37°C | 5.5 | Autoclave |
| Vit$B_6$ (pyridoxine) | Lactobaciluscasei Saccharomyces Carlsbergenesis | 28°C *To* 30°C | 5.0-5.2 | Autoclave |
| Vit$B_2$ | Lactobacillus Casei | 37°C | 6.8 | Autoclave |
| Nicotinic acid & Nicotinamide | Lactobacillus arabinoses Lactobacillus mesenteroid | 37°C | 6.8 | Autoclave |
| Folic acid | Terahymenagellii, Lactcasei, Strep fecalis | 37°C | | Autoclave |
| Pantothenic acid | Lactobacillus carlbergenesis | 30°C | 6.8 | Autoclave |
| Nicotonic acid | Lactobacillus arabinacos Lactobacillus mesenteroid | 37°C | 6.8 | Autoclave |
| Aneurine ($B_1$) | Lactobacillus fermentum | 37°C | 6.5 | Autoclave |

## 5.3 Preparation of Sera & Vaccines

Sera and antibody containing preparation which is made by the plasma of an immune person or animal contains a large number of antibodies which, if the blood is withdrawn an allowed to clot, than serum is separates.

A serum may contain anti-toxic, antibacterial or antiviral antibodies and accordingly it is called an anti-toxic, antibacterial or antiviral serum. Anti-toxic sera are known as "antitoxins". Most antitoxins or antisera are obtained from animals in which active immunity has been simulated artificially.

### Vaccine

Immunity can be acquired by the individual himself by the development of antibodies naturally or by the introduction of the antigen. The antigenic material producing immunization by stimulating an immune response is termed as a "Vaccine".

Following are some of the vaccines used in general.

**(i) Sterile Vaccines:**

Cholera vaccine

Pertussis vaccine

Plague vaccine

Typhus

**(ii) Living Vaccines:**

Bacillus Calmette-Guerin vaccine

Bacillus calmette-Percutaneous

Measles vaccine (Live attenuated)

Poliorivyelitis (oral) vaccine

Small-pox vaccine

Yellow fever vaccine

**(iii) Mixed Vaccines:**

Diphtheria and Pertussis vaccine

Diphtheria and Tetanus vaccine

Diphtheria, Tetanus, pertussis vaccine

Diphtheria, Tetanus, Pertussis and Poliomyelitis vaccine

**(iv) Inactivated vaccine:**

Influenza vaccine

Measles vaccine (Inactivated)

Rabies vaccine (Human cell culture)

Typhus vaccine

Japanese Encephalitis

**CLASS OF VACCINES**

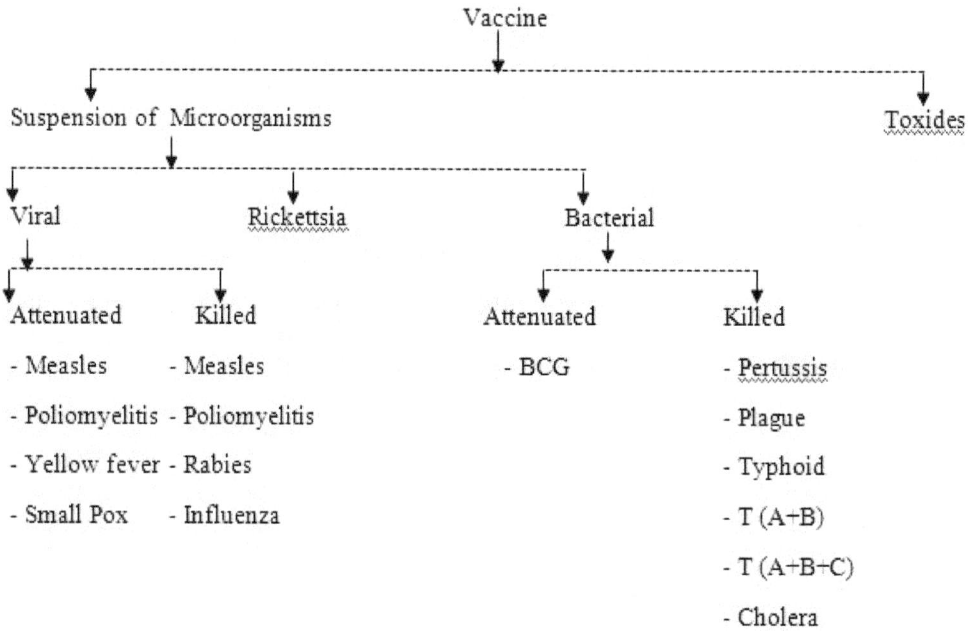


**Some important official antitoxins**

1. Diphtheria Antitoxin
2. Botulinum Antitoxin
3. Gas-gangrene Antitoxin
4. Staphylococcus Antitoxin
5. Tetanus Antitoxin

**Preparation by seed hot**

1. BCG
2. Polio
3. Japanese Encephalitis
4. Measles
5. Rabies (Human cell culture)

**Freeze dried vaccine**

1. BCG
2. Typhoid – Paratyphoid
3. Viper venom

**Aqueous Suspension**

1. Yellow fever 2. Polio

**Sterile Suspension**

1. Plague
2. Tetanus
3. Snake venom
4. Shick test
5. Rabies

**Passive immunising agent**

1. Viper venom
2. Snake venom
3. Scorpion venom
4. Tetanus antitoxin
5. Diphtheria antitoxin
6. Rabies antitoxin

## pH Range of Vaccines

Tetanus, Polio, DPT - 6 -7

Typhoid, Paratyphoid - 6 -7.4

Japanese Encephalitis - 6.8 – 7.4

Typhus - 6.6 – 8.5

Rabies - 7.2 ± 0.2

Shick test - 7.2 – 7.6

## Official Sera and Vaccine

| Name | Category | Composition |
|---|---|---|
| Japanese encephalitis (Human mouse brain) | Active immunising agent | Inactivated Japanese Encephalitis virus |
| Measles vaccine | Active immunisation agent | Live attenualid measles virus Aq. Suspension from<br>i) Chicken embryo cultura<br>ii) Immunogenic strain<br>iii) No human serum |
| Vaper venos | | Dried secretion obtained from poisonous glands Viperaerusselli |
| Yellow fever vaccine | Active immunisation agent | Aq. Suspension of chick embryo tissue infected with ITD strains of yellow fever virus |

**Table** *Contd...*

| Name | Category | Composition |
|---|---|---|
| Typhoid vaccine | Active immunisation agent | Strain of Salmonella typhi having component O.H. & VI antigens |
| Typhus vaccine | Active immunisation agent | Sterile suspension of killed rickttsial of strain of epidemic thypus (Rickettsia prowazake) |
| Typhoid para typhoid –A vaccine | Active immunisation agent | Freezed dried preparation from somonellatyphi& salmonella parayphi –A |
| Tetanus vaccine | Active immunisation agent | Sterile suspension prepared from hyper immune serum/ plasma of healthy horse having specific activity of neutralizing the toxin from C. diptheria |
| Cholera vaccine | Active immunising agent | Homogenous preparation of killed cholera vibrio's of two classical type of V. Cholera<br>i) Inaba<br>ii) Ogata |
| B.C.G Vaccine (Anti-TB) | Active immunising agent | It is a freeze dried live bacteria obtained from bacillus of calmette&guerin |

## Vaccines Obtained From

| Vaccines | OBTAINED FROM |
|---|---|
| Mumps | Chick embryo tissue culture |
| Measles | Chick embryo tissue culture |
| Rabies | Duck embryo |
| Small pox | Calf / Sheep lymph |
| Encephalitis | Chick embryo tissue culture |

## Toxins Botained from Microoraganisms

| TOXINS | MICROORAGANISMS |
|---|---|
| Clostridium toxin | C. prefringes |
| Botulinium toxin | C. botulinium |
| Tetanus toxin | C. tetani |

## Diagnostic and Confrirmatiory Tests for Various Diseases

| Test | Organism/ disease |
|---|---|
| Shick test<br>Elerk test | Diptheria |
| Dick test<br>Schultz – charlfow reagent test | Scarlet fever |
| Mc. Fadian test<br>Ascoli test | Anthrax |
| Weil felix reaction | Typhus fever |
| Brucellins test | Undulant fever |
| Widal test | Typhoid |
| Khan test<br>VDRL test<br>Wasserman test | Syphilis |
| Fries test | Lymphogranuloma venerum |

**Table** *Contd...*

| Test | Organism/ disease |
|---|---|
| Rapid plasma regent (RPR) | Syphilis |
| Western blot test<br>Elisa test | AIDS |
| Ames test | Cancer |
| Ducrey test | Determine sensitivity to Haemophilus ducreyi (Canchloid) |
| Brucellergin test | Allergy to determine Brucella |
| Trichinella test | Sensitivity to trichinella protein |
| Echinococcus test | Determine sensitivity to echinococcous protein |
| Tubercullin test | Allergy to tubercle bacillus |
| Lupromin reaction | Leprosy |
| Casoni test | Hydatoid disease |
| Mantoux test | Old tuberculin |
| Sham test | Pyrogen testing |
| Coagulase test | Virulent S. aureus |
| Rose water test | Rheumatoid arthritis |
| PautBunnet test | Infective mononucleosis |
| Coombs test | Non agglutinating antibodies |
| Nagler's reaction | Clostridium pretingens, clostridium tetani |
| Hem agglutination inhibition test | Rubella |
| Compliment fixation test | Pneumonial mycoplasma |
| Tine test plague` | Plague |
| Donovan bodies | Kala-azar |
| Viral capsid antigen (VCR) | IgG or IgM antibody |
| Bile solubility test | Pneumoccus |
| Microhemagglutination test | Treponema pallidum |
| Direct fluorescent antibody | Primary syphilis |
| Ghon's complex | T.B |
| Nemimoacent reaction | Rickettsia |
| Scratch test | Skin disease |
| Disk effusia test | Antibody sensitivity in bacteria |
| Schilling test | Vit$B_{12}$ absorption |
| Mc loney test | Determination of delayed hypersensitivity to diphtheria toxoid |
| Neufeld quelhong reaction | To determine type of pneumococcus pneumonia |
| Leshmanian test | Leshmaniasis |
| RIA | To determine HCG hormone in pregnancy |
| Ouchterlony | Smallpox |
| Radial immune diffusion (RID) | Influenza virus |
| Francis test | Pneumococci |
| Satcllitism | H.influenzae |
| String test, cholera redrn. | V. Chlorea |
| Straus reaction | Brucellosis |

## 5.4 Sterilization

| Sterilisation method | Mechanism |
|---|---|
| Dry heat | Oxidation of proteins |
| Moist heat | Denture & coagulation of proteins |
| Ethylene oxide | Alkylation of sulfhydryl, imino, carboxyl and hydroxyl groups of proteins |
| Formaldehyde | Alkylating agent as ethylene oxidase |
| Radiation UV Light | Nucleoprotein damage by UV of λ 256 μm & adjacent wave length |
| Ionizing radiation (High speed electrons) | Denaturation of essential cell constituents such as enzymes, DNA etc. |
| Filtration | Retention bacteria |

### Biological Indicators used in Sterilization

| Method of Sterilization | Organism | D.Value |
|---|---|---|
| Dry heat | B. subtilis, Clostridium tetani | 121 °C -- 0.8 minutes |
| Moist heat | Bacillus sterothermophils or Clostridium sporogensis | 121 °C -- 1.5 minutes |
| Filtration | Pseudmonasdiminuta | |
| Ethylene oxide sterilization | B. subtilis | |
| Radio sterilization | Spores of Bacillus pumilus | |
| Ionization radiation | B. pumilus | |

**D. Value:** (Decimal reduction value) is am measure of resistance of a micro-organism to a particular type of sterilization process. So the duration or absorbed doses regained to reduce the number enable microorganism to 10% of the original number.

**Expression of D. Values:**

**In case of steam sterilization**: Expressed in minutes at a definite temp. ie $D_{121}, D_{170}$, etc

**In case of radiation sterilization:** Expressed by the absorbed dose & subscripts are used to show the los ester used. Ie. $D_{10}$

**In case of ethylene oxide sterilization:** Expressed by the time are minutes.

**Z Value:** It is the change in temp required to after the D.value elates the resistance of a micro-organism to change temperature.

### Physical Indicatores used in Sterilization

| | Serial No. | Holding temperature | Steam Pressure in pounds | Time |
|---|---|---|---|---|
| Moist heat | 1. | 115° – 118°C | 10 | 30 minutes |
| | 2. | 121° – 124°C | 15 | 15 minutes |
| | 3. | 126° – 129°C | 20 | 10 minutes |
| | 4. | 134° – 138°C | 30 | 3 minutes |
| | | 180°C | | 2 hours |
| Dry heat | Plastic dosimeter | | | |
| Radio sterilization | Bubble point test | | | |

### Chemical Indicators used in Sterilization

| | |
|---|---|
| Moist heat | Brownie's tube type I & II colour change Red to Yellow to Green |
| Dry heat | Browne's tube |
| Radio sterilization | Disk which change colour on exposure to ionizing radiation |
| Ethylene oxide | A sachet which change colour on exposure to ehyleneoxide |

## Process of Sterilization of Drugs

| Material | Process |
|---|---|
| Tetracycline injection | Aseptic method |
| Insulin injection | Sterilized by bacterial filtration |
| Quinine injection | Sterilized by heating in autoclave |
| Morphine injection | Sterilized by heating with a bactericide |
| Hydrocortisone | Aseptic method |
| Paraldehyde | Sterilized by bacterial filtration |
| Phenol & glycerine | By dry heat |
| Rubber closures | Autoclave |
| Plastic syringes | Gaseous sterilization |
| Glass syringe | By dry heat |
| Needles (Disposable) | $\gamma$ – radiation |
| Glass wares | Autoclave, Hot air oven |
| Thermometer | Glutaraldehyde, Ethylene oxide |
| Rubber gloves | Moist heat |
| Elastic adhesive dressing | Ethylene oxide &$\gamma$- radiation |
| Dialysis machine | Formalin |
| Ampoule and sealed bottles | Autoclave, $\gamma$- Radiation |
| Operation theatre | UV radiation |
| Hospital blanket | Autoclave, Formalin treated |
| Culture media containing sugar gelatine | Autoclave, Tyndallisation |
| Antibiotic solution & toxin | Filtration |
| Serum | UV, Filtration |
| Talcum powder | Dry heat |
| Plastic wound dressing | Ethylene oxide &$\gamma$- radiation |
| Metal instruments | Autoclaving, hot air oven , IR |
| Heart lung machine | Ethylene oxide |
| Disposable instruments | Ethylene oxide &$\gamma$ – Radiation |
| Powder, Fat & oils | Dry heat |
| Administration sets | $\gamma$ – Radiation |
| Metal instruments | Dry heat |
| Ligature, suture & surgical cotton | Moist heat |

## List of Industrial Products

| Products | Micro-organisms |
|---|---|
| Citric acid | Aspergillus niger<br>Aspergillus wenter |
| Fumaric acid | Rhizophusnigricans |
| Gluconic acid | A. niger |
| Itaconic acid | Aspergillus terreus |
| Pectinases | A.wentii / A/ aureus |
| 11-α – hydroxyl progesterone | Rhizphusarrhizus<br>Rhizophusnigricans |
| Giblurellic acid | Fusarium moniliforme |
| Lictic acid | Rhizophusoryzal |
| Backers yeast | Saccharomyces cereviseiae |
| Soy sauce | Saccharomyces rouxii |
| Sour French bread | Candida unilleri |
| Commercial alchol | S. cerevisiae<br>Kluyvermoycesfragilis |
| Riboflavin | Eremotheciumashloyi<br>Ashbyagossypii |

**Table** *Contd...*

| Products | Micro-organisms |
|---|---|
| Microbial protein | Candida utilis<br>Sacchromyceslipolytica |
| Streptokinase<br>Streptodernase | Strep. Equisimillis |
| Bionesecticides | Bacillus thiuringenesis<br>Bacillus popillae |
| Insulin<br>Interferon<br>Somatostatin (Human growth harmone) | Recombinout DNA varieties of Coil |
| Microbial protein | Methane oxidizing bacteria |
| Actone – Butanol | Clostridium acetobutylicum |
| 2,3 – Butanediol | Bacillus polymyrea<br>Enterobacter aerogeues |
| Dihydroxyactone | Glucobactersuboxydans |
| 2-keto gluconic acid | Psendomorasspp<br>G. suboxydans |
| Bacterial amylase<br>Bacterial protease | Bacillus subtilis |
| Dextran | Luconostoemesenteroid |
| Sorbase | G. suboxydans |
| Cobalamine (Vit -$B_{12}$) | Streptommesenteroidolivaceus Propionibacterium |
| Glutamic acid | Mocrococcusglutamicus |

## Characters of Fermented Milk

| Cultured butter milk | Mixture of Streptococcus lactis or S. cremoris<br>+<br>Luconosticcitrovorum or L. dextramicur |
|---|---|
| Cultured sour cream | Streptococci + Lueconostoe |
| Bulgarim milk | Lactobacillus bulgaris |
| Acidophinus milk | L- acidophillus |

## Isolation Medium of Microbes

| MICROORGANISMS | MEDIUM |
|---|---|
| N. gonorrhoea | Thayer martin medium |
| Vibrio cholera | Thiosulphate – Citrate bile salt sucrose medium |
| M. tuberculosis | Lowenstein Tenses Agar |
| Corrybacterius diphtheria | Lofflers medium<br>Blood tellenite medium |
| Staph. Aureus | Sheep blood sugar |
| N. meningitides | Chokolate Agar & Muller titration medium |

## 5.5 Different Disease & Its Causative Organisms

### List of various bacterial disease & their causative organisms

| Disease | Causative Organism | Type |
|---|---|---|
| Strep throat<br>Scarlet fever | Streptococcus pyogens | G(+ve) capsulated |
| Diphtheria | Corynebacterium diphtheria | G(+ve) rod |
| Botulism | Clostridium Botulinum | G(+ve) spore, rod |
| Food poison | Staphylococcus aureus | G(+ve) Stph |

**Table** *Contd...*

| Disease | Causative Organism | Type |
|---|---|---|
| Anthrax | Bacillus anthracis | G(+ve) Spore, rod |
| Tetanus | Clostridium tetani | G(+ve) spore, rod , aerobic |
| Gas gangrene | Clostridum perfringens | G(+ve) spore, rod, aerobic |
| Staphylococcus skin infection | STephylococcus aureus | G(+Ve) stph |
| Pertuisis (Whooping cough) | Bordetella pertuosis | G(-Ve) rod |
| Meningococcal meningitis | N. meningitilis | G(-Ve) diplococcus |
| Haemophylus meningitis | Hemophylus influenza | G(-Ve) rod, capsule |
| Flavobactmeaningitis | Flavobacteriummaningosepticum | G(-Ve) rod |
| Atypical pneumonia | Mycoplasma pneumoniae | Mycoplasma |
| Klebsiella pneumonia | Klebsiella pneumoniae | G(-Ve) rod, capsule |
| Serratia pneumonia | Serratiamarcescens | G(-Ve) rod |
| Typhoid | Salomonellatyphi | G(-Ve) rod |
| Shigellosis | Shigella serotypes | G(-Ve) rod |
| Cholera | Vibrocholerae | G(-Ve) rod, curved |
| Brucellosis | Brucella spp | G(-Ve) rod |
| Bubonic plague | Yersienapestis (bipolar) | G(-Ve) rod, Bipolar rod |
| Gonerrhoea | N. gonorrea | G(-Ve) rod, diplococcus |
| Vaginitis | Grandnerella vaginalis | G(-Ve) rod |
| Conjunctivitis (Pink eye) | Haemophyllus influenza | G(-Ve) rod, capsule |
| Q- fever | Coxiellaburnetti | Rickettsia |
| Rocky mountain fever<br>Endemic typhus fever<br>Spotted fever | Rickettsia | Rickettsia |
| Typus fever | Rpowazekii | Rickettsia |
| Serub fever | R. tsutsugamushi | Rickettsia |
| Rickettsia pox | R. akari | Rickettsia |
| Tick borne fever | R. conorii | Rickettsia |
| Chlamydial urethritis | Chlamydia tachomatis | Chlamydia |
| Lymphogranuloma venerium | Chlamydia tachomatis | Chlamydia |
| Psitacosis | Chlamydia psittaci | Chlamydia |
| Trachoma | Chlamydia trachomoniasis | Chlamydia |
| Relapsing fever | Borrelia recurrent is | Spirochete |
| Syphillis | Treponema pallidim | Spirochete |
| Tuberoculosis | Mycibacteruimtuberoculae | AFB |
| Leprosy (Hassen's disease) | Mycobactriumlaprae | AFB |
| Mycoplasma urethritis | Mycoplasma hominis | Mycoplasma |

## Viral Disease

| | |
|---|---|
| Influenza | RNA |
| Resp. syncytial disease | RNA |
| Rhino virus infection | RNA |
| Measles (Rubella) | RNA |
| Mumps (Epidemic parotitis) | RNA |
| Yellow fever | RNA |
| Dangue fever | RNA |
| Hepatitis A | RNA |
| Gastro enteritis | RNA |
| Viral fever | RNA |
| AIDS | Retro virus (RNA) |

**Table** *Contd...*

| Rabies | RNA |
|---|---|
| Polio | RNA |
| Arboviral encephalitis | RNA |
| Hapatitis E,D,C | RNA |
| Cytomegalo virus | DNA |
| Adenovirus infection | DNA |
| Herpex simples | DNA |
| Chicken pox (Varicella ) | DNA |
| Small pox (Varicella) | DNA |
| Warts kawaslo disease | DNA |
| Hepatitis B | DNA |
| Show virus disease | |

## Fungal Disease

| Cryptococcus's | Cryptococcus neoformans |
|---|---|
| Candidiasis vaginitis | Candida albicans |
| Thrush, onychia Tinea pedis | Trichophyton spp |
| Tinea captis | Microsporuraspp |
| Tinea barhea | Blastomycesdermatitidis |
| Coccidiodomycosis | Coccidioidesimmitis |
| Aspergillosis Otto mycosis | Aspergillus fumigatus |

## Protozoal Disease

| Amoebasis | F. hystolytica |
|---|---|
| Primary amoebic meningo encephalitis | Naegleriaflowleri |
| Giadriasis | Giardia lambia |
| Trichomoniasis | Tricomonas vaginalis |
| Leishmaniasis | Leishmaniadonovani |
| Toxoplasmosis | Toxoplasma gonadii |
| Malaria | Plasmodium spp. |
| Babesiosis | Babesiamucroti |

## Multicellular Parasites – Flat Worms

| Chinese lever fluke | Clonorchissinensis |
|---|---|
| Intestinal fluke | Fasciolopsisbuski |
| Lunge fluke | Paragonimuswestermans |
| Liver fluke | Fasiola hepatica |
| Beef tape worm | Taneasaginata |
| Pork tape worm | Taneiasolium |
| Fish tape worm | Diphyllobothriumlatum |
| Swarf tape worm | Hymenolepsis nana |
| Dog tape worm | Echinococcus granulises |

## Different Worms

| | |
|---|---|
| Pin worm | Enterobiousvermicularis |
| Whip worm | Trichuristrichuria |
| Round worm | Ascarislumbricoids |
| Trichinosis | Trichinella spiralis |
| Filariasis | Wuchereriabonocrafti |
| Guinea worm | Drachunculusmedinesis |
| Eye worm | Loa loa |

## List of Uncommon Diseases

| | |
|---|---|
| Sporotrichosis | Sporothrixshenckii |
| South American blstomycosis | Paracoccidioidesbrasilensis |
| Moniliasis | Condidaalbicans |
| Balantidiasis | Balantidium coli |
| Kala azar | Leishmaniadonovani |
| Orenal sore | L. tropica |
| Espundia | L. Brasiliensis |
| Epidemophyton (skin, nail, finger infection) | E. floccosum |
| Epidemic ring worm of scalp of children | M. Audoccinni<br>M. gypseum |
| Parasite of hair | T. mentagrophytes |
| Ring worm | T. rubrum<br>T. megnine |
| Hair scalp infection | T. Tonsurans |
| Mice cancer | Polyma virus (Mouse polyoma) |
| Tumours | SV – 40 |
| Benign tumours | Papilloma virus |
| Encephalitis | Eastern equine encephalitis<br>Western equine encephalitis |
| Acute febrile illness | Venezuelan equine encephalitis |
| Fever rash joint pain | Rose river virus<br>West Nile virus |
| Haemorrhagic fever | Flavi virus |
| Cervical adenitis in young children | M. scrofulaceum |
| Plumonary disease | M. Szulgoni |
| Local abiscess at trauma site | M. fortuitum |
| Chronic respiratory disease | M. chelonei |
| Mild upper respiratory tract infection Erysipelas Puerperal fever | S. equisimilis |
| Meningitis tract infection in endocarditis | S. feacalis<br>S. fecium<br>S. durans<br>S.bovis |
| Endocarditis & dental carries | S. sangeuis<br>S. mutans<br>S. salivarius<br>S. mitis |
| Yaws (Skin disease) | Treponema pertenul |
| Non veneral endemic syphilis | T. evdemicum |
| Pinta (Skin disease) | T. carateum |
| Trench fever | Rocha limeaquintana |
| Murine typhus | Rickettsia typhi |
| Wound infection | Staphylo aureus |

**Table** *Contd...*

| | |
|---|---|
| Glanders | Pseudomonas mallei |
| Swine erysipelas | Erysipelothyixrhusiopathiae |
| Malta fever | Brucella spp |
| Chancroid | Hemophilusducreyi |
| Fool typhoid | Salmonella gallinzum |
| Bangis disease | Brucella abortus |
| Tula resnia | Francisellatularensis |

## 5.6 Bioconversions

| Type of Reaction | Micro Organism | Substrate-Product |
|---|---|---|
| Oxidation | Corynebacterium | Nepthalene → Salicylic acid |
| Reduction | Clostridium | α, β unsaturated carboxylic acid |
| Hydrolysis | Streptomcecsaureofacins | AnhydrotetracyclineTetracline |
| Condensation | Streptomyccesgriseus | Streptomycin → Streptomycin phosphate |
| Oxidation | Bacillus subtilis | 5- Hydroxytryptophan |
| Oxidation | Nocardia | ŋ- Dodecyl benzene → Phenyl acetic acid |
| Demethylation | Cynninghamellabalckeslens | 10, 11 – dimthoxyaporphine → Isoapocodein |
| Reduction | Saccharmoyces cerevisiae | Benzaldehyde → Benyl alcohol |
| Reduction | Streptomyces aureofacins | Pentachloroaniline |
| Glycosidation (Condensation) | E. coil | 6-Azauracil → 6- Azauracilniboside |
| N-Acylation | Kluyveracitrophila | 6APS + glycine methyl ester → Ampicillin |
| 11-α- Hydroxylation | Rhizopusnigricans | Progesterone → 11-α-Hydroxy progesterone |
| 1-Dehydrogenation | Anthrobacter simplex | Cortisol → prednisolone |
| Side chain spitting | Mycobacterium | β – Sitosterol → Androstadiendione |
| Side chain spitting | Anthrobacter simplex | Cholestrol → 1, 4- Androstadiene 3, 17 dione |
| Side chain splitting | | β – Bitosterol → Androstadiendione |

### Conversation / Substrate Products with the Microorganisms Involved

| Microorganisms | Conversation / substrate products |
|---|---|
| Acetobactersuboxydans Actobacterxylinum | Glycerol → Dihydroxyacetone |
| Aerobacteraerogenes | DDT → P-P' Dichloro diphenyl methane |
| Rhodotorulagracilis | Chlorobenzilate → 4,4' – Dichlorobenzophenone |
| Brevibacterium | 2,4,5 – trichlorophenoxy acetate → 3,5 – Dichlaro catechol |
| Anthrobacterium | 2-Chloro-2-hydrox propionate → Pyruvic acid |
| Artherbactersimplex | Prednisolone |
| Brevobacterium | 3,5 – dichloroacatechol |
| Rhizopusnigricans | II α – hydroxprogesterone |
| Micobacterium | β – Bitosterol |
| Rhodotorulagracilus | 4,4' Dichlorobenzophenone |
| Aerobacteraerogenes | P,P' – Dichlorodihenyl methane |
| Artherobacter simplex | II α- hydroxyprogesterone |
| Brevibacterium | 3, 5 - dichlorocatechol |

# Microbiology MCQs

1. The best medium for the production of penicillin is
   (a) Nutrient agar
   (b) Corn steep liquor
   (c) Sulphite waste liquor
   (d) Whey
2. food poisoning is caused by
   (a) clostridium tetani
   (b) clostridium welchi
   (c) diphtheria
   (d) clostridium batulinum
3. which of the following is called serum hepatitis?
   (a) HCV (b) HAV
   (c) HBV (d) HIV
4. Koplic's spots will develop in
   (a) HIV (b) Measels
   (c) Mumps (d) Rubella
5. Industrially important antibiotic producing organisms shall be isolated by
   (a) Disk plate method
   (b) Direct plate method
   (c) Serial dilution method
   (d) Crowded plate method
6. Industrial alcohol will be produced by using starter culture
   (a) Top yeast (b) Middle yeast
   (c) Bottom yeast (d) Feeder yeast
7. Which type of antibodies will associate in blood cell coagulation
   (a) IgE (b) IgA
   (c) IgM (d) IgG
8. Cold like symptoms will caused by which bacteria
   (a) Pseudomonas
   (b) E.coli
   (c) Haemophilus influenza
   (d) Haemophilus streptococcus
9. Lysol is a
   (a) Sterilent (b) Disinfectant
   (c) Antiseptic (d) Antifungul agent
10. "antagonism" is seen in
    (a) Log phase (b) Plasmids
    (c) Colplasmid (d) Both b and c
11. In streptococcus fecalis where the conjugation takes place
    (a) Pili (b) Cell membrane
    (c) Cell wall (d) flagella
12. The infected mad dogs may contain
    (a) Nergi bodies (b) Niagri bodies
    (c) Negri bodies (d) Neisser bodies
13. In which disease the nesser will produce
    (a) Mumps (b) rubella
    (c) Polio (d) measles
14. the first phase of growth curve is
    (a) log phase (b) lag phase
    (c) $\gamma$ phase (d) both a and b
15. The plasmids involved in
    (a) DNA replication
    (b) Protein synthesis
    (c) Cell wall synthesis
    (d) None of the above
16. Rancidity is spoiled foods is due to
    (a) Lipolytic organism
    (b) Protiolytic organism
    (c) Toxigenic microbes
    (d) Saccharolytic microbes
17. Which of the following is a neutral stain
    (a) Picric acid (b) Gmiemsa
    (c) Neutral red (d) Malachite green

18. Multiple antibiotic resistance is mediated by
    (a) Episome (b) Plasmid
    (c) Colplasmid (d) Both b and c
19. The genetic material in HIV in
    (a) Ds DNA (b) SsDNA
    (c) S-RNA (d) None
20. Mycoplasmas are bacterial cells that
    (a) Fail to reproduce on artificial media
    (b) Have a rigid cell wall
    (c) Are resistant to penicillin
    (d) Stain well with gram's stain
21. In gram positive and gram negative bacteria the electron transport contains
    (a) Naphthquinone (b) Plastoquinone
    (c) Ubiquinone (d) Both a and b
22. Protein particles which can infect are called
    (a) Virons (b) Prions
    (c) Nucleoida (d) none
23. Which virus was first observed
    (a) hepatitis virus
    (b) TMV
    (c) Cauliflower mosaic virus
    (d) none
24. Poly A tail is frequently found in
    (a) Histone in RNA (b) Bacterial RNA
    (c) Eukariotic RNA (d) TRNA
25. AIDS is caused by
    (a) Retrovirus (b) Prion
    (c) Rhabdovirus (d) retroprison
26. A major ingradient of penicillin production media is
    (a) Corn meal
    (b) Corn steep liquer
    (c) Cane steep liquer
    (d) none
27. peptone water medium is an example for
    (a) synthetic medium
    (b) semisynthetic medium
    (c) differntial medium
    (d) none of these
28. The etiologic agent of botulism is a
    (a) Neurotoxin (b) Endotoxin
    (c) Enterotoxin (d) All of the above
29. Which of the following is an example of live vaccine
    (a) Pertusis (b) Mumps
    (c) Cholera (d) rabies
30. The bacterial cells are at their metabolic peak during
    (a) Lag phase (b) Log
    (c) Stationary (d) decline
31. The method in which the cells are frozen dehydrated is called
    (a) Pasteurisation (b) Dessication
    (c) Disinfection (d) lypophilization
32. listeriosis was ----------disease
    (a) food borne (b) water borne
    (c) milk borne (d) air borne
33. Pus forming forms are called as
    (a) Pyoderm
    (b) Pyogenic
    (c) Pyrogen
    (d) None of the above
34. Elek's gel diffusion test is used for the detection of
    (a) Tetani toxin (b) Cholern toxin
    (c) Diophtheria toxin (d) toxoid
35. In ELISA technique the antibodies are labeled by
    (a) Acredine organe
    (b) Alkaline phosphate
    (c) Neutral red
    (d) Bromothymol blue
36. Spirulina belongs to
    (a) Xanthophyceae (b) Cyanophyceae
    (c) Rhodophyceae (d) pheophyceae
37. The first antibody to contact invading microorganism was
    (a) IgG (b) IgM
    (c) IgA (d) IgD

38. Temprature required for pasteurization is
    (a) Above 150°C (b) Below 100°C
    (c) 110°C (d) none
39. which of the following is pathogen to human
    (a) spirogyra (b) cephaleuros
    (c) prototheca (d) b and c
40. The viruses that live as parasites on bacteria are
    (a) Fungi (b) Commensets
    (c) Bacteriophages (d) none
41. The antrax disease is most frequently infected in
    (a) Cattle (b) Sheeps
    (c) Rats (d) A and b
42. Staining material of gram positive bacterium is
    (a) Fast green (b) Haematoxylon
    (c) Crystal violet (d) Safranin
43. Separation of a single bacterial colony is call
    (a) Isolation (b) Separation
    (c) Pure culturing (d) all
44. The pigment present in red algae is
    (a) Rhodochrom
    (b) Fucoxanthin
    (c) Chlorophyll only
    (d) Chlorophyll +phycobilin
45. Which of the following is ionizing radiation
    (a) UV rays (b) IR
    (c) $\gamma$- rays (d) none
46. Cell cycle regulated by
    (a) Cyclones (b) Cdks
    (c) Cyclones and Cdks (d) none
47. Melate dehydrogenase enzyme is a
    (a) Transferase (b) Hydrolase
    (c) Isomerase (d) oxidoreductase
48. In E.Coli att site is in between
    (a) Gal and biogenes
    (b) Bio and niacin genes
    (c) Gal and B genes
    (d) None of these
49. A cell becomes flaccid when placed in a
    (a) Isotonic solution
    (b) Hypertonic solution
    (c) Hypotonic solution
    (d) Normal solution
50. Salt and sugar preserve foods because they
    (a) Make them acid
    (b) Produce a hypotonic environment
    (c) Deplete nutrients
    (d) Produce a hypertonic environment
51. Citrus canker is caused by
    (a) Phytomonas (b) Salmonella
    (c) Lactobacillus (d) Hay basillus
52. In a floroscent microscope the objective lens is made of
    (a) Glass (b) Quartz
    (c) Polythene (d) none
53. fixation of atmospheric nitrogenis by means of
    (a) biological process (b) lightining
    (c) ultraviolet light (d) all of the above
54. In a antigen heptenes are
    (a) Immunogenic
    (b) Non immunogenic
    (c) Antigenic
    (d) None
55. Important class of respiratory enzymes
    (a) NAD (b) Cytochromes
    (c) ATPase (d) hydrolase
56. The best vector for gene cloning
    (a) Relaxed control plasmid
    (b) Stringent control plasmid
    (c) Both a and b
    (d) None
57. The antibody that is first formed after infection is
    (a) IgG (b) IgM
    (c) IgD (d) IgE
58. Erytrocytes will get its ATP energy only by
    (a) Glycolysis (b) Kreb's cycle
    (c) Electron transport (d) HMP shunt
59. Virus will contain
    (a) Cell membrane (b) Cell wall
    (c) DNA (d) DNA or RNA

60. The bacterial pili mainly contain
    (a) Carbohydrates (b) Lipids
    (c) Proteins (d) Minerals
61. The wonder drug of second world war is produced by
    (a) Algae (b) Fungi
    (c) Bacteria (d) plants
62. Role of bacteria in carbon cycle is
    (a) Photosynthesis
    (b) Chemosynthesis
    (c) Breakdown of organic compounds
    (d) Assimilation of nitrogen compounds
63. Centromere is that part of chromosome where
    (a) Nucleoli are formed
    (b) Crossing over takes places
    (c) Chromatds are attached
    (d) Naking occures
64. Somatic cell of the adult body are haploid in many except
    (a) Vertebrates (b) Invertibrates
    (c) Fungi (d) Vascular plant
65. Congencial diseases are
    (a) Diseases present at birth
    (b) Deficiency diseases
    (c) Occur during life
    (d) Spread from one individual to another
66. The enzyme needed in biological systems for joining two molecules is called
    (a) Lyases (b) Diastases
    (c) Polymerases (d) Hydrolase
67. Antibodies in our body are produced by
    (a) B- lymphocytes (b) T- lymphocytes
    (c) Monocytes (d) RBCs
68. Thylakoid is present in
    (a) Mitochondria (b) Chloroplast
    (c) ER (d) Golgi apparatus
69. Production of RNA from DNA is called
    (a) Translation (b) RNA splicing
    (c) Transcription (d) Transposition
70. Meosomes are the part of
    (a) Plasma membrane (b) ER
    (c) Lysosomes (d) golgi
71. monoclonal antibodies are produced by
    (a) hybridoma technology
    (b) biotechnology
    (c) fermentation technology
    (d) none
72. First line of body defense is ?
    (a) Antibody molecules
    (b) Unbroken skin
    (c) Antigen molecules
    (d) Phagocytic cells
73. The photorespiration involves
    (a) Calvin cycle (b) Hatch-slack cycle
    (c) Glycolate cycle (d) Kreb's cycle
74. Bioleaching is done by
    (a) Protozoa (b) Bacteria
    (c) Algae (d) All of the above
75. Yeast extract is an excellent source of
    (a) Avitamin (b) Proteins
    (c) B vitamin (d) carbohydrates
76. Example of anaerobic medium
    (a) Wilson blair medium
    (b) Mac conkey broth
    (c) Robertson's cooked meat
    (d) EMB agar
77. Syphilis is caused by
    (a) Staphylococcus aureus
    (b) Yercinia psdtis
    (c) Treponima pallidum
    (d) Streptococcus syphilitic
78. Analysis of protein antigen by
    (a) Southern blot (b) Northern blot
    (c) Western blot (d) None
79. ELISA test is used for the identification of
    (a) Jaundice (b) AIDS
    (c) Cancer (d) diebetis
80. Autoclaving is carried at
    (a) dry heat
    (b) atmospheric pressure
    (c) 120°C
    (d) All

81. The apparatus used to maintain a continuous culture
(a) Chemostate (b) Autostate
(c) Thermostate (d) A and c

82. The nucleic acid of polio viruses is
(a) DNA (b) RNA -(+)type
(c) t-RNA (d) m-RNA

83. Diphtheria is caused by
(a) Corynebacterium (b) Staphylococcus
(c) Streptococcus (d) none

84. The most infectious food borne disease is
(a) Tetanus (b) Dysentery
(c) Gas gangrene (d) Botulism

85. Temperature in pasteurization is
(a) 62.8°C (b) 35.7°C
(c) 68.2°C (d) 60.8°C

86. Genetic constitution of the cell is
(a) Phenotype (b) Genotype
(c) Cryptotype (d) histotype

87. Virions means
(a) infectious virus particle
(b) non infectious particle
(c) incomplete particles
(d) defective virus particle

88. Rabies virus is
(a) nake RNA virus
(b) naked DNA virus
(c) enveloped RNAvirus
(d) enveloped DNA virus

89. Example for DNA virus
(a) polio virus (b) adeno virus
(c) echo virus (d) poty virus

90. The cellular immune response is mediated by
(a) Bcells (b) Tcells
(c) BTcells (d) Endothelial cell

91. The test used for the detection of typhoid fever
(a) WIDAL test (b) ELISA test
(c) Rosewaller test (d) Western blotting

92. m- RNA synthesis from DNA is termed
(a) Transcription (b) Transformation
(c) Translation (d) Replication

93. Kinetosomes are observed in
(a) Algae (b) Fungi
(c) Protozoa (d) viruses

94. Father of Microbiology is
(a) Louis Pasteur (b) Lister
(c) A.V. leeuwenhock (d) Robert Koch

95. Rapid bacterial growth phase is called
(a) Log (b) Lag
(c) Lack (d) None

96. The major constituents in agar are
(a) Fats (b) Aminoacids
(c) Polysaccharides (d) Polypeptides

97. Reagenic type of antibody is
(a) IgG (b) IgA
(c) IgM (d) IgE

98. The term mutation was coined by
(a) Pasteur (b) Darwin
(c) Hugo devries (d) Lamark

99. blood group antigens are
(a) species specific (b) isospecific
(c) autospecific (d) organspecific

100. mycotoxins are formed during the end of
(a) lag phase (b) log phase
(c) death phase (d) stationary phase

## Answer Key Microbiology

1. b
2. d
3. c
4. b
5. d
6. c
7. c
8. c
9. b
10. d
11. c
12. c
13. d
14. b
15. d
16. a
17. c
18. b
19. a
20. c
21. a
22. b
23. b
24. c
25. a
26. b
27. b
28. a
29. c
30. b
31. d
32. a
33. b
34. c
35. b
36. b
37. b
38. b
39. c
40. c
41. d
42. c
43. a
44. d
45. c
46. c
47. d
48. a
49. b
50. d
51. a
52. c
53. d
54. b
55. b
56. a
57. b
58. a
59. d
60. c
61. b
62. c
63. c
64. c
65. a
66. c
67. a
68. b
69. c
70. a
71. a
72. b
73. c
74. b
75. c
76. c
77. c
78. c
79. b
80. c
81. a
82. b
83. a
84. d
85. a
86. b
87. c
88. c
89. b
90. a
91. a
92. a
93. c
94. c
95. a
96. c
97. d
98. c
99. b
100. a

# Chapter 6

# Biochemistry

## 6.1 Vitamins

### Introduction

Vitamins are the naturally occurring org. compounds which are required (in addition to fats, carbohydrates, proteins, mineral salts & water) in minute amounts by the animals, some bacteria and microorganisms for maintenance & normal growth of the life, as they cannot synthesized by them except vitamin-D.

- The bacterium E-coli doesn't require org .vitamin as it can synthesis the entire vitamin.
- Vitamins from other organic food stuffs in that.
  - (i) They don't enter into tissue structures, unlike proteins.
  - (ii) Do not undergo degradation for providing energy in like carbohydrate and lipids.
  - (iii) Several B-complex vitamins plays an important role as "coenzymes" in several energy transformation reactions in the body,
- Vitamins differ from hormones in not being produced within the organism and most of then have to be provided in the diet.

**Classification of Vitamins:**

1. Fat Soluble Vitamins e.gVit A. D, E, α- lipoic acid & K
2. Water soluble vitamins
   - A. Non B – complex e.gVit- C
   - B. B- complex
     - (i) Energy releasing e.g. $\mathbf{B_1}$, $\mathbf{B_2}$ ,$\mathbf{B_3}$, $\mathbf{B_6}$ ,$\mathbf{B_7}$Pantothenic acid
     - (ii) Hematopoietice.g. Folic acid,Vit. $\mathbf{B_{12}}$

**Note:** Some authors categorized niacin &pantothenic acid as BB & Bf respectively & some are categorized niacin & pantothenic acid as B, & B; respectively.

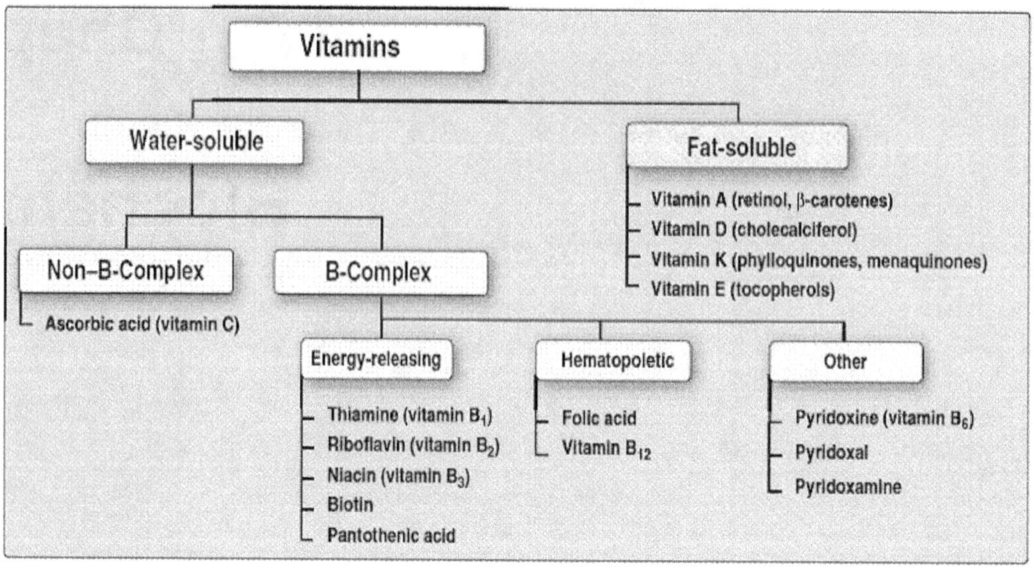


**Difference between fat soluble & water soluble vitamins:**

| S. No. | Fat soluble Vitamins | Water soluble vitamins |
|---|---|---|
| 1. | These are soluble in fats | These are soluble in water |
| 2. | Required bile salts & fats for absorption | These are easily absorbed |
| 3. | Normally these are not excreted in urine | These have a threshold for urinary excretion |
| 4. | Generally stored in lever | These are not stored in body except $\mathbf{B_{12}}$ |
| 5. | These are generally isoprenoid compound | These are not isoprenoid compounds |

These are some biological inactive compounds which are quite similar to vitamins in structure. They are known as provitamins as they are converted easily into active vitamins vivo. e.g carotenes & ergosterol are provitamins for Vit A &Vit$\mathbf{D_2}$respectively.

## Vitamin-A

### Biochemical functions

(Note: The Biochemical function of V it. A can be remembered in the term of TV BEMA)

T- It plays role in construction of normal teeth in deficiency of Vit.-A teeth becomes unhealthy due to thinning of enamel and chalky deposits on surfaces.

V- Role in vision: It plays a major role in visual system which occurs in a cyclic process known as Rhodopin cycle or walds visual cycle.

B- Role in Bone It plays role in construction of normal bone. Deficiency results is slower Of endochondral bone formation & decreased osteoblastic activity, The bone becomes cancellous losing their final structure.

E- Epithelial tissue Vit-A essential to maintain healthy epithelial tissue. This is due to fact that retinols retinoic acid is required to prevent Keratin synthesis.

M- Metabolism: Vit-A is also believed to be involved is the biosynthesis of mucopolysaccharides Such as chondrotin sulphates & metabolism of protein synthesis & also in metabolism of DNA.

A- Antioxidants: Carotenoids (most important β - carotene) function as antioxidant & reduce the risk of cancers initiated by the free radicals and strong oxidants.

**Deficiency of Vitamin-A**

(**Note:** The Deficiency of Vitamin-A can be remembered in the term of **X-Ray USG**)

X- Xerophthalmia or xerosis Severe deficiency of Vt-A leads to xerophlthmia& is characterized dryness of cornea, conjunctivitis &keratinizatlon or epithelial cells and contains areas of conjuctiva, white triangular plaques known as Biots spot are seen

**According to WHO classification:**

**Primary signs:**

'X' - **$X_1$A**- Conjunctivalxerosis

**$X_1$B**- Bitots spot appear in convectived on either side of cornea of the eye

**$X_2$** - Corneal Xerasis / Dryness

**$X_3$A**- Corneal ulcers (less than $1/3^d$ of cornea)

**$X_3$B**- Corneal ulcers (more than $1/3^d$ of cornea)

**Secondary sign:** corned scars nyetalopia (night blindness)

'R' - Reproduction - reproductive stem is adversely affected due to degeneration of germinal epithelial cells leads to sterility of male. Termination of pregnancy due to fatal death observed.

'U' - Urinary stone formation

'S' - Skin become rough and dry keratenization occurs.

'G'- Growth retardation occurs due to impairment of skeletal formation.

**Therapeutic uses**

1. Treatment of established Vit-A deficiency: 50,000 - 100,000 IU 1M or orally for 1-3 days followed by intermittent supplemental doses.
2. Prophylaxis of Vit-A deficiency during infancy, pregnancy, lactation, hepatobiliary disease, steatorthelo : 3000-5000 IU / day.
3. Skin disease: All trans retinoic. acid (Tretinoin) used topically for acne while 13-cis retinoic acid (Isotretinoin) used orally for acne .
4. Decreased risk of heart attacks, skin & lung cancers (by ß-carotenes).

## Vitamin D

**Biochemical function**

(Note: The Biochemical functions of Vit-D can be remembered in the term of IBK)

**'I'-** Intestine: Calcitriol (1 .25 DH cc) is the biologically active form of. Vit-D increase the

Intestinal absorption of calcium and phosphate.

**'B'-** Bone: In the osteoblast of bone, calcitriol stimulates calcium update for deposition as calcium phosphate

**'K;-** Kidney: Calcitriol involved in minimizing the excretion of calcium &phosphate through the kidney by decreasing their excretion & enhancing reabsorption.

**Deficiency:**

1. Rickets in children &osteomalacia in adult
2. Renal osteodystrophy. - Excessive bone turn over & structural change.

**Therapeutic use:**

1. prophylaxis ofVit-D deficiency
2. metabolic ricket
3. senile or post menopausal osteoporosis
4. Hypoparathyroidism
5. Franconia syndrome
6. In psoriasis, skin cancer & immunological disorder.

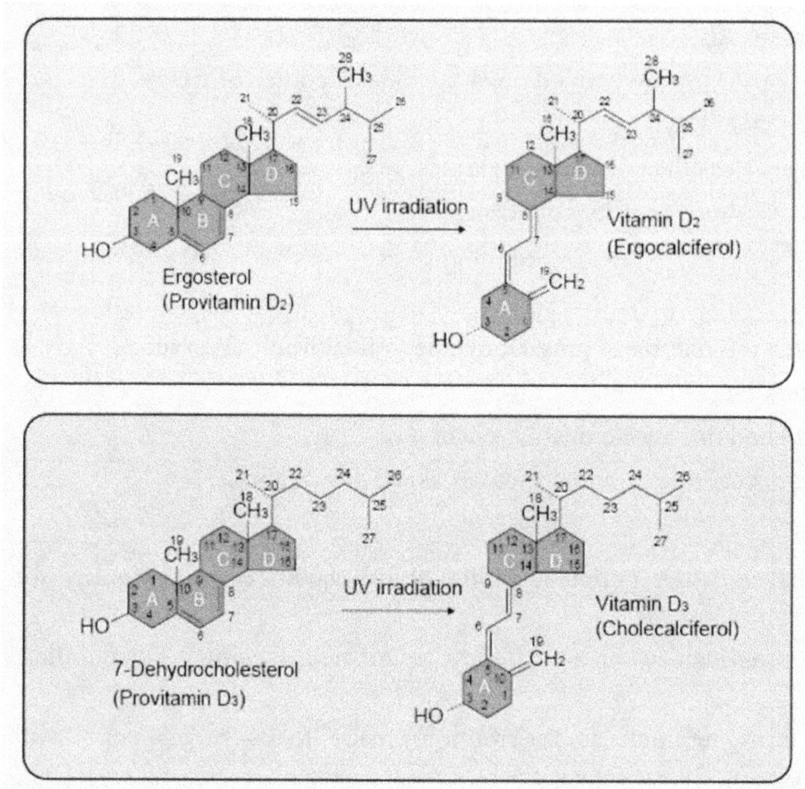


## Vitamin - E

Biochemical Function: RAM

1. **Role in reproduction:** Vit-E is closely associated: with reproductive functions and prevents sterility, V it-E preserves and maintains germinal epithelium of gonads for proper reproductive function.
2. **As on antioxidant:** The main role of Vitamin-E appears to be as a cellular antioxidant where it stabilizes poly unsaturated fatty acids thus certain fats, Vit-A, carotene of sulphur containing acids.
   - The presence of phenolic (hydroxyl) group at the positon 6 of
   - The presence of phenolic (hydroxyl) group at the position 6 of the chromane ring is the most important functional group for its antioxidant activity.
   - Vit E is the lipophlic in charter and is found in association with lipoproteins, fat deposits and cellular membrane. It protects the unsaturated fatty acid (PUFA) from peroxidation reaction. It acts as a scavengers gets itself oxidized to Quinone from) by free radicals K &spanes UFA, as

     Reaction showing the donation of H by Vitamin –E. Vitamin –E is oxidize to Quinone from.

**3. Metabolic Function**

- A tocopherolactone, a metabolite of tocopherol is believed to play a role in the biosynthesis of coenzyme Q(Ubiquinone) in certain tissues.
- Vitamin –E is involved in biological oxidation, most probably between Cytochrome b&c
- Vitamin –E plays some role in nucleic acid synthesis.
- Vit. E plays a role in heme synthesis by enhancing the actions of enzymes aminolevulinic acid (ALA) synthases & ALA dehydratase.
- Vit. E is required for proper storage of creatinine in skeletal muscles.

**Deficiency of Vitamin –E**

1. Muscular dystrophy
2. Hemolylic anaemia
3. Dietary hepatic necrosis
4. Sterility

**Table** Clinical & therapeutic case

| Disease | Mechanism of action of Vit -E |
|---|---|
| **Nocturnal muscle cramps (NMC)** | By Virtue of its antioxidant property vit-E prevents oxidation of certain radicals & ensures better utilization of oxygen in muscle tissue, thereby improving muscle metabolism. |
| **Intermittent claudication (IC)** | A decrease in circulating lactate level & increase in pyruvate level. Improvement of blood supply due to opening of new vessels improving circulation. |
| **Fibroblastic breast disease (FBD)** | Acts by correcting the deranged progesterone estragon ration in women of FBD |
| **Atherosclerosis** | Inhibits the formation of lipid peroxidase & restores PG - $I_2$ synthesis Inhibits platelets aggregation.,nElevates HDL – cholesterol level (increased scavenging action ↑ |

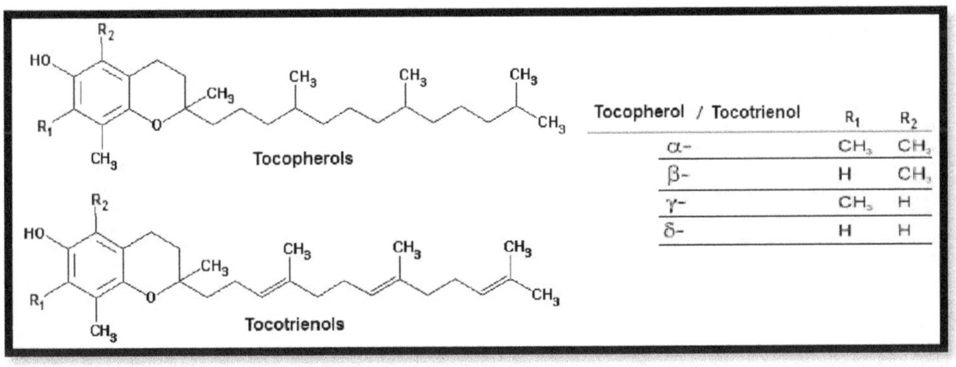


## Vitamin – K

**Biochemical Function:**

1. **Blood Coagulation:** The main function of Vit-K is promotion of blood coagulation by helping in the post – transcriptional modification of blood factors such as prothrombin, and factors II, VII, IX & X.

   Enzymes that forms γ carboxyl glutamate (GLA0 from glutamate is known as the carboxylase (microsomal). The same enzyme requires Vit-K as the coenzyme.

   Carboxylation: It was suggested that carboxylation reaction require the intermediate formation like 2, 3 epoxide derivatives of Vit-K.

2. **Calcium bending proteins:** Vit-K similarly is found to be carboxylate specific glutamate residues of calcium bending proteins of bones. Spleen placenta & kidneys. This enhance the capacity of those protein to deposit calcium in the tissue concerned.
3. **Role in oxidative phosphorylation:** Vit-K also plays important role as a cofactor in oxidative phosphorylation, taking places or the inner mitochondrial membranes.

**Deficiency symptoms**

1. The blood clotting time is increased.
2. In new born infants: Hypoprothrobinemia & bleeding in many tissue occur

## Vitamin – C (Ascorbic acid)

**Biochemical function:**

1. Role in collagen synthesis – Hydroxy proline & hydroxyl lysine are important constituents of collagen fibre.
2. Role in bone formation
3. Iron & Haemoglobin Metabolism
4. Tryptophan Metabolism
5. Tyrosine Metabolism
6. Absorption of iron
7. Cellular oxidation (Reduction process)

**Deficiency Sympion**

**Scurvy – Sympions**

- Sore & Spongy gums
- Loose teeth
- Anemia
- Fragile blood caplliancies
- Poor dentine formation
- Delayed wound healing

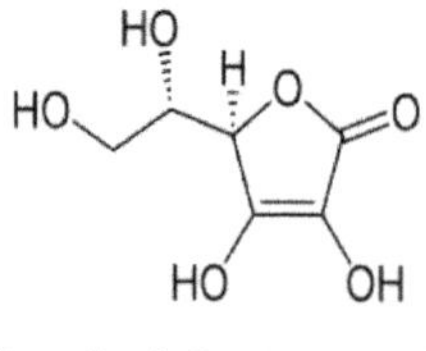


**Figure 1** Chemical Structure of Vitamin C

## Thiamine ($B_1$)

**Biochemical function:**

Biological active form – Thiamine pyrophosphate (TPP) acts as a coenzyme in several metabolic functions.

1. Acts as coenzyme to the enzyme pyruvate dehydrogenase complex (PDH) which convents pyruvic acid to acetyl CoA oxidative decarboxylation.
2. Acts as a coenzyme to $\alpha$ – oxgulatanate dehydrogenase complex & convents $\alpha$ – oxogulanatate to tosuccinyl CoA (Oxidative decarboxylation)
3. TPP also acts as a coenzyme with the enzyme transketolase in transketolase in reaction in HMP shunt pathway of glucose metabolism

4. Transmission of nerve impulses: TPP plays a major role is the transmission of nerve impulses because TPP essential for the synthesis of neurotransmeter Acetyocholine.

**Deficiency ymptoms of Thiamine ($B_1$)**

**Berry –Berry**

(a) Dry Berry – Berry Oedema is not associates, polyneuritis predominates .

(b) Wet Berry- Berry Cardiovascular as neurological symptoms oedema associated .

(c) Wrincke – knorsakoff syndrome: loss of memory, apathy & typical movements of eye wall

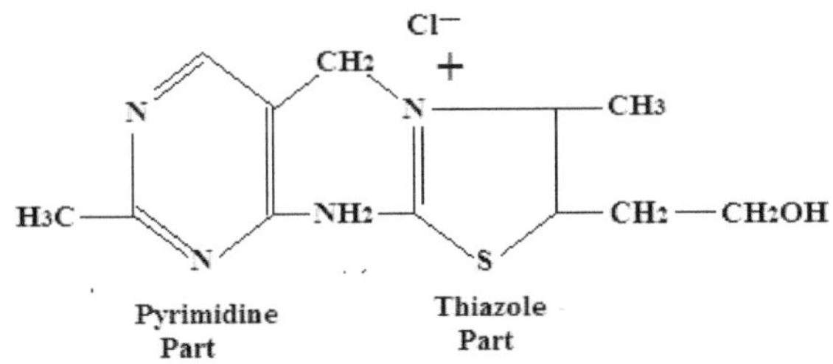


**Figure 2** Chemical Structure of Vitamin $B_1$

## Riboflavin ($B_2$ or Vitamin G)

**Biochemical Function:**

- The Biochemical active form of the cofactor FMN & FAD acts an cofactors in many numbers of the hydrogen transfer reaction in metabolism.

| Enzyme (FAD Dependent) | Reaction |
|---|---|
| **A. Carbohydrate metabolism** | |
| 1. Pyruvate dehydrogenase complex | Pyruvate → Acetyl CoA |
| 2. A- ketoglutrate dehydrogenase complex | α- ketogulatmate → Succinyl CoA |
| 3. Succinate dehydrogenase complex | Sccinate to formant |
| **B. Lipid Metabolism** | |
| 1. Acylo CoA dehydrogenase | Acetyl CoA → α, β unsaturated acyl Co |
| **C. Protein Metabolism** | |
| 1. Glycine oxidase | Glycine → glyoxylate + NH3 |
| 2. D-amino oxidase | D – amino acid → α keto acid + NH3 |
| **D. Purire Metabolism** | |
| 1. Xanthine oxidase | Xanthine → Hypoxanthine → Uric acid |

**FMN dependant**

1. Cytoichrome – C – Reductase → Cytochrome $C_1$Fection
2. L-amino acid oxidese → L – amino acid + α – ketoacid + NH3

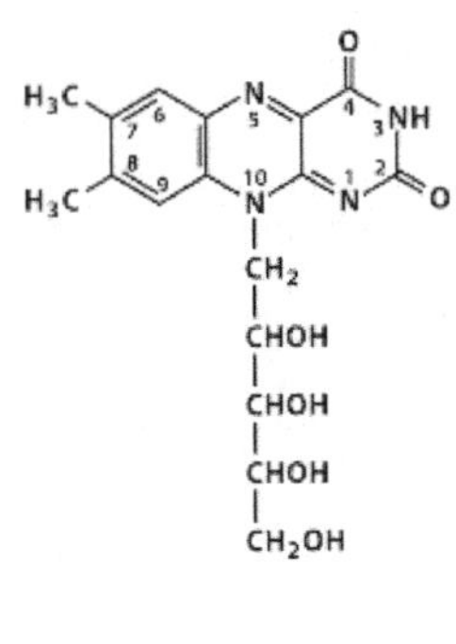

## 6.2 Enzyme and Hormones

Hormones and Enzymes play a vital role in our body by controlling and regulating many functions. Hormones are known as chemical messengers as they trigger many functions while enzymes are catalysts as they affect the rate of a reaction.

**Hormones -** Hormones are a group of biomolecules which are produced in the ductless glands and are carried to different parts of the body by the blood stream where they control various metabolic processes or show physiological activity. Example: insulin, glucagon etc.

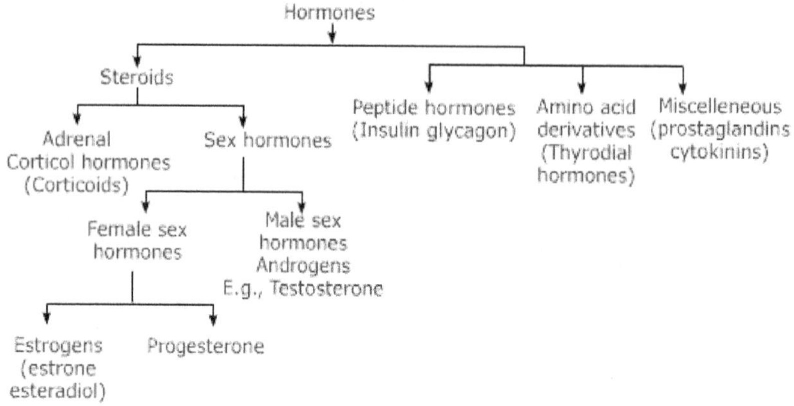


**Enzyme -** Enzymes can be defined as biological polymers that catalyze biochemical reactions."

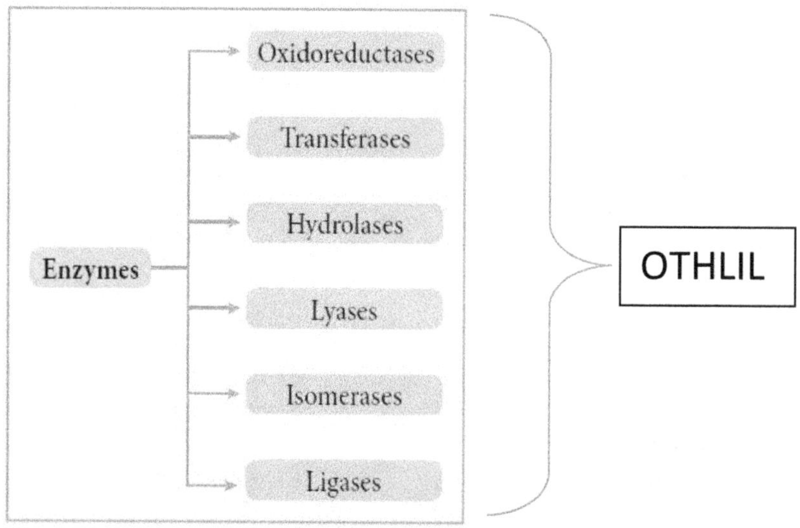


| Types | Biochemical Property |
|---|---|
| **Oxidoreductases** | The enzyme Oxidoreductase catalyzes the oxidation reaction where the electrons tend to travel from one form of a molecule to the other. |
| **Transferases** | The Transferases enzymes help in the transportation of the functional group among acceptors and donor molecules. |
| **Hydrolases** | Hydrolases are hydrolytic enzymes, which catalyze the hydrolysis reaction by adding water to cleave the bond and hydrolyze it. |
| **Lyases** | Adds water, carbon dioxide or ammonia across double bonds or eliminate these to create double bonds. |
| **Isomerases** | The Isomerases enzymes catalyze the structural shifts present in a molecule, thus causing the change in the shape of the molecule. |
| **Ligases** | The Ligases enzymes are known to charge the catalysis of a ligation process. |

**Biochemical Role of Enzymes**

Definition: Enzymes may be defined as biocatalysts synthesized by living cells. They are protein in natural (exception-RNA acting as ribozymes) colloidal &thermolabile in character & specific in their action.

**Classification of enzymes:**

Enzymes are classified under four board categories.

(a) Intracellular enzymes: They are functional within the cells where they are synthesized.

(b) Extracellular enzymes: They are active outside the cell e.g all digestive tract enzyme

(c) Constitutive enzymes: They are formed at constant rates & in constant amount regardless of the metabolic state of the cell or organism. E.g enzymes of glycolytic sequence.

(d) Inducible enzyme: They are present in very small amounts in a cell. When enzyme substrate is present. Enzyme concentration can increase threshold fold or more. e.g. β glactosidase Cyclooxygenase-2 (Cox-2)

According to IUB system enzymes are classified as follows

| Enzymes class | Example | Reaction catalysed |
|---|---|---|
| **Oxidoreductose** | Alcohol dehydraserase, cytochrome oxidase | $Oxd^n \rightarrow Red^n$ |
| **Transferases** | Hexokinase, Transaminase, transmethylase, phosphatase | Transfer of functioned group A-X+B → A+B-X |
| **Hydrolases** | Lipase, Cholineesterase , Urease, Phosphatase | Hydrolytic reaction<br>A-B + H2O → AH + BOH |
| **Leases** | Aldolase, histidase, fumarase | Group elimination to from double bonds & addition of groups to double bonds.<br>A-B + X-Y → A-X + BY |
| **Isomerases** | Retinolisomerease, glucose phosphate isomerase | Interconversion of isomers<br>A → A |
| **Ligases** | Glutominesynthetase succinate thiokinase | Bond formation coupled with ATP hydrolysis. |

**Note:** The word "OTHLIL" is used to recognize the six classes.

**Chemical nature & property of enzymes.**

- All enzymes are protein but few RNA molecules have function as enzymes.
- Ribozymes are also know as RNA enzyme or catalytic RNA (e.g RNA from E-Coil)
- The functional part of the enzyme is called holoenzyme
- Holoenzyme → Apoenzyme + Coenzyme
- (Active enzyme) (Protein Part) (non protein part)
- The coenzyme can be separated by dialysis, but the non-protein part which is very tightly bound to epoenzyme & cannot be separated by dialysis called prosthetic group.
- The monomeric enzyme is made up of a single polypeptide e.g. ribonuclear, tryspin, Oligmeric enzyme made up of more than one polypeptide chain e.g. locate dehydrogenase.
- Enzymes show all the general properties of proteins.

**Specificity of enzymes**

Enzymes are very specific in nature i.e. particular enzyme of lake only a particular substrate. Thus an enzyme can catalyse a small range of reaction or only one reaction. In general the stereo & substrate specificity is due to opoenzy me part of holoenzyme, while the reaction specificity in due to the coenzyme or prosthetic group. Three types of enzymes specificity are well recognized.

## Differences among Enzymes, Hormones & Vitamins

| Enzymes | Hormones | Vitamins |
|---|---|---|
| **These are specific catalytic** | These are regulatory substance | These are accessory substances |
| **All enzymes are proteinaceous** | Hormones are steroids Or Peptides (Insulin, Oxytocin)<br>Or Amino acid derivative<br>(e.g. thyroxine, adrenalin) | Vitamins belonge to nature (estradiol) diverse group chemically nutrients |
| **These are synthesized by the animal cell** | These are synthesized within some part of body | These are not synthesized by most animal cell. Plants can however synthesized them |
| **These can initiate and continue reaction** | Can not initiate reaction but can influence the rate at which they proceed. | - |
| **These are not consumed during growth** | Consumed during growth | - |
| **These are involved in coenzyme system** | These are not involved in coenzyme system | -involved |
| **These operate in biological System e.g Pepsin, Cytochrome Oxide,** | Only some hormones are involved in enzyme system e.g Estradiol, Adrenalin | Most vitamins are Involved in enzyme e.g. A,D,F,K,BVitamin&C |

## 6.3 Carbohydrates

Carbohydrates are the compounds which contain carbon, hydrogen & oxygen. They are commonly known as saccharides or sugars. Carbohydrates are widely distributed in nature in plants and animals. The most common carbohydrate found in plants is Starch. The carbohydrate found in animal is Glycogen. It is a storage form of carbohydrates found in liver and muscles.

**Chemical composition:** carbohydrate have an empirical formula Cn(H2O)n.

- Carbohydrates are compound containing Carbon, Hydrogen and Oxygen.
- Carbohydrates are actually sugars.
- They are also called Saccharides.
- Carbohydrates are carbonyl derivatives of poly hydroxyl alcohol.
- They are obtained on hydrolysis.
- Ratio of hydrogen and oxygen is 2:1.

Carbohydrates are naturally occurring organic compounds containing carbon, hydrogen,oxygen elements. Chemically Carbohydrates are Polyhydroxy aldehyde or Polyhydroxyketones or the compounds that produce these on hydrolysis. Carbohydrates are also referred as saccharide.

On the basis of sugar unit carbohydrate are classified into three major classes:

1. Monosaccharides
2. Oligosaccharides
3. Polysaccharides

1. **Mono saccharides:**

   Mono saccharides contain Single sugar unit. Also called simple sugars, cannot be hydrolyzed into smaller units. Depending upon no. of carbon in a unit, mono saccharides are subdivided into a dioses to decoses. More common subclasses of mono saccharides are:

**Aldoses:** Contain aldehyde as Funtional group

- Aldotrioses e.g. Glycerose,
- Aldotertroses e.g. Erythrose,
- Aldopentoses e.g. Ribose,
- Aldohexoscs e.g. Glucose (dextrose), Galatose (present in milk)
- Aldoheptose e.g. Glucoheptose.

**Ketoses:** Contain Ketone as functional group

- Ketotriosese.g Dihydroxyacetone,
- Ketotetrosese.gErythrulose,
- Ketopentosese.g Ribulose,
- Ketohexoses e.g. Fructose present in fruits honey
- Ketoheptose e.g. Scdoheptulose.

**Properties of Mono saccharides:**

1. Muta-rotation
2. Glycoside Formation
3. Reducing Power
4. Reduction
5. Oxidation with mild and strong oxidizing agent
6. Methylation / Esterification
7. Dehydration
8. Form osazone with phenyl hydrazine

2. **Oligosaccharide**: Oligosaccharides are polymers of mono saccharides containing two to ten mono saccharides:

   **1. Disaccharides:** Yield two mono saccharides on hydrolysis.

   **a. Reducing Disaccharides:** Contain hemiacetal or hemiketal group

   Example: Maltose (Glucose + Glucose) Germinating grain (used to make beer)

   Lactose (Galactose + Glucose), other examples are Isomaltose.

   **b. Non Reducing Disaccharides:** Contain no hemiacetal groups

   Example: Sucrose (Glucose + Fructose)

   **2. Tri saccharides:** Example: Raffinose (Glucose + Fructose + Galactose) found in cotton seed and sugar beet.

   **3. Tetra saccharides:** Yield 4 mono saccharides on hydrolysis. Example: Stachyose (Glucose + Fructose + Galactose + Galactose) (only tetra saccharide known to exist in plant e.g. Whole grains, peas, lentils)

3. **Polysaccharides:** Polysaccharides are polymer of monosaccharides. The long chain polymers are either straight chain or branched. They are also called glycanes. On hydrolysis produces monosaccharides. They are Non-sugar and tasteless. General formula $(C_6H_{10}O_5)_n$ Insoluble in water and form colloids with water. Example: Starch, Cellulose, Pectin

**Classification of Polysaccharides:**

✓ On the Basis of Function:

**(a) Storage** Example: Starch, Plant store glucose as starch. The cereal grain (wheat, rice, corn, oat, barley) as well as tuber (potato) rich in starch. Glycogen storage form of glucose in animal and human which is analogous to the starch in plant. Glycogen is synthesized and stored mainly in the liver and muscles.

**(b) Structural** Example: Cellulose, Pectin

✓ On the basis of composition:

a. **Homo Polysaccharides:** On hydrolysis gives single monosaccharide units
- Pentosan: Contains pentoses
- Hexosans: Contains hexoses subdivided in to
- Glucosans: Polymer or glucose e.g. Starch, Glycogen
- Fructosans: Polymer or fructose e.g. Inulin
- Galactans: Polymer of galactose e.g. Galactan
- Mannans: Polymer of mannose e.g. Mananas.

b. **Hetero Polysaccharide**: e.g. Hyaluronic acid, Chondroitin sulphates.

Gum: Consist of arabinose, rhamnose, galactose and glucoronic acid.

Agar: The sulphuric acid esters of galactans consists of galactose, galactouronic acid.

Pectins: Fundamental unit is pectic acid, consist of arabinosc, galactose, galactouronic acid.

**Functions of Polysaccharides:**

1. They serve as structural components of the cells
2. They serve as stored form of energy.
3. They serve as nutrient.

**Biological role of carbohydrate**

1. Most abundant dietary source of energy (4cal/g).
2. Serve as storage form of energy (glycogen) to meet the immediate energy demand of the body.
3. Precursor for synthesis of many compounds (Fatty acid and Amino acid).
4. Glycolipid and Glycoprotein participate in structure of cell membrane and cell function, cell growth, adhesion (cell to cell attachment), fertilization.
5. Structural component of many organisms. Cellulose in plant cell wall. Chitin in Exoskeleton of some insects. Cell wall of microorganism
6. Structural component: Pentose sugar (Deoxy ribose and ribose sugar) in DNA and RNA.

## Carbohydrate Metabolism

### Glycolysis

**Greek:** Glycose = Sweet Lysis = dissolution

**Definition:** It is the sequence of 10 enzyme catalysed reaction that converts glucose into pyruvate with the simultaneous production of ATP.

**Phase of Glycolysis:**

During glycolysis, the 6 carbon glucose is broken down into two mole of 3 carbon pyruvate via 10 enzyme catalysed sequential reaction. These reaction are grouped under two phase, phase I & phase II.

**Phase I or Preparatory phase:**

It consists of the first 5 step. In these reaction, glucose is enzymatically phosphorylated by ATP (first at carbon 6 & later at carbon I) to yield fructose 1, 6 diphosphate which is then split in half to yield 2 mole of the 3 carbon compound glyceraldehyde. 3 phosphate. The first phase of glycoses thus results in cleavage of the hexose chain. This phase requires an investment of ATP mole to active (or prime) the glucose mole @ prepare for its cleavage into two 3 – carbon pieces. Besides glucose, other hexoses such as as D-fructose, D-mannose may also convert into glyceraldehyde's 3-phosphate.

**Phase II or pay off phase:** The lose 5 reaction of glycolysis constitute this phase. This phase represents the payoff of glycolysis, in which the energy liberated during conversion of 3-moles of glyceraldehyde's 3-phosphate to 3-mole of pyruvate is converted by the coupled phosphorylation of 4 mole of ADP to ATP. Although 4 moles of ATP are formed in phase II the net overall yield is only 2 moles of ATP per mole of glucose is oxidised since 2 mole of ATP are invested in phase-I. The phase- II is thus energy conserving.

## Reaction Steps in Gluconeogenesis

### Cori Cycle

Under anaerobic condition the lactate formed from the oxygen of glucose is the important precursors of gluconeogenesis. The conversion of lactic acid to glucose occurs entirely in the liver through Cori cycle.

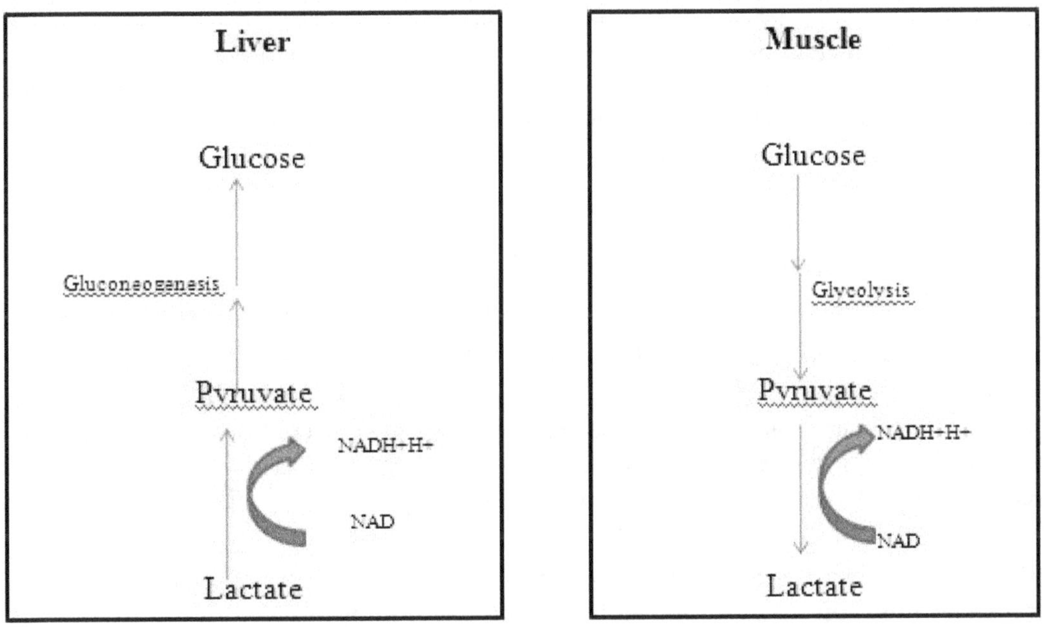


The cycle involving the synthesis of glucose is liver from the skeletal muscle lactate & the reuse of glucose thus synthesized by the muscle for energy purpose is known Cori Cycle.

### Glucose- Alanine Cycle

The glycogenic amino acids are transminated to TCA cycle intermediate which from oxaloacetate or pyruvate. Alinine is the major is the major substrate for glycogenosis which is released from mussel. Alquine is transported to form pyruvate, which is then converted to glucose. Glucose can enter is glycolysis formatting pyruvate, which can be trasminated to from alanine. This cycle i.eglcose alanine is of primary importance in starvation.

**Energy yield of the citric acid cycle**

A grand total of 12 ATP molecules is formed during complete oxygen of one mole of acetyl CoA i.e during one tur of citric acid cycle (However a total of 15 ATP moles is format when we start with the oxidation of 1 mol. Of pyruvate. This corresponds to a total of 38 ATP moles for the oxygen of 1 mole of glucose.

### Organ Function Test

### Liver Function Test

1. Tests based excretory function e.g – Bile salt, Bile pigment, Bromeslpthalein
2. Tests based on serum enzymeeg. – Determination of transaminases , Alakine phosphatase,5'- nucleotidase, γ- glutamyltranspeptidase,serumisocitrate dehydrogenase, Isoenzymes of lactate de

## 6.4 Proteins

"Proteins are nitrogenous organic compounds of high molecular weight which play a vital or prime role in living organisms."

### Introduction

The proteins are most abundant macro molecules in the cells and they constitute over half the dry weight of most of the organism. They are made up of 20 standard a-amino acids. They are mainly composed of C, H, O, N elements. Some proteins also contain S, P element also. Chemically proteins are polymers of L-α-amino acids. Amino acids are polymerized through formation of number of peptide linkages. Protein molecule consists of very long chains having about 100-1000 amino acids unit joined by Peptide linkages. Cell contains 100 or 1000 of different protein, each with different function and biological activity.

### Properties of Protein

1. Solubility: Form colloidal solution in water
2. Molecular weight: Majority of amino acid consist of 40-4000 amino acid. Molecular weight (4000- 44000).
3. Shape: Globular (Insulin, enzymes), Oval (Albumin), Fibrous/Elongated (Fibrinogen).
4. Isoelectric pH: Protein exists as Zwitter ion or dipolar ion. The pH at which a protein has equal number of positive and negative charges is known as isoelectric pH. When subjected to an electric field the proteins do not move either towards anode or cathode, hence this property is used to isolate proteins. The proteins become least soluble atIsoelectric pH and get precipitated. The Isoelectric pH of casein is 4.5 and at this pH thecasein in milk curdles producing the curd.
5. Precipitation of protein: By dehydration or neutralization.
6. Precipitation by salting out: Sodium sulphate and ammonium sulphate.
7. Precipitation by heavy metal: $Pb^{2+}$, $Hg^{2+}$, $Fe^{2+}$ ,$Zn^{2+}$, $Cd^{2+}$.
8. Precipitation by anionic or alkaloidal reagent: Tannic acid, Trichloro acetic acid and sulphosalicylicacd etc.
9. Denaturation: Partial or complete unfolding (disorganization) of the native (natural) protein structure is known as denaturation. This is caused by heat, acids, alkalies, alcohol, acetone, urea, beta- mercaptoethanol.
10. Coagulation: When proteins are denatured by heat, they form insoluble aggregates known as coagulum. All the proteins are not heat coagulable, only a few like the albumins, globulins are heat coagulable.

## Classification of Proteins

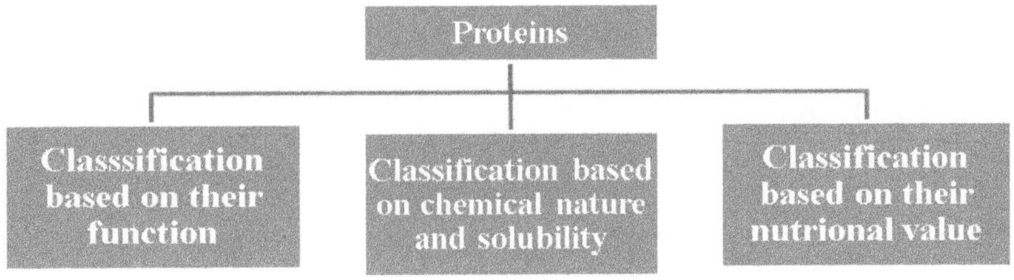


**A. Classification based on their Function –**

1. Structural Protein – keratin of hair and nails, collagen of bone.
2. Enzyme (catalytic protein) – Pepsin.
3. Transport Proteins – Hemoglobin.
4. Hormonal Protein – Insulin.
5. Contractile Protein – Actin and myosin.
6. Storage Protein – ovalbumine and glutelin.
7. Genetic Protein – Nucleoprotein.
8. Defense Protein – snake venoms and immunoglobulin.
9. Receptor Protein – Hormones.

**B. Classification based on chemical nature and solubility –**

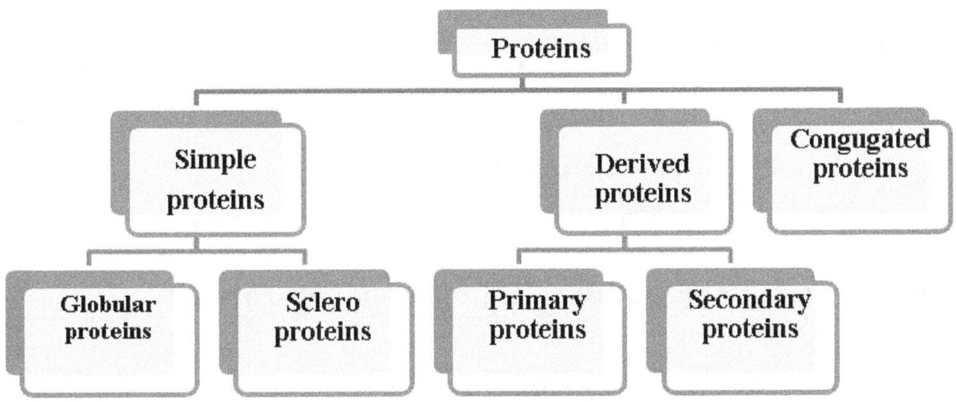


**A. Simple Proteins** – They contain only one amino acid.

**a. Globular Proteins**

**1. Albumins**

- Soluble in water and salt solution.
- Coagulated by heat.
- Ex- Serum albumin and Lactalbumine.

**2. Globulins**

- Soluble in neutral and dilute salt solution.
- Coagulated by heat.
- Ex – Serum globulins Ovoglobulin.

**3. Glutelins**

- Soluble in dilute acids and alkalies but Insoluble in water.
- Mostly found in plant.
- Coagulated by heat.
- Ex- Glutelin (wheat), Oryzenin ( rice)

**4. Prolamines**

- Insoluble in water but soluble in ethanol.
- Not coagulated by heat.
- Ex- Gliadin (wheat) and Zein (maize)

**5. Histones**

- Soluble in water but insoluble in dilute ammonium hydroxide.
- Not coagulated by heat.
- Ex – Thymus histones and Globin of heamoglobin and Histones of codefish sperm.

**6. Globins**

- These are generally consisting of histones.
- They are not precipitated by $NH_4OH$.

**7. Protamines**

- They are simplest and basic in nature.
- Soluble in water and $NH_4OH$.
- Not coagulated by heat
- Ex- Sardinine and Cryptinine.

**b. Scleroproteins – Also called Fibrous Proteins.**

**1. Collagen**

- Connective tissue protein.
- Collagens on boiling with water or dilute acid give gelatin.
- This gelatin is soluble and digestible.

**2. Elastins**

- These proteins are found in elastic tissues such as **tendon and arteries.**

**3. Keratins**

- These are present in exoskeletal structures.
- Ex – Hairs, Nails and Horns.

**B. Derived Proteins** – These are formed from simple and conjugated proteins.

**I. Primary Proteins**

1. **Coagulated proteins** – These are denatured proteins produced by agents such as- heat, acids and alkalis.
   **Ex** – cooked proteins, coagulated albumin.
2. **Proteans**– These are the earliest products of proteins hydrolysis by enzyme, dilute acid, alkalis etc. insoluble in water.
   **Ex** – fibrin formed from fibrinogen.
3. **Metaproteins** – These are the second stag products of protein hydrolysis obtained by treatment with slightly stronger acid and alkalies.
   **Ex-** acid and alkali albuminates.

**II. Secondary Proteins**

- They are formed by hydrolytic cleavage of proteins at their peptides linkage.
- **Ex- Protepses, Peptones, polypeptides and peptides.**

**C. Conjugated Proteins**

They are simple proteins combines with a non protein group called prosthetic group.

1. **Nucleoproteins** – They contain nucleic acid as the prosthetic group.
   **Ex-** Virus proteins.
2. **Glycoprotein's -** They contain carbohydrates as prosthetic group.
   **Ex** – mucin of saliva.
3. **Lipoproteins** –They contain lipids as prosthetic group.
   **Ex-**lipoproteins of blood and lipoproteins of egg yolk.
4. **Phosphoproteins** – They contain phosphoric acid as the prosthetic group.
   **Ex-** casein (milk) and vitelline ( egg).
5. **Chromoproteins–** They contain coloured substance as the prosthetic group.
   **Ex-**Heamoglobin.
6. **Metalloproteins** – They contain metal ions (Fe, Cu ,Mgetc ) as prosthetic group.
   **Ex-** ferritin which contain iron.

**D. Classification based on their nutrional value –**

1. **Complete Protein** – These proteins have all the ten essential amino acid in the required proportion by the human body to promote moderate growth.
   Ex- egg albumin.
2. **Partially incomplete proteins** – They have partially lacking one or more amino acid.
   Ex- Wheat and Rice proteins.
3. **Incomplete proteins -** They have completely lacking one or more amino acid.
   Ex –Gelatin.

**Structure of proteins**

Proteins are the polymer of L-α- amino acids. The structure of proteins is rather complex which can be divided into 4 levels of organization-

1. Primary structure
2. Secondary structure
3. Tertiary structure
4. Quaternary structure

**Primary structure**

- The primary structure of protein refers to the sequence of amino acids present in the polypeptide chain.
- Amino acids are covalently linked by peptide bonds.
- Each component amino acid in a polypeptide is called a "residue" or "moiety".
- By convention, the 10 structure of a protein starts from the amino- terminal (N) end and ends in the carboxyl-terminal (C) end.

**Secondary structure**

- Secondary structure refers to the coiling of the polypeptide chain into a helical structure.

- In this structure there is hydrogen bonding between neighboring amino acid which occurs at the sites where the peptide chain is folded to form a helix.
- Hydrogen bond occurs between the carbonyl oxygen and amide nitrogen.
- Three type of secondary structure are possible –
    1. α- helical structure
    2. Reverse turn
    3. Pleated structure

**Tertiary structure of proteins**

- Tertiary structure refers to the folding of the proteins chain to form a tight and compact three dimensional structure.
- The molecule are attached by following forces –
    1. Hydrophobic interaction- formed between non-polar side chains of amino acid.
    2. Hydrogen bonds- occur between the polar side chain
    3. Ionic bonds - formed between the oppositely charged polar side chains of amino acid such as acidic and basic.
    4. Disulfide bonds –they are S-S bonds between the SH group of two cysteine molecules.

**Quaternary structure**

- It is fourth level of organization in protein structure.
- It is shown by protein containing more than one poly peptide chain.
- These peptides are further strengthened by ionic bonds, hydrogen bond, hydrophibic bonds etc.
- This assembly as a whole is called **oligomer.**

**Proteins as nutrition**

1. Proteins are necessary for body building.
2. Proteins are necessary for repair and maintenance of body tissue.
3. They are necessary for synthesis of antibiotic.
4. They are necessary for hemoglobin, enzyme and hormones.
5. Proteins help in cell mediated immunity and bactericidal action of leucocytes.
6. They are source of energy.

**Source of proteins-** Proteins obtained from various source –

1. Animal source – like milk, meat, eggs, cheese, fish etc.
2. Vegetable source – like pulses, cereals, beans nuts, oils.

**Protein requirement** – For adult person 1gram/kg body weight.

**Biological value of proteins-** The quality of a protein is measured by its ability to supply essential amino acid. This is expressed as biological value. Biological value indicates the percentage of absorbed nitrogen which is retained in the body.

**Protein deficiency disease** -Various disease are caused by the dietary deficiency of proteins and amino acids. Some diseases are caused by abnormal metabolism of proteins.

1. **Marasmus**
    - It occurs in children in the second six month of life.
    - It occurs due to very low protein and calories in diet.
    - Generally it occurs due to early termination of beast feeding.

Symptoms

- ➢ The child is very thin with no subcutaneous fat.
- ➢ Muscles are severely wasted.
- ➢ Head is large and limbs are thin like sticks.
- ➢ Weight of the child is greatly reduced.
- ➢ Diarrhoea and dehydration
- ➢ Loose skin and old age appearance with curly hairs.

**2. Kwashiorkar**

- ➢ It is a protein energy malnutrition disease.
- ➢ It occurs in children due to low protein diet.

Symptoms

- ➢ Underweight with edema
- ➢ Difficult to feed
- ➢ Retarded growth
- ➢ Ulceration on limbs
- ➢ Anemiaand enlarge liver.
- ➢ Skin alteration like pigmentation and cracks.
- ➢ Vomiting and diarrhea

## Biological Role of Protein

1. Structural function

**Structural protein:** They give biological structure, strength or protection to the body tissue system. Example: Collagen, Gelatin, in bones and tendon, Elastin in ligaments and Keratin in epidermal tissue (skin, hair, nails)

**Contractile Proteins:** Fibrous protein functioning in the contractile system of skeletal muscles. Example: Myosin

**2. Dynamic Function:** Protein acting as enzyme, hormones, blood clotting factor, immunoglobulin.

**a. Enzymes :** Highly specialized protein, catalyze most of the chemical reactions of organic

Biomolecules in cell, tissue and systems Example: Pepsin, trypsin, hexokinase

**b. Transport protein:** Carry specific ions or molecules from one organ to another.

Example: Hemoglobin: carrier of oxygen and carbon dioxide.

Lipoprotein (Serum albumin): carrier of lipids from liver to the other organ.

Myoglobin (hemoglobin, serum albumin): Molecules and ions from one organ to the other.

**c. Nutrient and storage protein:** They store and provide nutrients. Example: Seed protein of wheat, corn and rice, albumin of egg white, casein of milk.

**d. Defense protein:** They defend (protect) the body from harmful foreign organisms, (bacteria, virus, foreign substance) Example: Immunoglobulin's

**e. Regulatory protein:** They help to regulate cellular or physiological activity, Example: Hormones like insulin, Pituitary, parathyroid, growth hormones etc.

## Qualitative Test for Proteins

| S. No. | Test | Observation | | Inference | |
|---|---|---|---|---|---|
| | | Positive | Negative | Positive | Negative |
| 1. | **Ninhydrine test**<br>2ml sample solution+ 2-3 drop of ninhydrine solution. Boil for 2 minute and cool. | Blue colour was produced. | No changes occur. | Protein may be present. | Protein may be absent. |
| 2. | **Xanthoproteic test**<br>2ml sample sol. + 1ml Con. $HNO_3$, boil than cool +40% NaOH drop wise. | Orange colour was produced. | No changes occur. | Protein may be present. (tyrosine, phenyl alanine and tryptophan) | Protein may be absent. |
| 3. | **Millions test**<br>2ml sample sol. +2 ml millons reagent, boil and cool+ add few drops of $NaNO_2$ solution. | Red ppt and solution appear red in color. | No changes occur. | Protein may be present. (tyrosine) | Protein may be absent. |
| 4. | **Aldehyde test**<br>2ml sample solution+2 ml millons reagent+ 1ml formaline + 2ml conc. $H_2SO_4$ from side of test tube. | Violet ring is formed at the junction. | No changes occur. | Protein may be present. (peptone) | Protein may be absent. |
| 5. | **Arginine test**<br>2ml sample sol. in 10% NaOH solution +5 drops of α-napthol +5 drops of sodium hypobromide solution. | Red colour produced. | No changes occur. | Protein may be present. (gelatin) | Protein may be absent. |
| 6. | **Sulphur test**<br>2ml sample sol.+ 2ml NaOH solution, few drop of lead acetate solution. | Black ppt | No changes occur. | Protein may be present. (peptone) | Protein may be absent. |

| S. No. | Test | Observation | | Inference | |
|---|---|---|---|---|---|
| | | Positive | Negative | Positive | Negative |
| 1. | **Precipitation by heavy metal** 2ml sample sol+5% $CuSO_4$ sol. | Bluish/ white ppt. was found | No changes occur. | Protein may be present. | Protein may be absent. |
| | 2ml sample sol+ 2/3 drops of 2% lead acetate sol. | White ppt. was found | No changes occur. | Protein may be present. | Protein may be absent. |
| | 2ml sample sol+ 2/3 drops of 5% mercuric nitrate sol. | Brownish ppt. was found | No changes occur. | Protein may be present. | Protein may be absent. |
| | 2ml sample sol+ 2/3 drops of 5% ferric chloride sol. | White ppt. was found | No changes occur. | Protein may be present. | Protein may be absent. |
| 2. | **Precipitation by alkaloid reagent**<br>2ml sample sol+ 2/3 drops of 20% sulphosalicylic acid. | White ppt. was found | No changes occur. | Protein may be present. | Protein may be absent. |
| | 2ml sample sol+ 1ml Esbachs reagent. | Yellow ppt. was found | No changes occur. | Protein may be present. | Protein may be absent. |
| | 2ml sample sol+ 2ml tannic acid. | White ppt. was found | No changes occur. | Protein may be present. | Protein may be absent. |
| | 2ml sample sol+ 2ml of 10% trichloroacetic acid | White ppt. was found | No changes occur. | Protein may be present. | Protein may be absent. |
| 3. | **Other protein**<br>2ml sample sol+ 3 drop C.P.R. indicator+ 1% of 1 ml acetic acid. | Ppt was produced | No changes occur. | Casein may be present. | Casein may be absent. |
| 3.a | **Hellers test**<br>2ml sample sol+ 2ml $HNO_3$ (nitric acid ). | Yellow colour is produced | No changes occur. | Casein may be present. | Casein may be absent. |
| 3.b | **Half saturation test**<br>2ml sample sol+5ml Ammonium sulphate solution. After 5 minute collect filtrate + add 2 ml NaOH solution of 40%+ 2 ml of $CuSO_4$ solution. | Violet colour | No changes occur. | Albumin | Globulin, gelatin, peptone may be present. |

# Biochemistry MCQs

1. Which type of antibodies will associatein blood cell coagulation
   (a) IgE (b) IgA
   (b) IgM (d) IgG
2. The best medium for the production of penicillin is
   (a) Nutrient agar (b) Corn steep liquor
   (c) Sulfite waste liquor (d) Whey
3. The infected mad dogs is may contain
   (a) Nergi bodies (b) Niagri bodies
   (c) Negri bodies (d) Neisser bodies
4. In most of purple bacteria the light harvesting centers are
   (a) B 850 & Fe – S (b) B 850 & B 875
   (c) B 845 & B 875 (d) B 850 & B 830
5. What will be population of bacteria after one hour in the case of bacteria culture havimg .
   (a) $1.6 \times 10$ cell / ml (b) $16 \times 10$cell /ml
   (c) $1.6 \times 10$ cell /ml (d) $4 \times 10$ cell /ml
6. The symptom " general feeling of illness and discomfort " is called
   (a) Cystitis
   (b) Malaise
   (c) Anaphylactic shock
   (d) Arthritis
7. In Elisas technique , the antibodies are labeled by
   (a) Acredine organe
   (b) Alkaline phosphate
   (c) Neutral red
   (d) Bromothymol blue
8. How would you distinguish pseudonmonas species from E-cloi ?
   (a) Gram staining
   (b) Morphology
   (c) Glucose fermentation vs Respiration
   (d) All of the above
9. Pick out the vector using in human genome project
   (a) Phagemid vector
   (b) Yeast artificial chromosomes
   (c) Cosmid vector
   (d) Yeast episomal plasmids
10. Which of the following change is a transition
    (a) ATGC –ATCC (b) ATGC –ATGG
    (c) ATGC –AGGC (d) None
11. Fixation of atmospheric nitrogen is by means of
    (a) Biological process (b) Lightining
    (c) Ultraviolet light (d) All of the above
12. Antibodies in our body are produced by
    (a) B –lymphocytes (b) T –lymphocytes
    (c) Monocytes (d) RBC s
13. How much of globulin is present in human serum?
    (a) 8 % (b) 12 %
    (c) 16 % (d) 4 %
14. Direct microscopic count can be done with the aid of
    (a) Neuberg chamber
    (b) Anaerobic chamber
    (c) Mineral oil
    (d) Olive oil
15. Syphilis is caused by
    (a) Staphylococcus aureuss
    (b) Yersinia psdtis
    (c) Treponema pallidum
    (d) Streptococcus syphilitis
16. Which of the following genera is most likely to contain organisms capable of surviving high temperature ?
    (a) Vibrio (b) Pseudomonas
    (c) Torula (d) coxiella

17. The suitable assay method for antibiotics is
    (a) enzymatic assay
    (b) turbidometric assay
    (c) end point determination assay
    (d) metabolic assay
18. An example of competitive inhibition of an enzyme is the inhibition of
    (a) Succinic dehydrogenase by malonic acid
    (b) Cytochrome oxidase by cyanide
    (c) Carbonic anhydrase by carbon dioxide
    (d) Hexokinase by glucose -6 -phosphate
19. Which one of the following mineral elements play an important role in biolo0gical nitrogen fixation
    (a) Copper (b) Magnesium
    (c) Zinc (d) molybdenum
20. one of the genes present exclusively on the x – chromosome in human is concerned with
    (a) Baldness
    (b) Red –green colour blandness
    (c) Facial hair /moustache in males
    (d) Night blindness
21. The following organisms have been proposed as sources of single cell protein
    (a) Bacteria (b) Yeasts
    (c) Algae (d) All the three
22. Koplic spots observed in the mucous membrane is characteristic feature of the disease
    (a) Rubella (b) Measles
    (c) Mumps (d) Influenza
23. Vrial genome can become integrated into the bacterial genomes are known as
    (a) Prophage (b) Tempertephage
    (c) Bacteriophage (d) Metaphage
24. Rancidity of stored food is due to the activity of
    (a) Toxigenic microbes
    (b) Proteolytic microbes
    (c) Saccharolytic microbes
    (d) Lipolytic microbes
25. All of the following are bacteriostatic chemotherapeutic agents except
    (a) Bacitracin
    (b) Chloramphgenicol
    (c) Novopbiocin
    (d) Tetracycline
26. DNA transfer from one bacterium to another through phages is termed as
    (a) Transduction (b) Induction
    (c) Transfection (d) Infection
27. Microorganisms usually make acetyle CO –A by oxidizing
    (a) Acetic acid
    (b) Pyruvic acid
    (c) $\alpha - {}^{1}$ketoglutaric acid
    (d) Fumaric acid
28. The most commonly used microorganism in alchohol fermentation is
    (a) A spergilus niger
    (b) Bacillus subtilis
    (c) Sacharomyces cerevisiae
    (d) Escherichia coli
29. Clostridium welchii spore formation can be induced only on specified media such as
    (a) Wilson – blair medium
    (b) Macconkey medium
    (c) Ellner medium
    (d) Thayee – martion medium
30. The orderly increase in the quantity of all of the cellular components is known as
    (a) Reproduction (b) Growth
    (a) Binary fission (d) None
31. β – lactum ring is present in
    (a) Erythromycin (b) Penicillin
    (c) Tetracyclins (d) Chromphenical
32. Intermediate group of pathogen between bacteria and viruses which are intracellular parasites are called
    (a) Mucoplasmas (b) Rickettsias
    (c) Prions (d) Virusoides

33. The percentage of O2 required by moderate anaerobe is
    (a) 0 % (b) < 0.5 %
    (c) 2 – 8 % (d) 5 -10 %

34. Lederberg and Tatum (1946) described the phenomena of
    (a) Conjunction (b) Transformation
    (c) Mutation (d) Plasmids

35. The size of virus particle may range
    (a) 0.02 to 0.2 μm (b) 0.5 to 10 μm
    (c) 0.015 to 0.2 μ m (d) 0.1 to 100 μm

36. To prepare vaccine for small pox , the material used by Edward Jenner is
    (a) Small pox material
    (b) Chicken pox material
    (c) Cow –pox material
    (d) Measles material

37. In the medium other than nutrient , if any substance is used in excess , that medium is
    (a) Enriched medium
    (b) Special medium
    (c) Enrichment medium
    (d) Nonc

38. The causative organism of rocky mountain spotted fever was first described by
    (a) Howard Ricketts (b) da Rocha – lima
    (c) a and b (d) Robert Koch

39. Cultures are prepared by penetrating the inoculation loop with suspension into the medium , they are
    (a) Stock cultures (b) Streaking
    (c) Sub cultures (d) None of these

40. Counter immunoelectrophoresis is useful for detection of
    (a) One antigen /antibody
    (b) Tow antigens / antibody
    (c) More than two
    (d) None

41. What is the technique for quantitative estimation of immunoglobulin ?
    (a) Single diffusion in one dimension
    (b) Single diffusion in two dimension
    (c) Double diffusion in one dimension
    (d) Double diffusion in two dimension

42. Patients suffering from AIDS have following immune abnormalities _
    (a) Decreased CD4 + T cells
    (b) Increased CD8 +t cells
    (c) CD4 +CD8 + ratio greater than 21
    (d) b & c

43. The most effect method for productive virus free plants
    (a) Meristem culture
    (b) Root culture
    (c) Floriculture
    (d) Somatic embryogenesis

44. Hybridoma technique is widely used for producing
    (a) Callus Culture
    (b) Organ cultures
    (c) Monoclonal antibodies
    (d) All

45. The etiological agent of infection mononucleosis also associated with a form of Brukitt,s lymphoids is
    (a) Vercella zoster virus
    (b) Epstein Barr virus
    (c) Picorna virus
    (d) Papovavirus

46. Food poisoning is caused by which bacteria
    (a) Clostridum tetani
    (b) Clostridium welchi
    (c) Diphtheria
    (d) Clostridium botulinum

47. The medium used in membrane filter technique was
    (a) EMB agar
    (b) EMR – Vp medium
    (c) Lactose broth
    (d) Endo agar

48. The infected mad dogs may contain
    (a) Nergi bodies (b) Niagri bodies
    (c) Negri bodies (d) Neisser bodies

49. Rancidity in spoiled food is due to
    (a) Lipolytic organisms
    (b) Proteolytic organisms
    (c) Toxigenic microbes
    (d) Saccharolytic microbes

50. Poly A tail is frequently found in
    (a) Histone in RNA (b) Bacteria RNA
    (c) Eukaryotic RNA (d) TRNA

51. Thermal death time is
    (a) Time required to kill all cells at a given temperature
    (b) Temperature that kill all cells in a given time
    (c) Time and temperature needed to kill all cells
    (d) All of a - c

52. Tumer inducing plasmids are extensively used in production of
    (a) Avirulent phases
    (b) Single cell proteins
    (c) Transgenic plants
    (d) Nitrogen fixing bacteria

53. Transgenic animals are produced when GH gene fused with
    (a) MT gene (b) GH
    (c) GRF (d) FIX

54. Which of the following is ionizing radiation
    (a) U.V. rays (b) IR
    (c) ¥ rays (d) None

55. The etiological agent of infection mononucleosis also associated with a form of Brukitt's lymphoma is
    (a) Vercella zoster virus
    (b) Epstein barr virus
    (c) Picorna virus
    (d) Papovavirus

56. Diversity in antibody molecules is brought about by
    (a) Post –traslational modifications
    (b) Gene rearrangements
    (c) Usage of special genetics codes
    (d) Multiple mutations in the polypeptide

57. Biological indicator serve to demonstrate the efficiency of ------
    (a) BOD incubatopr
    (b) Laminar air flow bench
    (c) Microorganism
    (d) Sterilization

58. Sight of infection of coliform bacilli is
    (a) Colon (b) Gall bladder
    (c) Urinary tract (d) Lungs

59. Which of the following disease is not an autoimmune disease
    (a) Multiple sclerosis
    (b) Grave's disease
    (c) Systemic iupus erythematosus
    (d) Dengue

60. Wasermann test of complement fixation is used for the diagnosis of
    (a) Smallpox (b) Syphilis
    (c) Typhoid (d) Rabbies

61. PAP smear test is used in diagnosis of
    (a) Syphilis (b) T. B.
    (c) Gonorrhea (d) Fibroid

62. Diagnostic test for the identification of primary syphilis ---
    (a) VDRL test
    (b) Treponema pallidum immobilization test
    (c) Kahn's test
    (d) Dark ground microscopic examination

63. Neil mooseri reaction is related to ---
    (a) Rickettsiae
    (b) Chlamydiae
    (c) Spirochaetes
    (d) Clostridium periringens

64. Pfeiffer phenomenon is related to
    (a) Vibrio cholera (b) anthrax
    (c) Rickettisial pro (d) All

65. Daisy head colony is associated with --
    (a) M .tuberculosis (b) diphtheria
    (c) Cl. Tetani (d) None

66. Cholera red reaction is identified by
    (a) Sulphuric acid (b) Nitric acid
    (c) Hydrochloric acid (d) Carbolic acid

67. Identify the obligate anaerobes
    (a) Salmonella (b) Vibrio cholera
    (c) Cl. Tetani (d) Sarcinae

68. The largest protozoa is
    (a) Balantidium coli
    (b) Entamoeba coli
    (c) Trichomonus vaginalis
    (d) Toxoplasma gondii

69. Hydatid disease is identified by ---
    (a) Schick test (b) Dick test
    (c) Casoni test (d) Freis test

70. Genetic information transfer DNA to RNA is called –
    (a) Transcriptase (b) Transduction
    (c) Transformation (d) Recombination

71. Premonition is particularly seen in –
    (a) Ascaris (b) Giardia
    (c) Plasmodium (d) None

72. ------- is used for detecting susceptibility of an individual to diphtheria toxin
    (a) Schick tests (b) Dick test
    (c) V-P test (d) Precipitin test

73. Cholera occurs in --------- form
    (a) Endemic (b) Epidemic
    (c) Sporadic (d) All
    (e) None

74. Statements applicable to human lice is ----
    (a) Cause pruritic skin lesions
    (b) Transmit epidemic typhus , relapsing fever and trench fever
    (c) Pediculus humanus and phthirus pubis are two species
    (d) All

75. Fungal disease in human is caused by –
    (a) Inhalation of conidia
    (b) Invasion of mucous membrane
    (c) Contamination of wounds with conidia or mycelia fragments
    (d) None

76. Rh factor of the blood was discovered by scientist –
    (a) Louis Pasteur
    (b) Landsteiner and weiner
    (c) Janskey
    (d) Moss

77. To be anaphylactic , the sensitizing substance should be –
    (a) Protein in nature
    (b) Should have a large molecular weight
    (c) Soluble in tissue fluids
    (d) All of the above

78. Staphylococcus aureus are characterized by
    (a) Formation of acid in sucrose , dextrose
    (b) Liquification of gelatin due to production of gelatinase
    (c) Strains are catalase positive
    (d) All

79. Dpneumoniae can be cultivated in
    (a) Glucose broth
    (b) Serum broth
    (c) Agar and blood agar
    (d) All

80. Cholera occurs in -- ------ form
    (a) Endemic (b) Epidemic
    (c) Sporadic (d) All

81. Organisms can be attenuated for inoculation by
    (a) Growing it at a temperature higher than optimum
    (b) By passage through animals of different species which are less susceptible to it
    (c) Any one of the above
    (d) None

82. The markers helpful in detecting anti – immunity are
    (a) Hyper gamma globulinaemia
    (b) Circulating antibodies
    (c) Response to cortisone and lymphoid hyperplasia
    (d) All

83. The agglutinin test is used for
    (a) Identification of i9solated bacteria
    (b) Typing of bacterial species
    (c) Study of antigenic structure of bacteria
    (d) All

84. Yellow fever is caused by
    (a) Bunya virus (b) Calci virus
    (c) Arbo virus (d) None
85. Vector for leishmaniasis is
    (a) Tick (b) Mite
    (c) Sand fly (d) Tsetse fly
86. Gonorrhea is
    (a) Air borne disease
    (b) Water borne disease
    (c) Sexually transmitted venereal disease
    (d) A and C
87. Bartholin cyst is caused by
    (a) Candida (b) Streptococcus
    (c) Staphylococcus (d) Gonococcus
88. Specific test for syphilis is
    (a) VDRL test (b) ELISA
    (c) FTA (d) None
89. Coagulase test is used for
    (a) Salmonella (b) Staphylococcus
    (c) Bordetella (d) Pneumococcus
90. Staphylococcus aureus was isolated by
    (a) Rosenbach
    (b) Louis Pasteur
    (c) Passet
    (d) Sir Alexander ogston
91. The causative agent of tetanus is
    (a) Clostridium botulinum
    (b) Cl. Tetani
    (c) Cl. Welchii
    (d) Cl. Perfringens
92. Culture medium for clostridia spp.
    (a) 76 lower stein jensen's medium
    (b) Mac conkey's medium
    (c) Robertson's cooked meat medium
    (d) None of these
93. Rabies virus can multiply in
    (a) The central nervous system only
    (b) The peripheral nerves
    (c) Muscle tissues
    (d) All the above
94. Brucella causes
    (a) Pertusis (b) Plague
    (c) Brucellosis (d) None
95. Lepromin test
    (a) Is negative in tubercular leprosy
    (b) Positive in lepromatous type
    (c) Indicated delayed hypersensitivity test
    (d) Indicates infection
96. Streptolysin 'S' is
    (a) Oxygen unstable (b) Thermostable
    (c) Oxygen stable (d) None
97. Acid fast bacteria are
    (a) Neisseria (b) Staphylococci
    (c) Mycobacteria (d) All of the above
98. Shigella was first isolated by
    (a) Shiga (b) Schmitz
    (c) Sonnei (d) Robert Koch
99. Prophylaxis of cholera is
    (a) Protected water supply
    (b) Environmental sanitation
    (c) Immunisation with killed vaccines
    (d) All of these
100. Primary mediators in anaphylaxis
    (a) Histamine (b) Serotonin
    (c) Heparin (d) All

# Answer Key Biochemistry

1. b
2. c
3. b
4. b
5. b
6. b
7. c
8. c
9. b
10. d
11. d
12. a
13. a
14. a
15. c
16. c
17. c
18. a
19. d
20. b
21. d
22. c
23. b
24. d
25. a
26. a
27. a
28. a
29. c
30. b
31. b
32. b
33. c
34. a
35. c
36. c
37. a
38. c
39. b
40. a
41. b
42. d
43. a
44. c
45. b
46. d
47. b
48. c
49. a
50. c
51. b
52. c
53. a
54. c
55. b
56. d
57. d
58. c
59. b
60. b
61. d
62. d
63. a
64. a
65. b
66. a
67. c
68. a
69. c
70. a
71. c
72. a
73. d
74. d
75. d
76. b
77. b
78. c
79. d
80. d
81. c
82. d
83. d
84. c
85. c
86. c
87. d
88. a
89. b
90. b
91. b
92. c
93. d
94. c
95. c
96. c
97. c
98. c
99. b
100. d

# Previous Years GPAT Solved Question Papers

## GPAT 2015

1. Which type of alkaloid is present in Vinca?
   (a) Ergot (b) Tropane
   (c) Indole (d) Quinoline
2. What is the biological source of Alexandrian Senna
   (a) Cassia aungustifolia
   (b) Cassia acutifolia
   (c) Cassia Bravifolia
   (d) Cassia Nerifolia
3. In the following drug find out the Potassium Sparing Diuretics
   (a) Milrinone (b) Thiazide
   (c) Spironolactone (d) Amilioride
4. How the wetting agent act in the suspension
   (a) Increase contact angle between substance and solvent
   (b) Reduce contact angle between substance and solvent
   (c) No change in contact angle between substance and solvent
   (d) None of the above
5. Which phase of suspension is reversible phase
   (a) Cracking (b) Creaming
   (c) Phase Inversion (d) Coalscence
6. Which eye infection is also called as 'Pink Eye' infection
   (a) Fungal keratitis (b) Viral keratitis
   (c) Conjunctivitis (d) Myopia
7. Match compound with the pathway they inhibit

| | |
|---|---|
| 1. Vancoycin | (P) Folate metabolism |
| 2. Rifampin | (Q) DNA synthesis |
| 3. Puramycin | (R) protin synthesis |
| 4. Ciprofloxacin | (S) RNA synthesis |
| | (T) Cell wall synthesis |

   (a) 1-T, 2-S, 3-R, 4-Q
   (b) 1-R, 2-S, 3-T, 4-P
   (c) 1-Q, 2-R, 3-T, 4-Q
   (d) 1-T, 2-Q, 3-P, 4-S
8. The given reaction in an example of
   (a) Arndt-Eistert homologation
   (b) Mannich reaction
   (c) Michael addition
   (d) Chichibabin amination reaction
9. What is the 6-methyl derivative of erythromycin
   (a) Azithromycin (b) Roxithromycin
   (c) Clarithromycin (d) Clindamycin
10. In the diagnosis of myasthenia gravis, only one of the following drugs will be used as a drug of choice
    (a) Neostigmine (b) Pyridostigmine
    (c) Physostigmine (d) Edrophoinum
11. Methyl [5(proopylthio)-1H-benzoimidazol-2yl] carbamate is Geneva name of which of the following drug
    (a) Mebendazole (b) Albendazole
    (c) Thibendazole (d) Triclabendazole
12. Which of the following is oil of fruit pulp
    (a) Arachis oil (b) Castor oil
    (c) Olive oil (d) Apricot oil
13. What is true about bioavailability
    (a) Amount of unbound drug (Free drug reaching systemic circulation)
    (b) Amount of bound Drug
    (c) Amount of metabolite drug
    (d) Amount of Excreted Drug

14. Polymorphs in pharmaceutical solids are detected by which technique
    (a) MS (b) LC-MS
    (c) Solid state NMR (d) Coulter counter
15. A series of alpha - acylureido penicillin's like azlocillin, mezloacillin, and piperacillin are superior because of
    (a) Reduced acid hydrolysis
    (b) Increased beta - lactmase resistance
    (c) Improved penetration through the cell envelop
    (d) Slow rate of metabolism
16. Bacillus subtilis is used in assay of which antibiotics
    (a) Penicillin (b) Cephalosporin
    (c) Vancomycin (d) Streptomycin
17. Which of the following titrations will always have an equivalence point at a pH > 7.00
    (a) Weak acid with a weak base
    (b) Strong acid with a weak base
    (c) Weak acid with a strong base
    (d) None of the above
18. Inadequate drying during coating of tablet leads to which coating defect
    (a) Chipping (b) Lamination
    (c) Mottling (d) Lamination
19. Match the crude drug with its biological source
    1. Pale catechu (P) Conium naculatum
    2. Clove (Q) Cymapsistetragonoloba
    3. Gaur bean (R) Uncariagambir
    4. Hemlock (S) Syzygiumaromaticum
    (a) 1-Q, 2-P, 3-S, 4-R
    (b) 1-Q, 2-S, 3-R, 4-P
    (c) 1-R, 2-S, 3-Q, 4-P
    (d) 1-R, 2-S, 3-P, 4-Q
20. Which of the following plot indicates the effects of antagonist on receptors
    (a) Michaelis-Menten plots
    (b) Line weaver burk Plots
    (c) Displacement plots
    (d) Schild plots
21. All of the following statements concerning zero-order degradation are true except
    (a) Its rate is independent of the concentration
    (b) A plot of con Vs time gives a straight line on reactilinear paper and a slope is a rate constant
    (c) Its half-life is a changing parameter
    (d) Its concentration remains unchanged with respect to time
22. The liquefaction time of cocoa butter of hydrogenated vegetable oil based suppositories is
    (a) 30-50 min (b) 30-40 min
    (c) 11-17 min (d) 3-7 min
23. Which of the following is most likely to undergo lysis
    (a) A cell losing water from its cytoplasm
    (b) A cell with inact, multilayer peptidoglycan cell wall
    (c) A cell with disturbed pentaglycine bridges in its cell wall
    (d) A cell a hydrophilic outermost layer in its cell wall
24. Match the drugs with the disease for which it is prescribed
    1. Bedaquline (P) Anitdiabetic
    2. Sitagliptin (Q) Anitiarrrhythmic
    3. Mexilitine (R) Antidipressant
    4. Paraoxitine (S) Antituberualr
    (a) 1-S, 2-P, 3-Q, 4-R
    (b) 1-S, 2-P, 3-Q, 4-R
    (c) 1-Q, 2-P, 3-R, 4-S
    (d) 1-R, 2-S, 3-P,4-Q
25. Which micro-organism used in hairy root culture
    (a) Agrobact rhiaogens
    (b) A. tumefaciens
    (c) N. tabacum
    (d) Solanum chrysotrichum
26. Delayed disintegration in tablet is a result of
    (a) Large force of compression
    (b) Small force of compression
    (c) Higher amount of granule
    (d) Low amount of granule
27. Match drugs with their receptor that they inhibit
    1. $5HT_{1A}$ agonist (P) Cisapride
    2. $5HT_3$ antagonist (Q) Ketanserine

3. $5HT_{2A}$ antagonist (R) Ondensetron
4. $5HT_4$ agonist (S) Buspiron
   (a) 1-S, 2-R, 3-Q,4-P
   (b) 1-R, 2-S, 3-T, 4-P
   (c) 1-Q, 2-R, 3-T, 4-Q
   (d) 1-T, 2-Q, 3-P, 4-S

28. Passive immunity in new born babies is due to
    (a) IgG (b) IgM
    (c) IgE (d) IgA

29. Upper consolute temperature and lower consolute temperature are related to
    (a) CMC temp (b) Kraft Temp
    (c) Cloud temp (d) Absolute temp

30. Compact size, low weight mass instrument is:
    (a) EI-TOF
    (b) MALDI-Quadrapole
    (c) MALDI-TOF
    (d) Ion-Trap

31. A Pharmaceutical company plans to market a generic version of a drug produce whose patent has expired has expire (d) Which type of documentation must be submitted to the FDA
    (a) IND
    (b) NDA
    (c) ANDA
    (d) SNDA & Letter of intent

32. Which of the following does not produce azeotropic mixture with water
    (a) Methanol (b) Ethanol
    (c) Propanol (d) Isopropanol

33. For a particular durg, the rate of absorption but not the extent of the absorption of GIT, is affected by presence of food in GIT then taking the drug with food will result in
    (a) Smaller area under the plasma drug concentration time curve
    (b) Smaller maximal plasma drug concentration
    (c) Smaller time at which the maximal plasma drug concentration occurs
    (d) Smaller fractional bioavailability and total clearance

34. According to USP Alcohol contains
    (a) 94.9 to 96% Ethanol
    (b) 94.9 to 96% Methanol
    (c) 50% Ethanol
    (d) 50% Methanol

35. What does in mean that a cell is polyploid
    (a) That is contains more than 2 copies of one or a few of its of chromosomes
    (b) That is contains more than 2 copies of a full set of homologous chromosomes
    (c) That is contains more than 2 copies of its sex chromosome
    (d) That is contains more than 2 copies of its autosomal chromosomes

36. Amount of dextrose in large volume infusion fluids
    (a) 5% w/v (b) 10% w/v
    (c) 25% w/v (d) 50% w/v

37. ............, Anthelmintics having Immunosuppressant activity.
    (a) Piperazine (b) Levamisole
    (c) Ivermectin (d) Niclosamide

38. Choose correct statement for PEGylation:
    (a) Used to enhance In-vivo half-life of smaller Peptides and proteins
    (b) Avoidance of Reticulo-endothelial (RES) clearance
    (c) Reduce clearance rate through kidney
    (d) All

39. Characteristics feature if hemorrhagic dengue fever is
    (a) Reduction in platelet count
    (b) Reduction in RBC count
    (c) Reduction in coagulation factors
    (d) Increased RBC

40. The carbonyl starching frequency for simple aldehydes, ketones, and carboxylic acids is about 1710 cm-1 , where as the carbonyl stretching frequency for esters is about cm-1
    (a) 1650 (b) 1700
    (c) 1750 (d) 1850

41. Plarographic method of analysis to obtain individual amounts of Cu2+ and Cd2+ in a given mixture of the two ions (Cu2+ and Cd2+) is achieved by measuring their
    (a) Half-wave potentials
    (b) Migration currents
    (c) Decomposition potentials
    (d) Diffusion currents

42. Consider the reaction: A + B = C
    The unit of the thermodynamic equilibrium constant for the reaction is
    (a) mol L-1 (b) L mol-1
    (c) mol2 L-2 (d) Dimensionless

43. ________________, system does not have orifice to release the drug.
    (a) Elementary Osmotic Pump
    (b) L-OROS
    (c) Sandwich Osmotic Pump Tablet
    (d) Controlled Porosity Osmotic Pump Tablet

44. Sanguinarine belongs to the subgroup of:
    (a) Morphinans
    (b) Benzyl isoquinolines
    (c) Phthalide isoquinolines
    (d) Benzophenanthrenes

45. Identify the IUPAC of dexamethasone
    (a) 2-Chloro-6α, 9α-difluoro-11α, 17, 21-trihydroxy-16α-methylpregna-1,4-dien-3, 20-dione
    (b) 9α-Fluoro-11β, 17α, 21-trihydroxy-16β-methylpregna-1, 4-diene-3, 20-dione
    (c) 9α-Fluoro-11β, 17α, 21-trihydroxy-16β-methylpregna-1, 4-diene-3, 20-dione
    (d) 6α-Fluoro-11α, 21-dihydroxy-16α-methylpregna-1, 4-diene-3. 20-dione

46. Tamoxifen is nonsteroidal drug acting at steroid receptor(s) It produces which type of effects
    (P) Androgen (Q) Antiestrogen
    (R) Antiprogestogen (S) Estrogen
    (a) P and Q (b) Q and S
    (c) Q and R (d) R and S

47. Which enzymes is used by the HIV to form DNA in the host cell
    (a) Restriction endonuclease
    (b) DNA-directed polymerase only
    (c) Reverse transcriptate only
    (d) Both (b)and (c)

48. 'Sparging' is the process where
    (a) Silanol groups react with trimethylsilyl group
    (b) An inert has is bubbled through the solvent reservoir to remove dissolved gases
    (c) Solvents are mixed together in a fixed ratio
    (d) Column is washed with solvents from nonpolar to polar and reverse

49. Morphine does not cause:
    (a) Constriction of pupil
    (b) CNS depression
    (c) Respiratory depression
    (d) Diarrhoea

50. Which of the following is not recommended in patients with renal insufficiency or cardiac dysfunction
    (a) Aloe
    (b) Bisacodyl
    (c) Isapghol
    (d) Magnesium hydroxide

51. Higuchi model is applicable to drug that isIn the formulation
    (a) Dissolved in formulation
    (b) Dispersed in formulation
    (c) Chemically bound to carrier in formulation
    (d) Osmotically controlled in the formulation

52. Which of the following in correct about parenteral nutrition
    (a) Parentral nutrition solutions are hypertonic solutionsand IV fluids are isotonic
    (b) Parentralnutribtion solutions and IV preparations are isotonic solutions
    (c) Parentrtal nutrition solutions are hypertonic solutions and IV fluids are isotonic
    (d) Parentral nutrition solutions can be supplemented with mediacations

53. Cyclic AMP (cAMP) is an important second messenger in signal transduction pathway(s)Which enzyme catalyzes the generation/accumulation of cAMP after a receptor – ligand interaction
    (a) Protein kinase A
    (b) cAMP phosphodiesterase
    (c) Guanylyl cyclase
    (d) Adenylate cyclase

54. Which of the following in not include in immunization programme as per WHO recommendations for all children
    (a) BCG (b) Oral polio
    (c) Measels (d) Typhoid

55. Match the given condition with appropriate drug used for its treatment

| | |
|---|---|
| 1. Pernicious anemia | (P) Erythropetin |
| 2. Meagaloblastic anemia | (Q) Oprelvekin |
| 3. Anemia associated Vitamin with chronic renal | (R) Ratenteral B12 failure |
| 4. Thrombocypeniadue to cancer chemotherapy | (S) Folic acid |

    (a) 1-P, 2-Q, 3-R, 4-S
    (b) 1-R, 2-S, 3-P, 4-Q
    (c) 1-R, 2-Q, 3-S, 4-P
    (d) 1-R, 2-P, 3-S, 4-Q

56. In mammals, The major fat in adipose tissue is:
    (a) Triglyceride
    (b) Cholesterol
    (c) Sphingophospholipids
    (d) Phospholipids

57. Plarographic method of analysis to obtain individual amounts of Cu2+ and Cd2+ in a given mixture of the two ions (Cu2+ and Cd2+) is achieved by measuring their
    (a) Half-wave potentials
    (b) Migration currents
    (c) Decomposition potentials
    (d) Diffusion currents

58. What is the objective of trademark
    (a) To claim exclusive properties of products or services
    (b) To claim innovation of products or services
    (c) To deal with market place of expressive ideas
    (d) To protect consumers from being misled

59. Turbulent flow is exhibited by fluids whose
    (a) Re<40' (b) Re>40'
    (c) Re=40 (d) All of the above

60. Characteristics of drug-protein binding:-
    (P) Often parallels drug lipid solubility
    (Q) Drug-plasma albumin binding tends to be relatively nonselective
    (R) Acidic drugs bind to albumin while basic drug bind to glycoproteins
    (S) In rheumatoid arthritis patients, increased alpha1- acidic glycoprotein tends to promote increased lidocaine protein binding
    (a) P and Q (b) P, Q and R
    (c) P, Q, R and S (d) P and R

61. C=O stretchings are very strong and easily observable bands in IR spectroscopy. However in the IR spectrum of glucose C=O absorption band is not seen. Why
    (a) In glucose, C=O group is not terminal
    (b) In glucose C=O group is absent
    (c) In glucose, hemiacetal group is present
    (d) In glucose, hemiketal group is present

62. What is the use of Phenol coeficient
    (a) To compare a disinfectant's killing efficacy to that of phenol
    (b) To determine the dilution at which the disinfectant is to be used
    (c) To determine the purity of disinfectant
    (d) All of the above

63. Arrange the following esters as per decreasing order of rate of saponification
    (i) Ethyl benzoate
    (ii) Ethyl p- methoxybenzoate
    (iii) Ethyl p- chlorobenzoate
    (iv) Ethyl p-nitrobenzoate
    (a) I>II>III>IV (b) IV>III>II>I
    (c) IV>III>I>II (d) II>IV>I>III

64. Which of the following statements about bentonite are CORRECT
    (P) Gycerin is used to pre-wet the bentonite prior to mixing with water to form its gel
    (Q) Aqueous bentonite suspensions retain their viscosity above pH 6 but are precipitated by acids
    (R) MgO increase gel formation while alcohol in significant amounts can precipitate bentonite gel
    (S) Betonite exhibits rheopexy
    (a) P and Q (b) Q and R
    (c) P,Q and R (d) P, Q, R and S
65. Acid insoluble ash of a leaf is called as
    (a) Earthy matter & silica
    (b) Inorganic content
    (c) Organic Content
    (d) All of the above
66. Grape fruit juice is P- glycoprotein and CYP40 enzyme inhibitor . if drug X is degraded by proteolytic enzymes, administration of grapefruit juice with X
    (a) Increase bioavailability of X
    (b) Decrease Bioavailability of X
    (c) Does not affect bioavailability of X
    (d) Cause unexpected action of X
67. Tannins give positive test for all of the following EXCEPT
    (P) Goldebeater skin test
    (Q) Phenazone
    (R) Biuret test
    (S) FeCl3
    (a) P and Q (b) Q and R
    (c) P, Q and R (d) P,Q and S
68. Vigabatrin is a GABA analogue that potentiates action of GABA in the brain because it
    (a) Binds to GABA receptor and acts as agonist
    (b) Inhibits GABA transaminase
    (c) Blocks NMDA receptor via the glycine binding site
    (d) Inhibits neuronal reuptake of GABA from synapses
69. Drug that increases systolic B.P. but reduces diastolic B.P.
    (a) Isoproterenol (b) Epinephrine
    (c) Nor Epinephrine (d) Propranol
70. Which of the following are characteristics for colloid mills
    (P) Due to centrifugal forces, the mill undergoes periodical vibratory movement
    (Q) Particles smaller than 1 μm can be obtained with them
    (R) The main types of colloid mills are hammer , turbine and dial mills
    (S) The principle of their operation is based on the abrasion of particles at high speed
    (a) Only, P, Q and R are correct
    (b) Only P and R are correct
    (c) Only Q and S are correct
    (d) P, Q, R and S are correct
71. Inflamation of soft tissue due to hyaluronidase is called as
    (a) Tendinitis
    (b) Bursitis
    (c) Cellulitics
    (d) Cumulative Injury Disorder (CID)
72. The hydroxyl derivative of cymene is called as what
    (P) Thymol (Q) Carvacrol
    (R) Menthol (S) Cumene
    (a) P, Q, R and S (b) P, Q , and R
    (c) P and Q (d) Only P
73. Which of the following are the correct properties of ferroin? Ferroin is
    (P) 1, 10-phnathroline
    (Q) A bidentate ligand complex
    (R) Red in reduced form
    (S) Blue in oxidized form
    (a) P and Q (b) R and S
    (c) P, R and S (d) P, Q, R and S
74. Each of the following is a glycosaminoglycan dengue fever is
    (a) Chondroitin and dermatan
    (b) Heparan and heparin
    (c) Hyaluronic acid and keratin
    (d) Keratin and chitin

75. If X is an equivalent of silver deposited is silver coulometer and Y is an equipment of copper deposited in copper coulometer when constant current is passed through the electrochemical cell for the same time which of the following is correct
   (a) X =Y (b) X = 2Y
   (c) X = Y/2 (d) 2X =Y
76. Which of the following classes of medication is the most common initial treatment of men with symptomatic benign prostatic hypertrophy (BPH)
   (a) Alpha-1 agonist (b) Alpha-1 blocker
   (c) Beta-1 agonist (d) Beta-1 blocker
77. Which of the following reagents can be used for alkaloid detection
   (P) Mayer reagent
   (Q) Kedde reagent
   (R) Dr4agendoff reagent
   (S) Alcoholic solution of 2, 4 dinitrophenyl-hydrazine
   (a) Only P and Q are correct
   (b) Only P and R are correct
   (c) Only P and Rare correct
   (d) Only R and S are correct
78. Which schedule Drugs & Cosmetics Act include Particulars to the shown in /manufacturing Records
   (a) Schedule A (b) Schedule V
   (c) Schedule U (d) Schedule W
79. All of the following statements about plasmodium falciparum are correct EXCEPT
   (a) Trohozoites, Schizonts and gametocytes are not seen in peripheral blood smear.
   (b) Is associated with recurrent relapses after initial treatment because of liver hypnozoites
   (c) More than one parasite/multiple infection can be seen within single RBC
   (d) Causes more severe disease in pregnancy
80. The chairman of the investigational new Drug (IND) committee in India is
   (a) Drugs controller General of India, Government of India
   (b) Secetary, Department of Health Reasearch, Government of India
   (c) Directorate General of Health Sciences, Government of India
   (d) Secretary, Department of Biotechnology, Government of India
81. In the filling of container what is the meaning of "overfill container"
   (a) Container filled to its minimum capacity
   (b) Container filled to its maximum capacity
   (c) Empty container
   (d) Cleaned container
82. What is the name of floor on which production work is done rather than administration
   (a) Administration area
   (b) Production area
   (c) Quality control area
   (d) Quarentine Area
83. Quinoline contains two basic rings. One of the rings in quinolone. It is attached to second ring via o one carbon bridge. Which in the second ring
   (a) 8-Azabicyclo [3.2.1] octane
   (b) 1-Azabicyclo [2.2.2] octane
   (c) 1, 4-Diazabicyclo [2.2.2] octane
   (d) Rubane
84. Which of the first drugs are potentiated by the second
   (a) Phenytoin – Ethinyloestradiol
   (b) Warfarin – Phenobarbitone
   (c) Lithium- Thaazide diuretics Potentiated due to reduced Lithium clearance
   (d) Bromorcriptine- Metpoclopramide
85. Which of the following is a long acting □2 agonist that can be given by nebulization and as well a dry powder inhaler for the treatment of COPD
   (a) Foramterol (b) Albuterol
   (c) Pulmicort (d) Fluticasone
86. Which anticholinergic drug mostly used as anti Parkinson drug
   (a) Procyclidin (b) Methinicol
   (c) Tacrin (d) Atropine

87. To create successful new product, a company understands consumers, markets, and competitors and develop a/an
    (a) Impressive advertising campaign
    (b) Strong wed site to push the product
    (c) Aggressive marketing strategy
    (d) Product that satisties consumers' needs

88. Which of the following method is an example of facilitated diffusion?
    (a) Passive diffusion
    (b) Endocytosis
    (c) Carrier mediated diffusion
    (d) Active transport

89. Which of the following causes arterial and bronchial constriction and platelet aggregation
    (a) Prostaglandin E2
    (b) Prostaglanding A2
    (c) Prostaglandin D2
    (d) Thromboxane A2

90. What is mechanism of action of carbamazepine
    (a) Inhibition of GABA transaminase
    (b) Blockade of sodium channel
    (c) Blockade of glutamate receptor
    (d) Blockade of GABA receptors

91. Passive diffusion follows which order of kinetics
    (a) Non selective and mixed order
    (b) Selective and first order
    (c) Non selective and first order
    (d) Selective and mixed order

92. Conc v/s time curve drown from single oral dose, which parameter can be calculated
    (a) Elimination constant
    (b) Rate constant
    (c) Absorption peak
    (d) Plasma conc.

93. If a basic drug reabsorbed significantly from kidney which of the following statement will be correct
    (a) Its renal clearance increases in basic urine
    (b) Its renal clearance decreases in basic urine
    (c) Its renal clearance increases in acidic urine
    (d) Its renal clearance decreases in acidic urine

94. o, m, p- isomers can be differentiated on the basis of:
    (a) Chemical shift
    (b) Coupling constant
    (c) Extinction coefficient
    (d) Dipole moment

95. Monitoring of plasma drug concentration is required while using:
    (a) Antihypertensive drugs
    (b) Levodopa
    (c) Lithium carbonate
    (d) MAO inhibitors

96. Bacterial endotoxin are mainly detected by
    (a) Pyrogen test (b) LAL test
    (c) Thermal test (d) Bacterial test

97. The shelf life of a medicine is defined as :
    (a) Time required for 10% degradation of drug
    (b) Time required for 50% degradation of drug
    (c) Time required for 90% degradation of drug
    (d) Time required for 100% degradation of drug

98. In which rearrangement reaction, Isocyanate is formed?
    (a) Curtious (b) Lossen
    (c) Both A & B (d) None

99. Chitin gets converted in to Chitosan upon:
    (a) Acetylation (b) Deacetylation
    (c) Oxidation (d) Reduction

100. Efficiency of drug is checked in modest population in
    (a) Clinical trail-phase1
    (b) Clinical trail-phase2
    (c) Clinical trail-phase3
    (d) Clinical trail-phase4

101. The mixed gland of our body which secrets both hormones and digestive enzyme, so pancreatic enzyme digest which substances
   (a) Lipids, Protein, Carbohydrate but not Nucleic acid
   (b) Protein, Carbohydrate, Nucleic acid but not Lipids,
   (c) Carbohydrate, Lipids, nucleic acid but not Protein
   (d) Lipids, Protein, Nucleic acid but not Carbohydrate

102. In which type of bacteria the cell wall is thicker
   (a) Gram +ve (b) Gram –ve
   (c) Both (d) None

103. Out of the following anti cancer drug cardio toxicity is seen in
   (a) Mitomycin-C
   (b) Doxorubicin
   (c) Methotraxate
   (d) Cyclophosphamide

104. Which of the following free radical is most dangerous free radical
   (a) O- (b) H+
   (c) H2O2 (d) Superoxide

105. The phosphate of a metal has the formula MHPO4. The formula of its Bromide would be:
   (a) MBr (b) MBr2
   (c) MBr3 (d) MBr4

106. Silicone based adhesive used in TDDS possess following properties:
   (a) Chemical and biological inertness
   (b) Low toxicity
   (c) Low sensitization and irritation
   (d) All

107. Schleuniger tester is used for the tablets to measure:
   (a) Roughness (b) Hardness
   (c) Dissolution (d) Friability

108. Creatinine clearance is used as a measurement of:
   (a) Passive renal absorption
   (b) Glomerular filtration rate
   (c) Renal excretion rate
   (d) All

109. 1-[2-[(2-chloro thienly)methoxy]-2-(2,4-dichlorophenyl)ethyl]-1Iimidazole is:
   (a) Oxiconazole (b) Sulconazole
   (c) Tioconazole (d) Miconazole

110. The drug of choice in prolonged febrile convulsions is:
   (a) Carbamazepine (b) Diazepam
   (c) Phenytoin (d) Paracetamol

111. Geometrical isomerism is possible in case of:
   (a) 2-Pentene (b) Pentane
   (c) Propene (d) Ethene

112. The loading dose (DL) of a drug is usually based on the:
   (a) Total body clearance of the drug
   (b) Percentage of drug bound to plasma proteins
   (c) Fraction of drug excreted unchanged in the urine
   (d) Apparent volume of distribution & desired drug concentration in plasma

113. Biologically active arachidonic acid is
   (a) All transeicosatetraenoic acid
   (b) All cis eicosatetraenoic acid
   (c) All transeicosatrienoic acid
   (d) All cis eicosatrienoic acid

114. Antidiabetic action of gliburidestart at molecular level by which mechanism
   (a) Phosphorylation of receptor
   (b) Binding to potassium ions
   (c) Decrease in potassium effiux
   (d) Increase in potassium effiux

115. Momordica charantia having blood sugar lowering activity due to:
   (a) Momordicin (b) Charantin
   (c) Momortin (d) Charantiamarin

116. Insulin stimulates glucose transport by promoting the translocation of:
   (a) GLUT 4
   (b) GLUT 2 & GLUT 4
   (c) GLUT 1 & GLUT 4
   (d) GLUT 2

117. Oral rehydration salt contains ionic electrolytes in concentration mmlo/L
   (a) Na+ 20, K+ 10 (b) Na+ 40, K+ 20
   (c) Na+ 53, K+ 40 (d) Na+ 60, K+ 20

118. In pinacol – pinacolone rearrangement, the final product is ketone. What is the starting compound for the rearrangement
   (a) 1, 1-diol (b) 1, 2-diol
   (c) 1, 3-diol (d) Geminal diol

119. Which of the following method is useful for measuring the number of viable cells in a culture
   (a) Plate count technique
   (b) Dry weight method
   (c) Petroff-Hauser counter
   (d) Light scattering in a spectrophotometer

120. Seeding involves the spread of cancer cells to
   (a) Blood vessels
   (b) Serious membranes of body cavities
   (c) Fascia surrounding muscles and bones
   (d) Dermis and subcutamneum of the skin

121. Barbiturates are being replaced by hypnotic benzodiazepines because of
   (a) Low therapeutic index
   (b) Suppression in REM sleep
   (c) High potential of physical dependence, abuse
   (d) All of the above

122. Adverse drug Event reporting in the responsibility of all of the following EXCEPT
   (a) Pharmacist and physician
   (b) Manufacturer
   (c) Consumer
   (d) Regulatory authorities

123. Time dependent dilatant behavior is knows as
   (a) Thixotrophy (b) Rheopexy
   (c) Rheomalaxis (d) Plastic

124. Chairman of DTAB is:
   (a) Health minister of India
   (b) Director general of Health services
   (c) Drug controller of India
   (d) President of AICTE

125. Plasmodesmata is:
   (a) Lignified element
   (b) Vascular element
   (c) Very fine protoplasmic thread
   (d) None

## Answer Key GPAT 2015

| 1-c | 2-b | 3-c | 4-b | 5-b | 6-c | 7-a | 8-b | 9-a | 10-d |
|---|---|---|---|---|---|---|---|---|---|
| 11-b | 12-c | 13-a | 14-c | 15-c | 16-d | 17-c | 18-a | 19-c | 20-d |
| 21-d | 22-d | 23-d | 24-a | 25-a | 26-a | 27-a | 28-a | 29-a | 30-b |
| 31-c | 32-c | 33-b | 34-a | 35-b | 36-a | 37-b | 38-d | 39-a | 40-c |
| 41-d | 42-d | 43-d | 44-b | 45-b | 46-b | 47-c | 48-b | 49-d | 50-d |
| 51-b | 52-a | 53-d | 54-a | 55-b | 56-a | 57-d | 58-c | 59-b | 60-c |
| 61-c | 62-a | 63-c | 64-c | 65-a | 66-b | 67-d | 68-b | 69-a | 70-c |
| 71-c | 72-c | 73-d | 74-d | 75-a | 76-b | 77-b | 78-c | 79-b | 80-a |
| 81-b | 82-b | 83-b | 84-c | 85-a | 86-a | 87-c | 88-c | 89-d | 90-b |
| 91-a | 92-b | 93-b | 94-b | 95-c | 96- b | 97- a | 98-c | 99-b | 100-b |
| 101-a | 102-a | 103-b | 104-d | 105-b | 106-d | 107-b | 108-b | 109-c | 110-b |
| 111-a | 112-d | 113-b | 114-c | 115-b | 116-c | 117-d | 118-b | 119-a | 120-b |
| 121-d | 122-d | 123-b | 124-b | 125-d | | | | | |

# GPAT 2016

1. What is the Carr's index of good flow powder property
   (a) 5-15 (b) 12-16
   (c) 18-21 (d) 28-35
2. Which microorganism is involved in the assay of Rifampicin
   (a) Bacillus subtilis
   (b) Micrococcus luteus
   (c) Bacillus pumilus
   (d) Bacillus cereus
3. Which percentage of dextrose is isotonic with the blood plasma
   (a) 5% (b) 10%
   (c) 15% (d) 20%
4. What is the biological source of Alexandrian Senna
   (a) Cassia aungustifolia
   (b) Cassia acutifolia
   (c) Cassia Bravifolia
   (d) Cassia Nerifolia
5. HLB of SPAN and TWEEN surfactants may be obtained from which of the following equations
   (a) HLB = E/5
   (b) HLB = (E+P)/5
   (c) HLB = 20 [(1- S)/A)]
   (d) HLB = (hydrophilic group numbers)-(lipophilic group numbers)+7
6. If the given drug is absorbed by passive what will be its absorption kinetics
   (a) Zero Order
   (b) First Order
   (c) Second order
   (d) Pseudo-zero Order
7. Which of the following is delayed type of her sensitivity reaction
   (a) Arthus reaction
   (b) Penicillin sensitivity
   (c) Tubercullin sensitivity
   (d) ABO incompatibity
8. Which of the following is NOT suitable as a post-coital contraceptive
   (a) Levonorgestrel 1.5mg
   (b) Ulipristal acetate 30 mg
   (c) Mifepristone 10-25 mg
   (d) Mestranol 1.5 mg
9. Which of the following properties are characteristics of tannis
   (P) They give a precipitate with alkaloids
   (Q) They give a yellow of bluish red color with iron (III) chloride
   (R) They transform hide into leather
   (S) They give a pale-pink precipipate with iodine
   (a) P, Q, S (b) P and Q
   (c) P and R (d) Only Q
10. dverse drug Event reporting in the responsibility of all of the following EXCEPT
    (a) Pharmacist and physician
    (b) Manufacturer
    (c) Consumer
    (d) Regulatory authorities
11. Time dependent dilatant behavior is knows as
    (a) Thixotrophy (b) Rheopexy
    (c) Rheomalaxis (d) plastic
12. Chairman of DTAB is:
    (a) Health minister of India
    (b) Director general of Health services
    (c) Drug controller of India
    (d) President of AICTE
13. Plasmodesmata is:
    (a) Lignified element
    (b) Vascular element
    (c) Very fine protoplasmic thread
    (d) None

14. Efficiency of drug is checked in modest population in
    (a) Clinical trial-phase1
    (b) Clinical trial-phase2
    (c) Clinical trial-phase3
    (d) Clinical trial-phase4

15. Which of the following statements is correct for gram positive becteria
    (a) Cell wall has a thin peptidoglycan layer
    (b) Cell wall lipid content is very low and smaller volume of periplasm
    (c) Lipopolysaccharide layer is present
    (d) Teichoic acid is present

16. The terms upper consulate temperature and lower consulate temperature are related to which phenomenon
    (a) Cloud point
    (b) Critical solution temperature
    (c) Kraft point
    (d) Phase inversion

17. Match the alkaloids with their synthesis precursors.

| | |
|---|---|
| (1) Pilocarpine | (P) Necleotide |
| (2) Connine | (Q) Tryptophan |
| (3) Caffine | (R) Histadine |
| (4) Yohimbine | (S) Acetate derived |

    (a) 1-S, 2-R, 3-P, 4-Q
    (b) 1-S, 2-Q, 3-P, 4-R
    (c) 1-P, 2-R, 3-S, 4-Q
    (d) 1-R, 2-S, 3-P, 4-Q

18. Which one of the following is a solid dosage form excipient which can play the role of a diluent, a disintegrant, a glidant, a lubricant and a pore/ channel former.
    (a) Lactose
    (b) Microcrystalline cellulose
    (c) Ethyl cellulose
    (d) Eudragit RL 100

19. What is the required floor area for running a pharmacy for wholesale or distribution
    (a) 6 sq meters (b) 10 sq meters
    (c) 15 sq meters (d) 30 sq meters

20. Bioavailability differences among drug's oral formulations are most likely to occur if it
    (a) Is freely water soluble
    (b) Is incompletely absorbed
    (c) Is completely absorbed
    (d) Undergoes little first-pass metabolism

21. Match the drug with their receptor profiles

| | |
|---|---|
| (1) Ergotamine | (P) 5-$HT_{2A}$ antagonist |
| (2) Ondansetron | (Q) 5-$HT_1$ partial agonist /antagonist |
| (3) Sumartriptan | (R) 5-$HT_3$ antagonist |
| (4) Ketanserin | (S) 5-$HT_{1D}$ agonist |

    (a) 1-R, 2-S, 3-Q, 4-P
    (b) 1-Q, 2-R, 3-S, 4-P
    (c) 1-R, 2-S, 3-P, 4-Q
    (d) 1-S, 2-R, 3-P, 4-Q

22. What strategy of drug design is frequently used on complex lead compounds derived from natural products
    (a) Extension
    (b) Simplication
    (c) Rigidication
    (d) Conformational block

23. Which type of photon detector is commonly microfabricated into arrays of 500 or More individual detectors
    (a) Photocell
    (b) Phototube
    (c) Photumultiplier tube
    (d) Photodiode

24. Which of the following is a phjse II drug metabolism reaction associated with genetic polymorphism
    (a) Glucuroinidation
    (b) Acytylation
    (c) Reduction
    (d) Glutathione conjugation

25. A gram-negative diplococcus associated with urinary tract infection , pelvic inflammatory disease and conjunctivitis, meningitis is
    (a) Neissria gonorrhoeae
    (b) Chlamdia Trachomatis
    (c) Hemophilus influenza
    (d) Streptococcus pneumonia

26. Pregnancy test kits are designed to detect
    (a) Estrogen
    (b) Human chorionic gonadotropin
    (c) Follicle-stimulating hormone
    (d) Luteinizing hormone

27. Drug Z is a depolarizing neuromuscular blocking agent effective for the treatment of pinworm. Identify drug Z
    (a) Phyrantel (b) Paramomycin
    (c) Integrase (d) Protease

28. Metheneamine used for UTI is a prodrug. How and to what is is converted into
    (a) At low pH of Urine, to formaldehye
    (b) At high pH of urine, to aminosalicylic acid
    (c) At low pH of Urine, to amonosalicylic acid
    (d) At high pH of urine,to formaldehyde

29. The correct order for the basic features of a mass spectrometer is
    (a) Acceleration, deflection, detection, ionization
    (b) Ionization, Acceleration, deflection, detection
    (c) Acceleration, ionization, deflection, detection
    (d) Acceleration, deflection, ionization, detection

30. Match the following enzymes/protein with specific functions in DNA replication

| | | | |
|---|---|---|---|
| (1) | Helicases | (P) | Processive unwinding of DNA |
| (2) | DNA Primses | (Q) | Seals the single strand |
| (3) | DNA ligases | (R) | Relieves torsional strain |
| (4) | Topiosomerases | (S) | Initates synthesis of RNA Primers |

    (a) 1-P, 2-Q, 3-R, 4-S
    (b) 1-P, 2-S, 3-Q, 4-R
    (c) 1-S, 2-Q, 3-P, 4-R
    (d) 1-P, 2-Q, 3-R, 4-S

31. Which is the first line drug for the treatment of generalized seizures
    (a) Valproic acid
    (b) Anhydortetracycline
    (c) Carbamazepine
    (d) Doxycycline

32. Tetracyline in basic solution is usstable and forms which product
    (a) Epithtracycline
    (b) Anhydrotetracycline
    (c) Isotetracycline
    (d) Doxycycline

33. The location of the blood-brain barrier is considered to be
    (a) At the level of the brain capillaries
    (b) At the level of gila
    (c) At the level of neurons
    (d) At the level of dendrites

34. The following drug metabolizing reaction in entirely non-microsomal:
    (a) Glucuronide conjugation
    (b) Acetylation
    (c) Oxidation
    (d) Reduction

35. Which of the following methods is used to determine whether a process functions properly for its intended use
    (a) Capacity (b) Inspection
    (c) Validation (d) Design Review

36. Match product, source and plant part form which they are obtained

| | | | |
|---|---|---|---|
| (1) | Bacosides | (P) | Aciacia catechu |
| (2) | Cutch | (Q) | Rubiatictorium(ii) Leaf |
| (3) | Henna | (R) | Bacopamonnieri |
| (4) | Alizarm | (S) | Lawsoniainternis |

    (a) 1-R-ii, 2-S-I, 3Q-Q-iii, 4-P-iv
    (b) 1-R-I, 2-P-iv, 3-S-ii, 4-Q-i
    (c) 1-Q-ii, 2-P-iii, 3-S-iv, 4-R-I
    (d) 1-S-ii, 2-R-iv, 3-P-I, 4-Q-i

37. What is the significance of term overfill
    (a) It is similar to overage
    (b) It is the excess volume to be field in containers as vials, ampoules to avoid loss by degradation
    (c) It is the excess filing of container as vials, ampoules to avoid the loss during case
    (d) It is violation of packaging regulation as per GMP

38. Identity the false statements
    (a) A characteristics of drugs eliminated by zero order kinetic process is that the half – life is not constrains
    (b) The plasma drug concertation versus time curve for a drug eliminated by zero order kinetics linear
    (c) A fundamental characteristics of all first order pharmacogenetics processes is that the rate of the process is proportional to drug concentration
    (d) A characteristics of absorption by lipid diffusion is its saturability at high drug concentrations

39. 2', 3'-Didehydro-3'-deoxy thymidine is the chemical name of which of following antiviral agents
    (a) Didenosine (b) Zidovudine
    (c) Stavudine (d) Zalcitabine

40. Oseltamivir is antiviral drug. It produces its action by inhibiting which enzymes
    (a) DNA polymerase (b) Neuraminidase
    (b) Praziquantel (d) Ivermectin

41. In NMR spectrum, a signal is observed as triplet. What will be the ratio of relative peak areas in this signal
    (a) 1:1:1 (b) 1:2:1
    (c) 1:3:1 (d) 1:4:1

42. Which problem can arise if the material to be compressed into tablet tends to adhere to die walls
    (a) Picking (b) Sticking
    (c) Capping (d) Marbling

43. What is the half life of Tc-99m
    (a) 66 years (b) 66 hours
    (c) 6 hours (d) 60 minutes

44. Eudragits are
    (a) Phthalate polymers
    (b) Cellulose polymers
    (c) Acrylate polymers
    (d) Amide polymers

45. Drugs (price control) order 1995 and related orders form time to time are enforeced by
    (a) NPPA (b) CSIR
    (c) DBT (d) ICMR

46. Match the drugs with plant from which they are isolated and their families

| | | |
|---|---|---|
| (1) Artemisinin | (P) Periwinkle | (i) Dioscoreaceae |
| (2) Diosgenin | (Q) May apple | (ii) Apocynaceae |
| (3) Etoposide | (R) Sweet wormwood | (iii) Berberidaceae |
| (4) Vinblastine and Vicnristine | (S) Maxican wild yam | (iv) Asteraceae |

    (a) 1-R-iv, 2-S-i, 3-Q-iii, 4-P-ii
    (b) 1-s-iv, 2-R-i, 3-Q-iii, 4-P-ii
    (c) 1-Q-iii, 2-R-ii, 3-Q-i, 4-P-iv
    (d) 1-R-iv, 2-S-iii, 3-Q-i, 4-P-ii

47. Which of the following is an irreversible phenomenonralated to stability of emulsion
    (a) Craking (b) Creaming
    (c) Coalescence (d) Flocculation

48. If a drug is highly bound to plasma proteins, what might be its reason or consequence
    (a) It most likely carried by α-glycorprotien
    (b) It has a high renal clearance
    (c) It has a large Vd
    (d) It is a likely candidate for drug interactions

49. In order to make a generic substitution; a pharmacist must do also act as a hydrogen bond acceptor
    (e) Notify the patient of the substitution
    (f) Charge the same or lower price for the generic
    (g) Place the brand name on the label and write "substitute for"
    (h) Obtain the physician's consent to substitute the product

50. Which of the following groups can form ionic interactions and also act as a hydrogen bond acceptor
    (a) Hydroxyl group (OH)
    (b) Carboxylate group (RCOO)
    (c) Aminononium group (RNH3+)
    (d) Ketone (C=O)

51. Which of the following drug does not give pink colour with ruthenium red
    (a) Agar (b) Guar gum
    (c) Pectin (d) Isabgol

52. The IUPAC name, 4-Amino-N(5,6-dimethoxy-4-pyrimidinly) benzenseulfonamide belong to which generic drug
   (a) Sulfadimidine (b) Sulfadoxine
   (c) Sulfalene (d) Sufamerazine

53. Method of inspections used to determine the absorption rate constants. It assumes that
   (P) Ka is at least five time grater activities
   (Q) Absorption in complete (i.e. > 95% complete) at the time of peak concentration
   (R) Both Absorption and elimination are first order processes
   (a) P and Q (b) Q and R
   (c) Q and R (d) P and R

54. The clinical trial registry in India is maintained by
   (a) World health organization, Delhi
   (b) Indian council of medical research, New Delhi
   (c) Institute of Clinical Research, New Delhi
   (d) Central drugs standard control Organization, New Delhi

55. What is the correct order for unsaturation in following fatty acids
   1) Palmitoleic Acid
   2) Linolenic
   3) Linoleic acid
   4) Arachidonic acid
   (a) 1>2>3>4 (b) 3>4>2>1
   (c) 4>3>2>1 (d) 4>2>3>1

56. Which of the following is an example of Diazonium ion
   (a) CH3+N3- (b) CH N +
   (c) H N-NH + (d) None of these

57. Which term describes 'The degree to which a set of inherent properties of a product system , of process fulfils requirements, the best'
   (a) Standard (b) Quality
   (c) Quality objective (d) State of control

58. What will be AUC value of lidocaine if the administered dose is 0.2 g and the total body clearance is 45 L/h
   (a) 4.44 h.mg/L (b) 0.0044 h.mg/L
   (c) 9.00 h.gm/L (d) 9000 h. mg/L

59. Toluene is converted of which compound in presence of CrO3 with acetic anhydride
   (a) Benzyl alcohol (b) Benzaldehyde
   (c) Benzoic acid (d) Benzoin

60. Match the antimalarial drugs with their modes of action
   (1) Artemisinin
      (P) Inhibition of parasite mitochondrial electron Tranport
   (2) Pyremethamine
      (Q) Inhibition of heme polymerase
   (3) Quinine
      (R) Generation of oxygen and carbon-centered redicals
   (4) Atovaquone/Proguanil
      (S) Inhibition of dihydrofolate reductase
   (a) 1-P, 2-S, 3-Q, 4-R
   (b) 1-Q, 2-S, 3-P, 4-R
   (c) 1-S, 2-R, 3-Q, 4-P
   (d) 1-R, 2-S, 3-Q, 4-P

61. Methyl ether of erythromycin is ___________
   (a) Clarithromycin (b) Dirithromycina
   (c) Azithromycin (d) Mithramycin

62. Ebullioscopicmethod is based on which of the following observation
   (a) Freezing point depression
   (b) Boiling point elevation
   (c) Osmotic pressure change
   (d) None of the above

63. How many fundamental svibrations can be expected for C2H5CL
   (a) 7 (b) 11
   (c) 14 (d) 18

64. Which of the antibodies provide passive immunity to newborn baby
   (a) lgG (b) lgM
   (c) lgA (d) lgE

65. Increased number of number mitosis may be present in the following tissue EXCEPT
   (a) Bone marrow cells (b) Nails
   (c) Hepatocytes (d) Intestinal Cells

66. To which chemical class the vinca alkaloids belong
    (a) Tropane (b) Indole
    (c) Tryptopha (d) Purine

67. An antibiotic thatn resembles the 3' end of a charged tRNA molecule is
    (a) Streptomycin (b) Vincamycin
    (c) Puromycin (d) Tetracycline

68. If the cohesive forces in between similar molecules are less than the adhesive forces between dissimilar\ molecules, a deviation in Raolt's law is observed . here witch deviation will be seen.
    (a) Positive
    (b) Negative
    (c) Absent
    (d) Either positive or negative

69. Phenylalanine, a precursor of most of the phenolics is higher plants is a product of which one of the following pathways
    (a) Shikimic acid pathway
    (b) Malonic acid pathway
    (c) Mevalonic acid pathway
    (d) Methylerhtritol pathway

70. Within how many days a pharmacist should dispense diluted aqueous mixtures
    (a) 7 days (b) 14 days
    (c) 21 days (d) 30 days

71. What molecular feature is penicillin G is said o mimic
    (a) Disaccharide of N-acetylmuranicanidN-actylgulcosamine
    (b) N-acetylneuraminic acid
    (c) The pentapeptide moiety of five glycine units
    (d) The dipeptide moiety D-ala-D-Ala

72. If a drug is known to be distributed into total body water, how many milligrams are needed to obtain an initial plasma level of 5mg/L in a patient weighting 70 kg
    (a) 210 (b) 150
    (c) 50 (d) 35

73. What does 'pharmacokinetical compartment' mean
    (a) Part of the body water which is located is the vascular system
    (b) Total body water
    (c) Plasma, intracellular fluid, together, anatomical water compartments where drug is absorbed
    (d) Part of the body water in which the change of a drug concentration has the same kinetics

74. The resistance to macrolide antibiotics by of gram positive organism is developed due to
    (a) Decreases uptake of antibiotics
    (b) Synthesis of esterase enzyme that hydrolyzes lactone ring of macrolide
    (c) Methylation of 50S subunit at the antibiotic binding site
    (d) Increased metabolism of antibiotic

75. The ethanolic solution contaminated with benzele showed absorbance of 0.69 at 260 nm in a 2 cm cell if the molar absorptivity of benzene in thanolis 230 M-1cm-1, what is the concentration of benzene in the solution
    (a) 0.003 M (b) 0.0015 M
    (c) 0.001M (d) 0.015M

76. The most effective agent for treating psychosis would be
    (a) Buspirone
    (b) Sertaline
    (c) Dextroamphetamine
    (d) Olanzapine

77. TGA is regulatory body of which country
    (a) Europe (b) Australia
    (c) Canada (d) UK

78. Which prostaglandins have a keto function at C-9 and a α- Hydroxyl group at C-11 in prostanoic acid backbone
    (a) PGA (b) PGI
    (c) PGE (d) PGF

79. When morphine is heated at 140oC under pressure, with strong HCL, it converts pnto:
    (a) Morphinone (b) Apomorphine
    (c) Codeine (d) Oxymorphine

80. All of the following are gram-negative rods EXCEPT
(a) Clostridium (b) Escherichia
(c) Salmanella (d) Shigella

81. The cells which secrets male sexhormone testosterone are:
(a) Crypts of lieberkuhn
(b) Escherichia
(c) Salmonella
(d) Shigella

82. If QA and QC are compared
(a) Both are literally the same
(b) QA is a higher activity in the management hierarchy
(c) QA is a higher activity in the management hierarchy
(d) QA is a done by the production person and QC is done by analyst

83. Bio availability of drug refers to
(P) The ratio of drug excreted unchanged in urine to that excreted as metabolites
(Q) Fraction of the drug reaching the target to produce the action
(R) The length of time an administered drug is available for action
(S) Percentages of administered dose that reaches systemic circulation in the unchanged form
(a) Only P (b) Q and R
(c) R and S (d) Only S

84. Following intravenous administration, drugs are distributed fastest to
(a) The skin, kidney, and brain
(b) The liver, kidney, and brain
(c) The liver, adipose, and brain
(d) The liver, kidney, and adipose

85. Which of the following agents act as hypoglycemic as ATP sensitive potassium channel blocker
(a) Mitiglinide (b) Pioglitazone
(c) Liraglutide (d) Sitagliptin

86. Carabilide shows strong IR absorption in which of the following range in cm-1
(a) 3200-3600 (b) 1640-1690
(c) 1000-1300 (d) 2210-2260

87. Match the drugs with their adverse effects

| | |
|---|---|
| (1) Cyclophosphamide | (P) Pulmonary fibrosis |
| (2) Doxorubicin | (Q) Nephrotoxicity, ototoxicity |
| (3) Bleomycin | (R) Acute hemorrhage cystitis |
| (4) Cisplatin | (S) Cardiotoxicity |

(a) 1-S, 2-R, 3-P, 4-Q
(b) 1-P, 2-Q, 3-S, 4-R
(c) 1-P, 2-S, 3-Q, 4-R
(d) 1-R, 2-S, 3-P, 4-Q

88. Which one of the following technique is used to determine glass transition temperature
(a) X-ray diffractometry
(b) Raman spectroscopy
(c) Differential scanning calorimetry
(d) Atomic forced microscopy

89. Match the schedules with the particulars they describe
(1) Schedule T
(P) Standards for patent or proprietary medicines
(2) Schedule U
(Q) Requirements/ guidelines to import &/or manufactures new Drug
(3) Schedule V
(R) GMP practices for Ayurvedic, siddha & Unani medicines
(4) Schedule Y
(S) Particulars to be shown in the manufacturing records
(a) 1-R, 2-S, 3-Q, 4-P
(b) 1-S, 2-Q, 3-P, 4-R
(c) 1-R, 2-S, 3-P, 4-Q
(d) 1-S, 2-R, 3-P, 4-Q

90. Which of the following UV rays cause cancer
(a) UVA (b) UVB
(c) UVC (d) All of the above

91. Which are the types of antibodies involved in hypersensitivity reactions
(a) LgG and LgD (b) LgG and LgM
(c) LgD and LgA (d) LgM and LgD

92. The term used to describe unequal distribution of colour on a tablet is
    (a) Chipping (b) Mottling
    (c) Lamination (d) Double impress
93. Why acetyl chloride undergoes nucleophilic substitution at a faster rate than methyl acetate
    (a) The ester is more sterically hindered than the acid chloride
    (b) The chloride ion is a better leaving group than methoxide
    (c) The acid chloride is more sterically hindered than the ester
    (d) The methoxide ion is a better leaving group than chloride
94. The key concept of Total Quality Managements (TQM) is
    (a) Total control of all quality related activities
    (b) Commitment of all employees to quality improvement and having team meetings
    (c) Top management's direct involvement
    (d) The Introduction ot the ISO 9000 Series
95. A drug of low water solubility when given orally is absorbed up to 90% of the administered does. The drug belongs to which class according to BCS classification
    (a) Class IV (b) Class III
    (c) Class II (d) Class I
96. Which of the following is NOT a component of evaporator
    (a) Heat exchange
    (b) Vacuum separator
    (c) Condenser
    (d) Cyclone separator
97. In parkinson's disease, there is a predominant loss of dopaminergic neurons
    (a) Substantia (b) Cerebellar
    (c) Cerebral cortext (d) Locus ceruleus
98. At equilibrium the receptor occupancy is related to drug concentration by
    (a) Henderson-Hasselbach equation
    (b) Hill- Langmuir equation
    (c) Lineweaver-Burk equation
    (d) Langmuir adsorption isotherm
99. Which method is not suitable to calculate area under the curve
    (a) Least square method
    (b) Weighing andplatometery
    (c) Trapezoid rule
    (d) Integration of curve
100. OROS is a technology developed for/as
    (a) Oral release rapid onset system
    (b) Orally rapid disintegrating tablets
    (c) Osmotic controlled oral drug delivery system
    (d) Transdermal drug delivery system
101. Match the events in tablet manufacturing process with the effects found in tables
    (1) Rapid drying of coated tablets after coaching
    (2) Use to highly viscous solution
    (3) Improper feed rate form hopper
    (4) Excessive compression force
    (a) 1-R, 2-S, 3-Q, 4-P
    (b) 1-R, 2-S, 3-P, 4-Q
    (c) 1-S, 2-R, 3-Q, 4-P
    (d) 1-R, 2-P, 3-S, 4-Q
102. At pH 5, the ratio of the protonated to unprotanated forms of morphine pKa 7 would be
    (a) 1:100 (b) 1:10
    (c) 10:1 (d) 100:1
103. What structure is formed if the acyl side chain of penicillin is hydrolysed
    (a) Penicellienic acids
    (b) Penillic acids
    (c) 7-Aminopenicillanic acid
    (d) 6-Aminopenicillanic acid
104. The clinical trial is being conducted with 1500 volunteers which may spans on period of 2 years as per protocol. The clinical trial is in which phase
    (a) Phase 1 (b) Phase 2
    (c) Phase 3 (d) Phase 4

105. Which of the following drug has not undergone a clinical trial for its use to decrease intracranial pressure
   (a) Dideoxyinosine (b) Zidovudine
   (c) Acetazolamide (d) Nicotine

106. Colloidal depression have which type of rheology
   (a) Newtonian (b) Pesudoplastic
   (c) Non- Newtonian (d) Dilatant

107. Which of the reactive oxygen species is most dangerous to cells
   (a) Singlet oxygen (b) Hydroxyl radical
   (c) Superoxide (d) Peroxide

108. The Gibb's Phase rule
   (a) Holds only for systems with more than components
   (b) Predicts that a maximum of three phase can exits in one components system
   (c) Does not count phase compositions as intensive variables
   (d) Does not count pressure and temperature as intensive variables

109. Nerve impulse from the cochlea arrive first in which region of the brain
   (a) Auditory cortex (b) Thalamus
   (c) Medulla oblongata (d) Inferior colliculus

110. The product of a Michael reaction of a ketone enolate to ana, b-unsaturated ketone is And addition reaction occurs in a/an
   (a) 1,5- deketone; 1,4-fashion
   (b) α-substituted acetate; 1,2 fashion
   (c) β - hydorxy keto; 1,3 – fashion
   (d) α, β - keto ester; 1,5 –fashion

111. Which of the following is a drug considered as potassium sparing diuretic
   (a) Trimatrine (b) Chlorthiazide
   (c) Mannitol (d) Furosemide

112. Which of the reagent from the given can be used to protect ketone group
   (a) Acidic methanol (b) Basic methanol
   (c) Methanol + KCN (d) Phenobarbitone

113. Which of the following drugs causes less inhibition or REM sleep
   (a) Zolpidem (b) Ethanol
   (c) Lorazepam (d) Phenobarbitone

114. The starting materials for synthesis of sulfamethoxazole are
   (a) 4- Aminobenzene-1-sulfonyl amide + 3-chloro-5-methyl isoxazole
   (b) 4- Aminobenzene-1-sulfonyl amide + 3-amino-5-methyl isoxazole
   (c) 4- Aminobenzene-1-sulfonyl amide + 3-amino-5-methyl isoxazole
   (d) 4- Aminobenzene-1-sulfonyl amide + 5-chloro-5-methyl isoxazole

115. Match the following plant product with their chemical class
   (1) b-amyrin (P) Alkaloid secondary alcohol
   (2) Sqaulene (Q) Alkaloid, phenol
   (3) Morphine (R) Triterpene, secondary alcohol
   (4) Ephedrine (S) Asyclic triterpene, polyene
   (a) 1-R, 2-S, 3-Q, 4-P
   (b) 1-S, 2-Q, 3-P, 4-R
   (c) 1-P, 2-S, 3-Q, 4-R
   (d) 1-R, 2-S, 3-P, 4-Q

116. All of the following except one are subject to therapeutic drug monitoring, Which one
   (a) Phenytoin (b) Lithium
   (c) Gentamicin (d) Losartan

117. Thiamine deficiency causes decreased energy production because
   (a) It is required for the process of transamination
   (b) It is a co-factor in oxidative reduction
   (c) It is a co-enzyme for transketolase is pentose phosphate pathway
   (d) It is a co-enzyme for pyruvate dehydrogenase & alpha ketoglutarate dehydrogenase

118. Which of the following drugs are often found in both prescription and over-the-counter nasal decongestands
   (a) Alpha 2 agonists (b) lpha 1 agonists
   (c) Alpha 1 antagonists (d) Beta 2 agonists

119. What is the surface tension of water of at 25oC
   (a) 58 dyne/cm (b) 68 dyne/cm
   (c) 72 dyne/cm (d) 82 dyne/cm

120. Acridine and xanthene rings are related to each other in that.........
   (a) Xanthene is oxygen isoster of acridine
   (b) Acridine is oxygen isoster of xanthene
   (c) Xanthene is nitrogen isoster of aciridine
   (d) Xanthene is sulfur isoster os acridine

121. Colligative properties depend on..............
   (a) Structural arrangement of atoms within the molecules of solute and solvent
   (b) The number of solute particles is solution
   (c) The physical properties of the solute particles dissolved is solution
   (d) Sum of the corresponding properties of individual atoms or functional group within the molecules

122. In polarography current must be blocked
   (a) Residual (b) Migration
   (c) Diffusion (d) None

123. The propellant commonly used in topical aerosols is
   (a) Trichloromonfluoromethane
   (b) Trifluromonfluroethane
   (c) Dichlordifluromthane
   (d) Isopropyl alcohol

124. Which of the following increase systolic and diastolic pressure in normal patient
   (a) Epineherine (b) Norepinephrine
   (c) Tyramine (d) Phenylephrine

125. A large Reynold number is indication of which type of flow
   (a) Smooth and stream line flow
   (b) Laminar flow
   (c) Steady flow
   (d) Highly turbulent flow

# Answer Key GPAT 2016

| 1-b | 2-a | 3-a | 4-b | 5-c | 6-b | 7-c | 8-d | 9-c | 10-d |
|---|---|---|---|---|---|---|---|---|---|
| 11-b | 12-b | 13-c | 14-b | 15-b | 16-b | 17-d | 18-b | 19-c | 20-b |
| 21-b | 22-b | 23-d | 24-b | 25-a | 26-b | 27-a | 28-a | 29-b | 30-b |
| 31-a | 32-c | 33-a | 34-b | 35-c | 36-b | 37-c | 38-d | 39-c | 40-b |
| 41-b | 42-b | 43-c | 44-a | 45-a | 46-a | 47-b | 48-d | 49-a | 50-d |
| 51-b | 52-b | 53-a | 54-b | 55-d | 56-b | 57-b | 58-a | 59-b | 60-d |
| 61-a | 62-b | 63-d | 64-c | 65-b | 66-b | 67-c | 68-b | 69-a | 70-b |
| 71-d | 72-a | 73-d | 74-b | 75-b | 76-d | 77-b | 78-c | 79-b | 80-a |
| 81-b | 82-b | 83-d | 84-b | 85-a | 86-b | 87-d | 88-c | 89-c | 90-b |
| 91-b | 92-b | 93-b | 94-c | 95-c | 96-d | 97-a | 98-b | 99-a | 100-c |
| 101-c | 102-c | 103-d | 104-c | 105-c | 106-c | 107-b | 108-b | 109-c | 110-a |
| 111-a | 112-a | 113-a | 114-b | 115-a | 116-a | 117-d | 118-b | 119-c | 120-a |
| 121-b | 122-b | 123-b | 124-c | 125-d | | | | | |

# GPAT 2017

1. In a free radical reaction, free radicals are formed at
   (a) Initiation step (b) Propagation step
   (c) Termination step (d) Both (a) and (b)

2. Which of the following dienes can undergo Diels–Alder reaction most readily

   (a) 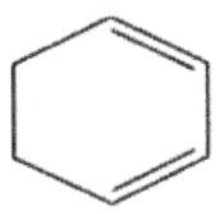 (b) 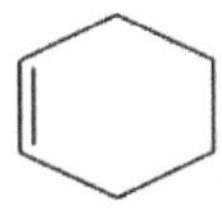

   (c) 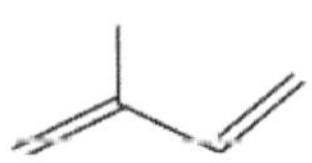 (d) 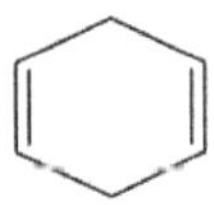

3. Separating techniques such as gas chromatography and liquid chromatography are not appropriate for separation of amino acids. Select correct reason from the following
   (a) Amino acids high polarity substances
   (b) Amino acids are low polarity substances
   (c) Amino acids are non polar substances
   (d) Amino acids lowly charges substances

4. When trans-2-butene is treated with bromine an anti-addition of bromine yields meso- 2,3-dibromobutane.

   Select the correct statement regarding the reaction from the following
   (a) The reaction is stereoselective as well as stereo specific
   (b) The reaction is stereoselective and not stereo specific
   (c) The reaction is nonstereoselective as well as non stereo specific
   (d) The reaction is stereo specific and not stereo selection

5. Reduction of imines to give amines in protic solvents can be carried out by one of the following reagents. Select the correct reagent
   (a) Sodium hydride
   (b) Sodium chloride and HCl
   (c) Lithium aluminium chloride
   (d) Sodium cyanoborohydride

6. In the reaction of 2-nitrotoluene with bromine in presence of iron, which of the product shown below is the most abundant (major) product

   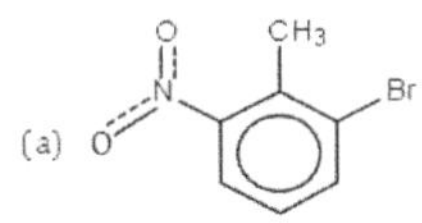 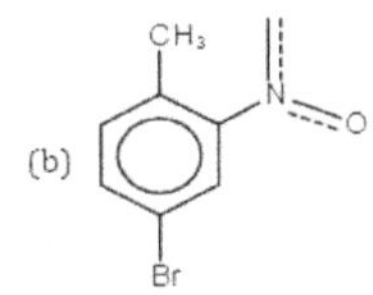

   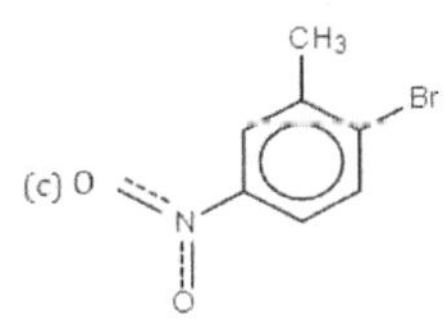 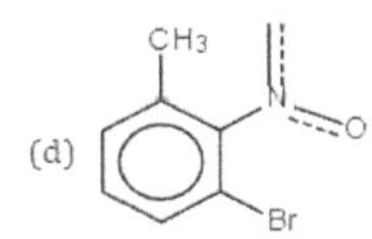

7. Which of the following cannot react as a nucleophile
   (a) $(CH_3)_4N^+$ (b) $CH_3NH_2$
   (c) $(CH_3)_2NH$ (d) $(CH_3)_3N$

8. Which of the following compounds will be oxidized by CrO3 in acid
   (a) 4-Methylcyclohexene
   (b) 3-Methyl 3-hydroxyclohexanone
   (c) 4,4-Dimethyl-1-methyl-1,3-cyclohexandiol
   (d) 2-Methylcyclohexanone

9. Which of the following compounds absorbs at the longest wavelength
   (a) 1,3,5-Hexatriene
   (b) 1,3,5,7-Octatetraene
   (c) 1,7-Diphenyl-1,3,5-heptatriene
   (d) 1,6-Diphenyl-1,3,5-heptatriene

10. Which of the following reagents will reduce a disubstituted alkyne to trans-alkene
    (a) Na and NH3 (b) LiAlH4
    (c) B2H6 (d) Pd and H2

11. Which of the following statement is true about following reaction

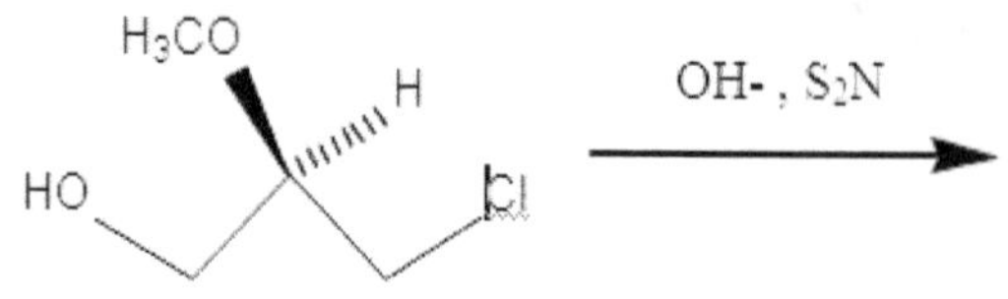

(a) The product will not have a stereo center
(b) The product will have R configuration
(c) The product will not have S configuration
(d) The reaction will happen with racemisation

12. Which functional group is present in the molecule shown below

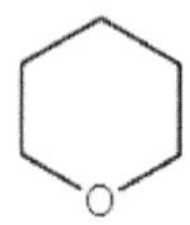

(a) Amide (b) Alcohol
(c) Ester (d) Ether

13. Match the following agents that cause cancer with the preferable sites for where it might cause

| | |
|---|---|
| 1. Arsenic | (a) Prostate |
| 2. Benzene | (b) Angiosarcoma |
| 3. Cadmium Compounds | (c) Leukemia |
| 4. Vinyl chloride | (d) Hemangiosarcoma |

(a) 1 - d; 2 - c; 3 - a; 4 -b
(b) 1 - b; 2 - a; 3 - c; 4- d
(c) 1 - c; 2 - d; 3 - b;4 - a
(d) 1 - a; 2 - b; 3 -d; 4 - c

14. If the pKa of lidocaine is 7.9 and pH of the infected tissue is 8.9, the fraction of drug in the ionized form will be

(a) 10% (b) 1%
(c) 90% (d) 99%

15. Which among the following are the salient features of Glucocorticoids

(a) Gets combined with highly specific cytosolic glucocorticoids
(b) They promote phagocytosis by macro-phages
(c) Releases of lytic enzymes
(d) Increases lipid eicosanoids and prosta-glandin gene

16. The most commonly used test of sensitivity to antimicrobial agent is

(a) Kirby- Bauer techniques
(b) Immunodiffusion techniques
(c) Qudin procedure
(d) Ouchter- Ion procedure

17. Bulk product is defined as

(a) Product completing all processing stages but not necessarily final packing
(b) A product ready for final dispatch
(c) Raw material used for making final dosage form
(d) A defined quantity of raw material from the same batch

18. Product,_and Promotion are four 'P's of marketing

(a) Price and Place
(b) Place
(c) Process
(d) Production, Process, Price, Production

19. Insulin and thyroxin arrive at an organ / tissue / cell at the same time. Thyroxine causes an effect on the organ but insulin does not because

(a) The organ cell have receptors for thyroxine but not for insulin
(b) Thyroxin is a lipid -soluble hormone and insulin
(c) The target cell in the organ have up-regulated for
(d) Thyroxin is local hormone and insulin is a circula

20. Which among the following is an incorrect statement with regard to the drug Dantrolene

(a) It is a pyrazoline derivative
(b) It is an imidazoline analogue
(c) It is a nitrophenylfurfurylidene derivative
(d) It is a skeletal muscle relaxant

21. Diazepam is not suitable for peroral sustained release form since

(a) Is not absorbed in lower intestine
(b) It has biological half life greater than twelve effects hour
(c) It has biological half life less than one hour
(d) It has undesirable side effects

22. Antioxidant used as blocking agent in sterile product is
    (a) Ascorbic acid esters
    (b) Sodium bisulphate
    (c) Ascorbic acid
    (d) EDTA
23. Many mediators have been implicated in the asthmatic response. The clinical efficacyof pharmacologic intervention with inhibitors or antagonist of the mediators involves following category - except
    (a) Platelet activating factors
    (b) Anticholinergics
    (c) Antihistaminics
    (d) Cytokine inhibitors
24. Match the following adrenergic drugs with their receptor affinity
    (1) Epinephrine
        (a) More alpha 1, no beta 1, beta 2 & dopamine
    (2) Noradreanline
        (b) More alpha 1 & beta 1, less beta 2, no dopamine
    (3) Phenylephrine
        (c) More beta 1 & Beta 2, no alpha 1 and dopamine
    (4) Dobutamine
        (d) More alpha 1 & beta 1 , no beta 2 & dopamine
    (a) a - 2; b - 4; c - 1; d -3
    (b) a - 1; b - 3; c - 4; d- 2
    (c) a - 3; b - 1; c - 2;d - 4
    (d) a - 4; b - 2; c -3; d - 1
25. If the drug substance has been substituted wholly or in part by another orsubstance it is called as
    (a) Spurious drug (b) Adulterated drug
    (c) Misbranded drug (d) Mixed drug
26. One of the principle upon which HPLC detector functions is
    (a) Redox property of solute is the basis for functioning of Electrochemical detectors
    (b) Fluorimetric detector has high selectivity and low sensitivity
    (c) Small difference in Refractive Index of mobile phase permit precise measurements in Refractive index detectors
    (d) UV detector function based on its ability to detector
27. Methanolic extract of a crude drug powder when treated with magensium turnings and concentrated hydrochloric acid turned the solution magenta coloured. The test is termed as
    (a) Shinodatest (b) Van Urk's Test
    (c) Keller Killiani test (d) Vitali Morin Test
28. Etoposide and Teniposide are the semisynthetic derivatives of
    (a) Myrrhabolic acid (b) Podophyllotoxin
    (c) Abietic acid (d) Umbelliferone
29. The thymus secretes several hormones related to the immunity. These hormones promote the maturation of T lymphocyte cells. These hormones are
    (1) Thymosin
    (2) Thymichumoral factor
    (3) Thymic factor
    (4) Interleukins
    (a) Only 1, 2 (b) 1, 2 and 3
    (c) only 3 (d) Only 4
30. For the measurement of particle size of powders, the distance measured between two tangents on opposite sides of the particle parallel to some fixed direction is called
    (a) Feret diameter
    (b) Martin diameter
    (c) Projected area diameter
    (d) Edmundson diameter
31. Beta oxidation of fatty acids takes place in
    (a) Mitochondria (b) Cytoplasm
    (c) Nucleus (d) Choroplast
32. Which of the following genera is not the source for tropane alkaloids
    (a) Datura (b) Duboisia
    (c) Nicotiana (d) Atropa

33. The useful variable from in vitro dissolution test data for IVIVC includes
    (a) t50 % - t63.2
    (b) Sampling interval
    (c) Sample volume
    (d) Volume of dissolution fluid

34. In respect of female reproductive cycle, which of the following statements are correct
    (1) The female reproductive cycle consists of menstrual phase, a pre-ovulatory phase, ovulation and a post ovulatory phase
    (2) During the menstrual phase, small secondary follicles in the ovary begin to enlarge while the uterus is shedding its lining
    (3) During the pre-ovulatory phase, a dominant follicle continues to grow and begins to secret estrogen and inhibin while the uterine lining begins to rebuild
    (4) Ovulation results in the release of an ovum and the shedding of the uterus lining tonourish and support the release ovum
    (5) After ovulation, a corpus luteum forms the ruptured follicles and begins to secreteprogesterone and estrogen, which it will continue to do throughout pregnancy if the egg is fertilized
    (6) If pregnancy does not occur, then the corpus luteum degenerates into a scar known as corpus albicans and uterine lining is prepared to be shed again
    (a) 1, 2, 3 and 6 (b) 2, 3, 4and 6
    (c) 1, 2, 4 and 5 (d) 1, 4, 5 and 6

35. Apparent volume of distribution will be highest in case of the drug with % plasmaprotein binding
    (a) 10 (b) 89
    (c) 50 (d) 68

36. To rule out the probability of dose dumping from an oral CR dosage form, USP hasincluded which sampling time point for in vitro dissolution test where D is normal dosing interval
    (a) 0.50D (b) 0.25D
    (c) 50-1.0D (d) 1.0-2.0D

37. Which of the following statement regarding cerebral hemisphere is true
    (a) The right and left hemisphere are symmetrical
    (b) This right more important for spoken and written language
    (c) The left hemisphere is more important for musical and artistic awareness
    (d) Hemispheric lateralization is more pronounced in male than in female

38. Which among the following is a Class-I method, used for rendering a solution of drug isotonic with body fluids
    (a) Cryoscopic method
    (b) White-Vincent method
    (c) Sprowlsmethod
    (d) Hammarlund method

39. (Weight in pounds/150) * Adult Dose = Child dose. The above formula is known as in Posology
    (a) Youngs formula (b) Dillings formula
    (c) Clarkes formula (d) Frieds formula

40. The type of particle diameter obtained by microscopic method of evaluation is
    (a) Projected diameter
    (b) Surface –volume diameter
    (c) Volume - surface diameter
    (d) Stokes diameter

41. Naphazoline
    (a) Is used for relief ofnasal congestion
    (b) Exhibits peripheral beta-adrenoceptor stimulant
    (c) Is a pyrazolinederivative
    (d) Chemically, is 1H Imidazole, 3,4 -dihydro-2 –(3-naphthylmethyl) monohydrochloride

42. A patient receiving warfarin develops rheumatoid arthritis. Which one of the following drugs would be Contraindicated
    (a) Ibuprofen (b) Tolmetin
    (c) Aurothioglucose (d) Aspirin

43. A crude drug powder was heated with ferric chloride, water and concentrated hydrochloric acid followed by extraction with chloroform. The chloroform layer was treated with ammonia, the ammonical layer turned pink. The test indicates presence of____ phytoconstitutent
(a) Anthraquinone-C-glycosides
(b) Flavanones
(c) Cardiac glycosides
(d) Saponin glycosides

44. The first vaccine was discovered by
(a) DeBary (b) Paul Ehrlich
(c) Robert Koch (d) Edward Jenner

45. Type IV dissolution apparatus as per USP is
(a) Flow through cell
(b) Paddle type apparatus
(c) Reciprocating cylinder
(d) Paddle over dsk apparatus

46. Hoeppler viscometer is a type of
(a) Falling sphere viscometer
(b) Capillary viscometer
(c) Cup and Bob viscometer
(d) Cone and plate viscometer

47. Following are the list of various inherited metabolic disorders that can affect functioning of liver
(a) Primary biliary cirrhosis
(b) Glycogen storage disease
(c) Gilbert's syndrome
(d) Haemochromatosis
(e) Wilson's disease
(a) a, b, c, d (b) b, c, d, e
(c) a, c, d, e (d) a, b, d, e

48. In relation to buccal and sublingual route of administration which of the following statement is incorrect
(a) Absorption through epithelium is not affected by partition coefficient of the Drug
(b) Drug absorption by these routes by pass first pass metabolism
(c) There is an optimum log P for sublingual absorption
(d) These are preferred routes for anti-anginal drug

49. Which among the following statements describing surface activity for surfactants is incorrect
(a) Increase in length of hydrocarbon chain decreases surface activity
(b) Increase in ethylene oxide chain of polyoxy ethyl alcohol Increase in surface activity
(c) Increase in surface activity results in decrease length of hydrocarbon chain
(d) Relationship between hydrocarbon chain length andhydrphobicity

50. Surface tension is categorized as a/an factor
(a) Capacity (b) Intensive
(c) Extensive (d) Tolerance

51. Which of the following gums is obtained from endosperm
(a) Guar gum (b) Acacia gum
(c) Tragacanth gum (d) Sterculia gum

52. High lightening differences among brands within the same product category is ______
(a) Product brand
(b) Brand launch
(c) Product differentiation
(d) Branding

53. Hot stage microscopy is an important tool in preformulation studies for the study of
(a) Pseudopolymorphism
(b) Paricle size measurement
(c) Microbial contamination
(d) Compaction behavior

54. In Bismuth subgallate suppositories B.P.C, when no strength of the drug is specified, B.P.C directs ______________bismuth subgallate per suppository
(a) 300 mg (b) 200 mg
(c) 100 mg (d) 400 mg

55. The Michaehis-Menten hypothesis
(a) Postulates the formation of an enzymesubstrate complex
(b) Enables us to calculate the isoelectric point of an enzyme

(c) States that the rate of a chemical reaction may be independent of substrate concentration
(d) States that the reaction rate is proportional tosubstrate concentration

56. The largest gene in human is _______
(a) Dystrophin
(b) Titin
(c) Insulin
(d) Phosphofructokinase

57. Which of the following techniques is not useful to detect polymorphs
(a) DSC
(b) HPLC
(c) PXRD
(d) Melting point determination

58. Which of the following constituents is responsible for colour of shellac
(a) Shelloic acid (b) Laccaic acid
(c) Aleurotic acid (d) All of the above

59. Match the following drugs with alteration they produces in structural-functional of kidney
(1) Aminoglycoside Anitibiotics
(A) Glomerular abnormality
(2) ACE inhibitors
(B) Tubalar epithelial cell Demage
(3) Methotrxate
(C) Hemodynamic Mediated kidney injury
(4) NSAIDs
(D) Obstructure nephrophathy
(a) 1 - B; 2 -C ; 3 - D; 4 -A
(b) 1 - A; 2-B; 3 - C; 4- D
(c) 1 - C; 2-D; 3 - A; 4- B
(d) 1 - D; 2-A; 3 - B; 4- C

60. Hixon Crowell's cube root law of dissolution states that
(a) There is a change in particle size and surface area during dissolution of drug
(b) Dissolution process is controlled by diffusion of molecules/ions
(c) High free energy of activation is required for solution
(d) Renewal of surface fluid layer around drug particle

61. All of the following statements regarding estrogen therapy in postmenopausal women are true EXCEPT
(a) It restores the loss of bone mass due to osteoporosis
(b) It may be useful to treat vasomotor symptoms
(c) Administration in a regimen including a progestin
(d) It is useful in the treatment of atrophic vaginities

62. Chapter IV of which law states that experiments on animals are avoided wherever it is possible to do so; as for example; in medical schools, hospitals, colleges and the like, if other teaching devices such as books, models, films and the. like, may equally suffice. Also, that experiments on larger animals are avoided when it is possible to achieve the same results by experiments upon small laboratory animals like guinea- pigs, rabbits, frogs and rats
(a) The prevention of cruelty to animal act,1960
(b) The Pharmacy Act, 1948
(c) Drugs and Cosmetics Act, 1940
(d) Medicinal and Toilet Preparations Act, 1955

63. Which among the following rules about spin - spin coupling and bond multiplicities are correct with regard to NMR spectra
(a) Coupling constant rarely exceeds 20 cps whilechemical shifts are over 1000 cps
(b) Spin - Spin interactions are dependent of strength of the applied field
(c) Coupling constants increase with distance
(d) Equivalent nuclei interact with each other to show interaction

64. Most accepted mechanism for developing bacterial resistance to sulphonamides is
(a) An alternative metabolic pathway for synthesis of essential
(b) An increasing capacity to metabolize the drug
(c) Increased antagonism of drug
(d) An alteration in enzyme that utilizes PABA

65. All the dopaminergic agonists having affinity for D2 receptors are clinically used in following conditions except
   (a) Obsessive-compulsive disorder
   (b) Hyperprolactinemia
   (c) Acromegaly
   (d) Parkinsonism

66. The labelling instruction "To be diluted 20 times its volume with water" indicates the dispensed product is a
   (a) Mixture (b) Elixir
   (c) Linctus (d) Mouthwash

67. Which among the following is a structural variant of GABA and is used as a muscle relaxant
   (a) Metocurine (b) Tybamate
   (c) Baclofen (d) Cyclobenzaprine

68. A steroidal phyto constituent lowering blood sugar is obtained from
   (a) Momordica charantia
   (b) Quillaja saponaria
   (c) Dioscorea deltoidea
   (d) Glycyrrhiza glabra

69. Which of the following drug is associated with the reaction of extreme photosensitivity
   (a) Niacin
   (b) Digitalis
   (c) Tetracycline
   (d) Fluoroquinolones

70. Which among the following statements related to Ceric sulphate as oxidizing agent, as titrant are correct
   (a) Ce (IV) during reaction exists as an anionic complex in media of sulphuric acid
   (b) Ionic equation is $Ce3+ \rightarrow Ce2+ + e-$
   (c) Formal potential of Ce(III) Ce (II) couple is 1
   (d) Ce (IV) does not permit use of HCl as reducing media

71. A labeled piece of DNA that is complementary to the sequence of DNA you are interested in, say the gene you are trying to put into cells, is called as
   (a) A probe (b) A receptor
   (c) A epitope (d) A target

72. As per first schedule of Drugs and Cosmetics Act ,1940, following is name of the book under Siddha system of medicine
   (a) Arka Prakasha (b) Yog Ratnakar
   (c) Nagamuni (d) Vrinda Chikitsa

73. Amantidine is helpful in Parkinson's disease because
   (a) It liberates dopamine from nerve endings
   (b) It decreases cholinergic activity
   (c) It is metabolized into dopamine
   (d) It increases adrenergic activity

74. An intermediate 3- Chloroaniline 4, 6 - disulphonamide on heating with formic acid yields a compound
   (a) 6 chloro 2H -1,2,4benzothiadiazine 7 sulphonamide
   (b) 3 chloro-2H 1,2,4- benzothiadiazine 7 sulphonamide
   (c) Used in treatment of urinary tract infections
   (d) Used as antibacterial

75. Acetyl Choline is hydrolyzed by enzyme
   (a) Acetylase
   (b) Cholinasc
   (c) Acetylcholinesterase
   (d) Transferase

76. Rubella virus is associated with disease
   (a) Progressive encephalitis
   (b) Enterovirus infection
   (c) Yellow fever
   (d) Brucellosis

77. Which among the following electronic systems are not involved in the origin of UV spectrum
   (a) s and p shell electrons
   (b) sigma and pi electrons
   (c) Charge transfer electrons
   (d) d and f shell electrons

78. Which of the following is not a thermoplastic resin
   (a) Phenolic plastic resin
   (b) Polystyrene
   (c) Polyethylene
   (d) Polypropylene

79. Choose the right combination from the following
    (1) Diacytic stomata and sessile Trichome
        (A) Datuar
    (2) Paracytic stomata and Unicellular and multi cellular
        (B) Vasaka
    (3) Anomocytic stomata and Unicellular and multi cellular
        (C) Senna Trichome
    (4) Anisocytic stomata and Multicellular covering trichome
        (D) Digitalis
    (a) 1-B, 2-C, 3-D, 4-A
    (b) 1-C, 2-D, 3-A, 4-B
    (c) 1-A, 2-D, 3-B, 4-C
    (d) 1-D, 2-B, 3-A, 4-C

80. Pharmaceutical alternatives possess
    (a) Indentical therapeutic moiety/precursor but not in the same amount/dosage form
    (b) Same amount of therapeutic moiety
    (c) Same dosage form
    (d) Same formulation ingredients in exactly same amount of dose

81. Topical application of timolol to the eye would be expected to induce which of the following
    (a) Decreased formation of aqueous humor
    (b) Miosis
    (c) Mydriasis
    (d) Increased outflow of aqueous humor

82. The major component of liquid glucose isand is prepared from
    (a) Maltose, Pectin (b) Dextrin, Starch
    (c) Dextrose, Starch (d) Glucose, Starch

83. Which of the following formulations under ASU system are offered infinite period of shelf life in D and C Act
    (a) Asava&Arishta (b) Churna
    (c) Ghutika (d) Kwatha

84. Which of the following is an example of hemiesters anionic surfactant for pharmaceutrical emulsions
    (a) Sulfosuccinates (b) Sarcosinates
    (c) Taurates (d) Lactylates

85. The major differences between the prokaryotic and eukaryotic protein synthesis mechanisms are in which part of the process
    (a) The initiation of synthesis
    (b) The chain elongation process
    (c) The chain termination process
    (d) None of the above

86. In DNA replication the newly added nucleotide is joined to the growing DNA strand by an enzyme
    (a) DNA polymerase
    (b) DNA ligase
    (c) Restriction endonuclease
    (d) Reverse transcriptase

87. Glycosides are condensation products of
    (a) Protein + aglycone (b) Sugar + Protein
    (c) Sugar + aglycone (d) Fats + aglycone

88. Which of the following dosage form of digoxin will provide greater bioavailability based onvalue of F
    (a) F equals 1.0 (b) F equals 0.32
    (c) F equals 0.62 (d) F equals 0.77

89. The process by which the formed elements of blood develop is call as hemopoiesis. In the process of hemopoiesis the stem cells are converted in to myeloid stem cell and subsequently differentiated and are developed into precursor cells. Match the following precursor cells with the formed elements of blood from which they are formed.
    (1) Reticulocyte (A) Platelets
    (2) Megakaryoblast (B) Macrophages
    (3) Myeloblast (C) Erythrocytes
    (4) Monoblast (D) Neutrophils
    (a) 1-C, 2-A, 3-D, 4-B
    (b) 1-A, 2-C, 3-B, 4-D
    (c) 1-B, 2-D, 3-C, 4-A
    (d) 1-D, 2-B, 3-A, 4-C

90. Using Young's rule, calculate the dose for a 5 year old child if the adult dose is 340mg
    (a) 200 mg (b) 100 mg
    (c) 400 mg (d) 800 mg

91. Which among the following statements on electro analytical methods are correct
    (a) Measures conductance between two electrodes with AC powered Wheatstone bridge
    (b) Polarography involves plotting of conductance – voltage
    (c) Potentiometry involves application of Ilkovic equation
    (d) Coulometry involving application of Nernst law relating equivalence between quantity of electricity passed and amount of compound generated at electrodes

92. Chemical interferences are common than spectral interferences due to
    (a) Formation of compounds of low volatility
    (b) Ionization in flames
    (c) Increase in rate of atomization
    (d) No shift in ionization equilibrium

93. Phase 0 studies means
    (a) In vitro studies
    (b) Part of phase I studies of clinical trials
    (c) First in human microdosing studies
    (d) Studies carried out on small number of animals

94. Condensation product of Ethyl isopentyl ester of diethyl malonic acid with urea and sodium ethoxide yields
    (a) Amylobarbitone (b) Phenobarbitone
    (c) Pentobarbitone (d) Quinobarbitone

95. Clavulanic acid is
    (a) Inactivates bacterial - lactamase
    (b) Protien inhibitor of peptidoglycan synthesis
    (c) Specific for gram negative bacteria
    (d) Inhibitor of 50S ribosomal subunit

96. The method by which different constituents of a liquid mixture can be separated without decomposition of the constituents is
    (a) Distillation under reduced pressure
    (b) Molecular distillation
    (c) Steam distillation
    (d) Fractional distillation

97. The preferred rheological behavior of Pharmaceutical suspensions is that of
    (a) Pseudoplasticity and thixotrophy
    (b) Pseudoplasticity
    (c) Dilatancy and thixotrophy
    (d) Pseudoplasticity and rheopexy,

98. An inventory turnover of a year is considered satisfactory
    (a) Four to six times, Six
    (b) To eight times
    (c) One to two times
    (d) None of the above

99. The number of glucopyranose units in the structure of alpha cyclodextrins are
    (a) 8 (b) 9
    (c) 7 (d) 6

100. The compound 2 - (Diethylamino) ethyl [bicyclohexyl] - 1-carboxylate hydrochloride is
    (a) Dicycloverine
    (b) Diphenhydramine
    (c) Both nicotinic and specific antispasmodic,
    (d) Diagonistic agent for diagnosis of thyroid gland,

101. In new product development process, after analysis of business next step to be taken is
    (a) Test marketing
    (b) Penetration marketing
    (c) Brand marketing
    (d) Individual marketing

102. Which of the following alkaloid (form) is used to treat migrane
    (a) Vinca (b) Coca
    (c) Ergot (d) Belladonna

103. Free flowing powders show a flatter cone and have
    (a) Smaller angle of repose
    (b) Larger angle of repose,
    (c) Intermediate angle of repose
    (d) None of the above,

104. The WIPO is the specialized agency of the United Nations. It promotes protection of throghout the world
    - (a) Intellectual properties
    - (b) World properties
    - (c) Pharmaceutical organizations
    - (d) Finace companies

105. Herpesviruses are large encapsulated viruses that have double stranded DNA genome that encodes approximately 70 proteins. It causes acute infection followed by latent infection in which virus persists in noninfectious form with periodic reactivation and shedding of infectious virus. Following are the examples of such herpesvirus –except
    - (a) Epstein-Barr Virus (b) Herpes simplex
    - (c) Varicella Zoster (d) Cytomegalovirus

106. A fatty acid not synthesized in human body and has to be supplied in diet is
    - (a) Stearic acid (b) Oleic acid
    - (c) Palmitic acid (d) linolenic acid

107. Chemical class of drugs that are susceptible to oxidation are
    - (a) Esters (b) Lactam
    - (c) Sterols (d) Carbamates

108. The only analgesic acting centrally is
    - (a) Methadone (b) Naloxane
    - (c) Tramadol (d) Naloxane

109. Neuropathy is adverse effect of
    - (a) Isoniazid (b) Ethambutol
    - (c) Pyrazinamide (d) Dapsone

110. As per I.P. if the solubility range of a solute is 30 to 100 parts, it will be
    - (a) Soluble (b) Freely soluble
    - (c) Sparingly soluble (d) Slightly soluble

111. SDS is used in PAGE of a mixture of proteins for their efficient separation on the gel. SDS, in the experiment is used to
    - (a) Have uniform charge density on the proteins
    - (b) Stabilize the proteins
    - (c) Decrease the surface tension of buffer
    - (d) Solubilize the proteins

112. Indicate which of the following statements is true
    - (e) A weakly acidic drug is unionised when pH of the solution is at last 2 pH units below its pKa
    - (f) Acidic drugs are noninonized at pH 9
    - (g) Acidic drugs are less soluble in alkaline solution
    - (h) The higher the pKaof a weak acid, the stronger is acid

113. Dissemination of cancer occurs through one of the following pathway - except
    - (a) Migration
    - (b) Direct seeding
    - (c) Lymphatic spread
    - (d) Hematogenous spread

114. Which of the following alkaloids has hypotensive activity
    - (a) Emetine (b) Quinine
    - (c) Reserpine (d) Papaverine

115. Which of the following is a characteristic of cytochrome P-450
    - (a) Catalyzes aromatic and aliphatic hydroxylations
    - (b) Located in the lipophilic environment of mitochondrial membrane
    - (c) Catalyzes O-, S-, N methylation reactions
    - (d) Catalyzes conjugation reactions

116. The Michalis-Menten equation for standard for saturated active transport system is-
    - (a) $V_{max} = k_{cat}[E_0]$ (b) $V_{max} = k_m$
    - (c) $V_{max} = k_m[S]$ (d) None

117. Which among the following describe the characteristic features of Tetracyline
    - (a) Undergoes epimerization in solutions having intermediate pH range
    - (b) Forms Anhydroustetracycline in presence of acidic
    - (c) Forms Minocycline in basic medium
    - (d) Forms stable chelate complexes with potassium ions

118. Cells that contribute for immune system are
(1) T Lymphocytes
(2) Eosinophil
(3) B Lymphocytes
(4) Dendritic cells
(5) Erythrocytes
(6) Natural killer cells
(a) 1, 3, 4 and 6 (b) 1, 2, 4 and 6
(c) 1, 3, 5 and 6 (d) 1, 2, 5 and 6

119. Dielectric constant of Ethanol at room temperature is almost equal to
(a) 24 (b) 48
(c) 54 (d) 72

120. Foaming during liquid filling can be reduced by following ways, except
(a) Increase in speed of the filling line
(b) Minimised product turbulence
(c) Closed system filling
(d) Defoaming device

121. If the excitation energy of the resonance level is 2.10 eV (when hc=12,330) then the wave-length of resonance line of sodium atoms is
(a) 577.2 nm (b) 587.2 nm
(c) 567.2 nm (d) 597.2 nm

122. After vascular injury, platelets encounter extracellular matrix constituents such as collagen and adhesive glycoprotein. On contact with these proteins platelets undergo
1. Adhesion
2. Secretion
3. Aggregation
4. Degradation
(a) 1, 2 and 3 (b) 1, 2 and 4
(c) 1, 2, 3 and 4 (d) 1, 2 and 4

123. A reporting relationship in which an employee receives orders from, and reports to, only one supervisor is known as
(a) Unity of command (b) Centralisation
(c) Decentralisation (d) Line of authority

124. In humans end product of purine catabolism is
(a) Uric acid (b) Urea
(c) Purine oxide (d) Xanthine

125. Which of the following adverse effects is caused by thioridazine
(a) Tardive dyskinesia
(b) Constipation
(c) Orthostatic hypotension
(d) All of the above

# Answer Key GPAT 2017

| 1-d | 2-a | 3-a | 4-a | 5-d | 6-b | 7-a | 8-c | 9-d | 10-a |
|---|---|---|---|---|---|---|---|---|---|
| 11-a | 12-d | 13-a | 14-c | 15-a | 16-a | 17-a | 18-a | 19-b | 20-a |
| 21-b | 22-a | 23-a | 24-a | 25-a | 26-a | 27-a | 28-b | 29-b | 30-a |
| 31-a | 32-c | 33-a | 34-a | 35-a | 36-b | 37-c | 38-a | 39-c | 40-a |
| 41-a | 42-d | 43-a | 44-d | 45-a | 46-a | 47-b | 48-a | 49-a | 50-b |
| 51-a | 52-c | 53-a | 54-c | 55-a | 56-a | 57-b | 58-b | 59-a | 60-a |
| 61-a | 62-a | 63-a | 64-a | 65-a | 66-d | 67-c | 68-a | 69-c | 70-a |
| 71-a | 72-c | 73-a | 74-a | 75-c | 76-a | 77-a | 78-a | 79-a | 80-a |
| 81-a | 82-c | 83-a | 84-a | 85-a | 86-a | 87-c | 88-a | 89-a | 90-b |
| 91-a | 92-a | 93-c | 94-a | 95-a | 96-b | 97-a | 98-a | 99-d | 100-a |
| 101-a | 102-c | 103-a | 104-a | 105-a | 106-d | 107-c | 108-a | 109-a | 110-c |
| 111-a | 112-a | 113-a | 114-c | 115-a | 116-a | 117-a | 118-a | 119-a | 120-a |
| 121-b | 122-a | 123-a | 124-a | 125-d | | | | | |

# GPAT 2018

1. A technique of using very small metal particles coated with desired DNA in the gene transfer is called:-
   (a) Microinjection
   (b) Biolistic
   (c) Liposome mediated
   (d) Electroporation
2. Arrange the following steps in sequence of their order for production of recombinant Insulin:-
   (a) Fusion of A and B chains for disulphide bond.
   (b) Cynogen bromide treatment to remove methi onine and â galactosidase.
   (c) Introduction of A and B chain in the plasmid containing â galactosidase g ene.
   (d) Synthesis of A and B chain in E coli.
   (a) a → b → d → c
   (b) d → c → a → b
   (c) c → d → b → a
   (d) b → a → d → c
3. Motif is represented by
   (a) Commas repeated on the lattice
   (b) 3D translational periodic arrangement of points
   (c) Geometric shapes of lattice
   (d) Centre of symmetry in lattice
4. Statement 1: Vortex formation can be minimized by push pull mechanism.

   Statement 2: Vortex formation reduces the mixing intensity by increasing the velocity of impeller.
   (a) True, False (b) True, True
   (c) False, False (d) False, True
5. Which of the following fluid can be considered as an ideal fluid?
   (a) Viscous fluid
   (b) Non-viscous fluid
   (c) Compressible fluid
   (d) All of these
6. Which of the following agencies is not classified as an 'executive agency' for administration of the act under the provision of Drugs and Cosmetics Act 1940?
   (a) Licensing authority
   (b) Drug inspectors
   (c) Drugs Consultative Committee
   (d) Customs collectors
7. As per Factories Act 1948, in CHAPTER VI dealing with working hours of adults, no adult worker shall be required or allowed to work in a factory for more than ___ __ _ ___ hours in a week.
   (a) 30 (b) 40
   (c) 48 (d) 56
8. Henri Fayol's principle "Espirit de corps" means:-
   (a) Corporate objective (b) Group objective
   (c) Team activity (d) Team spirit
9. How customer's bias about the product will influence the marketing communication?
   (a) Positive effect
   (b) Negative effect
   (c) No effect
   (d) Both positive and Negative
10. Which of the following is not patentable in India as per The Patents Act 1970?
    (a) New product
    (b) New process
    (c) New use of existing drug
    (d) New process for existing drug

11. Match the following enzymes in Column I with their respective functions under Column II

| Column I | Column II |
|---|---|
| i. DNA ligase | (p) Synthe size a DNA copy of RNA |
| ii. Alkaline phosphatase | (q) Forms a bond between 3' – OH and 5'-$PO_4$ |
| iii. Reverse transcriptase | (r) Removes terminal $PO_4$ from 3' or 5'end of DNA |
| iv. Polynucleotide kinase | (s) Adds phosphate to 5' –OH end |

(a) i-r, ii-s, iii-p, iv-q
(b) i-p, ii-q, iii-r, iv-s
(c) i-q, ii-r, iii-p, iv-s
(d) i-s, ii-p, iii-q, iv-r

12. Which of the following replacement of amino acid in a protein may produce greatest change in its conformation?

(a) Ser → Thr (b) Glu → Val
(c) Gln → Tyr (d) Phe → Ile

13. The hexose monophosphate pathway produces distinctively two useful products. Identify these products with the ratio in which they are produced.

(a) One NADPH to two ribose-6-phosphate
(b) Two NADPH to one ribose-5-phosphate
(c) Two NADPH to one ribulose-5-phosphate
(d) Two NADPH to one fructose-6-phosphate

14. The correct statement about Vitamin D is:-

(a) The oral administration of 1, 25-dihydoxycholecalciferol is required in chronic renal failure
(b) 25-Hydroxycholecalciferol is the active form of the vitamin
(c) Vitamin D antagonizes the effects of parathyroid hormone
(d) A deficiency of vitamin D causes an increase in calcitonin secretion

15. All of the following enzymes are used in ELISA except:-

(a) Glucose oxidase
(b) Alkaline phosphatase
(c) Coagulase
(d) β-galactosidase

16. Which of the following equilibrium suggests noncompetitive inhibition of enzyme E for conversion of substrate S to product P with inhibitor I?

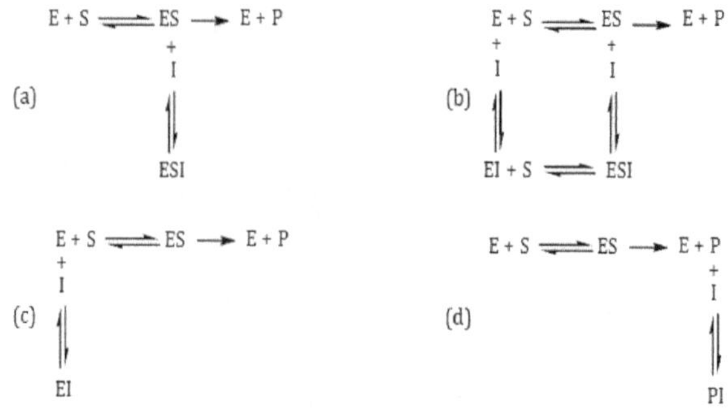


17. Which method is used for the Limit test for arsenic?

(a) Gutzeit method
(b) Oswald method
(c) Arrhenius method
(d) Karl-Fischer method

18. The agent used to prevent the dental carries is:-

(a) Sodium fluoride
(b) Strontium chloride
(c) Zinc chloride
(d) Dicalcium phosphate

19. Which of the following definitions of an asymmetric reaction is the most accurate?

(a) A reaction that creates a new chiral centre in the product
(b) A reaction that involves a chiral reagent
(c) A reaction which creates a new chiral centre with selectivity for one enantiomer/ diasatereoisomer over another
(d) A reaction that is carried out on an asymmetric starting material

20. What software programme is used to determine the Verloop steric parameter in QSAR?

(a) Alchemy (b) Chem3D
(c) Sterimol (d) Chem-Draw

21. The oral oligosaccharide hypoglycemic agent, which is administered at the start of the meal is:-

(a) Pioglitazone (b) Miglitol
(c) Acarbose (d) Glimepride

22. Which functional group is crucial for anti-malarial activity of artemisinin?
    (a) Aldehydic functional group
    (b) Ethylene bridge
    (c) Ketonic functional group
    (d) Peroxide bridge

23. Select the drug which exhibits dual alpha and beta adrenergic receptor agonists activity.
    (a) Terbutaline (b) Clonidine
    (c) Metaproterenol (d) Dobutamine

24. Appropriate hybridization schemes for the C atoms in molecule CH3CO2H are:-
    (a) $sp^3$ and sp (b) $sp^3$ and $sp^2$
    (c) $sp^2$ and sp (d) $sp^3$ and $sp^3$

25. In Universal indicators, a pH of 7 is shown with:-
    (a) Yellow color (b) Green color
    (c) Blue color (d) Pink color

26. Which statement regarding Hückel's rule is FALSE?
    (a) There must be (4n + 2) pi ($\pi$) electrons
    (b) The molecule must be planar
    (c) The molecule must be cyclic
    (d) Each of the pi ($\pi$) electrons must be associated with a conjugated double bond

27. Anthracene is isomeric with:-
    (a) Phenanthrene (b) Naphthalene
    (c) Benzene (d) Azulene

28. The molecular formula of phenanthrene is:-
    (a) C14 H10 (b) C12 H10
    (c) C14 H14 (d) C14 H8

29. In electrophilic substitution of pyridine, reaction of pyridine with H2O2 in acetic acid leads to formation of:-
    (a) 1,4-Dihydropyridine
    (b) 2-Hydroxypyridine
    (c) 2-Pyridone
    (d) Pyridine-N-oxide

30. Which compound is most basic?
    (a) 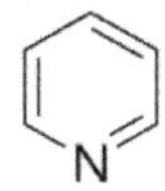
    (b) 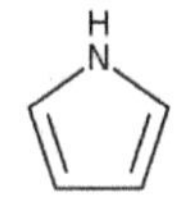
    (c) 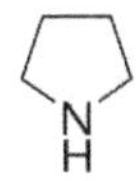
    (d) 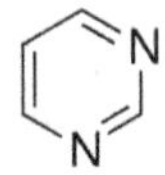

31. Correct Nomenclature for the following bridged bicyclic ring system is:-

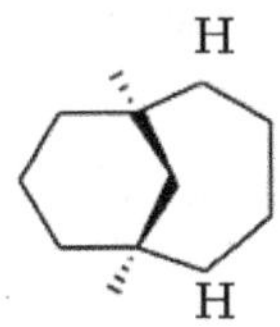

    (a) bicyclo[4.4.0]decane
    (b) bicyclo[4.3.0]decane
    (c) bicyclo[4.3.1]decane
    (d) bicyclo[4.4.1]decan

32. Which among the following correctly defines Diastereomer?
    (a) These have same magnitude but different signs of optical rotation
    (b) Nonsuperimposable object mirror relationship
    (c) These differ in all physical properties
    (d) Separation is very difficult

33. Galactose and Glucose are:-
    (a) Epimers
    (b) Anomers
    (c) Isomers
    (d) Ketose-Aldose isomers

34. Which among the following is a non-essential amino acid?
    (a) Lysine (b) Threonine
    (c) Serine (d) Histidine

35. Which of the following is a 3,3-sigmatropic reaction which converts a 1,5-diene to an isomeric 1,5 diene?
    (a) Cope rearrangement
    (b) Claisen rearrangement
    (c) Photochemical [2+2] reaction
    (d) Diels-Alder reaction

36. What quantity of an indicator solution shall be added when quantity is not mentioned in an assay or test?
    (a) 0.1 ml (b) 0.05 ml
    (c) 0.2 ml (d) 0.5 ml

37. In Kjeldahl method, sample containing nitrogen is digested with
    (a) Concentrated sodium hydroxide
    (b) Fuming nitric acid
    (c) Concentrated sulphuric acid
    (d) Strong ammonia solution

38. 0.5What is the concentration of paracetamol in a 0.1 N sodium hydroxide solution, whose absorption in a 1 cm cell at its lambda max, 257 nm, was found to be 0.825? The A (1%, 1 cm) in the IP monograph of paracetamol is given as 715 at 257 nm
    (a) 1.1 g/100 ml
    (b) 0.0011 mg/100 ml
    (c) 0.0011 g/100 ml
    (d) 0.0011μg/100 ml

39. The unit for specific absorbance A (1%, 1cm) is:-
    (a) μg/mL (b) mg/L
    (c) liter $mole^{-1}$ $cm^{-1}$ (d) dl $g^{-1}$ $cm^{-1}$

40. What is the nuclear magnetic resonance frequency of 1H in a 7.05 Tesla magnetic field strength?
    (a) 300.0 MHz (b) 200.0 MHz
    (c) 60.0 MHz (d) 100 MHz

41. What is Hydrogen Deficiency Index (HDI) value for toluene?
    (a) 1 (b) 2
    (c) 3 (d) 4

42. In NMR, the aromatic proton resonate in a characteristic narrow range at:-
    (a) δ 6.5 – δ 8.0 (b) δ 11.0 – δ 12.0
    (c) δ 2.0 – δ 4.0 (d) δ 0.7 – δ 1.3

43. The difficulties of long elution time and poor resolution of complex mixtures are observed in elution analysis. These difficulties can be overcome by modification of elution analysis, known as:-
    (a) Isocratic-elution analysis
    (b) Gradient-elution analysis
    (c) Displacement analysis
    (d) Frontal analysis

44. Materials whose consistency depends on the duration of shear, as well as on the rate of shear, exhibit:-
    (a) Rheopexy (b) Thixotropy
    (c) Viscoelasticity (d) Plasticity

45. Which of the following solutions are more likely to have the same osmotic pressure? Solutions of:
    (a) Diluted nonelectrolytes with the same molal concentration
    (b) Concentrated nonelectrolytes with the same molal concentration
    (c) Diluted electrolytes with the same molal concentration
    (d) Concentrated electrolytes with the same molal concentration

46. Which statements are correct for the micelle formation?
    (p) Micelles are dynamic structures that are continually formed and broken down in solution.
    (q) The typical micelle diameter is about 2–3 μm and so they are visible under the light micro scope.
    (r) Micelle formation is a spontaneous process.
    (s) When the surfactant concentration is increased above the CMC, the number of micelles increases and the free surfactant concentration decreases below CMC.
    (a) P and Q (b) P and R
    (c) P and S (d) R and S

47. Which equation is used to predict the stability of a drug product at room temperature from experiments at accelerated temperature?
    (a) Higuchi equation
    (b) The Arrhenius' equation
    (c) Hildebrand equation
    (d) The Hixson-Crowell equation

48. Which statement correctly describes Hess's Law?
   (a) The enthalpy of all reactants in their standard states is defined as zero
   (b) Enthalpy changes can be calculated only if one or more of the reactants is/are element
   (c) The enthalpy change of a reaction can be calculated only at 1 atm pressure and 25 °C
   (d) The enthalpy change of a reaction is independent of the route of reaction

49. Identify the starting material A and B in the synthesis of Clomifene.

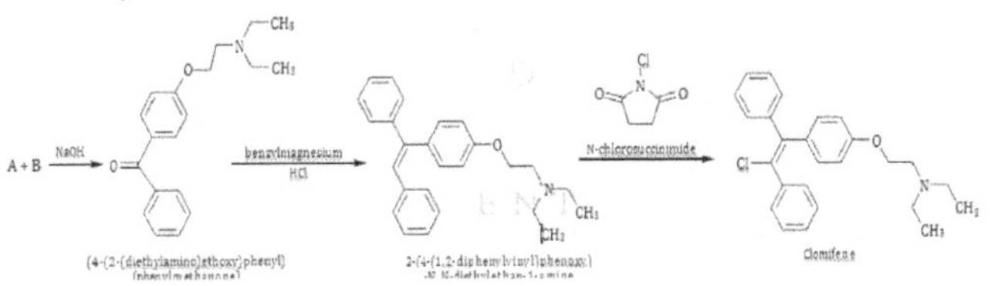

   (a) Where A 4-hydroxy-benzophenone and B 2-diethylamino-ethyl chloride
   (b) Where A 4-hydroxy benzaldehyde and B 4-methoxy aniline
   (c) Where A 4-hydroxy-benzophenone and B 4-methoxy aniline
   (d) Where A 4-hydroxy-benzophenone and B benzaldehyde

50. The role of glutathione in tissues includes all except:-
   (a) Participate in decomposition of hydrogen peroxide
   (b) Participate in activation of methionine
   (c) Participate in detoxification reactions
   (d) Biologically active in oxidized form

51. When Ke is constant and Ka is larger:-
   (a) $C_{max}$ is more and $t_{max}$ is longer
   (b) $C_{max}$ is lesser and $t_{max}$ is longer
   (c) $C_{max}$ is lesser and $t_{max}$ is short
   (d) $C_{max}$ is more and $t_{max}$ is short

52. When considering drug delivery to the brain which of the following is false?
   (a) The cells in the blood vessels that supply the brain are tightly connected which restricts drug absorption
   (b) Only relatively small lipophilic molecules readily, passively diffuse in to the brain
   (c) Drugs with a low log P value show improved passive diffusion into the brain (P: oil / water partition coefficient)
   (d) Polar molecules can be taken up into the brain through active transport

53. IVIVC utilizes the principles of statistical moment analysis:-
   (a) Level A (b) Level B
   (c) Level C (d) Level D

54. The systems that follows, Weibull Mathematical Model used to describe drug release kinetics are:-
   (a) Swellable polymeric devices
   (b) Diffusion matrix formulation
   (c) Erodible matrix formulation
   (d) Transdermal system

55. Which method is used by pharmacists for complete blending of potent powders with large quantities of diluents?
   (a) Spatulation
   (b) Levigatio
   (c) Trituration
   (d) Geometric dilution

56. Substance used to reduce friction during tablet compression and facilitate ejection of tablets from the die cavity is called as:-
   (a) Lubricant (b) Glidant
   (c) Anti-adherent (d) Humectant

57. What quantities of 95% v/v and 45% v/v alcohols are to be mixed to make 800 mL of 65% v/v alcohol?
   (a) 480 mL of 95% and 320 mL of 45% alcohol
   (b) 320 mL of 95% and 480 mL of 45% alcohol
   (c) 440 mL of 95% and 360 mL of 45% alcohol
   (d) 360 mL of 95% and 440 mL of 45% alcohol

58. The proportion of NaCl liquid to give 1.5% solution of drug isotonic with blood plasma is:- (The freezing point of 1% w/v solution of drug is -0.122 and NaCl is -0.576 °C)
   (a) 0.79% (b) 0.585%
   (c) 0.9% (d) 0.5%

59. Which of the following statement is NOT TRUE about prokaryotes?
    (a) Nucleus is not bounded by nuclear membrane
    (b) Cell wall contains peptidoglycan
    (c) 80S ribosomes are distributed in cytoplasm
    (d) It is Haploid in nature

60. Match the following diseases under column I with the respective causative organisms under Column II.

| Column I | Column II |
|---|---|
| i. Creutzfeldt-Jacob disease | (p) Yersinia pestis |
| ii. Typhus | (q) Prions |
| iii. Syphilis | (r) Rickettsia prowazekii |
| iv. Plague | (s) Treponema palladium |

    (a) i-r, ii-s, iii-p, iv-q
    (b) i-p, ii-q, iii-r, iv-s
    (c) i-q, ii-r, iii-s, iv-p
    (d) i-s, ii-p, iii-q, iv-r

61. As the dielectric constant values increases, the polarity of the solvents _ .
    (a) Decreases
    (b) Increases
    (c) Remains constant
    (d) Decreases and then remains constant

62. The angle of repose is calculated by _.
    (a) $\tan \alpha$ = Radius/Height
    (b) $\tan \alpha$ = 1+Radius/Height
    (c) $\tan \alpha$ = 1- Radius/Height
    (d) $\tan \alpha$ = Height/Radius

63. Spray drying / spray congealing method is generally used to prepare _ .
    (a) Tablets (b) Microcapsule
    (c) Capsules (d) Ointments

64. HLB value of tragacanth is:-
    (a) 4.7 (b) 8.7
    (c) 13.2 (d) 14.3

65. Vials and bottles are regularly not subjected to following test:-
    (a) Sterility test
    (b) Clarity test
    (c) Leaker (chamber) test
    (d) Pyrogen test

66. As per USP, test limit for treated soda lime glass with container size of 200 ml is:-
    (a) 0.70ml of 0.02N Acid
    (b) 1.0ml of 0.2N Acid
    (c) 0.20ml of 0.02N Acid
    (d) 0.70ml of 0.2N Acid

67. In plasma, phenobarbital is present as ionized and unionized forms in equal amount because:-
    (a) It is weakly acidic drug
    (b) It is weakly basic drug
    (c) pH of plasma is 6.8
    (d) pKa of the phenobarbital is 7.4

68. A material which is insoluble and inert and used in matrix tablet formulation is:-
    (a) Polyethylene
    (b) Stearyl alcohol
    (c) Polyethylene glycol
    (d) Triglycerides

69. Which test is done for USP Type-I glass containers for injections?
    (a) Water attack test
    (b) Powdered glass test
    (c) Powdered glass followed by water attack test
    (d) Water attack followed powdered glass test

70. Isoelectric point of Type A gelatin is .
    (a) pH 7.0 (b) pH 4.7
    (c) pH 9.0 (d) pH 7.4

71. What is the effective ratio of methyl paraben and propyl paraben for anti-microbial activity?
    (a) 1:1 (b) 5:1
    (c) 2.5:1 (d) 10:1

72. Which of the following formula is used to determine shelf life as per first order reaction?
    (a) $T_{90}$ 0.693/k (b) $t_{90}$ 0.104/k
    (c) $t_{1/2}$ 0.693/k (d) $t_{1/2}$ 0.105/k

73. Following are endogenous carriers use for targeted drug delivery except:-
    (a) Lipoprotein (b) Serum Albumin
    (c) Erythrocyte (d) Microparticulates

74. The friability issue of the tablet can be solved by different ways except:-
   (a) Increasing the upper punch pressure of tablet machine
   (b) Addition of more tablet binder to granules
   (c) Increasing the moisture content of granules
   (d) Adjusting the lower punch pressure of tablet machine

75. What are the specific surface per unit volume Sv of spherical particles with density of 3 gm/cm3 and volume surface diameter, dvs of 2.57μm?
   (a) 7.78 × 103 cm2/cm3
   (b) 2.33 × 103 cm2/cm3
   (c) 1.55 × 103 cm2/cm3
   (d) 1.00 × 103 cm2/cm3

76. In a free-flowing powder, the bulk density and tapped density would be close in value, therefore, the Carr index would be:-
   (a) Small (b) Medium
   (c) Large (d) None

77. Buffer capacity is also referred to as:-
   (a) Buffer index (b) Buffer value
   (c) Buffer efficiency (d) All of these

78. Keesom interactions has a force of:-
   (a) 0.5- 1 kcal/mol (b) 1-7 kcal/mol
   (c) 1-3 kcal/mol (d) None of these

79. Dipole - induced dipoles are also known as:-
   (a) London forces
   (b) Keesom forces
   (c) Debye forces
   (d) Hydrogen bonding

80. The interfacial tension of Oleic acid against water at 20oC is:-
   (a) 15.6 (b) 52.3
   (c) 428 (d) 8.51

81. Suspensions of starch in water exhibit:-
   (a) Plastic flow
   (b) Psudoplastic flow
   (c) Dilatant flow
   (d) None of these

82. Very weak bases having pKa < 5:-
   (a) Are ionized in the entire pH range of GIT
   (b) Absorbed only in stomach
   (c) Are unionized at all pH values
   (d) None of these

83. During determination of absorption rate constant by method of residual, flip-flop phenomenon occurs when (Ka absorption rate constant and KE overall elimination rate constant).
   (a) $K_E/Ka \geq 3$ (b) $Ka/K_E \geq 3$
   (c) $K_E/Ka \leq 3$ (d) $Ka/K \leq 3$

84. Which of the following disinfectant effectively destroys vegetative bacterial cells including Gram positive and Gram negative bacteria, bacterial endospores, fungi, and viruses?
   (a) 8% formaldehyde + 70% alcohol
   (b) 70% Alcohol
   (c) 0.1% Phenol aqueous
   (d) 0.1% Iodine aqueous

85. Which of the following are obligatory intracellular parasites?
   (P) Virus
   (Q) Fungus
   (R) Mycoba cterium
   (S) Rickettsia
   (a) All (b) (P), (Q) and (R)
   (c) (R) and (S) (d) (P) and (S)

86. Select the correct statement.
   (a) Acids salt corresponding to an insoluble salt will be more water soluble than original salt
   (b) Hydroxides and oxides of compounds other than alkali metal cations and the common ions are generally water soluble
   (c) Sulphides are water soluble except for their alkali metal salts
   (d) Ammonium and Quaternary ammonium salts are water insoluble

87. What is the viscosity of resulting liquid after mixing 300mL of liquid A (η=1.0 cP) with the 200mL of liquid B (η=3.4 cP)?
   (a) 2.2 cP (b) 1.4 cP
   (c) 1.6 cP (d) 1.8 cP

88. A compound now increasingly used as standard practice for enhancing the flow of rubber latex by spraying on to the scraped bark of the rubber tree increasing the latex yields from 36% to 130% is:-
    (a) Brassinosteroids (b) Abscisic acid
    (c) Ethephon (d) Kinetin

89. The constituent of Cochineal is:-
    (a) Cantharidin (b) Hirudin
    (c) Tannic acid (d) Carminic acid

90. The sweet taste and odour of fennel is due to:-
    (a) Anethole (b) Fenchone
    (c) Eugenol (d) Phellandrene

91. Catechu is used in medicine as an:-
    (a) Antidiabetic (b) Anti cance
    (c) Antipyretic (d) Astringent

92. Tropane alkaloids are biosynthesized from amino acid.
    (a) Phenylalanine (b) Tyrosine
    (c) Ornithine (d) Leucine

93. One mg of Lycopodium contains an average of:-
    (a) 97000 spores (b) 96000 spores
    (c) 95000 spores (d) 94000 spores

94. Charaka, a physician belonged to which system of medicine?
    (a) Ayurveda (b) Unani
    (c) Siddha (d) Homeopathy

95. The CCCN code indicating the botanical drugs is:-
    (a) 2211 (b) 1122
    (c) 1211 (d) 1311

96. Uncaria gambir belongs to the family:-
    (a) Rubiaceae (b) Combretaceae
    (c) Punicaceae (d) Rosaceae

97. Alkanna tinctoria (Boraginaceae) roots are used in:-
    (a) Dandruff
    (b) Tooth paste
    (c) Facial cleansing wash
    (d) Lipstick formulations and hair dyes

98. Identify the clotting factor which is known as Stuart factor or thrombokinase.
    (a) Clotting factor - IV
    (b) Clotting factor - VIII
    (c) Clotting factor - X
    (d) Clotting factor - XII

99. Which part of the eye is light sensitive (photosensitive)?
    (a) Iris (b) Sclera
    (c) Lens (d) Retina

100. Identify the specific site where maturation of sperm takes place.
    (a) Spermatic cord (b) Epididymis
    (c) Testis (d) Vas deference

101. Identify the hormone that stimulates sperm production in testes and ovulation in females.
    (a) Prolactin
    (b) Luteinising hormone
    (c) Follicle stimulating hormone
    (d) Adrenocorticotropic hormone

102. Identify the correct pair from the following:-
    (a) Sympathetic stimulation: Bronchoconstriction
    (b) Parasympathetic stimulation: Secretion of gastric juice
    (c) Sympathetic stimulation: Contraction of pupil
    (d) Parasympathetic stimulation: Dilatation of pupil

103. The number of subjects required in a phase- 1 clinical trial is:-
    (a) 20 to 100
    (b) Upto several hundred
    (c) 300 to 3,000
    (d) Several thousands

104. To obtain a more effective bronchodilation, the drugs that are combined along with beta-adrenoceptor agonists are:-
    (a) Cholinergic antagonists
    (b) Cholinergic agonists
    (c) Beta-adrenoceptor antagonists
    (d) Alpha-adrenoceptor antagonists

105. Which of the following antipsychotic drugs, at low doses, is combined with antidepressants in treatmentresistant depression?
(a) Chlorpromazine (b) Haloperidol
(c) Risperidone (d) Fluphenazine

106. The management of Type-B adverse drug reaction is:-
(a) To reduce the dose
(b) To withhold the dose and avoid in future
(c) To increase the dose
(d) To reintroduce and withdraw slowly

107. Abatacept, a fusion protein, and a co-stimulation blocker used in the treatment of Rheumatoid arthritis blocks the:-
(a) Activation of T-cells
(b) Inhibition of T-cells
(c) Activation of B-cells
(d) Inhibition of B-cells

108. Hemophilia A is a disease characterized by deficiency of:-
(a) Factor VIII (b) Factor II
(c) Factor VII (d) Factor V

109. The enzyme HMG-CoA reductase is involved in the pathogenesis of:-
(a) Atherosclerosis (b) Renal failure
(c) Alzheimer disease (d) Parkinson disease

110. Rheumatic heart disease is caused by:-
(a) Streptococcal infection
(b) Excessive lipid consumption
(c) Abnormal lipid metabolism
(d) Atherosclerosis

111. Which of the following is NOT a gene associated with breast cancer?
(a) BRCA1 (b) HER2
(c) BRCA2 (d) CHRM1

112. Which of the following is NOT true about the Ebola Virus Disease (EVD)?
(a) Spreads through human-to-human transmission via direct contact
(b) Antiviral drugs are approved by FDA to mitigate the infection
(c) Diagnostic tests include ELISA
(d) The virus is named after a river

113. Hypodermoclysis refers to which route of drug administration?
(a) Sublingual (b) Intradermal
(c) Subcutaneous (d) Intravenous

114. Which of the following is a shortest acting cholinersterase inhibitors enlisted below?
(a) Neostigmine (b) Pyridostigmin
(c) Edrophonium (d) Physostigmine

115. Which of the following is a suitable antidote for mercury poisoning?
(a) Atropine (b) Dimercapro
(c) Naloxone (d) Nalorphine

116. Histamine concentration is highest in:-
(a) Beta cells (b) Mast cells
(c) Lymphocytes (d) Adipocytes

117. Select the â-lactamase inhibitor.
(a) Griseofulvin (b) Clavulanic acid
(c) Sulfamethoxazole (d) Tetracycline

118. The mechanism of action of ciprofloxacin is:-
(a) Inhibition of protein synthesis by interacting with 30s ribosome
(b) Inhibition of protein synthesis by interacting with 50s ribosomes
(c) Inhibition of DNA synthesis by interacting with topoisomerase
(d) Inhibition of cell wall synthesis

119. Which of the following is NOT CORRECT for myasthenia gravis?
(a) Down regulation of nicotinic receptors (Nm) leads to myasthenia gravis
(b) Tubocurarine is used to treat myasthenia gravis
(c) It is an autoimmune disorder
(d) Thymectomy is treatment option for myasthenia gravis

120. Which of the following describes the effect of Sodium cromoglycate?
(a) Mast cell degranulation
(b) Mast cell stabilization
(c) Leukotriene antagonism
(d) Glucocorticoid receptor agonism

121. Which of the following side effect of ACE inhibitors result from inhibition of bradykinin breakdown?
   (a) Analgesia (b) Hyperglycaemia
   (c) Productive cough (d) Dry cough

122. Identify antihistamine drug with additional serotonin receptor blocking activity and good appetite stimulant property.
   (a) Cyproheptadine
   (b) Cimetidine
   (c) Ranitidine
   (d) Chlorpheniramine

123. Which of the following are the mechanisms of action of digitalis glycosides?
   i. Inhibition of $Na^{+}$-$K^{+}$ ATPase enzyme.
   ii. Reduction in the auriculo-ventricular conduction rate.
   iii. Increase in the cardiac output.
   iv. Acceleration of auriculo-ventric ular conduction rate.
   (a) Only iii (b) i, ii and iii
   (c) ii, iii and iv (d) Only i

124. The following is NOT true for Furosemide:-
   (a) Causes hypokalemia
   (b) Causes hypouricemia
   (c) Causes hypomagnesemia
   (d) Acts by inhibiting sodium reabsorption

125. Which of the following about the Varicella-Zoster Virus (VZV) is NOT true?
   (a) Varicella develops after an individual is exposed to VZV for the first time
   (b) Herpes zoster develops from reactivation of the virus later in life
   (c) There are no vaccines for this virus
   (d) The infection results in post-herpetic neuralgia

# Answer Key GPAT 2018

| 1-b | 2-c | 3-a | 4-a | 5-b | 6-c | 7-c | 8-d | 9-d | 10-c |
|---|---|---|---|---|---|---|---|---|---|
| 11-c | 12-b | 13-b | 14-a | 15-c | 16-b | 17-a | 18-a | 19-c | 20-c |
| 21-c | 22-d | 23-d | 24-b | 25-b | 26-d | 27-a | 28-a | 29-d | 30-c |
| 31-c | 32-c | 33-a | 34-c | 35-a | 36-a | 37-c | 38-c | 39-d | 40-a |
| 41-d | 42-a | 43-b | 44-b | 45-a | 46-b | 47-b | 48-d | 49-a | 50-d |
| 51-d | 52-c | 53-b | 54-c | 55-d | 56-a | 57-b | 58-b | 59-c | 60-c |
| 61-b | 62-d | 63-b | 64-c | 65-c | 66-c | 67-d | 68-a | 69-b | 70-c |
| 71-d | 72-b | 73-d | 74-d | 75-b | 76-a | 77-d | 78-b | 79-c | 80-a |
| 81-c | 82-c | 83-a | 84-a | 85-d | 86-a | 87-b | 88-c | 89-d | 90-a |
| 91-d | 92-c | 93-d | 94-a | 95-c | 96-a | 97-d | 98-c | 99-d | 100-b |
| 101-c | 102-b | 103-a | 104-a | 105-c | 106-b | 107-a | 108-a | 109-a | 110-a |
| 111-d | 112-b | 113-c | 114-c | 115-b | 116-b | 117-b | 118-c | 119-b | 120-b |
| 121-d | 122-a | 123-b | 124-b | 125-c | | | | | |

# GPAT 2019

1. As per US FDA, NDA'S for new chemical entities are classified as either :
   (a) 'P' for product review or 'S' for standard review
   (b) 'P' for priority review or 'S' for standard review
   (c) 'P' for product review or 'S' for safety review
   (d) 'P' for priority review or 'S' for safety review
2. In preformulation study polymorphs can be detected by:
   (a) Counter –current chromatography
   (b) Retractometry
   (c) High performance liquid chromatography
   (d) Differential scanning colorimetry
3. The following technique is /are used to determine the amount of drug bound to a protein:
   (a) Equilibrium dialysis
   (b) Solubility
   (c) pH titration
   (d) distribution method
4. In tablet hydroxyl propyl methyl cellulose is used as:
   (a) Diluents (b) Film former
   (c) Disintegrant (d) Binder
5. Dakin's solution is a synonym for:
   (a) Ammonium acetate solution
   (b) Chlorinated soda solution
   (c) Chloroxylenlol solution
   (d) Alluminium acetate solution
6. MEDLINE,EMBASE,EBM AND IDI's are:
   (a) Drug databases
   (b) New compendia specification of drugs
   (c) Chronicles of drug standards
   (d) source for drug patents
7. Theories of emulsification are characterized by one of the following except:
   (a) film formation
   (b) phase inversion
   (c) monomolecular adsorption
   (d) Solid particle adsorption
8. When two brands of a drug product give same clinical results, it is termed as:
   (a) Therapeutic equivalence
   (b) Bio equivalence
   (c) Pharmaceuticals equivalence
   (d) Clinical equivalence
9. Soda ash is also known as:
   (a) Lime stone
   (b) Sodium carbonate
   (c) Pure silica
   (d) Calcium carbonate
10. Microcrystalline cellulose is also called as:
    (a) Sugar tab (b) Nutab
    (c) Emdex (d) Avicel
11. Which of the following statement is NOT true regarding bulkiness?
    (a) The reciprocal of bulk density is bulkiness
    (b) Bulkiest substance will require container larger than required for less bulki substance
    (c) Smaller particle shift between larger ones ind increases bulkiness
    (d) Bulkiness increases with decrease in particle size
12. A mixture of emulsifier A and emulsifier B with H.L.B. values of 4 and 14 respectively are to be mixed in proportion to get a mixture with required HLB 12What is the weight of individual emulsifier that is to be taken to have a total weight of 7 gm?
    (a) A= 5.8 gm and B= 1.2gm
    (b) A = 1.4 gm and B= 5.6 gm

(c) A= 5.6 gm and B = 1.4 gm
(d) A = 1.2 gm and B= 5.8 gm

13. Which of the following oxide is not used for achieving Amber color to glass :
(a) Manganese (b) Iron
(c) Cobalt (d) carbon

14. In case of one compartment open model intravenous infusion Css(Steady state plasma concentration) is equal to:
(a) [Plasma concentration][infusion rate] / clearence
(b) [C max] [ infusion rate]/ Clearance
(c) [t max] [infusion rate] /clearance
(d) infusion rate /clearance

15. In case of suppository base , SFI stands for:
(a) solidified fatty acid indices
(b) solid fluid indices
(c) solidified fatty acid incline
(d) Solid fat index

16. If mean volume – number diameter of a powdered sample is 2.41 μm, density is 3gm/cm, the number of particles /gm will be :
(a) 5.38 × 10 10 (b) 3.68 × 10 10
(b) 4.55 × 10 10 (d) 4.70 × 10 10

17. Which polymorphic form of a drug candidate has highest melting point :
(a) Unstable (b) Metastable
(c) Hydrates (d) Stable

18. For bitter drugs in pediatric formulations excellent flavouring agent will be :
(a) Raspberrysyrup
(b) Orange syrup
(c) Lemon syrup
(d) Black current syrup

19. The co-administration of erythromycin with cyclosporine:
(a) Increase bioavailability , due to inhibition of hepatic metabolism
(b) Increase bioavailability , due to inhibition of microflora in intestine
(c) Decrease bioavailability , due to complex formation
(d) Decrease bioavailability , due to induction of hepatic metabolism

20. Essentially hospital formulary system provide mechanism to :
(a) streamline prescription writing
(b) Improve quality
(c) avoid brand and therapeutic duplication
(d) Improve surgical procedure

21. Volume of blood that flow per unit time per unit volume of the tissue is :
(a) residence time
(b) elimination rate
(c) gastric emptying rate
(d) perfusion rate

22. leaching by immersion of crude material in a solvent is also known as:
(a) maceration (b) precipitation
(c) evaporation (d) crystallization

23. The protein toxin that have been modified to reduce the toxicity without significantly altering the immunogenicity are known as:
(a) Sera (b) Antisera
(c) Toxoids (d) Vaccines

24. Which of the following is NOT a mechanism for achieving gastroretention?
(a) Osmosis (b) Floating
(c) Mucoadhesion (d) Swelling

25. The phase contrast microscopy is valuable in studying living cells which are :
(a) Stained
(b) Unstained
(c) treated with fluorescent dye
(d) treated with fluorescent antibody

26. The size of Lycopodium spores is :
(a) 45 μm (b) 15 μm
(c) 35 μm (d) 25 μm

27. Regholarrhenine A-F have been isolated from :
(a) Veratrums (b) Areca
(c) Aconite (d) Kurchi

28. Pungency of Zingiber officinale rhizome is due to the:
(a) Citral (b) gingerol
(c) commiphoric acid (d) Gingerol

29. The principle cultivation areas of pyrethrum flowers are in :
    (a) Sri Lanka (b) Malaysia
    (c) India (d) Kenya
30. In cassia angustifolia short term drought:
    (a) increases the concentration of sennosides A+B
    (b) decreases the concentration of sennosides A+B
    (c) causes loss of leaf biomass
    (d) Causes death of the plant
31. The glycoside scilliroside in red sqrill acts as:
    (a) Insecticide (b) Rodenticide
    (c) Acaricide (d) Molluscide
32. Shellac is a resinous substance prepared from a secretion that encrusts the bodies of a scale insect:
    (a) Viverra civet
    (b) karria lacca
    (c) Acipenser huso
    (d) Alverites moschiferus
33. All members of this order are trees or shrubs; mostly evergreen with needle – like leaves ; monoecious or dicious- sporophylls usually in cones. Resin ducts occure in all parts :
    (a) cycadales (b) ginkgoales
    (c) taxales (d) coniferae
34. In Gambir fluorescin test the petroleum spirit layer shows strong :
    (a) Green Fluorescence
    (b) Blue Fluorescence
    (c) Yellow Fluorescence
    (d) Red Fluorescence
35. Antiviral action of Neem in due to:
    (a) kaemferol (b) nelanin
    (c) nimbin (d) Azadirachitin
36. Characteristic microscopic features observed in Alzheimers decrease is
    (a) Epidural heamoregic patches
    (b) depigmentation of substantia nigra
    (c) Demyelination of neurons in spinal cord
    (d) presence of nueritic plaques containing Aβ-amyloid:
37. Cardiac output is :
    (a) volume of blood ejected by the auricle per minute
    (b) volume of blood ejected by the left ventricle per beat
    (c) volume of blood ejected by the left ventricle per minute
    (d) volume of blood ejected by the auricles per beat
38. What are satures?
    (a) cartilaginous joints
    (b) Non fibrous joints
    (c) synovial fluid
    (d) Fibrous joints of the skull
39. Following are the facts regarding clinical application of muscarinic receptor blocking drugs. Identify the false statement:
    (a) used in the treatment of Parkinson's disease is often an exercise in polypharmacy, since no single agent is fully effective.
    (b) Marked reflex vagal discharge may stimulate sinoatrial or atrioventricular node to improve cardiac output.
    (c) Mydriasis produced greatly facilitates opthalmoscopic examination of the retina and measurement of refractive error in uncooperative patient.
    (d) Scopolamine is one among the old remedies used to treat sea sickness.
40. Which of the following cells are called scavenger cells:
    (a) Neutrophils (b) Natural killer cells
    (c) Macrophages (d) Mast cells
41. Which is NOT true about calsitriol:
    (a) it is active form of Vit D3
    (b) it enhances reabsorption of calcium and phosphate from bone
    (c) it prevents tubular reabsorption of calcium and phosphate
    (d) enhances absorption of calcium and phosphate from intestine

42. Production of an abnormal igG immunoglobulin in grave's disease causes:
    (a) multinodular goitre
    (b) hypothyroidism
    (c) thyrotoxicosis
    (d) Rhumatoid arthritis

43. metabolic acidosis does not occure during:
    (a) starvation
    (b) chronic renal failure
    (c) wound healing
    (d) uncontrolled diabetes mellitus

44. Glucocorticoids have following effects EXCEPT:
    (a) stimulation of immune responses
    (b) resistence to stress
    (c) lipolysis
    (d) protein breakdown and glucose formation

45. which one of the following is NOT the role of nitric oxide
    (a) relaxing vascular smooth muscle
    (b) mediating microbicidal action of macrophages
    (c) serving as neurotransmitter in CNS
    (d) inducing platelate aggregation

46. identify the drug which is not useful the treatment of tuberculosis
    (a) pyrazinamide (b) gentamycin
    (c) streptomycin (d) ciprofloxacin

47. what is anaplasia?
    (a) morphological and functional alteration/changes, that are different from normal cells
    (b) morphological and functional resemblance to normal cells
    (c) increase in size of cells
    (d) lack of growth of cells

48. Match the following liver abnormalities with consequences :

| | |
|---|---|
| (a) steatosis | (M) raised bilirubin level |
| (b) cholestasis | (N) slight rise in serum trans-aminase level |
| (c) hepatits | (O) Accumulation of fat droplets within liver cells |
| (d) Fibrosis | (P) Elevated liver function test(LFT'S) |

    (a) a)-(N), b)-(P) ,c)-(M),d)-(O)
    (b) a)-(O), b)- (M), c)- (P), d)-(N)
    (c) a)-(N), b)-(O), c)-(P), d)-(M)
    (d) a)-(P), b) -(O), c)-(N), d)-(M)

49. Numerous isomers of human liver p450 enzymes have been identified. It is not worthy that ----------alone is responsible for the metabolism of over 50% of the priscription drugs metabolized by liver:
    (a) CYP3A4 (b) CYP1A2
    (c) CYP1A11 (d) CYP2B6

50. which of the following directly inhibits factor Xa?
    (a) dabigatron (b) warfarin
    (c) bivalirudin (d) rivaroxaban

51. which of the following anticonvulsants have both inhibition of excitatory glutametergic synapse and facilitation of GABA mediated cl- channel opening action:
    (a) Valproate (b) Ethosuximide
    (c) Topiramate (d) Phenytoin

52. which of the following is NOT a cardioselective β blocker?
    (a) bisoprolol (b) Nebivolol
    (c) acebutolol (d) pindolol

53. The term "aneurysm" refers to
    (a) permanent blockage of blood vessels
    (b) permanent abnormal dilatation of blood vessels
    (c) abnormal connections in blood vessels
    (d) abnormal growth of neurons near blood vessels

54. The antiemetic activity of glycopyrronium is related to potent inhibition of ------recepter both peripherally and centrally.
    (a) 5HT3 (b) D2
    (c) M1 (d) H1

55. Identify the false statement about benzodiazepines from the following
    (a) Benzodiazepines cause reduction of anxiety
    (b) Benzodiazepines cause convulsions
    (c) Benzodiazepines produce muscle relaxation and loss of motor co-ordination
    (d) Benzodiazepines are useful in insomnia

56. which of the following 5-alpha reductase inhibitor?
    (a) Gliclazide (b) Sildenafil
    (c) Finasteride (d) Polythiazide

57. several different chemicals released by microbes and inflamed tissue attract phagocytes this phenomenon is called as--------
    (a) Phagocytosis (b) Integrins
    (c) Chemotaxis (d) Emigration

58. Hematocrit 65% to70% indicates:
    (a) Hemophilia (b) Polycythemia
    (c) Hypoxia (d) Anaemia

59. The advers reaction associated with β-2 agonists administered by inhalation or nebulisation in the management of asthma does not include-----
    (a) Peripheral vasodilation
    (b) Hypertension
    (c) Tachycardia
    (d) Fine tremor

60. Select the ulcer protective drug from the following
    (a) Oxyphenonium (b) Metronidazole
    (c) Misoprostol (d) Sucralfate

61. Disturbances of oestrogen/progesterone balance could cause a relative deficiency of ---------- leading to disturbances in production of dropamine and serotonin. This contributes for emotional disturbances and depression.
    (a) Enzyme decarboxylase.
    (b) Tyrosine.
    (c) Pyridoxine phosphate
    (d) Co-factorA

62. Testing of chemicals by OECD guideline no. 420 refers to which of the following:
    (a) Acute oral toxicity by acute toxic class method
    (b) Acute oral toxicity by up and down procedure
    (c) Repeated dose 28-days toxicity study in rodents
    (d) Acute oral toxicity by fixed dose procedure

63. Which of the following is true?

    Excessive use of diuretics can lead to:
    (a) Hypervolemic shock
    (b) Neurogenic shock
    (c) Hypovolemic shock
    (d) Cardiogenic shock

64. As per the Medical Termination of Pregnancy Act and Rules, the safe custody of "forms" is with:
    (a) standing committee
    (b) registerd medical practitioner
    (c) owner of the approved place
    (d) chief medical officer

65. For protein detection most commonly used probe is:
    (a) interferon (b) Antibody
    (c) lectin (d) antigen

66. Consumers who are loyal to two or three brands are known as:
    (a) split loyals (b) switcher loyals
    (c) semicore loyals (d) shifting loyals

67. choose the CORRECT statement with respect to "the pharmacy act 1948"
    (a) education regulation 1991 does not prescribe the minimum qualification for the registration as pharmacist
    (b) section 12 of the act deals with approval of course of study under chapter -2 therof
    (c) section 12 of the act deals with the approval of course of study and examination under chapter-2 therof
    (d) state govt.is authorized to make any rules with respect to course of study

68. ELISA is based upon :
    (a) antigen protein interaction
    (b) antibody protein interaction
    (c) antigen antibody interaction
    (d) lectin antibody interaction

69. The relation between emissive power of the surface and its absorptivity is given by :
   (a) Stefan Boltzmann law
   (b) Darcy law
   (c) Fourier's law
   (d) Kirchhoff's law

70. In India the patent office has its head office at Kolkata and branch offices at:
   (a) Dibrugarh, indore and vapi
   (b) Kashmir, ahmedabad and Trivandrum
   (c) Chandigarh, Hyderabad and goa
   (d) Mumbai, Chennai and New delhi

71. Penalty for the cultivation of any cannabis plant to produce, sell, purchase transport in contravention of narcotic drugs and psychotropic substances act and rules on first conviction is:
   (e) Rigorous imprisonment up to 10 years or fine up toRs. 10 lakhs
   (f) Rigorous imprisonment up to 10 years or fine up to Rs. 1 lakhs
   (g) Rigorous imprisonment up to 6 month
   (h) fine up to Rs.10 lakhs

72. In direct, contact or jet condencers ,barometric leg serves one of the following functions :
   (a) To remove the condensate /cooling water mixture
   (b) To measure the pressure difference across the tube
   (c) To heat the liquid feed to its boiling point
   (d) To transfer the feed in to the evaporating chamber

73. which of the following is considered as differentiated product ?
   (a) Ranitidine (b) Zantac
   (c) Isoniazid (d) Paracetamol

74. Harding mill is a variant of:
   (a) Fluid energy mill (b) Ball mill
   (c) Hammer mill (d) Rotary cutter mill

75. Retention hyperbilirubenamia is caused due to--
   (a) Choleric jaundice
   (b) Non clearance of bilirubin
   (c) Reflux of bilirubin into blood stream
   (d) Over production of bilirubin

76. What will be the heat of vaporization of 1 mole of water, when it has the entropy change ($\Delta s$) of 35.2cal/mole.deg(at 25°C)?
   (a) 1.408 cal/mole (b) 10489 cal/mole
   (c) 8465 cal/mole (d) 880 cal/mole

77. Identify the name of drug with the following structure :
   (a) Esmolol (b) Betaxolol
   (c) Bisaprolol (d) Metaprolol

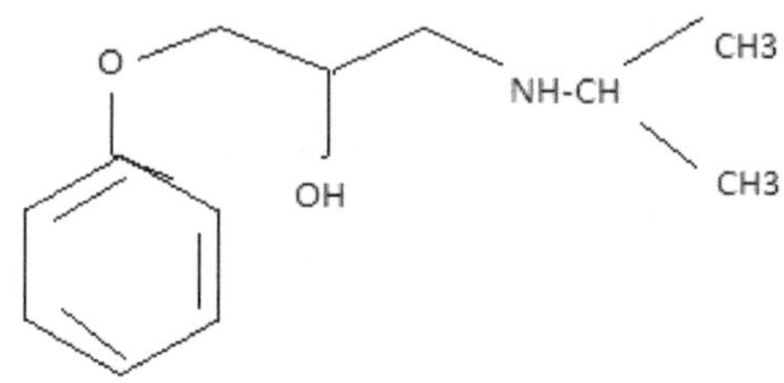


78. The following ACE inhibitor used in treating cardiovascular disorder is synthesized from the natural amino acid L-alanine and L-proline :
   (a) Ramipril (b) Enalapril
   (c) Lisinopril (d) Captopril

79. The infrared absorpsion peaks of nujol is due to vibrations involving:
   (a) S-Hstr and S-Hdef
   (b) O-Hstr and O-Hdef
   (c) C-Hstr and C-Hdef
   (d) N-Hstr and N-Hdef

80. Permitted tolerance limit for a 100ml class B volumetric flask and 1000ml class B volumetric flask according to BS 1792 specification respectively are-------------ml :
   (a) 0.15 and 0.80 (b) 0.80 and 0.30
   (c) 1.00 and 10.00 (d) 0.15 and 1.5

81. Predict λmax for a $\pi \rightarrow \pi^*$absorption band in the UV spectrum of following compo

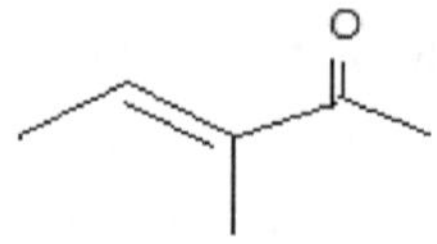


   (a) 237nm (b) 215nm
   (c) 241nm (d) 240nm

82. One of the following is a most commonly used protecting group for amines:
(a) Para methyl benzyl(PMB)
(b) t-butyloxy carbonyl (t-BOC)
(c) Methoxy methylene(MOM)
(d) Tetra hydro pyranyl oxy(THP)

83. Choose the correct sequence of process during atomization in atomic absorption spectroscopy:
(a) Desolvation → nebulization → dissociation → volatilization →ionization
(b) Nebulization→ desolvation → volatilization → dissociation → ionization
(c) Desolvation → nebulization → volatilization → dissociation →ionization
(d) Nebulization → volatilization → desolvation → dissoceation →ionization

84. Which among the following carrier gases has the highest thermal conductivity:
(a) Nitrogen (b) Oxygen
(c) Helium (d) Compressed air

85. Phase solubility analysis curve is not a good tool for :
(a) Complex formation
(b) Bioavailability determination
(c) Polymorph detection
(d) Impurity detection

86. Identify the named reaction

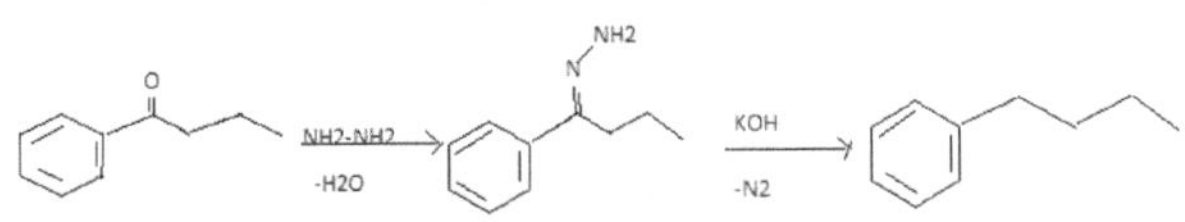


(a) Curtius rearrangement
(b) Clemmensen reduction
(c) Wolf kishner reduction
(d) Wolf rearrangement

87. Which of the following inactive clotting factor is activated by the vitamin –K as a co-enzyme?
(a) I,II,III,IV (b) II,V,IX,X,
(c) II,V,VI,VIII (d) II,VII,IX,X

88. Identify the molecule which will not exhibit Dipole moment?
(a) Carbon dioxide (b) Carbon monoxide
(c) Chloroform (d) Ammonia

89. the following combination of drugs are used in treating severe travelers diarrhea:
(a) Pyrimethamine and sulfadiazine
(b) Trimethoprim and sulfadiazine
(c) Pyrimethamine and sulfamethoxazole
(d) Trimethoprim and sulfamethoxazole

90. reaction of an α-halo ester with an aldehyde or ketone in the presence of a base like NaNH2 gives α,β-epoxy carboxylic ester .this reaction is referd as:
(a) Willgerodt rearrengment
(b) Bamford steven reaction
(c) Darzen's glycidic synthesis
(d) Bayer villiger rearrangement

91. amylopectin, a component of starch gives ----------colour with iodine :
(a) No colour (b) Green
(c) Blue (d) Red purple

92. anti-addition of bromine to trans-2 butene yields:
(a) Enantiomer and racemic mixture
(b) Only racemic mixture
(c) Only enantiomer
(d) Only meso compound

93. convertion of aryldiazonium chloride to arylchloride can be achived in the presence of ;
(a) Copper(II)chloride
(b) Copper(I) chloride
(c) Sodium chloride
(d) Calcium chloride

94. Von gierke's glycogen storage disease is due to defect of which enzyme :
(a) Phosphofrutokinase
(b) Glucosyl 4-6 transferase
(c) Glycogen phosphorylase
(d) Glucose-6-phosphatase

95. the chief product obtained by the reaction of neo-pentyl bromide under E1 reaction condition:
(a) Neopentyl alcohol
(b) 2-methyl 1-2 butene
(c) 2-methyl 1-1,3 butadiene
(d) 2methyl butane

96. RNA molecules having intrinsic catalytic activity are called as :
    (a) mRNAs (b) Ribozymes
    (c) Sn RNAs (d) rRNAs

97. this semisynthetic derivative of penicillin is synthesized by acylation of 6-APA with p-hydroxy phenyl glycine:
    (a) Becampicillin (b) Amoxicillin
    (c) Ampicillin (d) Cabenicillin.

98. chosse the correct product of the following reaction :

    HNO3 +2H2SO4 $\rightleftharpoons$ ?

    (a) H3O++2HSO4- +NO2+
    (b) H2O+2HSO4-+NO2+
    (c) H3O++2HSO4+NO2+
    (d) OH-+2HSO4-+NO2-

99. Oxazole is prepared the condensation of α – amino carbonyl compound with :
    (a) Amino acid (b) Isocyanide
    (c) Aminoether (d) Iminoester

100. select the correct order of ortho/para directing ability of the functional groups from those given below:
    (strogest first ,weakest last)

    (a) -NHCOR> $-OH > -C6H5 > I$
    (b) -NHCOR> $-NH2 > -C6H5 > I$
    (c) -NHCOR> $-NR2 > -C6H5 > I$
    (d) -NHR> $-NHCOR > -C6H5 > I$

101. Blockade in β-oxydation results in :
    (a) Von gierk's desease.
    (b) Scurvy
    (c) Sudden infant death syndrome
    (d) Taruli disease

102. The basic ring system present in the anti-hypertensive and antiglaucoma drug "timolol" is:
    (a) 1,3,5-thiadiazole and morpholine
    (b) 1,3-thiazole and morpholine
    (c) 1,2,5-thiadiazole and morpholine
    (d) 1,2,4-thiadiazole and morpholine

103. Dehydration of dicarboxylic acid to obtain corresponding anhydride is difficult due to stereochemical arrangement
    (a) Malic acid (b) Fumaric acid
    (c) Glutaric acid (d) Succinic acid

104. Which of the following pair of drugs is considerd as selective α1 blockers?
    (a) Timolol and metuprolol
    (b) Parazosin and terazosin
    (c) Formoterol and levalbuterol
    (d) Yohimbine and carynanthine

105. Calculate the accurate osmotic pressure at 0°C Of a blood serum sample using lewis equation having freezing point- 0.53°C :
    (a) 0.636 atm (b) 6.39atm
    (c) 574.28atm (d) 0.0441atm

106. Kinetically x/a(a-x)=kt is the expression for:
    (a) First order reaction
    (b) Second order reaction
    (c) Pseudo first order reaction
    (d) Fractional order reaction

107. Conversation of a carbonyl functionality directly to its hydrocarbon in basis media can be achieved by:
    (a) Lithium aluminium hydride reduction.
    (b) Clemmensen reduction
    (c) Sodium borohydride reduction
    (d) Wolf kishner reduction

108. Which of the following second generation β-1 selective blockers contains 1,3,5-thiadiazole ring in its structure?
    (a) Sotalol (b) Timolol
    (c) Penbutolol (d) Pindolol

109. The structural features present in anti-cancer antibiotics (doxorubicin, daunorubicin, ldarubucin and epirubicin) are----
    (a) naphthalene nucleus connected with amino suger via glycosidic linkage
    (b) anthracene nucleus fused to cyclohexane ring that is subsequently connected with amino sugar via glycosidic linkage:

(c) quinoline nucleus connected with amino sugar via a glycosidic linkage.
(d) Phenanthrene nucleus fused to cyclohexen ring that is subsequently connected with amino sugar via glycosidic linkage

110. When 50ml of sodium hydroxide (0.1 M)is added to 100 ml of 0.1 M acetic acid ,PH of the resultant solution is ---------

Ka of acetic acid =1.82×10-5

(a) 8.58 (b) 7.42
(c) 4.74 (d) 7.06

111. Gabriel ring closure method is employed for the synthesis of:
(a) 1,4-oxazine (b) Aziridine
(c) Oxirane (d) Oxaziridine

112. "shake well" label must be placed on on the containers of :
(a) Ophthalmic suspension
(b) Occuserts
(c) Ophthalmic solution
(d) Opthalmic gel

113. In case of aerosol testing,valve delivering acceptance criteria for a volume of 54 μl or less is:
(a) ± 75% (b) ± 5%
(c) ± 10% (d) ± 15%

114. containers may be rendered free from pyrogens by adequate cleaning and by:
(a) Autoclaving at 121°C for 15 minutes.
(b) Heating at 210 °Cfor 3-4 hours
(c) Autoclaving at 121°C for 1 hours
(d) Heating at 100°C for 3-4 hours

115. GMP regulation are pertaining to minimum requirements to be met by industry when ;
(a) Manufacturing, packaging and holding of human drugs and veterinary drugs
(b) Manufacture of human drugs and veterinary drugs.
(c) Manufacture and packaging of human drugs and veterinary drugs
(d) Manufacture and holding of human drugs and veterinary

116. Which one of the following viscometers can be used for characterizing non-newtonian system?
(a) Falling sphere viscometer
(b) Cup and bob viscometer
(c) Capillary viscometer
(d) Hoeppler viscometer

117. For drugs substances with highly variable pharmacokinetic characteristics the following bioequivalence study design is used:
(a) Parallel design
(b) Non-parallel design
(c) Non-parallel design
(d) Replicate design

118. Roll- tube technique is the modification of :
(a) Pour plate technique
(b) The streak plate technique
(c) Micromanipulator technique
(d) Spread plate technique

119. Which mechanism of metabolism of drug is not affected by weight change of patient:
(a) Conjugative metabolism
(b) Acetylation metabolism
(c) Hydrolytic metabolism
(d) Oxidative metabolism

120. 21 CFR part 211 of USFDA describes:
(a) Current good clinical practice
(b) Current good packaging practice
(c) Current good manufacturing practice
(d) Current good laboratory practice

121. In treating immunodeficiency disease the goal is to maintain IgG lelels at about :
(a) 100mg/dL (b) 400MG/dL
(c) 200mg/dL (d) 300mg/dL

122. Which one of the following is the property of micro emulsion?
(a) They have particle size more than 1 micron
(b) They have poor stability
(c) They exhibit a viscoelastic gel phase, when internal phase is added in excess
(d) They have milky yellow colour

123. The rheological and functional properties of synovial fluid are impaired due to
   (a) Increase in the content of mucus
   (b) Decrease in the content of mucus
   (c) Increase in the content of hyaluronic acid
   (d) Decrease in the content of hyaluronic acid

124. Movement of a charge particle through a liquid under the influence of an applied potential difference is known as
   (a) Sedimentation potential
   (b) Streaming potential
   (c) Electrophoresis
   (d) Electroosmosis

# Answer Key GPAT 2019

| | | | | | | | | | |
|---|---|---|---|---|---|---|---|---|---|
| 1-b | 2-d | 3-a | 4-b | 5-b | 6-a | 7-b | 8-a | 9-b | 10-d |
| 11-c | 12-b | 13-c | 14-d | 15-d | 16-c | 17-d | 18-a | 19-a | 20-c |
| 21-d | 22-a | 23-c | 24-a | 25-b | 26-d | 27-d | 28-b | 29-d | 30-a |
| 31-b | 32-b | 33-d | 34-a | 35-c | 36-d | 37-c | 38-d | 39-b | 40-c |
| 41-c | 42-c | 43-c | 44-a | 45-d | 46-b | 47-a | 48-b | 49-a | 50-d |
| 51-a | 52-d | 53-b | 54-c | 55-b | 56-c | 57-c | 58-b | 59-b | 60-b |
| 61-c | 62-d | 63-c | 64-c | 65-b | 66-a | 67-c | 68-c | 69-d | 70-d |
| 71-b | 72-a | 73-b | 74-b | 75-d | 76-b | 77-c | 78-b | 79-c | 80---- |
| 81-a | 82-b | 83-b | 84-c | 85-b | 86-c | 87-d | 88-a | 89-d | 90-c |
| 91-d | 92-d | 93-b | 94-d | 95-b | 96-b | 97-b | 98-a | 99-d | 100-d |
| 101-c | 102-c | 103-b | 104-b | 105-a | 106-b | 107-d | 108-b | 109-b | 110-c |
| 111-b | 112-a | 113-d | 114-b | 115-a | 116-b | 117-d | 118-b | 119-d | 120-c |
| 121-c | 122-c | 123-d | 124-c | | | | | | |

# Mock Tests

# Mock Test I

**NOTE:**

- The question paper consists of the multiple choice questions **(MCQ's).**
- Total of **125 questions** will be asked in the exam which will be of total **500 marks**.
- The time duration to complete the examination is of **3 hours**.
- For every correct response **4 marks** will be allotted.
- For every incorrect answer, **1 mark** will be deducted.

1. Bethanecol is a ......................compound
   (a) Muscarnic agonist
   (b) Muscarnic antagonist
   (c) Nicotinic agonist
   (d) Nicotinic antagonist
2. Which compound below is H2 receptor antagonist and used in treatment of ulcers
   (a) Animophenazine (b) Phenylepeherine
   (c) Procaine (d) Cimetidine
3. The function of ion channel protein is
   (a) Allow electron to cross membrane
   (b) Allow ion to cross membrane
   (c) Allow protein to cross membrane
   (d) None of the above.
4. Which of the following is NOT an endogenous compound
   (a) Adrenaline (b) Fluoxetine
   (c) Serotonin (d) Testosterone
5. Which of the following drugs is isolated from a natural source.
   (a) Aspirin
   (b) Morphine
   (c) Isoniazid
   (d) Diamorphine (Heroin)
6. What term is used for the chemical which is chiefly responsible for the biological activity of a natural extract.
   (a) Active drug (b) Prime drug
   (c) Active principle (d) Prime principle
7. Dragendorff's reagent is a solution of
   (a) Potassium mercuric iodide
   (b) Potassium cadmium iodide
   (c) Potassium bismuth iodide
   (d) Picric acid
8. Which one of these tests is specific for tropane alkaloids
   (a) Vitali morin test (b) Ehrlich test
   (c) Baljet test (d) Fiehe's test
9. Indication for aspirin administration are the following, EXCEPT:
   (a) Inflammatory conditions
   (b) Decreasing the incidence of transient ischemic attack, unstable angina, coronary artery thrombosis with myocardial infarction, and thrombosis after coronary artery bypass grafting
   (c) Relieving severe visceral pain (myocardial infarction, cancer pain condition, renal orbiliary colic)
   (d) Reducing elevated body temperature

10. Cyclohexyl nitrile and N, N-diethylamino is used as starting product in the synthesis of
    (a) Glycopyrrolate (b) Dicyclominec.
    (c) Homatropine (d) Cyclopentolate
11. Which of the following ring is present in Amiloride
    (a) Pyramidine ring (b) Pteridine
    (c) Pyrazine ring (d) Pyridine ring
12. Diphenhydramine belongs to histamine class of
    (a) Ethylene diamine (b) Amino alkyl ether
    (c) Alkyl amine (d) Phenothiazine
13. Phenytoin is
    (a) 5, 5-diphenylimidazoline 2, 4-dione
    (b) 4, 4-diphenylimidazoline 2, 4-dione
    (c) 4, 4-diphenylimidazoline 3, 5-dione
    (d) 5, 5-diphenylimidazoline 3, 5-dione
14. Keller kiliani test is used for identification of:
    (a) Fructose (b) Maltose
    (c) Deoxy sugar (d) Glucose
15. Which is not used as an adulterant for clove?
    (a) Mother clove (b) Blown clove
    (c) Clove stalk (d) Pale clove
16. Exhuasted fennel is identified by absence of:
    (a) Fenchone (b) Anethol
    (c) Carvone (d) Cineol
17. Monoterpenes contains number of isoprene units:
    (a) One (b) Three
    (c) Two (d) Four
18. Oleo gum resins are mixture of:
    (a) Volatile oil + Gum + Resins
    (b) Fixed oil + Gum + Resin
    (c) Fats + Gum + Resin
    (d) Gum + resins
19. Stomatal Index in Indian senna is in the range of:
    (a) 17 to 20 (b) 20 to 23
    (c) 23 to 26 (d) 26 to 29
20. Presence of star spots is the characteristic of drug:
    (a) Cascara (b) Senna
    (c) Aloe (d) Rhubarb
21. Hepa filter is made up of
    (a) Cellulose acetate (b) Porcelain
    (c) Asbestos (d) Borosilicate glass
22. Bloom strength is used to check the quality of
    (a) Lactose (b) Ampoules
    (c) Hardness of tablets (d) Gelatin
23. Which filler can NOT be used for the preparation of tablets for amine containing basic drugs to avoid discoloration of the tablets?
    (a) Dicalcium phosphate
    (b) Microcrystalline cellulose
    (c) Starch
    (d) Lactose
24. Codeine is
    (a) Monomethyl ether of morphine.
    (b) Aamide of apomorphine.
    (c) Acetyl derivative of morphine.
    (d) Dimethyl ether of papaverine.
25. In which of the following techniques the sample is kept below triple point?
    (a) Lyophilization (b) Spray drying
    (c) Spray congealing (d) Centrifugation
26. Dielectric constant is related to thickness of double layer
    (a) Directly (b) Indirectly
    (c) It is not related (d) Proportionally
27. Sodium carboxymethyl cellulose used in injectable preparation in the concentration
    (a) 0.1 % (b) 0.5 %
    (c) 1 % (d) It is not used
28. HLB value for ideal solubilizing agent is
    (a) 3-6 (b) 6-9
    (c) 9-15 (d) 15-18
29. Povidone K-30 is used for
    (a) Tablet coating
    (b) Tablet disintegrates
    (c) Tablet antiadherent's
    (d) Tablet diluents
30. Concentration of plasticizers or polymers are evaluated by
    (a) Turret --Burman method
    (b) Plackett-Burman method

(c) Kirbay Burman method
(d) None

31. Identify the drug which is NOT used in the treatment of malaria caused by Plasmodium falciparum :
(a) Artemisinin (b) Primaquine
(c) Quinine (d) Mefloquine

32. Which one of the following drugs does NOT act through G-Protein coupled receptors?
(a) Epinephrine (b) Insulin
(c) Dopamine (d) TSH

33. Which one of the following drugs is most effective in preventing transmission of HIV virus from the mother to the foetus?
(a) Lamivudine (b) Zidovudine
(c) Indinavir (d) Ribavirin

34. Identify the one rational combination which has clinical benefit:
(a) Norfloxacin – Metronidazole
(b) Alprazolam - Paracetamol
(c) Cisapride – Omeprazole
(d) Amoxycillin - Clavulanic acid

35. Stevens Johnson sjmdrome is the most common adverse effect associated with one of the following category of drugs
(a) Sulphonamides (b) Macrolides
(c) Penicillins (d) Tetracyclines

36. Streptomycin can NOT be given orally for treatment of tuberculosis because
(a) It gets degraded in the GIT
(b) It causes severe diarrhea
(c) It causes metallic taste in the mouth
(d) It is not absorbed from the GIT

37. Geriatric population should be included in the following Phase of clinical trials
(a) Phase I (b) Phase II
(c) Phase III (d) Phase IV

38. Indicate the HPLC detector that is most sensitive to change in temperature:
(a) PDA detector
(b) Refractive Index detector
(c) Electrochemical detector
(d) Fluorescence detector

39. One of the following statements is NOT true:
(a) Accuracy expresses the correctness of measurement
(b) Precision represents reproducibility of measurement
(c) High degree of precision implies high degree of accuracy also
(d) High degree of accuracy implies high degree of precession

40. Glass transition temperature is detected through
(a) X-Ray diffractometery
(b) Solution calorimetry
(c) Differential scanning calorimeter
(d) Thermogravimetric analysis

41. In Gas-Liquid Chromatography, some of the samples need to be derivatized in order to increase their
(a) Volatility
(b) Solubility
(c) Thermal Conductivity
(d) Polarizability

42. The given antibiotic is an example of ansamycins:
(a) Roxythromycin (b) Adriamycin
(c) Aureomycin (d) Rifamycin

43. The effects observed following systemic administration of levodopa in the treatment of Parkinsonism have been attributed to its catabolism to dopamine. Carbidopa, can markedly increase the proportion of levodopa that crosses the blood-brain barrier by
(a) Increasing penetration of levodopa through BBB by complexation with it
(b) Decreasing peripheral metabolism of levodopa
(c) Decreasing metabolism of levodopa in the CNS
(d) Decreasing clearance of levodopa from the CNS

44. Ethambutol molecule has
(a) Two chiral centers and 3 stereoisomers
(b) Two chiral centers and 4 stereoisomers
(c) Two chiral centers and 2 stereoisomers
(d) One chiral center and 2 stereoisomers

45. The characteristic of non-linear pharmacokinetics include:
    (a) Area under the curve is proportional to the dose
    (b) Elimination half-life remains constant,
    (c) Area under the curve is not proportional to the dose
    (d) Amount of drug excreted through remains constant

46. Which one of the following drugs is withdrawn from the market due to *torsade de pointes?*
    (a) Chlorpromazine (b) Astemizole
    (c) Haloperidol (d) Domperidone

47. Cell-wall biosynthesis is inhibited by antibiotics by inhibiting the biosynthesis of which of the following?
    (a) Lipopolysaccharide (b) Cellulose
    (c) Peptidoglycan (d) Proteins

48. Benzyl penicillin is the chemical name for which of the following penicillin?
    (a) Penicillin G (b) Penicillin V
    (c) Penicillin F (d) Phenethicilin

49. Streptomycin is produced by which of the following organisms?
    (a) Stretomyces noursei
    (b) Streptomyces nodosus
    (c) Streptomyces fradiae
    (d) Streptomyces griseus

50. Which of the following inhibits protein synthesis by combining with the 50S subunit ribosome?
    (a) Streptomycin (b) Tetracycline
    (c) Chloramphenicol (d) Penicillin

51. Oxidative phosphorylation involves
    (a) Electron transport system
    (b) Substrate level phosphorylation
    (c) Reaction catalyzed by succinic thiokinase in TCA cycle
    (d) None of the above

52. Which of the following is not a type of ion detector used in mass spectrometers?
    (a) Electron multiplier
    (b) Flame emission detector
    (c) Faraday cup collector
    (d) Photographic plates

53. Beer Lambert's law gives the relation between which of the following?
    (a) Reflected radiation and concentration
    (b) Scattered radiation and concentration
    (c) Energy absorption and concentration
    (d) Energy absorption and reflected radiation

54. Which of the following is a source used in spectroscopy?
    (a) Laser
    (b) Tube light
    (c) Sodium vapour lamp
    (d) Tungsten lamp

55. Which of the following options are correct in terms of wavelength for the different types of IR spectrometer?
    (a) Near IR: 0.8 – 2.5 nm
    (b) Mid IR: 0.8 – 2.5 nm
    (c) Far IR: 2.5 – 50 nm
    (d) Mid IR: 50 – 100 nm

56. The concentration of sucrose in simple syrup BP is
    (a) 85% w/w (b) 60.70% w/w
    (c) 66.70% w/w (d) 40.74% w/w

57. The HLB value of sodium laurylsulphate is
    (a) 6.5 (b) 13.8
    (c) 25.0 (d) 40.0

58. Oily injection are sterilized by
    (a) Dry heat sterilization
    (b) Tyndallisation
    (c) Autoclaving
    (d) U.V. radiation

59. Water attack test is used to identify alkalinity in
    (a) Type-I glass (b) Type-II glass
    (c) Type-III glass (d) All of the above

60. Which of the following is the formula for pH calculation?
    (a) log10 [H+] (b) -log10[H+]
    (c) log2[H+] (d) -log2[H+]

61. Shrinkage of gel by extrusion of liquid is called as
    (a) Syneresis (b) Dilatancy
    (c) Plasticity (d) Ebullition

62. Carbamazepine is a tricyclic antidepressant. It is classified as
    (a) Benzodiazepine
    (b) Arylalkanolamine
    (c) Iminostilbene
    (d) Benzimidazole

63. Sulfa drugs can be conveniently estimated using the reagent
    (a) 4,4-Dithiobis-(2-nitrobenzoic acid)
    (b) Tris-(hydroxy methyl) amino-menthane sodium nitrate
    (c) N-(1-napthyl) ethylenediamine
    (d) N-ethylmalcimide

64. Ehlrich's reagent is
    (a) Bismuth iodide solution
    (b) p- Dimethyl aniline solution in alcohol
    (c) p-Dimethyl amino benzaldehyde solution
    (d) p-Dimethyl aniline solution in methamol

65. Resolution of a monochromator is the ability to distinguish
    (a) As separate entities adjacent spectral features
    (b) Seperation of different colours
    (c) seperation of UV light and visible light
    (d) Dispersing characteristics

66. Important activities noticed in Testosterone
    (a) Androgenic, Myotropic and Anabolic
    (b) Progestational, Myotropic and Anabolic
    (c) Estrogenic, Myotropic and Anabolic
    (d) Androgenic, Optometric and katabolic

67. The UV visible region in the electromagnetic spectrum of radiation is
    (a) 200- 400nm (b) 300-660nm
    (c) 400-800nm (d) 200- 800nms

68. The Mantoux test uses
    (a) Old tuberculin
    (b) Diptheria toxin
    (c) Serum antigen
    (d) Polysaccharide antigen

69. The volume of distribution of a drug is
    (a) An expression of total body volume
    (b) A measure of total fluid volume
    (c) A relationship between the total amount of drug in the body and the concentration of the drug in the blood
    (d) Proportional to bioavailabillity of the drug

70. Vitamin D2 is
    (a) 22, 23- Dihydro- 5, 6 – cis – ergocalciferol
    (b) 5,6 –cis – chloecalciferol
    (c) 7- dehydrocholesterol
    (d) 21-24 – dihydro – 5,6- cis-ergocalciferol

71. R.W.C. is used to identify the strength of an
    (a) Antibiotic
    (b) Antipyretic
    (c) Antiseptic
    (d) Anti-inflammatory

72. The essential structrural unit for the anthelmintic activity of mebendazole is
    (a) Benzoyl group (b) Benzimidazole
    (c) Methylcarbamate (d) Imidazole

73. Most accepted mechanism for developing bacterial resistance to sulphonamides is
    (a) An increasing capacity to inactivate or destroy the drug
    (b) An alternative metabolic pathway for synthesis of an essential metabolite
    (c) An increased product of drug antagonist
    (d) An alternation in enzyme that utilizes PABA

74. C 17 α-β unsaturated lactone ring is a common fearure in
    (a) Digitalis and squill glycosides
    (b) Digitalis and strophanthus glycosides
    (c) Digitalis and senna glycosides
    (d) Digitalis and amygdalin

75. License to sell drug specified in Schedule C and C1 is given in form number
    (a) 19 (b) 18
    (c) 21 (d) 24

76. Liquid paraffin exhibits
    (a) Plastic flow
    (b) Newtonian flow
    (c) Pseudoplastic flow
    (d) Dilatant flow

77. The temperature at which the solubility of the surfactant is equal to CMC is
    (a) Kraft point (b) Boiling point
    (c) Melting point (d) (a) and (b)

78. Hcl gas is soluble in water due to
    (a) Hydrogen bonding
    (b) Chemical bond
    (c) Sulphur bond
    (d) None of the above

79. Which one of the equation is used to identify the drug release from a dossage from.
    (a) Henderson – Hasselbatch
    (b) Higuchi
    (c) Noyes – Whitney
    (d) Hixson – Cromwell

80. Dilatant flow is exhibited by
    (a) Flocculated suspension
    (b) Deflocculated suspension
    (c) Sodium alginate in water
    (d) None of the above

81. When a series of steps are involved in a reaction, the 'overall rate' of a reaction depends Upon the rate(s) of
    (a) All steps
    (b) All steps which follow the slowest step
    (c) All steps which precede the slowest step
    (d) The slowest step

82. The time required for the complete degradation of a drug in solution is a finite value. The order of that reaction is
    (a) First (b) Pseudo First
    (c) Second (d) Zero

83. Penicillin G is prepared as a salt of procaine penicillin G. Now the rate of decomposition of penicillin G will be
    (a) Increased (b) Reduced
    (c) Unchanged (d) Unpredictable

84. Aspirin undergoes decomposition in a formulation. It can be prevented by
    (a) Adding a chelating agent
    (b) Adding an antioxidant
    (c) Protecting it from light
    (d) Suppressing its solubility

85. Which one of the following (forms) creates more difficulties regarding dissolution?
    (a) Amorphous form (b) Anhydrous form
    (b) Crystalline form (d) Metastable form

86. Which one of these drugs diffuses easily through the membrane at intestinal portion of the GIT?
    (a) Aspirin (b) Chloroquin
    (b) Paracetamol (d) Tolbutamide

87. Near critical micelle concentration, micelles of the surfactant molecules assume the shape of
    (a) Cylindrical (b) Layered
    (c) rod-shaped (d) spherical

88. Polysorbate 80 (Tween 80) is a surfactant of type
    (a) Amphi-ionic (b) Anionic
    (c) Cationic (d) Non-ionic

89. Gegenions means
    (a) Amphiphiles
    (b) Ions having a charge opposite to the potential determining ions
    (c) Ions having same charge as that of potential determining ions
    (d) Potential determining ions

90. The drug Hydroxyzine comes under
    (a) Phenothiazine derivative
    (b) Tricyclic ring system
    (c) Piperidine ring system
    (d) Diphenyl Methane derivatives

91. MAO- Inhibitors are
    (a) Sedatives & hypnotics
    (b) General anaesthetics
    (c) Anticonvulsants
    (d) None of the above

92. Ethosuximide has
    (a) Pyrrolidinedione ring
    (b) Pyrrole ring system
    (c) Pyrazole ring
    (d) Thiazole ring

93. The drug Triamterene has
    (a) 1,3,7-triamino group
    (b) 2,4,7- triamino group

(c) 2,2,3- triamino group
(d) 2,4,8- triamino group

94. Theophylline is
(a) 1,3,7- trimethyl xanthine
(b) 1,7- dimethyle xanthine
(c) 1,3- dimethyl xanthine
(d) 3,7- dimethyl xanthine

95. The drug which has diethyl amino acetyl side chain is
(a) Lignocaine (b) Procaine
(c) Cocaine (d) None of these

96. The drug 'Acetazolamide', chemically is
(a) 5-acetamido, 1,3,4-thiadiazole-2-sulphonamide
(b) 3-aceto 1,3,4-thiadiazole 2-sulphonamide
(c) 1-acetamido 1,2,4-thiadiazole 4-sulphonamide
(d) All of these

97. The drug, which comes under 5 pyrazolone derivative is
(a) Antipyrine (b) Phenylbutazone
(c) Sulfinpyrazone (d) Acetamidophen

98. Phenobarbital is
(d) short acting barbiturate
(e) Long acting barbiturate
(f) Intermediate acting barbiturate
(g) Ultra short acting barbiturate

99. Hydrallazine HCL can be assayed by
(a) Non aqueous method
(b) Titration with M/20 mercuric acetate
(c) Gravimetric method
(d) Titration with M/20 KIO3

100. ........... is used in Pellagra
(a) Nicotinic acid (b) Nicotinamide
(c) Both (a) & (b) (d) Either (a)or (b)

101. Isoniazid is assayed by (official method)
(a) Adding N/10 Bromine & excess determined using Kl & N/10 Na2S2O3
(b) Adding N/10 iodine & excess determined using Kl & N/10 Na2S2O3
(c) Titration with N/10 Hcl
(d) Non aqueous method

102. Chloroquine is a
(a) 4-amino quinoline
(b) 8- amino quinoline
(c) 6- amino quinoline
(d) 6- methoxy quinoline

103. If therapy with multiple drugs causes induction of drug metabolism in your asthma patient, it will
(a) Result in increased smooth endoplasmic reticulum
(b) Result in increased rough endoplasmic reticulum
(c) Result in decreased enzymes in the soluble cytoplasmic fraction
(d) Require 3-4 months to reach completion

104. Which of the following is a phase II drug-metabolizing reaction
(a) Acetylation (b) Deamination
(c) Hydrolysis (d) Oxidation

105. A child has swallowed the contents of two bottles of a nasal decongestant whose primary ingredient is a potent alpha adrenoceptor agonist drug. The signs of alpha activation that may occur in this patient include
(a) Bronchodilation
(b) Cardioacceleration(tachycardia)
(c) Pupillary dilation (mydriasis)
(d) Vasodepression (vasodilation)

106. "Nicotinic" sites include all of the following except
(a) Bronchial smooth muscle
(b) Adrenal medullary cells
(c) Parasympathetic ganglia
(d) Skeletal muscle

107. A direct- acting cholinomimetic that is lipid-soluble and often used in the treatment of glaucoma is
(a) Acetylcholine (b) Bethanechol
(c) Physostigmine (d) Pilocarpine

108. Propranolol is useful all of the following except
(a) Angina
(b) Familial tremor
(c) Hypertension
(d) Partial atriovertricular heart block

109. Which one of the following is characteristic of captopril and enalapril
   (a) Competitively blocks angiotensim II at its receptor
   (b) Decrease angiotensim II concentration in the blood
   (c) Decrease rennin concentration in the blood
   (d) Increase sodium and decrease potassium in the blood

110. The biochemical mechanism of action of digitalis is associated with
   (a) A decrease in calcium uptake by the sarcoplasmic reticulum
   (b) An increase in ATP synthesis
   (c) A modification of the actin molecule
   (d) An increase in systolic intracellular calcium levels

111. Which of the following situation constitutes an added risk of digoxin toxicity
   (a) Starting administration of captopril
   (b) Starting administration of quinidine
   (c) Hyperkalemia
   (d) Hypernagnesemia

112. When used as an antiarrhythmic drug, Lidocaine typically
   (a) Increases action potential duration
   (b) Increases contractility
   (c) Increases PR interval
   (d) Reduces abnormal automaticity

113. A-50-year-old man has a history of frequent episodes of renal colic with high-calcium renal stones. The most useful agent in the treatment of recurrent calcium stones is
   (a) Mannitol
   (b) furosemide
   (c) Spironolactone
   (d) Hydrochlorothiazide

114. The instrument used to measure particle volume is
   (a) Coulter counter
   (b) Microscope
   (c) Hempel burette
   (d) Helium densitometer

115. Xenon arc lamp is the source of light in
   (a) Spectrofluorimeter
   (b) IR Spectrometer
   (c) Flame photometer
   (d) Calorimeter

116. The method of expressing magnetic field strength is
   (a) Cycles/sec (b) Pulses/sec
   (c) Debye units (d) Gauss

117. A solvent used in NMR studies is
   (a) Chloroform
   (b) Acetone
   (c) Carbontetrachloride
   (d) Methanol

118. Isoniazid is a primary antitubercular agent that
   (a) Requires pyridoxine supplementation
   (b) Causes occular complications that are reversible if the drug is discontinued
   (c) Is ototoxic and nephrotic
   (d) Should never be used due to hepatotoxic potential

119. The common attributes of ascorbic acid, an antiscorbutic vitamin, are
   (P) Exist in nature in both reduced an oxidised form and in a state of reversible equilibrium
   (Q) Has a keto-enol system in the molecule
   (R) Has an aldehyde group since it gives positive Schiff's reaction
   (S) Salt forming properties are due to the presence of free carboxyl group
   (a) P,R (b) Q,R
   (c) R,S (d) P,Q

120. Two properties of Radiopharmaceuticals are
   (P) Slow localization in target tissue
   (Q) Very long half-life to provide enough exposure to get imaging information
   (R) Short half-life to minimize radiation exposure yet long enough to get imaging information
   (S) Rapid localization in target tissue and quick clearance from non-target organs
   (a) P,Q (b) Q,R
   (c) R,S (d) P,S

121. Which of the following is an example for a trisaccharide?
(a) Verbascose (b) Stachyose
(c) Raffinose (d) Sucralose

122. Chrysolaminarin is ________.
(a) A storage polysaccharide of green algae
(b) A storage polysaccharide of brown algae
(c) A storage polysaccharide of red algae
(d) A storage polysaccharide of diatoms

123. Which of the following is an example for an artificial sweetener of saccharide origin?
(a) Sucralose (b) Saccharin
(c) Stachyose (d) All of these

124. In a chemical reaction 'X' is able to convert $Cu^{2+}$ ions to $Cu^{+}$ ions. If 'X' is a carbohydrate, which of the following best explains to be the 'X'?
(a) 'X' is a reducing sugar
(b) 'X' is a non-reducing sugar
(c) 'X' is a monosaccharide
(d) Both (a) and (c)

125. Which of the following is a reducing sugar?
(a) Glucose in closed ring form
(b) Glucose in open chain form
(c) Sucrose
(d) All of the above

## Answer Key Mock Test I

| 1-a | 2-b | 3-b | 4-b | 5-b | 6-c | 7-c | 8-a | 9-c | 10-b |
|---|---|---|---|---|---|---|---|---|---|
| 11-c | 12-b | 13-a | 14-c | 15-d | 16-a | 17-c | 18-a | 19-a | 20-d |
| 21-c | 22-d | 23-d | 24-a | 25-a | 26-b | 27-b | 28-d | 29-a | 30-b |
| 31-b | 32-b | 33-b | 34-d | 35-a | 36-d | 37-c | 38-b | 39-c | 40-c |
| 41-d | 42-d | 43-b | 44-b | 45-c | 46-b | 47-c | 48-a | 49-d | 50-c |
| 51-a | 52-b | 53-c | 54-d | 55-a | 56-c | 57-d | 58-a | 59-d | 60-b |
| 61-a | 62-c | 63-c | 64-c | 65-a | 66-a | 67-a | 68-a | 69-c | 70-a |
| 71-c | 72-b | 73-d | 74-b | 75-c | 76-c | 77-a | 78-a | 79-c | 80-a |
| 81-c | 82-d | 83-b | 84-d | 85-c | 86-b | 87-d | 88-d | 89-b | 90-d |
| 91-d | 92-a | 93-b | 94-c | 95-a | 96-a | 97-a | 98-b | 99-d | 100-d |
| 101-a | 102-a | 103-a | 104-c | 105-c | 106-a | 107-d | 108-d | 109-b | 110-d |
| 111-b | 112-d | 113-d | 114-a | 115-a | 116-d | 117-c | 118-a | 119-d | 120-c |
| 121-c | 122-d | 123-d | 124-d | 125-b | | | | | |

# Mock Test II

**NOTE:**

- The question paper consists of the multiple choice questions **(MCQ's).**
- Total of **125 questions** will be asked in the exam which will be of total **500 marks**.
- The time duration to complete the examination is of **3 hours**.
- For every correct response **4 marks** will be allotted.
- For every incorrect answer, **1 mark** will be deducted.

1. D-glucose reacts with molecular oxygen ($O_2$) in the presence of the enzyme glucose oxidase to form D-glucono-δ-lactone and ___________.
   (a) $H_2O$ (b) $H_2O_2$
   (c) $H_2$ (d) $O_3$
2. Most prominent carbohydrate component of hemicellulose is
   (a) Pectin (b) Arabinose
   (c) Arabinoxylan (d) Suberin
3. Which of the following is an example for heteropolysaccharide?
   (a) Hyaluronic acid (b) Gelatin
   (c) Glycogen (d) Both (a) and (b)
4. Glucose on oxidation with bromine water forms
   (a) Glucuronic acid
   (b) Glucosaccharic acid
   (c) Gluconic acid
   (d) Mannose
5. Dextrin is a branched bacterial homo polysaccharide of ________ linked D-glucose with ______ branches.
   (a) α-1 – 6 and α-1 – 3
   (b) β-1 – 6 and β-1 – 3
   (c) β-1 – 6 and α-1 – 3
   (d) α-1 – 6 and β-1 – 3
6. Laminarin is_____
   (a) A storage polysaccharide of red algae
   (b) A storage polysaccharide of brown algae
   (c) A structural polysaccharide of red algae
   (d) A structural polysaccharide of brown algae
7. Which of the following statements are true about agarose?
   (a) It is a branched polysaccharide
   (b) It is a linear polysaccharide
   (c) It is made up of arabinose
   (d) Agarose is one of the principal components of agar
8. Caramelization of sucrose yields
   (a) Glucose
   (b) Fructose
   (c) Glucose and Fructose
   (d) Charcoal
9. Which of the following reaction is called "Maillard reaction"
   (a) Reaction between amino group and hydroxyl group
   (b) Reaction between amino group and keto group
   (c) Reaction between amino group and aldehyde group
   (d) Reaction between amino group and carboxylic group
10. Bial's test is used to detect the presence of _____
    (a) Triose (b) Tetrose
    (c) Pentose (d) Hexose

11. Which of the following animal possess cellulose?
    (a) Coelenterates (b) Sponges
    (c) Tunicates (d) Protozoans
12. Glucose residues in amylose are linked by
    (a) α 1 – 4 (b) β 1 – 4
    (c) α 1 – 6 (d) β 1 – 6
13. Chitin is a_______
    (a) Homopolysaccharide of N acetyl glucosamine
    (b) Heteropolysaccharide of N acetyl glucosamine and N acetyl muramic acid
    (c) A complex polymer of many sugars
    (d) A branched homopolysaccharide of N acetyl glucosamine
14. The branch points of amylopectin are connected by
    (a) α 1 – 4 (b) β 1 – 4
    (c) α 1 – 6 (d) β 1 – 6
15. Which of the following is an example for homopolysaccharide?
    (a) Cellulose (b) Starch
    (c) Glycogen (d) All of these
16. Shrinkage of gel by extrusion of liquid is called as
    (a) Syneresis (b) Dilatancy
    (c) Plasticity (d) Ebullition
17. Carbamazepine is a tricyclic antidepressant. It is classified as
    (a) Benzodiazepine
    (b) Arylalkanolamine
    (c) Iminostilbene
    (d) Benzimidazole
18. Sulfa drugs can be conveniently estimated using the reagent
    (a) 4,4-Dithiobis-(2-nitrobenzoic acid)
    (b) Tris-(hydroxy methyl) amino-menthane sodium nitrate
    (c) N-(1-napthyl) ethylenediamine
    (d) N-ethylmalcimide
19. Ehlrich's reagent is
    (a) Bismuth iodide solution
    (b) p- Dimethyl aniline solution in alcohol
    (c) p-Dimethyl amino benzaldehyde solution
    (d) p-Dimethyl aniline solution in methamol
20. Resolution of a monochromator is the ability to distinguish
    (a) As separate entities adjacent spectral features
    (b) Seperation of different colours
    (c) Seperation of UV light and visible light
    (d) Dispersing characteristics
21. Important activities noticed in Testosterone
    (a) Androgenic, Myotropic and Anabolic
    (b) Progestational, Myotropic and Anabolic
    (c) Estrogenic, Myotropic and Anabolic
    (d) Androgenic, Optometric and katabolic
22. The UV visible region in the electromagnetic spectrum of radiation is
    (a) 200- 400nm (b) 300-660nm
    (c) 400-800nm (d) 200- 800nms
23. The Mantoux test uses
    (a) Old tuberculin
    (b) Diptheria toxin
    (c) Serum antigen
    (d) Polysaccharide antigen
24. The volume of distribution of a drug is
    (a) An expression of total body volume
    (b) A measure of total fluid volume
    (c) A relationship between the total amount of drug in the body and the concentration of the drug in the blood
    (d) Proportional to bioavailabillity of the drug
25. Vitamin D2 is
    (a) 22, 23- Dihydro- 5, 6 – cis – ergocalciferol
    (b) 5,6 –cis – chloecalciferol
    (c) 7- dehydrocholesterol
    (d) 21-24 – dihydro – 5,6- cis-ergocalciferol
26. R.W.C. is used to identify the strength of an
    (a) Antibiotic
    (b) Antipyretic
    (c) Antiseptic
    (d) Anti-inflammatory

27. The essential structrural unit for the anthelmintic activity of mebendazole is
    (a) Benzoyl group
    (b) Benzimidazole
    (c) Methylcarbamate
    (d) Imidazole
28. Most accepted mechanism for developing bacterial resistance to sulphonamides is
    (a) An increasing capacity to inactivate or destroy the drug
    (b) An alternative metabolic pathway for synthesis of an essential metabolite
    (c) An increased product of drug antagonist
    (d) An alternation in enzyme that utilizes PABA
29. C 17 α-β unsaturated lactone ring is a common fearure in
    (a) Digitalis and squill glycosides
    (b) Digitalis and strophanthus glycosides
    (c) Digitalis and senna glycosides
    (d) Digitalis and amygdalin
30. License to sell drug specified in Schedule C and C1 is given in form number
    (a) 19 (b) 18
    (c) 21 (d) 24
31. Liquid paraffin exhibits
    (a) Plastic flow (b) Newtonian flow
    (c) Pseudoplastic flow (d) Dilatant flow
32. The temperature at which the solubility of the surfactant is equal to CMC is
    (a) Kraft point (b) Boiling point
    (c) Melting point (d) (a) and (b)
33. HCl gas is soluble in water due to
    (a) Hydrogen bonding
    (b) Chemical bond
    (c) Sulphur bond
    (d) None of the above
34. Which one of the equation is used to identify the drug release from a dossage from.
    (a) Henderson – Hasselbatch
    (b) Higuchi
    (c) Noyes – Whitney
    (d) Hixson – Cromwell
35. Dilatant flow is exhibited by
    (a) Flocculated suspension
    (b) Deflocculated suspension
    (c) Sodium alginate in water
    (d) None of the above
36. When a series of steps are involved in a reaction, the 'overall rate' of a reaction depends Upon the rate(s) of
    (a) All steps
    (b) All steps which follow the slowest step
    (c) All steps which precede the slowest step
    (d) The slowest step
37. The time required for the complete degradation of a drug in solution is a finite value. The order of that reaction is
    (a) First (b) Pseudo First
    (c) Second (d) Zero
38. Penicillin G is prepared as a salt of procaine penicillin G. Now the rate of decomposition of penicillin G will be
    (a) Increased (b) Reduced
    (c) Unchanged (d) Unpredictable
39. Aspirin undergoes decomposition in a formulation. It can be prevented by
    (a) Adding a chelating agent
    (b) Adding an antioxidant
    (c) Protecting it from light
    (d) Suppressing its solubility
40. Which one of the following (forms) creates more difficulties regarding dissolution?
    (a) Amorphous form (b) Anhydrous form
    (c) Crystalline form (d) Metastable form
41. Which one of these drugs diffuses easily through the membrane at intestinal portion of the GIT?
    (a) Aspirin (b) Chloroquin
    (c) Paracetamol (d) Tolbutamide
42. Near critical micelle concentration, micelles of the surfactant molecules assume the shape of
    (a) Cylindrical (b) Layered
    (c) rod-shaped (d) Spherical

43. Polysorbate 80 (Tween 80) is a surfactant of type
    (a) Amphi-ionic (b) Anionic
    (c) Cationic (d) Non-ionic

44. Gegenions means
    (a) Amphiphiles
    (b) Ions having a charge opposite to the potential determining ions
    (c) Ions having same charge as that of potential determining ions
    (d) Potential determining ions

45. The drug Hydroxyzine comes under
    (a) Phenothiazine derivative
    (b) Tricyclic ring system
    (c) Piperidine ring system
    (d) Diphenyl Methane derivatives

46. MAO- Inhibitors are
    (a) Sedatives & hypnotics
    (b) General anaesthetics
    (c) Anticonvulsants
    (d) None of the above

47. Ethosuximide has
    (a) Pyrrolidinedione ring
    (b) Pyrrole ring system
    (c) Pyrazole ring
    (d) Thiazole ring

48. The drug Triamterene has
    (a) 1,3,7-triamino group
    (b) 2,4,7- triamino group
    (c) 2,2,3- triamino group
    (d) 2,4,8- triamino group

49. Theophylline is
    (a) 1,3,7- trimethyl xanthine
    (b) 1,7- dimethyle xanthine
    (c) 1,3- dimethyl xanthine
    (d) 3,7- dimethyl xanthine

50. The drug which has diethyl amino acetyl side chain is
    (a) Lignocaine (b) Procaine
    (c) Cocaine (d) None of these

51. The drug 'Acetazolamide', chemically is
    (a) 5-acetamido, 1,3,4-thiadiazole-2-sulphonamide
    (b) 3-aceto 1,3,4-thiadiazole 2-sulphonamide
    (c) 1-acetamido 1,2,4-thiadiazole 4-sulphonamide
    (d) All of these

52. The drug, which comes under 5 pyrazolone derivative is
    (a) Antipyrine (b) Phenylbutazone
    (c) Sulfinpyrazone (d) Acetamidophen

53. Phenobarbital is
    (a) Short acting barbiturate
    (b) Long acting barbiturate
    (c) Intermediate acting barbiturate
    (d) Ultra short acting barbiturate

54. Hydrallazine HCL can be assayed by
    (a) Non aqueous method
    (b) Titration with M/20 mercuric acetate
    (c) Gravimetric method
    (d) Titration with M/20 KIO3

55. ............. is used in Pellagra
    (a) Nicotinic acid (b) Nicotinamide
    (c) Both (a) & (b) (d) Either (a)or (b)

56. Isoniazid is assayed by (official method)
    (a) Adding N/10 Bromine & excess determined using Kl & N/10 Na2S2O3
    (b) Adding N/10 iodine & excess determined using Kl & N/10 Na2S2O3
    (c) Titration with N/10 Hcl
    (d) Non aqueous method

57. Chloroquine is a
    (a) 4-amino quinoline
    (b) 8- amino quinoline
    (c) 6- amino quinoline
    (d) 6- methoxy quinoline

58. If therapy with multiple drugs causes induction of drug metabolism in your asthma patient, it will
    (a) Result in increased smooth endoplasmic reticulum
    (b) Result in increased rough endoplasmic reticulum

(c) Result in decreased enzymes in the soluble cytoplasmic fraction
(d) Require 3-4 months to reach completion

59. Which of the following is a phase II drug-metabolizing reaction
(a) Acetylation (b) Deamination
(c) Hydrolysis (d) Oxidation

60. A child has swallowed the contents of two bottles of a nasal decongestant whose primary ingredient is a potent alpha adrenoceptor agonist drug. The signs of alpha activation that may occur in this patient include
(a) Bronchodilation
(b) Cardioacceleration(tachycardia)
(c) Pupillary dilation (mydriasis)
(d) Vasodepression (vasodilation)

61. "Nicotinic" sites include all of the following except
(a) Bronchial smooth muscle
(b) Adrenal medullary cells
(c) Parasympathetic ganglia
(d) Skeletal muscle

62. A direct- acting cholinomimetic that is lipid-soluble and often used in the treatment of glaucoma is
(a) Acetylcholine (b) Bethanechol
(c) Physostigmine (d) Pilocarpine

63. Propranolol is useful all of the following except
(a) Angina
(b) Familial tremor
(c) Hypertension
(d) Partial atriovertricular heart block

64. Which one of the following is characteristic of captopril and enalapril
(a) Competitively blocks angiotensim II at its receptor
(b) Decrease angiotensim II concentration in the blood
(c) Decrease rennin concentration in the blood
(d) Increase sodium and decrease potassium in the blood

65. The biochemical mechanism of action of digitalis is associated with
(a) A decrease in calcium uptake by the sarcoplasmic reticulum
(b) An increase in ATP synthesis
(c) A modification of the actin molecule
(d) An increase in systolic intracellular calcium levels

66. Which of the following situation constitutes an added risk of digoxin toxicity
(a) Starting administration of captopril
(b) Starting administration of quinidine
(c) Hyperkalemia
(d) Hypernagnesemia

67. When used as an antiarrhythmic drug, Lidocaine typically
(a) Increases action potential duration
(b) Increases contractility
(c) Increases PR interval
(d) Reduces abnormal automaticity

68. A-50-year-old man has a history of frequent episodes of renal colic with high-calcium renal stones. The most useful agent in the treatment of recurrent calcium stones is
(a) Mannitol
(b) furosemide
(c) Spironolactone
(d) Hydrochlorothiazide

69. The instrument used to measure particle volume is
(a) Coulter counter
(b) Microscope
(c) Hempel burette
(d) Helium densitometer

70. Xenon arc lamp is the source of light in
(a) Spectrofluorimeter
(b) IR Spectrometer
(c) Flame photometer
(d) Calorimeter

71. The method of expressing magnetic field strength is
   (a) Cycles/sec  (b) Pulses/sec
   (c) Debye units  (d) Gauss

72. A solvent used in NMR studies is
   (a) Chloroform
   (b) Acetone
   (c) Carbontetrachloride
   (d) Methanol

73. Isoniazid is a primary antitubercular agent that
   (a) Requires pyridoxine supplementation
   (b) Causes occular complications that are reversible if the drug is discontinued
   (c) Is ototoxic and nephrotic
   (d) Should never be used due to hepatotoxic potential

74. The common attributes of ascorbic acid, an antiscorbutic vitamin, are
   (P) Exist in nature in both reduced an oxidised form and in a state of reversible equilibrium
   (Q) Has a keto-enol system in the molecule
   (R) Has an aldehyde group since it gives positive Schiff's reaction
   (S) Salt forming properties are due to the presence of free carboxyl group
   (a) P,R  (b) Q,R
   (c) R,S  (d) P,Q

75. Two properties of Radiopharmaceuticals are
   (P) Slow localization in target tissue
   (Q) Very long half-life to provide enough exposure to get imaging information
   (R) Short half-life to minimize radiation exposure yet long enough to get imaging information
   (S) Rapid localization in target tissue and quick clearance from non-target organs
   (a) P,Q  (b) Q,R
   (c) R,S  (d) P,S

76. The volatile oils are complex mixtures of······
   (a) mono- and sesquiterpenes and phenylpropane derivatives
   (b) mono- and diterpene alcohols and ethers
   (c) sesquiterpenes and other aromatic compounds
   (d) monoterpene acids and lactones
   (e) monoterpene ethers and aldehydes

77. Which of the following are known as balsams?
   (a) Resins dissolved in volatile oil
   (b) A mixture of volatile oils with sesquiterpenes
   (c) Resins dissolved in water
   (d) Polysaccharides mixed with volatile oil
   (e) Juices evaporated to dryness

78. Alkaloids are naturally occurring compounds which contain .............in their molecules.
   (a) one or more N atoms
   (b) two heterocyclic rings
   (c) a side-chain on one of the benzene rings
   (d) one or more N atoms originating from amino acids
   (e) one or more O atoms

79. Tick the synthetic vasoconstrictor having an adrenomimic effect:
   (a) Noradrenalin
   (b) Adrenalin
   (c) Phenylephrine
   (d) Angiotensinamide

80. Indicate the group of drugs influencing the cerebral flow:
   (a) Ca-channel blockers
   (b) Derivatives of GABA
   (c) Derivatives of Vinca minor plant
   (d) All the above

81. Vasopressin possesses the following:
   (a) Antidiuretic property
   (b) Vasodilatation property
   (c) Release of a thyroid hormone into the plasma
   (d) Diuretic property

82. The action of insulin is potentiated by:
   (a) Sulphonylureas
   (b) Glucagon
   (c) Biguanides
   (d) None of the above

83. Which of the following glucocorticoids is a short- to medium-acting drug?
(a) Prednisolon (b) Dexamethasone
(c) Triamcinolone (d) All of the above

84. Which of the following NSAIDs is a propionic acid derivative?
(a) Ibuprofen
(b) Indomethacin
(c) Metamizole (Analgin)
(d) Diclofenac

85. Which category of histamine H1 antagonists is recognized for as second-generation antihistamines?
(a) Alkylamines (propylamines); i.e. Brompheniramine
(b) Piperidines; i.e. Loratadine, Fexofenadine
(c) Ethylenediamines; i.e. Suprastine
(d) Phenothiazines; i.e. Promethazine

86. Which one of the following non-narcotic agents inhibits mainly cyclooxygenase (COX) in CNS?
(a) Paracetamol
(b) Ketorolac
(c) Acetylsalicylic acid
(d) Ibuprofen

87. For which of the following conditions could aspirin be used prophylactically?
(a) Noncardiogenic pulmonary edema
(b) Peptic ulcers
(c) Thromboembolism
(d) Metabolic acidosis

88. Indicate the nonopioid agent of central effect with analgesic activity:
(a) Reserpine (b) Propranolol
(c) Clopheline (d) Prazosin

89. Which of the following nonopioid agents is an antidepressant with analgesic activity?
(a) Fluoxetine (b) Moclobemide
(c) Tranylcypramine (d) Amitriptyline

90. Indicate the atypical antipsychotic drug:
(a) Haloperidol (b) Clozapine
(c) Thioridazine (d) Thiothixene

91. Which of the following antipsychotic drugs is typical?
(a) Clozapine (b) Quetiapine
(c) Haloperidol (d) Olanzapine

92. Which of the following antipsychotic drugs has high affinity for D4 and 5-HT2 receptors?
(a) Clozapine (b) Fluphenazine
(c) Thioridazine (d) Haloperidole

93. Select the agent, which is preferred in the treatment of the drug-induced form of parkinsonism:
(a) Levodopa (b) Bromocriptine
(c) Benztropine (d) Dopamine

94. Which of the following agents is the precursor of dopamine?
(a) Bromocriptine (b) Levodopa
(c) Selegiline (d) Amantadine

95. Indicate the antipsychotic drug having a muscarinic-cholinergic blocking activity:
(a) Chlorpromazine (b) Clorprothixene
(c) Risperidone (d) Haloperidol

96. Which of the following antipsychotic agents is used in combination with an opioid drug fentanyl in neuroleptanalgesia?
(a) Haloperidol (b) Droperidol
(c) Chlorpromazine (d) Clozapine

97. Lithium carbonate is useful in the treatment of:
(a) Petit mal seizures
(b) Bipolar disorder
(c) Neurosis
(d) Trigeminal neuralgia

98. Block of which type of Monoamine Oxydase might be more selective for depression?
(a) MAO-A
(b) MAO-B
(c) Both MAO-A and MAO-B
(d) MAO-C

99. Which of the following benzodiazepines has the shortest duration of action?
(a) Triazolam (b) Clorazepate
(c) Prazepam (d) Clordiazepoxide

100. Indicate the anesthetic, which is used intravenously:
(a) Propofol (b) Halothane
(c) Desflurane (d) Nitrous oxide

101. Most of drugs are antacids EXCEPT:
(a) Misoprostol (b) Maalox
(c) Mylanta (d) Almagel

102. Indicate an antiemetic agent which is related to neuroleptics:
(a) Metoclopramide
(b) Nabilone
(c) Tropisetron
(d) Prochlorperazine

103. Glober is a radiation source used in the IR it is made up of-
(a) Tungsten (b) Nichrome
(c) Silicon carbide (d) None of these

104. Potassium element show which colour in flame
(a) Apple green (b) Crimson red
(c) Yellow (d) Violet

105. Coupling causes the peaks in $^{1}H$ NMR spectra to be split into
(a) two peaks
(b) multiple peaks equal to the number of hydrogens on surrounding atoms
(c) multiple peaks equal to the number of surrounding carbon atoms
(d) multiple peaks equal to the number of hydrogen on surrounding atoms, plus one

106. All hydrogen atoms
(a) have the same resonance frequency
(b) resonate at different frequencies depending on their environment
(c) are attached to carbon
(d) resonate at about the same frequency as carbon

107. Why is it important to use a deuterated solvent?
(a) NMR uses least of this solvent
(b) So the spectrometer can lock onto the sample to prevent the spectrum from drifting during acquisition
(c) Expensive solvents work best with NMR
(d) They dissolve polymer the fastest

108. What is the relationship between wavelength and wave number?
(a) Wavenumber = 1 / wavelength in centimeters
(b) Wavenumber - wavelength in nanometers = 1
(c) Wavelength in nanometers x wavenumber = 1
(d) None of the above

109. Why must the radiation source for fluorescence spectrometry be more powerful than for absorption spectroscopy?
(a) Because the magnitude of the output signal is proportional to the power of the incident radiation
(b) Because the sample won't fluoresce if the incident radiation is of low power
(c) To allow for scattering by the sample
(d) None of the above

110. Why do fluorescence spectrometers often use double-beam optics?
(a) So a reference solution can be used
(b) To compensate for beam attenuation by the monochromator
(c) To compensate for power fluctuations in the radiation source
(d) All of the above

111. For a molecule to absorb IR, why must the molecule's vibrations cause fluctuations in the dipole moment of the molecule?
(a) Because a change in dipole moment lowers the energy required for electronic transitions
(b) Because for absorption to occur, the radiation must interact with the electric field caused by changing dipole moment
(c) Because fluctuations in the dipole moment allow the molecule to deform by bending and stretching
(d) All of the above

112. Why phosphorescence measurements are usually made at a low temperature?
(a) To prevent thermal degradation of the phosphorescent species
(b) To promote phosphorescence by slowing the rate of radiation less transfer processes

(c) To increase the efficiency of the detector
(d) To decrease the efficiency of detector

113. Which of the following is the principal chromophore in an azo-dye?
(a) N=N (b) C Ξ N
(c) N Ξ N (d) C=N

114. An aqueous solution of a dye has a strong absorption with $\lambda_{max}$= 464 nm. The colour of the solution is:
(a) Green (b) Orange
(c) Colourless (d) Purple

115. In gas chromatography, the basis for separation of the components of the volatile material is the difference in
(a) partition coefficients
(b) conductivity
(c) molecular weight
(d) molarity

116. In reverse phase chromatography, the stationary phase is made
(a) non-polar
(b) polar
(c) either non-polar or polar
(d) none of these

117. Ion exchange chromatography is based on the
(a) electrostatic attraction
(b) electrical mobility of ionic species
(c) adsorption chromatography
(d) partition chromatography

118. A combination of paper chromatography and electrophoresis involves
(a) partition chromatography
(b) electrical mobility of the ionic species
(c) both (a) and (b)
(d) none of these

119. The eluent strength is a measure of
(a) solvent adsorption energy
(b) solvent absorption energy
(c) solvent diffusivity
(d) solvent mixing index

120. The value of wet point for 10 % additive concentration range from
(a) 10-15 (b) 15-45
(c) 45-90 (d) 50-250

121. Hofmeister or Lyotropic series rule applied to
(a) Hydrophilic particles
(b) hydrophobic particles
(c) Both
(d) Charged particles

122. Dielectric constant is related to thickness of double layer
(a) directly (b) indirectly
(b) It is not related (d) proportionally

123. Pluronics are
(a) Fatty acid esters of sorbitol anhydride
(b) Higher weight polyethylene glycols
(c) polyoxyethylene ethers
(d) Molecular combination of polyoxyethylene and polyoxypropylene

124. Surfactant and protective colloids differs in
(a) protective colloide do not reduce surface tension
(b) They used in higher concentration
(c) They increase zeta potential
(d) All

125. Sodium carboxymethyl cellulose used in injectable preparation in the concentration
(a) 0.1 % (b) 0.5 %
(c) 1 % (d) It is not used

# Answer Key Mock Test II

| 1-b | 2-c | 3-a | 4-c | 5-a | 6-b | 7-b | 8-c | 9-d | 10-c |
|---|---|---|---|---|---|---|---|---|---|
| 11-c | 12-a | 13-a | 14-c | 15-d | 16-a | 17-c | 18-c | 19-c | 20-a |
| 21-a | 22-a | 23-a | 24-c | 25-a | 26-c | 27-d | 28-d | 29-b | 30-c |
| 31-c | 32-a | 33-a | 34-c | 35-b | 36-c | 37-d | 38-b | 39-d | 40-c |
| 41-b | 42-d | 43-d | 44-b | 45-d | 46-d | 47-a | 48-b | 49-c | 50-a |
| 51-a | 52-a | 53-b | 54-d | 55-d | 56-a | 57-a | 58-a | 59-c | 60-c |
| 61-a | 62-d | 63-d | 64-b | 65-d | 66-b | 67-d | 68-d | 69-a | 70-d |
| 71-d | 72-c | 73-a | 74-d | 75-c | 76-a | 77-a | 78-a | 79-c | 80-d |
| 81-a | 82-c | 83-a | 84-a | 85-b | 86-a | 87-c | 88-c | 89-d | 90-b |
| 91-c | 92-a | 93-c | 94-b | 95-a | 96-b | 97-d | 98-a | 99-a | 100-a |
| 101-a | 102-d | 103-c | 104-d | 105-d | 106-b | 107-b | 108-a | 109-a | 110-c |
| 111-b | 112-b | 113-a | 114-b | 115-a | 116-a | 117-a | 118-c | 119-a | 120-b |
| 121-a | 122-b | 123-d | 124-d | 125-b | | | | | |

# Mock Test III

**NOTE:**

- The question paper consists of the multiple choice questions **(MCQ's).**
- Total of **125 questions** will be asked in the exam which will be of total **500 marks**.
- The time duration to complete the examination is of **3 hours**.
- For every correct response **4 marks** will be allotted.
- For every incorrect answer, **1 mark** will be deducted.

1. Which of the following is an accurate description of the phospholipid bilayer in cell membranes?
   (a) It is made up of two layers of phospholipid polymers.
   (b) It is made up of two layers of phospholipid molecules with the tails pointing away from each other.
   (c) It is made up of two layers of phospholipid molecules with the tails lying parallel to each other.
   (d) It is made up of two layers of phospholipid molecules with the tails interacting with each other.

2. Which of the following statements is true regarding the phospholipid bilayer in cell membranes?
   (a) Water and ions are unable to cross the bilayer due to the charges present in the head groups.
   (b) Water and ions are unable to cross the bilayer due the hydrophobic tails of the phospholipid molecules.
   (c) Water and ions are encouraged to cross the bilayer by interacting with the charges present in the head groups.
   (d) The molecules in the bilayer are fluid, and so the cell membrane is porous allowing the passage of ions and water across the cell membrane.

3. Which of the following statements is true?
   (a) Drugs and drug targets generally have similar molecular weights.
   (b) Drugs are generally smaller than drug targets.
   (c) Drugs are generally larger than drug targets.
   (d) There is no general rule regarding the relative size of drugs and their targets.

4. What is meant by a binding site?
   (a) The area of a macromolecular target that is occupied by a drug when it binds.
   (b) The portion of the drug to which a drug target binds
   (c) The functional groups used by a drug in binding to a drug target.
   (d) The bonds involved in binding a drug to its target.

5. Which of the following binding interactions is likely to be the most important *initial* interaction when a drug enters a binding site?
   (a) van der Waals interactions
   (b) hydrogen bond
   (c) ionic
   (d) induced dipole-dipole interactions

6. Which of the following underlined atoms is likely to be the strongest hydrogen bond acceptor?
   (a) amide nitrogen ($R\underline{N}HCOR'$)
   (b) aniline nitrogen ($Ar\underline{N}H_2$)
   (c) amine nitrogen ($R\underline{N}H_2$)
   (d) carboxylate oxygen ($RC\underline{O}_2^-$)

7. Which of the following underlined protons is likely to be the strongest hydrogen bond donor?
   (a) alcohol (RO<u>H</u>)
   (b) amine (RN<u>H</u>$_2$)
   (c) phenol (ArO<u>H</u>
   (d) ammonium ion (RN<u>H</u>$_3$$^+$)

8. Which of the following functional groups is most likely to participate in a dipole-dipole interaction?
   (a) Aromatic ring (b) Ketone
   (c) Alcohol (d) Alkene

9. Which of the following statements is untrue?
   (a) Desolvation is an energy expensive process that involves the removal of water from polar functional groups prior to a drug binding to its binding site.
   (b) Water molecules surrounding a hydrophobic region of a drug form an ordered layer of molecules with low entropy.
   (c) Interaction between the non-polar regions of a drug and the non-polar regions of a target require the removal of an ordered water coat and represents a gain in binding energy due to increased entropy.
   (d) An increase in entropy results in a greater positive value of $\Delta G$ and a greater chance of binding

10. Which ONE of the following is the best description of a protogenic solvent?
    (a) A protogenic solvent accepts electron lone pairs
    (b) A protogenic solvent neither accepts or donates protons
    (c) A protogenic solvent donates protons
    (d) A protogenic solvent donates or accepts electron lone pairs

11. For an aqueous solution of hydrochloric acid (HCl) the pH was found to be 4.18 units. What is the concentration of HCl in this solution?
    (a) $1.4\text{x}10^{-3}$ M (b) $1.4 \text{ x } 10^{-3}$ M
    (c) $3.2\text{x } 10^{-4}$ M (d) $6.6 \text{ x } 10^{-5}$ M

12. What is the pH of a 0.015 M solution of potassium hydroxide (KOH)?
    (a) 1.8 (b) 12.2
    (c) 5.6 (d) 8.8

13. A solution of the weakly basic drug erythromycin (pKb = 5.2) is buffered to pH 7.4. What percentage of the drug will be ionised at this pH?
    (a) 25% (b) 72%
    (c) 75% (d) 96%

14. A solution of diclofenac ($pK_a = 4.15$) is buffered to pH 5.5. How much diclofenac will be ionised at this pH?
    (a) 100% (b) 96%
    (c) 50% (d) 22%

15. A buffer solution contains 0.36 M sodium acetate ($CH_3COONa$) and 0.45 M acetic acid ($CH_3COOH$), $pK_a = 4.8$. What is the pH of this buffer solution?
    (a) 4.7 (b) 5.2
    (c) 3.8 (d) 6.1

16. 250 mL of a buffer contains 0.05 mol acetic acid ($CH_3COOH$) and 0.03 mol sodium acetate ($CH_3COONa$). What is the maximum buffer capacity of this buffer?
    (a) 0.46 mol $L^{-1}$ pH unit$^{-1}$
    (b) 0.18 mol $L^{-1}$ pH unit$^{-1}$
    (c) 0.22 mol $L^{-1}$ pH unit$^{-1}$
    (d) 1.84 mol $L^{-1}$ pH unit$^{-1}$

17. What is the isoelectric point for phenylalanine given the $pK_a$ for the COOH group is 1.83 and the $NH_3^+$ group is 9.13?
    (a) 2.43 (b) 4.83
    (c) 5.48 (d) 9.13

18. Which one of the following statements is true?
    (a) A strong electrolyte solution is a solution that always contains a high concentration of an acid or base.
    (b) The strength of an acid can be influenced by the solvent into which it is placed
    (c) In aqueous solution a strong acid will dissociate to form a strong conjugate base and together these form a conjugate pair.
    (d) pH 7 is considered to be neutral pH at all temperatures

19. Which one of the following statements concerning active pharmaceutical ingredients (APIs) is false?
   (a) The degree of ionisation of an API is dependent upon its $pK_a$ or $pK_b$.
   (b) The degree of ionisation of an API is dependent upon the pH of the surrounding solution.
   (c) The extent to which an API may be absorbed is influenced by the extent of its ionisation
   (d) APIs pass through biological membranes more readily when they are ionised

20. Choose the drugs which contain alkaloids derived from ornithine.
   (a) Hellebori rhizome
   (b) Henbane leaf
   (c) Cocae leaf
   (d) Ribes nigri leaf

21. Which statements are correct concerning with proazulens?
   (a) Proazulens show orange spot on TLC by spraying with cc. ammonium hydroxyde.
   (b) Proazulens give blue colour with EP reagent on heating.
   (c) Proazulens give red colour on ninhydrine reagent.
   (d) The proazulens give yellow precipitate with resorcinole.

22. The following properties are characteristic for saponins:
   (a) They give precipitate by shaking with water.
   (b) They are diterpenes.
   (c) They cause haemolysis on erythrocytes.
   (d) They give negative Keller-Kiliani test.

23. Which of the following properties are characteristic for tannins?
   (a) They give precipitate on alkaloids.
   (b) They give yellow or bluish-red color on iron-III-chloride.
   (c) They are 3-phenylbenzopyrane-derivatives.
   (d) They give pale pink precipitate on iodine.

24. Choose the antraquinone containing drugs.
   (a) Betulae folium
   (b) Graminis rhizome
   (c) Rhei rhizome
   (d) Herniariae herba
   (e) Rubi ideae folium

25. Galenicals prepared from Cinchona bark are used as ............. .
   (a) Abortive (b) bitter tonic
   (c) Stomachic (d) emetic

26. Pilocarpin the alkaloid of Jaborandi folium has.................. .
   (a) antagonist effect of atropine
   (b) agonist effect of atropine
   (c) sedative effect
   (d) diuretic activity

27. Which of the following compounds are C-glycosides:
   (a) Arbutin (b) vitexin
   (c) Gentiopicrine (d) hypericine

28. Choose the drugs containing purine derivatives.
   (a) Capsicum fuictus (b) Pasta guarana
   (c) Colae semen (d) Pyrethri flos

29. Choose the alkaloids derived from tryptophan.
   (a) ephedrine (b) chinin
   (c) vinchrystin (d) protoveratrin

30. The alkaloid found in calabar bean
   (a) physostigmine (b) Cocaine
   (c) colchicines (d) emetine

31. Devil's dung used as a carminative, and anti-spasmodic.
   (a) jalap (b) gamboges
   (c) asafetida (d) witch hazel

32. The following is/are the properties of nonhydrozable tannins except:
   (a) They give a bluish to black color with ferric chloride.
   (b) They usually contain phloroglucinol nucleus in part.
   (c) They are usually precipitated by bromine water TS.
   (d) They yield catechol when heated.

33. This does not possess narcotic properties and is therefore sometimes called anarcotine.
   (a) noscapine (b) hydrocodone
   (c) papaverine HCI (d) hydromorphone

34. Parts of this plant that are used as condiments, except:
   (a) Bawang (b) makabuhay
   (c) siling labuyo (d) luya

35. The hallucinogen derived from egrot:
   (a) THC (b) ETO
   (c) EDTA (d) LSD

36. The undissolved portion of the drug that remains after extraction:
   (a) solute (b) marc
   (c) solvent (d) active drug

37. Which of the following is an example for a trisaccharide?
   (a) Verbascose (b) Stachyose
   (c) Raffinose (d) Sucralose

38. Chrysolaminarin is ________.
   (a) A storage polysaccharide of green algae
   (b) A storage polysaccharide of brown algae
   (c) A storage polysaccharide of red algae
   (d) A storage polysaccharide of diatoms

39. Which of the following is an example for an artificial sweetener of saccharide origin?
   (a) Sucralose (b) Saccharin
   (b) Stachyose (d) All of these

40. In a chemical reaction 'X' is able to convert $Cu^{2+}$ ions to $Cu^{+}$ ions. If 'X' is a carbohydrate, which of the following best explains to be the 'X'?
   (a) 'X' is a reducing sugar
   (b) 'X' is a non-reducing sugar
   (c) 'X' is a monosaccharide
   (d) Both (a) and (c)

41. Which of the following is a reducing sugar?
   (a) Glucose in closed ring form
   (b) Glucose in open chain form
   (c) Sucrose

42. D-glucose reacts with molecular oxygen (O2) in the presence of the enzyme glucose oxidase to form D-glucono-δ-lactone and __________.
   (a) $H_2O$ (b) $H_2O_2$
   (c) $H_2$ (d) $O_3$

43. Most prominent carbohydrate component of hemicellulose is
   (a) Pectin (b) Arabinose
   (c) Arabinoxylan (d) Suberin

44. Which of the following is an example for heteropolysaccharide?
   (a) Hyaluronic acid (b) Gelatin
   (c) Glycogen (d) Both (a) and (b)

45. Glucose on oxidation with bromine water forms
   (a) Glucuronic acid
   (b) Glucosaccharic acid
   (c) Gluconic acid
   (d) Mannose

46. Dextrin is a branched bacterial homo polysaccharide of ________ linked D-glucose with ______ branches.
   (a) α-1 – 6 and α-1 – 3
   (b) β-1 – 6 and β-1 – 3
   (c) β-1 – 6 and α-1 – 3
   (d) α-1 – 6 and β-1 – 3

47. Laminarin is_____
   (a) A storage polysaccharide of red algae
   (b) A storage polysaccharide of brown algae
   (c) A structural polysaccharide of red algae
   (d) A structural polysaccharide of brown algae

48. Which of the following statements are true about agarose?
   (a) It is a branched polysaccharide
   (b) It is a linear polysaccharide
   (c) It is made up of arabinose
   (d) Agarose is one of the principal components of agar

49. Agar is obtained from green algae
   (a) A, B and C (b) B, C and D
   (c) C, D and E (d) D, E and A

50. Caramelization of sucrose yields
   (a) Glucose
   (b) Fructose
   (c) Glucose and Fructose
   (d) Charcoal

51. Which of the following reaction is called "Maillard reaction"
   (a) Reaction between amino group and hydroxyl group
   (b) Reaction between amino group and keto group
   (c) Reaction between amino group and aldehyde group
   (d) Reaction between amino group and carboxylic group

52. Bial's test is used to detect the presence of _____
   (a) Triose (b) Tetrose
   (c) Pentose (d) Hexose

53. Which of the following animal possess cellulose?
   (a) Coelenterates (b) Sponges
   (c) Tunicates (d) Protozoans

54. Glucose residues in amylose are linked by
   (a) $\alpha$ 1 – 4 (b) $\beta$ 1 – 4
   (b) $\alpha$ 1 – 6 (d) $\beta$ 1 – 6

55. Chitin is a_______
   (a) Homopolysaccharide of N acetyl glucosamine
   (b) Heteropolysaccharide of N acetyl glucosamine and N acetyl muramic acid
   (c) A complex polymer of many sugars
   (d) A branched homopolysaccharide of N acetyl glucosamine

56. The branch points of amylopectin are connected by
   (a) $\alpha$ 1 – 4 (b) $\beta$ 1 – 4
   (c) $\alpha$ 1 – 6 (d) $\beta$ 1 – 6

57. Which of the following is an example for homopolysaccharide?
   (a) Cellulose (b) Starch
   (c) Glycogen (d) All of these

58. Tubocurarine is a lead compound for a class of medicinally useful compounds. What feature of the above structure is crucial to its activity?
   (a) The phenol ring
   (b) The isoquinoline rings
   (c) The aromatic ring
   (d) The two positively charged nitrogen atoms

59. Which feature of acetylcholine interacts with the binding site of cholinergic receptors by hydrogen bonding?
   (a) The acyl methyl group
   (b) The ester
   (c) The quaternary nitrogen
   (d) All three N-methyl groups

60. What sort of receptor is the muscarinic receptor?
   (a) A G-protein coupled receptor
   (b) A kinase linked receptor
   (c) An intracellular receptor
   (d) An ion channel

61. Atropine has been used to decrease gastrointestinal motility and to counteract anticholinesterase poisoning. What function does this molecule have?
   (a) Muscarinic agonist
   (b) Muscarinic antagonist
   (c) Nicotinic agonist
   (d) Nicotinic antagonist

62. Which of the following is a clinical use for a muscarinic agonist?
   (a) Treatment of myasthenia gravis
   (b) 'Switching off' the gastrointestinal tract prior to surgery
   (c) 'Switching on' the urinary tract after surgery
   (d) Increasing heart muscle activity in certain heart defects

63. Which of the following statements is consistent with an electronic absorption being broad?
   (a) An electronic absorption includes vibrational and rotational structure.
   (b) The absorption of a photon is slower than the timescale of molecular vibrations.

(c) Hydrogen bonding causes an electronic absorption to be broad.

(d) Electronic transitions are always localized on a single atomic centre.

64. What term is applied to a drug which is effective against a relatively rare medical problem?

(a) New chemical entity

(b) Orphan drug

(c) Lead compound

(d) Parent drug

65. All of the following statements regarding angiotensin II are true EXCEPT:

(a) It is a peptide hormone

(b) It stimulates the secretion of aldosterone

(c) Angiotensin I is almost as potent as angiotensin II

(d) It is a potent vasoconstrictor

66. This drug is contraindicated in patients with bronchial asthma:

(a) Propranolol (b) Clonidine

(c) Enalapril (d) Nifedipine

67. An aqueous solution of a dye has a strong absorption with λmax= 464 nm. The colour of the solution is:

(a) green (b) orange

(c) colourless (d) purple.

68. Which of the following is the principal chromophore in an azo-dye?

(a) N=N (b) C≡N

(c) N≡N (d) C=N

69. How do values of λmax for the $\pi^* \leftarrow \pi$ transitions vary among a series of conjugated polyenes?

(a) Values shift to longer wavelength as the number of C=C double bonds increases.

(b) Values vary but in no particular pattern

(c) Values vary very little.

(d) Values shift to shorter wavelength as the number of C=C double bonds increases.

70. All of the following statements regarding verapamil are true EXCEPT:

(a) It blocks L-type calcium channels

(b) It increases heart rate

(c) It relaxes coronary artery smooth muscle

(d) It depresses cardiac contractility

71. Choose the unwanted effects of clonidine:

(a) Parkinson's syndrome

(b) Sedative and hypnotic effects

(c) Agranulocytosis and aplastic anemia

(d) Dry cough and respiratory depression

72. The reason of diuretics administration for hypertension treatment is:

(a) Block the adrenergic transmission

(b) Diminishing of blood volume and amount of Na+ ions in the vessels endothelium

(c) Depression of rennin-angiotensin-aldosterone system

(d) Depression of the vasomotor center

73. If the PKa of Phenobarbitone is 7.4.what fraction of drug would be ionized at pH 8.4?

(a) 0.01 (b) 0.50

(c) 0.90 (d) 1.00

74. The following is the example of cationic surfactant

(a) Benzalkonium chloride

(b) Polysorbate 80

(c) SLS

(d) Sorbitan monooleate

75. The type of particle diameter that is obtained by microscopic method of evaluation is

(a) Projected (b) Stokes'

(c) Volume (d) Volume-surface

76. Inversion sucrose in syrup due to heat is known as

(a) Isomerization (b) Epimerization

(c) Tautomeriation (d) Caramelization

77. Carnauba wax is used in the following step of sugar coating of tablet:

(a) Seal coating (b) Polishing

(c) Sub-coating (d) Syrup coating

78. One of the following diluent may discolour in the presence of amine containing drugs:

(a) Avicel (b) DCP

(c) Lactose (d) Talc

79. A sustained release tablet delivers 10mg of the drug every hour. The percentage of drug to be released in 300 mg tablet after six hours is approximately
    (a) 24%  (b) 30%
    (c) 80%  (d) 50%

80. A pharmacokinetics parameter that gives in estimation of renal function is
    (a) Serum creatinine
    (b) Blood urea nitrogen
    (c) Creatinine clearance
    (d) Urine creatinine

81. Effect of moderate consumption of alcohol on plasma lipoproteins is:
    (a) Raising serum levels of high-density lipoproteins
    (b) Increasing serum concentration of low-density lipoproteins
    (c) Decreasing the concentration of high-density lipoproteins
    (d) Raising serum levels of very low-density lipoproteins

82. Morphine causes the following effects EXCEPT:
    (a) Constipation
    (b) Dilatation of the biliary duct
    (c) Urinary retention
    (d) Bronchiolar constriction

83. Which one of the following non-narcotic agents inhibits mainly cyclooxygenase (COX) in CNS?
    (a) Paracetamol
    (b) Ketorolac
    (c) Acetylsalicylic acid
    (d) Ibuprofen

84. Neuroleptics are used to treat:
    (a) Neurosis
    (b) Psychosis
    (c) Narcolepsy
    (d) Parkinsonian disorders

85. Atypical antipsychotic agents (such as clozapine) differ from typical ones:
    (a) In reduced risks of extrapyramidal system dysfunction and tardive dyscinesia
    (b) In having low affinity for D1 and D2 dopamine receptors
    (c) In having high affinity for D4 dopamine receptors
    (d) All of the above

86. Which of the following antidepressants is a selective serotonin reuptake inhibitor?
    (a) Phenelzine  (b) Desipramine
    (c) Maprotiline  (d) Fluoxetine

87. Which of the following features do MAO inhibitors and tricyclic antidepressants have in common?
    (a) Act postsynaptically to produce their effect
    (b) Can precipitate hypotensive crises if certain foods are ingested
    (c) Increase levels of biogenic amines
    (d) Are useful for the manic phase of bipolar disorder

88. Inhaled anesthetics and intravenous agents having general anesthetic properties:
    (a) Directly activate GABAA receptors
    (b) Facilitate GABA action but have no direct action on GABAA receptors
    (c) Reduce the excitatory glutamatergic neurotransmission
    (d) Increase the duration of opening of nicotine-activated potassium channels

89. Rhizomes of *Zingiber officinale* contain some sesquiterpene hydrocarbons. Some hydrocarbons are given below:
    [P] β-Bisabolene  [Q] Gingerone A
    [R] Gingerol  [S] Zingiberene
    Identify the correct pair of constituents present in the rhizomes.
    (a) P and S  (b) P and Q
    (c) Q and S  (d) Q and R

90. Listed below are the chemical tests used to identify some groups of phytoconstituents. Identify the test for the detection of the purine alkaloids
    (a) Keller-Killani Test
    (b) Murexide Test
    (c) Shinoda Test
    (d) Vitali-Morin Test

91. Non-ionic surfactant vesicles relates to..........
    (a) Liposomes (b) Niosomes
    (a) Nanoparticles (d) a and b both

92. Which of the following is non-competitive inhibitor of citric acid cycle enzyme called α-ketoglutarate dehydrogenase?
    (a) Fluoroacetate (b) Arsenite
    (c) Melonate (d) Lithium

93. The heterocyclic ring present in dipyridamole is..........
    (a) Pyridine (b) Piperidine
    (c) Pyarazine (d) Piperazine

94. Which form no is used for import of biological drugs( C/C1)............
    (a) 9 (b) 12-A
    (c) 11-A (d) 24-A

95. Anorgasmia side effect produced by.............
    (a) Selective serotonin reuptake inhibitor
    (b) Tricyclic antidepressant
    (c) Monoamine oxidase inhibitors
    (d) All of the above

96. Which of the following problems associated with glass containers?
    (p) Weathering (q) Corrosion problem
    (r) Flaking (s) Breathing
    (a) p,q (b) p,r
    (c) p,s (d) r,s

97. Sodium nitroprusside is one of the most potent blood pressure lowering drugs. Its use is limited because of –
    (a) Its short duration of action
    (b) Ineffective in oral use
    (c) Very long duration of action
    (d) None of the above

98. True statement regarding inverse agonist is
    (a) Binds to the receptor and causes intended action
    (b) Binds to the receptor and causes opposite action
    (c) Binds to the receptor and causes no action
    (d) Binds to the receptor and causes submaximal action

99. Elimination after 4 half lives in first order kinetic is –
    (a) 84.2% (b) 93.7%
    (c) 80.5% (d) 75.1%

100. One of the following types of adverse drug reactions is not believed to be dose related phenomenon -
    (a) Side effects and toxic reactions
    (b) Toxic reactions and hypersensitivity
    (c) Side effects and hypersensitivity
    (d) Hypersensitivity and idiosyncrasy

101. Choose the statement which is incorrect –
    [P] Darcy equation is used to study Evaporation test
    [Q] Psychomatric chart is related to fluid flow measurement
    [R] Reynold number is rlated to flow rate
    (a) P & Q (b) P & R
    (c) Q & R (d) R only

102. Anti-cancer drug dactinomycin acts by mechanism
    (a) Inhibit RNA and protein synthesis
    (b) Intercalate between DNA strands
    (c) Inhibits DNA polymerase
    (d) Inhibits DHFRase

103. Ingestion of which of the following vitamin should be avoided by a patient taking an oral anticoagulant –
    (a) Vitamin A (b) Vitamin D
    (c) Vitamin K (d) Vitamin E

104. The only macrolide antibiotic which is having significant activity against M. laprae is-
    (a) Erythromycin (b) Clarithromycin
    (c) Azithromycin (d) Roxithromycin

105. A. Oxymel is a preparation in which the vehicle is a mixture of acetic acid and honey
    B. Infusion is a concentrated preparation containing active principles of vegetable or animal drugs
    (a) Both A and B are correct
    (b) A is correct and B is incorrect
    (c) A is incorrect and B is correct
    (d) Both are incorrect

106. The medicinal value of cod liver oil which is obtained from fish Gadus morrhria is due to
(a) Vit A and D (b) Vit A and K
(c) Vit D and E (d) Vit E and K

107. Imipenam is –
I. Obtained from chromobacterium violaceum
II. It is given with cilastatin
III. It is monocyclic
IV. Obtained from streptomyces cattelya
(a) I, II (b) II, IV
(c) III, IV (d) II, III

108. Ideal suppository base acid value ,saponification value, iodinification value are respectively –
(a) Below 0.2, 200-245, less than 7
(b) Below 0.2, 300-500, less than 8
(c) Above 0.2, 200-500, more than 7
(d) Above 0.1, 300-500, more than 7

109. Bitterness value is:
(a) Units eq. to bitterness of std solution of quinine hydrochloride
(b) Units eq. to bitterness of std solution of quinidine hydrochloride
(c) Units eq. to bitterness of std solution of quinine sulphate
(d) Units eq. to bitterness of std solution of quindine sulphate

110. Red shift is a –
(a) Shifting of $\lambda_{max}$ to a shorter wave length
(b) Shifting of $\lambda_{max}$ to a longer wave length
(c) Increase in intensity of $\lambda_{max}$
(d) Decrease in intensity of $\lambda_{max}$

111. Clavulanic acid is -
(a) Potent Inhibitor of cell wall transpeptidase
(b) Inactivates bacterial β-lactamases
(c) Specific for gram -ve organisms
(d) Specific for bacterial infection

112. Which is used as reference standard in NMR for aqueous solution?
(a) Euforium
(b) TMS
(c) DSS
(d) Lanthanide derivatives

113. Aspartame has main disadvantage as
(a) Carcinogenic
(b) Bitter after taste
(c) Less sweeter than sucrose
(d) Hygroscopic in nature

114. Tailing of peak in GLC include
(a) imethyl silane
(b) Tetramethyl silane
(c) Hexamethyl disilane
(d) None of these

115. Which anabolic steroid had been taken by cricketers?
(a) Nandrolones (b) Clomiphene
(c) Nafarelin (d) Goserelin

116. Which types of bark is present in Kurchi?
(a) Flat (b) Double quill
(c) Channeled (d) Recurve

117. All amino acids are optically actives except
(a) Tryptophan (b) Phenylalanine
(c) Valine (d) Glycine

118. Select a fat-soluble vitamin:
(a) Ascorbic acid (b) Tocopherol
(c) Thiamine (d) Riboflavin

119. Which of the following antienzymes is an aldehyde dehydrogenase inhibitor?
(a) Tazobactam (b) Sulbactam
(c) Aminocaproic acid (d) Disulfiram

120. This drug increases lipoprotein lipase (LPL) activity in adipose tissue:
(a) Cholestyramine (Questran)
(b) Lovastatin (Mevacor)
(c) Nicotinic acid (Niacin)
(d) Gemfibrozil (Loprol)

121. Which of the following synthetic steroids shows predominantly mineralocorticoid action?
(a) Hydrocortisone (b) Spironolactone
(c) Dexamethasone (d) Fludrocortisone

122. Direct effects on the heart are determined largely by:
(a) Alfa1 receptor (b) Alfa2 receptor
(c) Beta1 receptor (d) Beta2 receptor

123. Distribution of alfa adrenoreceptor subtypes is associated with all of the following tissues except those of:
   (a) Heart
   (b) Blood vessels
   (c) Prostate
   (d) Pupillary dilator muscle

124. Which of the following drugs causes bronchodilation without significant cardiac stimulation?
   (a) Isoprenaline (b) Terbutaline
   (c) Xylometazoline (d) Methoxamine

125. Which of the following sympathomimetics is a beta2-selective agonist?
   (a) Terbutaline (b) Xylometazoline
   (c) Isoproterenol (d) Dobutamine

# Answer Key Mock Test III

| 1-d | 2-b | 3-b | 4-a | 5-c | 6-d | 7-d | 8-b | 9-d | 10-c |
|---|---|---|---|---|---|---|---|---|---|
| 11-d | 12-b | 13-d | 14-b | 15-a | 16-b | 17-c | 18-b | 19-d | 20-d |
| 21-d | 22-b | 23-c | 24- | 25-d | 26-a | 27-d | 28-d | 29-d | 30-a |
| 31-c | 32-a | 33-a | 34-a | 35-d | 36-b | 37-c | 38-d | 39-d | 40-d |
| 41-b | 42-b | 43-c | 44-a | 45-c | 46-a | 47-b | 48- | 49-b | 50-c |
| 51-d | 52-c | 53-c | 54-a | 55-a | 56-c | 57-d | 58-d | 59-b | 60-a |
| 61-b | 62-c | 63-a | 64-b | 65-c | 66-a | 67-b | 68-a | 69-a | 70-b |
| 71-b | 72-b | 73-c | 74-a | 75-a | 76- | 77-b | 78-a | 79-c | 80-c |
| 81-a | 82-b | 83-a | 84-b | 85-d | 86-d | 87-c | 88-a | 89-a | 90-b |
| 91-b | 92-b | 93-b | 94-a | 95-a | 96-b | 97-a | 98-b | 99-b | 100-d |
| 101-a | 102-b | 103-c | 104-a | 105-a | 106-a | 107-b | 108-a | 109-a | 110-b |
| 111-b | 112-b | 113-a | 114- | 115-a | 116-d | 117-d | 118-b | 119-d | 120-d |
| 121-d | 122-a | 123-a | 124-b | 125-a | | | | | |

www.ingramcontent.com/pod-product-compliance
Lightning Source LLC
Chambersburg PA
CBHW080158170726
48282CB00005B/64
*9789395039178*